2020

School Nurse Resource Manual

A GUIDE TO PRACTICE TENTH EDITION

I. CLINICAL GUIDELINES

II. CLINICAL PROCEDURES

III. SCHOOL NURSE MANAGEMENT

IV. MANAGEMENT of VULNERABLE POPULATIONS

EDITORS
VICKI TALIAFERRO
CHERYL RESHA

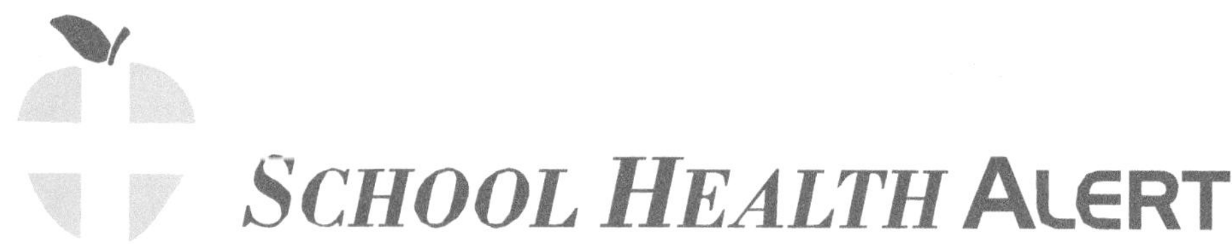

SCHOOL HEALTH ALERT
P.O. Box 150127
Nashville, TN 37215

SCHOOL NURSE RESOURCE MANUAL 2020

NOTICES

Nursing, including school nursing, is a dynamic, constantly changing field. The publisher, editors and contributors have made a diligent effort to ensure any guidelines, procedures or recommendations outlined in this manual are accurate, based on latest evidence, and in accordance with accepted school nursing practices at the time of publication. It is, of course, necessary for readers to apply their professional judgment, experience, knowledge of the patient, and any new research to determine the best treatment for a specific case. Additionally, it is the responsibility of the school nurse to adhere to their individual state nurse practice act when administering any treatment or medication.

Several websites are included in this manual to provide additional information, resources and references on a particular topic. However, listing these websites does not imply endorsement. Note that with any internet site, addresses and content may change, and information therein updated.

Mentions of any specific products within this book are for informational purposes and also do not constitute endorsements.

ISBN-13: 978-0-9792497-5-4 ISBN-10: 0-9792497-5-9

Phone: 866-370-7899
Fax: 615-370-9993

Table of Contents

Table of Contents

CLINICAL GUIDELINES INDEX

CLINICAL GUIDELINES INDEX

ABOUT THIS MANUAL

School nursing, a specialized practice of nursing, protects and promotes student health, facilitates optimal development, and advances academic success. School nurses, grounded in ethical and evidence-based practice, are the leaders who bridge health care and education, provide care coordination, advocate for quality student-centered care, and collaborate to design systems that allow individuals and communities to develop their full potential. [1] School nursing services uniquely address health and safety needs of students individually, as a population, and as a subspecialty of community/public health nursing.

School nurses' work is framed using five pillars of practice: standards of practice, care coordination, leadership, quality improvement, and community/public health nursing which incorporate many areas.[2] School nurse services require diverse knowledge including, but not limited to, pediatric and adolescent health, infectious diseases, mental health, chronic diseases, and emergency care. School nurses can influence health and safety aspects of schools and can provide leadership to a district's or campus' whole school, whole community, whole child (WSCC) approach that in addition to health services, health education, and the school environment addresses mental health and social services, nutrition services, physical activity, family and community involvement, and staff health promotion.

This resource serves as a quick reference for school nurses and can assist them, their administrators, and consulting physicians to develop policies and procedures for safe student care. This manual offers brief summaries of conditions that most school nurses encounter but is not intended to be a substitute for any comprehensive pediatric or emergency care textbook.

The *school nurse guidelines* were developed through cooperative efforts of school nurses and physicians. We strongly recommend a similar process at the district or system level with adaptations that account for state laws and regulations as well as the unique needs of students in a school district. The registered nurse plans student health services, however, vocational/practical nurses, or unlicensed staff such as office personnel or health clinic assistants may perform certain tasks within state nursing practice guidelines. The registered nurse is responsible for training persons assigned to perform a delegated nursing task, monitoring their performance, and ensuring their compliance with the procedures. State school nurse consultants are an invaluable resource regarding laws, regulations and nurse practice acts in each state.

PHYSICIAN/HEALTHCARE PROVIDER (MD or APRN) CONSULTATION

The availability of a physician's or healthcare provider's services to schools varies across communities. Some large districts have full-time medical advisor or consultant, while others have part-time healthcare provider services. Small districts may engage a healthcare provider to consult for a set number of hours or on-call. Some providers volunteer as a community service.

---

[1] National Association of School Nurses. (2017). *Definition of school nursing*. http://www.nasn.org/RoleCareer

[2] National Association of School Nurses. (2016). *Framework for 21st century school nursing practice: National Association of School Nurses*. https://doi.org/10.1177/1942602X15618644

Regardless of the arrangement, it is sound medical-legal practice for the school nurse to have written guidelines to standardize assessment and management decisions. Such guidelines with input from the school healthcare provider complement professional school nursing practice standards and the nursing process and should incorporate accepted pediatric care recommendations.

We suggest that students who have conditions that are likely to require treatment or emergency care during school hours or activities, have individual written orders from their own healthcare provider. These orders should be reviewed and updated at least each school year or as necessary and incorporated into the student's individualized healthcare plan. The most common individual orders are for students with asthma, life threatening allergies, or diabetes. Some students with seizure disorders, migraine headaches, or other chronic conditions also need individual orders each school year.

DESCRIPTION OF SCHOOL NURSE GUIDELINES

We offer an outline format so that important features of each condition and guidelines for action can be seen at a glance. Each guideline includes a definition or etiology of the disease or condition, presenting signs and symptoms, management strategies and follow- up. This format provides the registered nurse a quick reference for student care and offers information to educate and train staff who may assist the school nurse.

Registered nurses apply their professional skills and judgment in the management of each individual case, but each school and district or system should provide care for all students in a consistent manner guided by local policies and procedures, e.g., criteria for referral or exclusion and return to class.

Usual procedures, such as Standard (Universal) Precautions, parent notification, record keeping, confidentiality, etc. may not be repeated in all guidelines but is understood to be a standard practice in all aspects of care.

DESCRIPTION OF SCHOOL NURSE MANAGEMENT AND MANAGEMENT OF VULNERABLE POPULATIONS TOPICS

Like the school nurse guidelines section, we offer an outline format so that the important features and management needs of each content area can be seen at-a-glance. Each chapter begins with an overview of the topic and then discusses anticipated concerns/problems, management, follow-up and resources. These topics are not meant to provide a treatment plan for a specific condition like the guideline section; rather how the school nurse and school district manage particular vulnerable populations or population–based needs.

STANDING ORDERS

Although standing orders are not addressed in this edition, the distinction between the two types of orders should be understood.

General orders are written by a physician or consulting healthcare provider, often the identified as the school medical advisor, which apply to all students for whom the order may be applicable.

They should be reviewed annually and updated when necessary. It is not necessary for the school medical advisor to have previously examined the student. Dosage is based on weight or age. Common examples of general orders are acetaminophen for fever, ibuprofen for minor headache, etc. These orders are issued with the understanding that a registered nurse will administer these medications after an assessment of the child.

Some state boards of nursing do not allow general standing orders in school settings. Other boards may allow a "physician directed nursing protocol" which requires signatures of both a healthcare provider and a nurse (usually a nursing administrator or manager). If the administration of nonprescription products is permitted, the school's policy (for discretionary medications) should be in writing and parents must be informed. Parents should sign a written request for each school year indicating that their child may receive any of the named medications in the discretionary medication policy from school personnel according to the district's policy.

Specific orders are written and signed by a healthcare provider for *an individual child.* The parents should also sign a medication authorization form for school personnel to administer any medicine at school. These specific orders contain the drug or treatment, dose, route, time and duration of administration. For example, for a child with diagnosed with ADHD: "Methylphenidate 20 mg (one tablet) by mouth daily between 11 A.M. and noon after lunch or with food through December 20, 2016". Most districts require that individualized orders be renewed annually.

Each school/district should have a medication policy that guides medication administration and documentation of both specific, individual orders for medication and for any discretionary medications orders by the school healthcare provided as allowed.

We welcome your suggestions for future editions and wish you success in caring for our nation's children. You may contact us on the Internet at *www.schoolnurse.com*.

Robert Andrews, Publisher
School Health Alert
P.O. Box 150127, Nashville, TN 37215
(866) 370-7899
www.schoolnurse.com

STUDENT SERVICES/MULTI-DISCIPLINARY TEAM

DEFINITION/ETIOLOGY:
Research has shown that a collaborative approach is essential to learning and health.[1] Student services in secondary school environments are therefore ideal settings where collaboration and multi-disciplinary team approaches can provide successful academic outcomes and support the development of the "whole child".[2]

Student services refers to services, supports, programs and practices that assist students in achieving or enhancing their academic goals. Student services vary and are based on individual student as well as student population needs. Disciplines within school environments that provide student services include school nurses, school medical advisor (e.g., physician or advanced practice registered nurse), school psychologist, school social worker, school counselors, pupil services directors, and special education coordinators. These disciplines, using a multi-disciplinary, whole child approach, work with educational staff, students and families to ensure "that each student is healthy, safe, engaged, supported, and challenged, sets the standard for comprehensive, sustainable school improvement and provides for long-term student success".[3]

Multi-disciplinary team refers to professionals in school communities who work collaboratively with students and their families in the decision–making and goal-setting processes toward achieving successful individual or student population outcomes. Multi-disciplinary teams rely on the expertise, knowledge and experience of individual team members to develop plans and provide effective supports that are aligned with students' goals. School nurses, as the health experts in school environments, are therefore integral members of multi-disciplinary teams, as their perspective assists educators with better understanding the impacts of and supports that may be offered to students based on their health and medical status, conditions, concerns or diagnosis.

Multi-disciplinary Team Members
The following professionals who may be included in a multi-disciplinary team:

School Nurse
School nurses support student success. They are an integral part of school multi-disciplinary teams, bridging the gap between health and wellness, and learning. School nurses identify student health-related concerns and make accommodations and/or interventions to support learning. They also focus on early detection and correction of health problems. School nurses promote and protect the optimal health of students. They work with families, healthcare providers, and students to develop individualized healthcare plans for students with special health needs. Health counseling is provided to students and their families, as well as school staff. They identify and report school environmental concerns. The school nurse determines which nursing services can be delegated and provides supervision for the staff to whom he or she delegates.

STUDENT SERVICES/MULTI-DISCIPLINARY TEAM *(continued from previous page)*

School Psychologist

School psychologists are members of school teams whose expertise in social emotional health, mental health, and cognition, assists students in achieving their academic goals. Their collaborations with the school community, including families, teachers, administrators, school nurses, and other school staff, assists in the creation of supportive learning environments where students, with their families, can achieve life skills in- and out-side of the classroom and beyond elementary and secondary years. "School psychologists provide direct support and interventions to students, consult with teachers, families, and other school-employed mental health professionals (i.e., school counselors, school social workers) to improve support strategies, work with school administrators to improve school-wide practices and policies, and collaborate with community providers to coordinate needed services".[4] In order to improve student and school outcomes, including the use of best practices and equal opportunity for all school children, school psychologists are instrumental in the implementation of assessment and accountability systems (including standardized testing), school improvement and support systems and in improving school climate, school safety and access to high quality comprehensive learning supports.[5]

School Medical Advisors

School medical advisors support school districts' health and wellness programs. Their expertise in pediatric practices assist local boards of education and school administration with the planning, development, review and evaluation of school health programs, policies, and procedures. Their consultation, communication and coordination with school nurse supervisors and school nurses are vital to better understanding school and district-wide student health issues, concerns and statuses. Their roles and responsibilities further include participation in school health activities, such as the school wellness committee, health council, select planning and placement team meetings and other appropriate committees or meetings.[6]

School Counselor

School counselors assists students in maximizing their academic goals in elementary and secondary and in planning for post-secondary educational and other options. "Their expertise include providing: individual student academic planning and goal setting; school counseling classroom lessons based on student success standards; short-term counseling to students; referrals for long-term support; collaboration with families/teachers/ administrators/community for student success; advocacy for students at individual education plan meetings and other student-focused meetings; and data analysis to identify student issues, needs and challenges".[7]

School Social Worker

School Social Workers provide students with social and emotional supports to empower them in achieving their academic and personal goals. Through collaborations with students, families, school and community resources, school social workers assist in promoting a safe school environment where students are encouraged to advocate for themselves and others. School social workers' foci includes student culture and character development, parent outreach, professional development to support school districts' identified social and emotional needs, and student counseling.[8]

STUDENT SERVICES/MULTI-DISCIPLINARY TEAM *(continued from previous page)*

Pupil Services Directors

Pupil services directors are members of the education team who provide supervision and leadership for services and programs that support the needs of all students. Their work includes the coordination and monitoring of all special education programs and supporting the academic and social emotional needs of all students. Their expertise includes knowledge of: special education laws and processes; Section 504 planning; extended school year; co-teaching; gifted education; and pupil registration and enrollment policies and procedures. Most pupil services directors assume responsibilities for supervising, implementing and monitoring the following school programs: health services; speech; occupational and physical therapy; and related services.

Special Education Coordinators

Special education coordinators are focused on supporting, implementing and monitoring programs and services that provide educational assistance to students who qualify for special education. Special education coordinators are highly trained and experienced teachers with specialized certification, and who work under the direction of pupil services directors. Their roles and responsibilities include: actively facilitating the planning and placement team processes for special education; assisting special education teachers and related services professionals with technical assistance and professional development activities; and participating in the hiring processes of special education teachers, teacher assistants and related services staff.

REFERENCES

[1] Centers for Disease Control and Prevention. (2010). *The association between school based physical activity, including physical education, and academic performance*. US Department of Health and Human Services. https://www.cdc.gov/healthyyouth/health_and_academics/pdf/pa-pe_paper.pdf

[2] ASCD. (2019). *Whole child*. http://www.ascd.org/whole-child.aspx

[3] Ibid. Page 1.

[4] National Association of School Psychologists. (2019). *About school psychology*. Page 1. https://www.nasponline.org/about-school-psychology

[5] National Association of School Psychologists. (2019). *ESSA overview for school psychologists.* https://www.nasponline.org/research-and-policy/policy-priorities/relevant-law/the-every-student-succeeds-act/essa-implementation-resources/essa-overview-for-school-psychologists-x34810

[6] Connecticut State Department of Education. (2019). *School medical advisors: Recommendations for the qualifications, selection process and roles in the implementation of school health services programs in Connecticut schools*. Page 2. https://portal.ct.gov/-/media/SDE/School-Nursing/Publications/suggested_recommendations_for_school_medical_advisors.pdf

[7] American School Counselor Association. (2019). *Who are school counselors?* Page 1. https://www.schoolcounselor.org/asca/media/asca/Careers-Roles/SCInfographic.pdf

[8] School Social Work Association of America. (2019). *School social work*. Page 1.https://www.sswaa.org/

ACKNOWLEDGMENTS

This 10th Edition was edited by Vicki Taliaferro, BSN, RN, NCSN and Cheryl Resha, EdD, MSN, RN, FNASN.

CONTRIBUTORS

Andrea Adimando, DNP, MS, PMHNP-BC, BCIM

Andrea Adimando is an Assistant Professor of Nursing at Southern CT State University, teaching in the BSN and MSN programs. She has over 14 years of experience as a Board-Certified Psychiatric Nurse Practitioner, specializing in child and adolescent mental health assessment and treatment in inpatient, outpatient, community, and school settings.

Patricia K. Bednarz, RN, MN, FNASN

Patricia Bednarz is a health and education consultant. Ms. Bednarz had a 25-plus year career of diversified experience as a school nurse, project manager and nursing educator. She has managed state and federal grants that included writing and contributing to proposals as well as grant implementation, fiscal management and evaluation. In 2010, Patricia was named a Fellow in the National Academy of School Nurses. Ms. Bednarz has published articles in peer-reviewed journals, chapters in books and presented at state and national school nurse conferences. Currently, Ms. Bednarz is consulting for the Michigan Department of Health and Human Services in the School Wellness Program.

Mary Blackborow, MSN, RN, NCSN

Mary Blackborow has over 40 years' experience as a registered nurse. Her nursing experience included public health nursing and case management with 20 years' experience as a school nurse. Her school nursing experience includes middle and high school students as well as special needs students from 3 to 21. She has held leadership positions in school nursing organizations at the local, state and national levels. In 2015, she became a Johnson and Johnson School Health Leadership Fellow.

Kristen S. Borgognone, DNP, RN, NEA-BC, CIC

Kristen Borgognone is an Assistant Professor of Nursing at Southern Connecticut State University. She has over 33 years of experience as a registered nurse. Her nursing experience includes adult and pediatric critical care, emergency medicine and psychiatry. Her experience also includes infection prevention and patient safety. Her current research is focused on the health behaviors of college students and HPV prevention activities.

Jane Borr, BSN, RN, NCSN

Jane Borr is a school nurse and school nurse educator for a hospital funded school nurse program that partners with area school districts for nursing services in the schools. She currently serves on the Michigan Association of School Nurses board as Membership Chair and was treasurer from 2010 - 2014 and 2018-2019. She was a member of the Michigan School Nurse Task Force from 2011 - 2014 where she co-chaired the data and staffing committee. She is a nationally certified school nurse.

Jane Boyd, MSN, RN, NCSN

Jane Boyd is a retired State School Nurse Consultant with over 33 years of experience as a registered nurse and over 19 years as a school nurse. Her school nursing experiences includes elementary, middle and high school. From 2016-2019 she was the Delaware State School Nurse Consultant and participated on state-level committees and leadership positions.

Hendrina Cupery, RN, MSN, NCSN

Hendrina Cupery works as the Manager of the School Nurse and Faith Community Nurse Programs in Holland Michigan. She has worked in nursing for the past 25 years, fifteen of which have been in school nursing. She serves as the Treasurer of the Michigan Association of School Nurses. She is a nationally certified school nurse.

Sandra J. Delack, MEd, BSN, RN, NCSN, FNASN

Sandi Delack is a School Health Consultant and educator with 31 years of experience as a certified school nurse-teacher, where she served as District Coordinator for a suburban school district. She is a Past President of the National Association of School Nurses (NASN), Past President of the National Board for Certification of School Nurses (NBCSN), and former board member of ANA-RI. Sandi has also held numerous leadership positions at the state level and has been involved in policy and regulation development. She is currently a national presenter as well as an adjunct faculty member at Providence College.

Stephanie G. Denya, RN, BSN, MPH

Stephanie Denya is currently a Deputy Health Director for the city of Meriden Department of Health and Human Services in Connecticut. In addition, she supervises the school health and clinic programs. She has over 30 years of nursing experience, several of which include working as a public health nurse in a school setting. She has collaborated with state/local agencies on disaster preparedness trainings, improving immunization rates, and lead poisoning awareness for which she began a school lead screening initiative requiring all pre-K and Kindergarten students to have a lead screening prior to school entry. She is also a member of several local task forces which work together to assist children and families improve their health, access to care, and quality of life.

Bonnie Edmondson, EdD

Bonnie Edmondson is an Associate Professor and Graduate Coordinator of the School Health Education Program at Southern Connecticut State University. She has over 35 years of experience as an educator, coach, and former professional athlete. Dr. Edmondson has served on expert panels for the CDC and the U.S. Department of Health and Human Services, has written numerous documents on school health policies and practices, is a peer reviewer for numerous professional publications and journals, and is a well-known speaker on health and education policy and athletic coaching. In addition, she is a two-time national champion and former world ranked hammer thrower. She is active with USA Track and Field (USATF) serving as the head women's coach for the 2019 IAAF World Championships, the women's throwing events coach for the 2016 United States Olympic Team and six IAAF World Championship teams. Bonnie is Chair of the USATF Women's Commission. She holds an EdD in Educational Leadership, an MS in School Health Education, and a BA in English.

Patricia Fato, BSN, CPN

Patricia Fato is currently a Clinical Nurse at PACT. PACT is a daycare for medically fragile children and affiliated with Kennedy Krieger Institute. Patricia has over 12 years of Pediatric Nursing experience. She has a bachelor's degree in Nursing and is also a Certified Pediatric Nurse.

Susan Hoffmann, MSN, RN, NCSN

Susan Hoffmann is currently a School Nurse Consultant with over 35 years of nursing experience and over 25 years' experience in school nursing practice. Her school nursing experience includes providing direct services for elementary general education and special needs students with severe emotional and behavioral challenges, district lead nurse, mentoring, nursing education project management and leadership positions at both the state and national levels.

Bethanne Johnston, RN, MSN, CPNP

Bethanne Johnston is currently a Nephrology Pediatric Nurse Practitioner at Riley Hospital for Children, in Indianapolis, IN, with over 30 years of experience as a registered nurse and over 10 years as a nephrology nurse practitioner. Her nursing experience includes Pediatric ICU, Pediatric Emergency Medicine, and Pediatric Dialysis nursing. She currently manages children with varying stages of chronic kidney disease in the state of Indiana including those who are pre end-stage renal disease, pre-renal transplant, and children with end stage renal disease receiving hemodialysis and peritoneal dialysis. She is actively involved with the National Kidney Foundation of Indiana including serving on their board and participating in outreach programs. She is additionally involved in a program to mentor new advanced practice nurses for the IU Health System.

Stephanie G. Knutson, EdD, RN

Stephanie G. Knutson is an accomplished leader and educator with over 22 years of experience in diverse educational settings advocating for students of all ages and their families. As the School Health Administrator and Education Consultant for School Nursing and School Health Education for Connecticut State Department of Education, she provides state-wide educational leadership and facilitate policy development in the areas of school health education, and students' physical and mental health. Her deep understanding of the role of health in the growth and cognitive development in children, individual student achievement and closing the achievement gap, lends to her evaluation of school health services. Dr. Knutson promotes physical and mental health to maximize students' educational opportunities within secondary and higher educational institutions in Connecticut, where she creates and provides opportunities for professional development and enhancement of school staff, including school nurses, school medical advisors, health educators, principals, teachers, pupil services directors and other school staff.

Suzanne Levasseur, MSN, APRN

Suzanne Levasseur is the Supervisor of Health Services for the Westport Public Schools District in Connecticut. She is an Advanced Practice registered nurse and a Certified Pediatric Nurse Practitioner and is on staff at Danbury Hospital in Danbury, Connecticut. She is currently the President for the Association of School Nurses of Connecticut and is the editor of the texts, *Pediatric Nursing Secrets* and *Perinatal Nursing Services*.

Kristi Maynard, MSN, APRN, FNP-BC, CNE

Kristi Maynard is an assistant professor at Quinnipiac University. She is an Advanced Practice registered nurse, a Certified Family Nurse Practitioner, and a Certified Nurse Educator. She has clinical experience in primary and urgent care with patients of all ages.

Susan Nokleby, MS, RN, NCSN, FNASN

Susan Nokleby is an independent School Nurse Consultant in Minnesota. As a Licensed School Nurse, Susan has worked in a special education district and as an Administrator of Health Services. She is the past President of the School Nurse Organization of Minnesota and of the National Board for Certification of School Nurses. Sue authored a chapter on homelessness in the 2nd edition of the *Individualized Healthcare Plans for the School Nurse* and was a member of the working group for the revisions of ANA/NASN *School Nursing: Scope and Standards* (2017).

Barbara Obst, MSEd, BSN, RN, NCSN

Barbara Obst is the co- coordinator of the Specialized School Health Interagency Program at the Kennedy Krieger Institute, serving as the co- coordinator for the past 20 years. She has published articles in the NASN School Nurse and was a reviewer for the 3rd edition of *School Nursing a Comprehensive Text*. She has been a speaker on various topics related to children with special needs statewide, and nationally for school nurses and educators.

William (Bill) Patterson Jr., MPA, RN

Bill Patterson is a state level registered professional nurse for the State of Hawaii, Department of Education (HIDOE). Prior to joining the HIDOE, Bill worked for the State of Hawaii Department of Health as a Supervisor of the Children with Special Health Needs Program and a field public health nurse. Through public health nursing, Bill first encountered school health and school nursing issues which became his “cause” or passion. Professionally, Bill has twenty (20) plus years of experience in the clinical/medical and nursing fields and is a chapter contributor for *Legal Resource for School Health Services*. Bill is an active member of both the National Association of School Nurses (NASN) and the National Association of State School Nurse Consultants (NASSNC).

Yann B. Poncin, MD

Yann Pontin is an Assistant Professor and Vice Chairman for Safety and Quality at the Yale Child Study Center. He has administrative, supervisory, and clinical experience working across the care continuum from outpatient to inpatient care, which includes intensive outpatient, partial hospitalization, emergency services, residential care and in-home services. He has 15 years' experience consulting to public, private and therapeutic schools.

Julianna Putman, MS, CCC-SLP, TSLI

Julianna Putman is an ASHA certified speech and language pathologist. She received her Bachelor of Arts in Communicative Sciences and Disorders at Michigan State University. She then received her Master of Science in Speech and Language Pathology from The University of Tulsa. She is in her eighth year of school-based speech language pathology. Her focus is currently on students with Autism Spectrum Disorder, moderate-severe cognitive and/or physical impairments.

Cheryl Resha, EdD, MSN, RN, FNASN

Cheryl Resha is currently Department Chair and Professor of Nursing at Southern Connecticut State University (SCSU). She holds a Doctorate in Educational Leadership. Prior to joining SCSU, Dr. Resha worked for the Connecticut State Department of Education as a manager and state school nurse consultant; and for a large suburban school district as the school nurse supervisor. With over 20 years' experience in the field of school nursing, Dr. Resha has provided leadership and advocacy for school nurses, safe school nurse practice and quality school health programs. Professionally, Dr. Resha has also been a member of ASNC and NASN since 1998. As an active member of NASN for several years, Dr. Resha was inducted as a Fellow in the National Academy of School Nursing in June 2012. Dr. Resha has co-edited, authored and contributed to articles and publications regarding school nursing, such as the *Scope and Standards of Professional School Nurse Practice and* the *Legal Resource for School Health Services.*

Megan Roesler, MSN, RN, CPN

Megan Roesler is a nurse educator with the Specialized Health Needs Interagency Collaboration (SHNIC) program at the Kennedy Krieger Institute. She is a certified pediatric nurse with over 10 years of nursing experience. She conducts training and presentations throughout Maryland and has published various articles in NASN School Nurse magazine to support students with special health care needs. Megan also maintains clinical practice as a pediatric nursing clinical instructor at a local pediatric rehab hospital.

Vicki L. Taliaferro, BSN, RN, NCSN

Vicki L. Taliaferro is a school nurse consultant and editor of *School Nurse Digest* and *Administrator's Risk*. She is co-editor of the last 4 editions of the *School Nurse Resource Manual*. She has authored articles, school nurse text chapters, position papers and state and local guidelines on school health topics and initiatives. She has recently served as a consultant to the National Association of School Nurses as their coordinator of professional practice documents. As State School Nurse Consultant with the Maryland State Department of Education for 10 years, she provided technical advice to state school nursing leadership; developed state guidelines & policies and assisted with the development of Board of Nursing curriculums for delegation and medication administration. Additionally, she is a member of the National Assn. of State School Nurse Consultants having served as president and in other officer positions.

Antoinette Towle MSN, PNP BC, SNP BC

Antoinette Towle is presently an Associate Professor of Nursing at Southern Connecticut State University (SCSU) teaching across the curriculum nursing to undergraduate, RN to BSN, Accelerated and graduate nursing students. She has over 35 years' experience as a registered nurse, and over 15 years' experience as an Advanced Practice registered nurse. She holds a Doctorate in Nursing Education, is ANCC board certified as a Pediatric and School Health Nurse Practitioner. Dr. Towle has extensive experience working in school health, in a variety of roles, school nurse, school nurse practitioner, and the Director of Health Services.

Kara Ventura, PNP, FNP, DNP

Kara Ventura is the manager of Clinical Operations for the Adult Liver and Pediatric Liver and Kidney Transplant Programs at Yale New Haven Hospital. She is a Certified Pediatric Nurse Practitioner, a Certified Adult Nurse Practitioner and holds a Doctorate in Nursing Practice. She has practiced in transplant since 1997 and is involved Nationally and Locally on Transplant Committees. She currently is also a portfolio advisor for students enrolled in the DNP program and Columbia University School of Nursing.

Kim Walker, MSN, APRN, PMHCNS-BC

Kim Walker has been a practicing school nurse for over 20 years for the San Francisco Unified School District. She is a pediatric nurse practitioner and is board certified as a psychiatric clinical nurse specialist. She is the current secretary for the Bay Coast section of CSNO. She also has a small private practice in parent coaching.

Susan F. Zacharski, MEd, RN, FNASN

Susan Zacharski is currently a School Nurse Consultant with over 40 years of experience as a registered nurse and over 27 years' experience as a school nurse. Her school nursing experience includes Department Head of Health Services in an urban school district, preschool – 8th grade general education with a focus on special needs students including the medically fragile, participation in state level committees and leadership positions at both the state and national level. She was a member of the Michigan School Nurse Task Force from 2011–2014 where she co-chaired the school nurse practice committee.

REVIEWERS

Andrea Adimando, DNP, PMHNP-BC, BCIM
Assistant Professor of Nursing
Southern CT State University
Connecticut

Becky Bailey, BNSc, RN, NCSN
Coordinator
Custer Health
North Dakota

Julie Bartoy, MSN, RN
Macomb Community College
Department of Health and Human Services
Nursing Faculty-Pediatrics
Michigan

Jane Boyd, MSN, RN, NCSN
Education Specialist
School Support Services
Student Support Team
Delaware Department of Education
Delaware

Christie M. Butler, BSN, RN
School Nurse Consultant
Coordinated School Health | Whole Child Initiatives
Tennessee

Joan Cagginello, MS, BSN, RN
Nurse Administrator, Retired
Milford Board of Health, Chairman
Connecticut

Elizabeth Chau, SRN (UK), RN
Past NASN Exec Board
Past PPSN Chair
School Nurse, Retired
Nevada

Ann M. Connelly, MSN, RN, LSN, NCSN
Public Health Nurse Supervisor
School Nursing and Early Childhood Health Programs
Ohio Department of Health
Ohio

Michael Corjulo, APRN, CPNP, AE-C, PMHS
Clinical Director
Pediatric Resource Center
Connecticut

Linda Davis-Alldritt, MA, BSN, RN, FNASN, FASHA
Past President, National Association of School Nurses
School Nurse & School Health Services Consultant
Finland

Marie DeSisto, MSN, RN
Instructor
Cambridge College
Massachusetts

Nancy Dube, MPH, RH
Retired State School Nurse Consultant
Maine

Mary Freeland, RN
School Nurse
Independence High School
Arizona

Jessica Gerdes, MS, RN, NCSN, IL Licensed School Nurse
(Retired) State School Nurse Consultant, Illinois State Board of Education
(Current) adjunct faculty, Lewis University (IL) school nurse certificate program
Illinois

Kathleen A. Hassey DNP, MEd, BSN, BA, RN
Director of the School Health Academy
Northeastern University
Massachusetts

Evilia Janowski, MSA, BSN, RN
State School Nurse Consultant
Michigan Department of Education/Michigan Department of Health and Human Services
Michigan

Linda Khalil, MSEd, BSN, RN, SNT
Director, NYS Center for School Health, Contract Office for the NYS Education Department
State School Nurse Consultant
New York

Rebecca King, MSN, RN, NCSN
Retired Nursing Director Delaware Division of Public Health
Board Member, Mom's House of Wilmington
Founding Board of Directors "atTAcK addiction"
Delaware

Nicole Klein, PhD, RN-BC, NCSN, AE-C
Health Services Program Supervisor
Office of Superintendent of Public Instruction
Washington

Donna Kosiorowski, MS, RN, NCSN-E
School Health Consultant
Connecticut

Pat Krin, MSN, RN, FNP-BC-Retired, NCSN-E, **FNASN**
School Health Consultant
School Health Consulting Services
Connecticut

Natalie A. Kwit, DVM, MPH
State Public Health Veterinarian,
Vermont Department of Health
Vermont

Victoria Ladd, MSN, RN
State School Nurse Consultant
Division of Children's Health and Perinatal Services
S.C. Dept. of Health & Environmental Control
South Carolina

Teri B. Lawler, MA, LPCMH
Education Associate
Trauma-Informed Practices and Social and Emotional Learning
Office of Innovation and Improvement
Delaware Department of Education
Delaware

Suzanne Levasseur, MSN, APRN
Supervisor of Health Services
Westport Public Schools
Connecticut

Cheria McDonald, BSN, RN, NCSN
State School Nurse Consultant
Arkansas Department of Education
Division of Elementary and Secondary Education
School Health Services
Arkansas

Keisha Simons Major MSN-Ed, RN, NCSN
Nurse Manager, Office of School Health
Prince George's County Public Schools System
Maryland

Patricia McCain, ADN, RN, BS
Retired School Nurse
Michigan

Marques Mazyck, M.F.A.
Sickle Cell Advocate
Florida

Alicia Mezu, MSN/Ed, BSN, BS, RN
Lead Health Services Specialist
State School Nurse Consultant
Maryland State Department of Education
Maryland

Claire Molner, RN, MEd, NCSN
School Nurse/Health Educator
Proctor Junior Senior High School
Vermont

Kathy Neelon, MS, BSN
Nurse Coordinator
Wallingford Public Schools
Connecticut

Lynnette Ondeck, MEd, BSN, RN, NCSN
Vice President
National Association of School Nurses
School Nurse Corps Administration
Northwest Educational Service District
Washington

Emily Poland, MPH, RN
School Nurse Consultant
Team Leader, Coordinated School Health
Maine Department of Education
Maine

Deborah Pontius, MSN, RN, NCSN, FNASN
School Nurse Consultant and CE Instructor
Nationally Certified School Nurse
Fellow, National Academy of School Nurses
Nevada

Jessica R. Porter, BSN, RN, NCSN
Nationally Certified School Nurse
SCASN Webmaster
Iowa

Suzanne Putman, R.N., B.S.N., M.Ed.
POHI Nurse
Warren Woods Tower High School
Michigan

Darla Rebowe R.N., BSN, CSN
School Nurse
School Nurse Consultant
LSNO Vice President
Louisiana

Kathy L. Reiner, MPH, BA, BSN, RN
School Nurse Specialist
Colorado Department of Education
Board of Directors
Colorado

Deb Robarge, BSN, RN, NCSN
Indiana Association of School Nurses
Executive Director
Retired Health Center Director - Indiana School for the Deaf
Indiana

Linda M. Sawyer, Ph.D., MSN, RN, CNE
Professor of Nursing – Pediatrics
Macomb Community College
Michigan

Sally Schoessler, MSEd, BSN, RN
Director of Education, Allergy & Asthma Network
Virginia

Sharonlee Trefry, MSN, RN, NCSN
State School Nurse Consultant
Maternal and Child Health Division
Vermont Department of Health
Vermont

Anita Wheeler, MSN, RN
School Health Coordinator/ School Nurse Consultant
School Health Program
Diabetes and School Health Branch
Health Promotion and Chronic Disease Prevention Section
Texas Department of State Health Services
Texas

Susan Zacharski, MEd, BSN, RN, FASN
School Nurse Consultant
Michigan

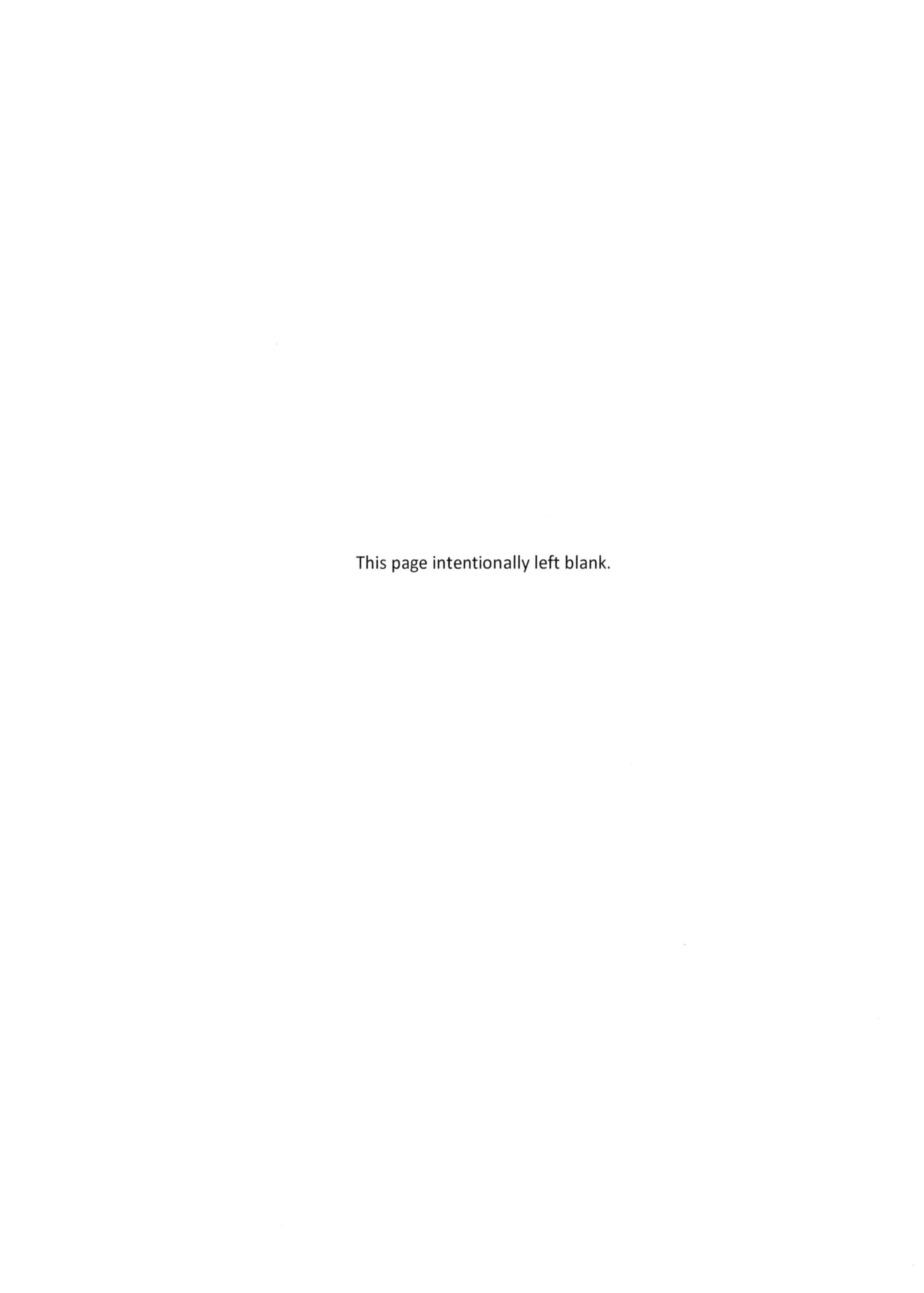

This page intentionally left blank.

SECTION I

CLINICAL GUIDELINES

ABDOMEN: Blunt Injury

DEFINITION/ETIOLOGY:
Following a hard blow to abdomen (by rock, fist, bicycle handlebar, etc.), an internal organ may be ruptured and bleed into the abdominal cavity slowly but continuously. Injured abdominal organs may include the spleen, liver, retroperitoneum, small intestines, colorectal, bladder, kidney, diaphragm or pancreas. Blunt abdominal injuries become apparent within nine hours.[1]

SIGNS AND SYMPTOMS:[2, 3]

- History of blow to abdomen
- Possible bruise visible
- Pain and tenderness to mild pressure
- Abdominal distention
- Vomiting
- Rapid, weak pulse with low blood pressure
- If kidney is bruised or torn, there may be blood in urine shortly after trauma or next day (more likely, if injury is to the lumbar area of the back)
- Shoulder pain (Kehr's sign). Kehr's sign is pain at the tip of the shoulder due to internal bleeding in the abdominal cavity. A positive Kehr's sign is a medical emergency. **Call Emergency Medical Services (EMS) immediately!**[4]
  - If spleen is ruptured there may be complaints of left shoulder pain.
  - If liver is injured there may be complaints of right shoulder pain.
  - If there is a small intestinal tear the pain is minimal at first but worsens steadily.
- Gradual onset of shock and coma.
- Symptoms may appear a day or two following the blow.

MANAGEMENT/TREATMENT:[5]

1. Identification of trauma may not be obvious with initial evaluation.
2. Assessment should include vital signs, abdominal status, visual inspection, listen for bowel sounds, palpate painful and non- painful areas, check for rebound tenderness and rigidity.
3. Do not give fluids or food until the cause of pain is determined or pain subsides.
4. Notify parent. Tell what to watch for in the next 48 hours.
5. Keep in clinic for 15 minutes after blow to abdomen.
6. Allow to rest in position of comfort.
7. Monitor pulse and blood pressure.
8. If student has none of the above symptoms, may return to class. Send a note to the teacher to have the student return to health room/clinic before close of school and sooner, if symptoms appear.
9. Reassess the student.
10. If any symptoms ensue, refer to emergency room or healthcare provider.
11. Complete injury report, including information and instructions given to parent/guardian.

ABDOMEN: Blunt Injury *(continued from previous page)*

FOLLOW-UP:

Check student again on following day.

POTENTIAL COMPLICATIONS:[6]

- Missed diagnosis.
- Delay in diagnosis.
- Delay in treatment.
- Ruptured spleen: can be life-threatening without immediate treatment.
- Hypovolemic shock: symptoms include rapid pulse, cold-moist-clammy skin, alteration of consciousness, low blood pressure.

NOTES:

- Anatomical differences and underdeveloped muscles in children make them more susceptible to abdominal injuries with less force. Anatomically, the abdomen begins nipple level.[7]
- *Bicycle handlebar injury:*
  Abdominal injury may occur when handlebars are turned so they punch the abdomen with force. Bicycle handlebar injuries are often considered trivial; alarming symptoms may not develop for 24 hours. Symptoms of serious injury are severe pain, vomiting or collapse.
- Children who fall on bicycles shortly after eating are at greater risk for problems.[8]

REFERENCES

[1] Jones, E. L., Stovall, R. T., Jones, T. S., Bensard, D.D., Cothren, C., Burlew, C. C., Johnson, J.L., Jurkovich, G.J., Barnett,C.C., Pieracci, F.M., Biffl, W.L., & Moore, E.E. (2014, April). Intra-abdominal injury following blunt trauma becomes clinically apparent within 9 hours. *Journal of Trauma and Acute Care Surgery.,76*(4), *1020–1023.* https://www.ncbi.nlm.nih.gov/pmc/articles/PMC4091734/

[2] Legome, E.L., & Geibel, J. (2019). Blunt abdominal trauma. *Medscape*. http://emedicine.medscape.com/article/1980980-overview#a2

[3] Merck Manual Professional Version. (2018). *Overview of abdominal trauma.* https://www.merckmanuals.com/professional/injuries-poisoning/abdominal-trauma/overview-of-abdominal-trauma?query=blunt%20abdominal%20trauma

[4] Emergency Medical Paramedic. (n.d.). *What is kehr's sign?* http://www.emergencymedicalparamedic.com/what-is-kehrs-sign/

[5] Crosby, M.F., Lyons, E., & Prestidge, L. (2019). Students with acute illness. In Selekman, J., Adair, R., & Yonkaitis, C. (Eds.), *School nursing: A comprehensive text* (3rd ed., pp. 432-33). F.A. Davis.

[6] Legome, E.L., & Geibel, J. (2019). Blunt abdominal trauma. *Medscape.* http://emedicine.medscape.com/article/1980980-overview#a2

[7] Saxena, A. & Grehal, H. (2017). *Pediatric abdominal trauma.* https://emedicine.medscape.com/article/1984811-overview

[8] Daley, B., Raju, R., & Lee, S. (2015). *Considerations in pediatric trauma.* https://emedicine.medscape.com/article/435031-overview#a3

ABDOMEN: Blunt Injury *(continued from previous page)*

OTHER REFERENCES CONSULTED

Daley, B., Raju, R., & Lee, S. (2015). *Considerations in pediatric trauma.* https://emedicine.medscape.com/article/435031-overview#a3

Bravo, A., & Lopez, H. (2017). *Case report, The challenge of blunt abdominal trauma in children: Report of a case and review of management.* file:///C:/Users/Susan/AppData/Local/Packages/Microsoft.MicrosoftEdge_8wekyb3d8bbwe/TempState/Downloads/2901-17096-1-PB%20(1).pdf

Carnet, K.P., & Roswell, K. (2018). Emergencies & injuries. In W.W. Hay, M.J. Levin, R. R. Deterding, & M. J. Abzug (Eds.), *Current diagnosis and treatment: Pediatrics* (24th ed., pp. 309-330). McGraw Hill Education.

U.S. National Library of Medicine, National Institute of Health. (2012). *Recognition and management of abdominal events at athletic events.* International Journal of Sports Physical Therapy Medicine. https://www.ncbi.nlm.nih.gov/pmc/articles/PMC3414076/

ABDOMINAL PAIN/APPENDICITIS

OVERVIEW/DEFINITION:
Pain or discomfort located between the bottom of the diaphragm and the top of the pelvic region. Acute abdominal pain: short term develops in hours over weeks. Chronic recurrent abdominal pain: can be weeks, months or even years.[1]

Abdominal pain may be due to a variety of conditions, including but not limited to:

Intra-abdominal causes:[2,3]

<u>Gastrointestinal tract</u>

- Dietary (excessive or inappropriate intake, food-borne pathogens)
- Constipation
- Appendicitis
- Lactose intolerance (recurrent)
- Irritable bowel syndrome (discomfort for at least 12 weeks within past 12 months plus at least two of the following: altered frequency and/or appearance of bowel movements, pain relief with bowel movement)
- Peptic ulcer (recurrent)
- Incarcerated inguinal hernia
- Celiac disease (recurrent)

<u>Liver/Gall Bladder/Spleen</u>

- Hepatitis
- Pancreatitis
- Cholecystitis (inflammation of the gall bladder) and cholelithiasis (gall stones)
- Contusion/rupture spleen (trauma)
- Sickle cell anemia (recurrent)

<u>Urinary Tract</u>

- Cystitis (inflammation or infection of the bladder)
- Glomerulonephritis
- Kidney stone

<u>Ovaries, Fallopian Tubes and Uterus</u>

- Dysmenorrhea (menstrual cramps) (recurrent)
- Rupture of ovarian follicle at ovulation (mittelschmerz)
- Pelvic inflammatory disease (PID)
- Complication of pregnancy (ectopic pregnancy/abortion)
- Sexual abuse

ABDOMINAL PAIN/APPENDICITIS *(continued from previous page)*

Extra-abdominal causes:

- Abdominal migraine
- Diabetic ketoacidosis
- Functional abdominal pain (emotional or psychosocial)
- Group A streptococcal pharyngitis ("strep throat")
- Hypoglycemia
- Lead poisoning
- Leukemia
- Lower lobe pneumonia
- Rheumatic fever

Common causes by age of students:[4]

1. Preschool: constipation, gastroenteritis, viral infection, urinary tract infection, pneumonia, trauma, lactose intolerance, sickle cell episode.
2. School age: gastroenteritis, viral infection, constipation, appendicitis, trauma, urinary tract infection, pneumonia, lactose intolerance, sickle cell pain episode.
3. Adolescent: Early adolescence is prime time for occurrence of appendicitis, mittelschmerz (ovulation pain), pelvic inflammatory disease (PID), dysmenorrhea, complication of pregnancy.

SIGNS AND SYMPTOMS:

Symptoms vary depending on the etiology of the pain. A good assessment will help to differentiate the cause of the abdominal pain.

- Mildly ill: pain interferes minimally with normal activities.
- Moderately ill: interferes with normal routine or signs of infection or systemic illness.
- Severely ill: signs of peritonitis or intestinal obstruction or mental change.

ASSESSMENT:

History:[5]

- Onset, location, duration, frequency, severity and pattern of the pain.
- Associated symptoms such as fever, vomiting, diarrhea, red or dark red blood in stool, urinary symptoms, weight loss, jaundice, arthritis or cough and sore throat.
- Precipitating factors including constipation, trauma, underlying diseases (sickle cell anemia), menstruation, medication and diet history.

Physical examination:[6,7]

- Check temperature; assess circulation and hydration status.
- Enlarged liver, spleen or abdominal mass can be identified with palpitation of the lower quadrants.
- Guarding (tensing of the abdominal muscles to **guard** inflamed organs within the abdomen from the pain) can be elicited with gentle palpitation and rebound without deep palpation.

ABDOMINAL PAIN/APPENDICITIS *(continued from previous page)*

ASSESSMENT *(continued)*

- Note signs of emergency surgical conditions:
  - peritonitis: includes guarding and rigidity of the abdominal muscles, rebound tenderness, decreased/absent bowel sound, abdominal distention or shock.
  - intestinal obstruction: distention, hyperactive bowel sounds and persistent vomiting.
  - appendicitis:[8, 9, 10]
    - low fever at to begin but may progress and appendicitis progresses
    - nausea, vomiting
    - anorexia
    - vague diffuse epigastric or periumbilical pain, over several hours pain becomes more intense and shifts to right lower quadrant, rebound tenderness, release of pressure on left lower quadrant of abdomen elicits pain in right lower quadrant of abdomen (Rovsing sign)
    - decreased bowel sounds
    - prefers to lie on left side/right knee flexed
    - **If suspect appendix, perform auscultation, percussion, followed by palpation**
  - complication of pregnancy (female with history of delayed menstrual period) includes lower abdominal pain, pallor or shock, abnormal vaginal bleeding.

Assess location and severity of the pain:

Potential medical conditions according to pain location (list is not inclusive):[11]

- Diffuse abdominal pain: associated with diabetic ketoacidosis, food poisoning, gastroenteritis, intestinal obstruction, pancreatic disease, peritonitis, pharyngitis and sickle cell anemia.
- Epigastric pain: associated with duodenal/gastric/peptic ulcers, esophagitis, gastritis, gastroenteritis, GERD/hiatal hernia, myocardial infarction, irritable bowel disease, liver conditions and ulcerative colitis.
- Right lower quadrant: associated with appendicitis, ectopic pregnancy, gastroenteritis, inguinal hernia, irritable bowel syndrome (IBS), kidney stone, ovarian conditions, pelvic inflammatory disease and testicular torsion.
- Right upper quadrant: associated with acute pancreatitis, gallbladder conditions, kidney stone, duodenal ulcer, liver conditions and lower lobe pneumonia.
- Left upper quadrant: associated with bowel obstruction, constipation, IBS, kidney stone, left lower lobe pneumonia, leukemia, pyelonephritis, splenic conditions and ulcerative colitis.
- Left lower quadrant: associated with constipation, ectopic pregnancy, inguinal hernia, irritable bowel syndrome (IBS), kidney stone, ovarian conditions, pelvic inflammatory disease, sigmoid colon and testicular torsion.
- Suprapubic region: associated with dysmenorrhea, endometriosis, pelvic inflammatory disease, sexually transmitted disease, and urinary tract infection/bladder infections.

ABDOMINAL PAIN/APPENDICITIS *(continued from previous page)*

ANTICIPATED CONCERNS/PROBLEMS:
- Ruptured appendix requires surgery.

MANAGEMENT/POTENTIAL INTERVENTIONS:
- If signs of appendicitis (the most common serious condition) or moderate-severe illness notify the parent/guardian immediately and refer to the student's healthcare provider.
- If mild, may rest for 15-30 minutes. If symptoms persist, refer for evaluation. If symptoms subside, return student to class.
- No food or drink by mouth. May sip small amount of plain water.

FOLLOW-UP:
- If student returns to classroom, re-evaluate within 2-4 hours.
- If referred to healthcare provider, verify that evening or next day students was seen.[12]
- If student requires surgery, upon the student's return, follow healthcare provider's instructions regarding athletic or PE participation.

REFERENCES

[1] Mayo Clinic. (2019). *Abdominal pain.* https://www.mayoclinic.org/symptoms/abdominal-pain/basics/definition/sym-20050728

[2] Merck Manual Professional Version. (2018). *Acute abdominal pain.* http://www.merck.com/mmpe/sec02/ch011/ch011b.html

[3] Alder, A., & Minkes, R. (2018). Pediatric appendicitis. *Medscape.* https://emedicine.medscape.com/article/926795-overview

[4] Ruest, C. E., & Williams, A. (2016, May). Acute abdominal pain in children. *American Family Physician,* 93(10), 830-837. https://www.aafp.org/afp/2016/0515/p830.html

[5] Merck Manual Professional Version. (2018). *Acute abdominal pain.* http://www.merck.com/mmpe/sec02/ch011/ch011b.html

[6] Ruest, C E., & Williams, A. (2016, May). Acute abdominal pain in children. *American Family Physician, 93*(10), 830-837. https://www.aafp.org/afp/2016/0515/p830.html

[7] Cosby, M.F., Lyons, E., & Prestidge, L. (2019). Students with acute illness and injury. In J. Selekman, R. Adair Shannon, & C. F. Yonkaitis (Eds.), *School nursing: A comprehensive text* (3rd ed., pp. 442-43). F.A. Davis.

[8] Merck Manual Professional Version. (2018). *Acute abdominal pain.* http://www.merck.com/mmpe/sec02/ch011/ch011b.html

[9] Alder, A., & Minkes, R. (2018). Pediatric appendicitis differential diagnosis. *Medscape.* https://emedicine.medscape.com/article/926795-differential

[10] Mayo Clinic. (2019). *Appendicitis.* https://www.mayoclinic.org/diseases-conditions/appendicitis/symptoms-causes/syc-20369543

[11] Merck Manual Professional Version. (2018). *Acute abdominal pain.* http://www.merck.com/mmpe/sec02/ch011/ch011b.html

[12] Cosby, M.F., Lyons, E., & Prestidge, L. (2019). Students with acute illness and injury. In J. Selekman, R. Adair Shannon, & C. F. Yonkaitis (Eds.), *School nursing: A comprehensive text* (3rd ed., pp. 442-43). F.A. Davis.

ABRASIONS

DEFINITION/ETIOLOGY:
An abrasion is a denuded area of skin (epidermis) resulting from a scrape on a hard or rough surface. Abrasions can occur on any part of the body, but most often occur on bony areas, such as the hands, forearms, elbows, knees, shins, and face. Abrasions often result from falls or friction accidents.[1]

SIGNS AND SYMPTOMS:

- Most abrasions are superficial (involve only the dermis layer).
- There is usually minimal bleeding and may ooze serosanguinous fluid. The amount of bleeding is greater when deeper layers of skin are scraped off.
- Abrasions can contain particles of dirt, or other foreign materials.

MANAGEMENT/TREATMENT:

- Wash gently under running tap water with antibacterial soap to remove foreign material. If feasible, allow a running stream of lukewarm water to pour over the wound.
    - During wash, if necessary, try to remove debris or other foreign materials by gently rubbing with 4x4 gauze pads.
    - Do not scrub a wound imbedded with dirt or other foreign material/debris. Instead, refer to healthcare provider.
- Assess and document tetanus immunization status.
- Do **NOT** use povidone-iodine, Dakin's solution and hydrogen peroxide for cleansing wounds. These solutions can damage normal tissue and hinder neodermal development necessary for healing. Only use antibiotic creams/ointments.
- Small abrasions may be left open to the air.
- Cover larger abrasions with a sterile, non-adherent bandage.
- After partial thickness abrasions are cleaned, a moist wound dressing can be applied within two hours of injury.[2] This dressing can be a hydrogel or hydrocolloid dressing and can be any of a variety of brand-name products. This dressing must stay in place at least forty-eight hours and up to seven days to enhance optimal wound healing. Moist wound dressings allow rapid resurfacing or re-epithelialization of wound surfaces and allow for migration of proteins necessary for wound healing.
- Notify parent/guardian if the abrasion is more extensive or deeper than a superficial abrasion. Complete the assessment/treatment section of the injury report if the abrasion was the result of an injury or fall at school. **Note**: Work with the school staff who observed the incident and document the incident per state, school or district protocol.
- The Bates-Jensen Wound Assessment Tool[3] can be used by a registered nurse to re-evaluate a partial thickness abrasion.
- Once re-epithelialization has occurred, no further dressing is needed.

ABRASIONS *(continued from previous page)*

FOLLOW-UP: Partial thickness and deeper abrasions

- Instruct the parent/guardian and student that the dressing is to remain in place until wound is healed. Wrap the dressing with plastic for bathing. The student may be given an extra dressing to take home if his/her dressing falls off or is damaged and needs replaced.
- The student should have a daily wound and dressing recheck; replace dressing as needed.
- Refer the student to his/her healthcare provider if the laceration or abrasion is not healing.
- Repeat cleansing at least daily, more often if necessary, to keep wound clean until healed.

POTENTIAL COMPLICATIONS:

1. Infection:
   - Pus on abrasion itself, usually located under crusts.
   - Cellulitis: spreading redness immediately around the abrasion.
   - Lymphangitis: red streaks radiating out from abrasion. (Sometimes this is mistakenly referred to as blood poisoning. It is actually an infection of the lymph channels.)
   - Regional lymph nodes enlarged; if abrasion on arm, nodes will be in axilla; if on leg, nodes will be in groin.

2. Scarring:
   - Minor abrasions: scar very superficial, usually regains pigmentation and blends with surrounding skin.
   - Deep abrasions: scar usually deeper and permanent. (May require later management for cosmetic reasons).

NOTES:[4]

- If no improvement in ONE day, refer to healthcare provider.
- For lymphangitis, refer to healthcare provider immediately.
- Nurse practitioners or other nurses with prescriptive authority may order amoxicillin or other antibiotics.

REFERENCES

---

[1] Healthline. (2019). *Everything you should know about skin abrasions.* https://www.healthline.com/health/abrasion

[2] Merck Manual. (2019). *Abrasions.* https://www.merckmanuals.com/professional/injuries-poisoning/lacerations-and-abrasions/abrasions

[3] Healthline. (2019). *Everything you should know about skin abrasions.* https://www.healthline.com/health/abrasion

[4] Merck Manual. (2019). *Abrasions.* https://www.merckmanuals.com/professional/injuries-poisoning/lacerations-and-abrasions/abrasions

OTHER REFERENCES CONSULTED

Ball, J., Binder, R., & Cowen, K. (Eds.). (2017). Alterations in skin integrity. Principles of Pediatric Nursing: Caring for Children (7th ed., pp.941-1041). Pearson Education, Inc.

ACUTE FLACCID MYELITIS

DEFINITION/ETIOLOGY:

Acute flaccid myelitis (AFM) is a condition affecting the motor neurons in the spinal cord; more specifically the gray matter of the spinal cord that controls the body's muscles and reflexes. AFM was first recognized in 2010 but has gained attention after the large outbreak in 2014.[1] The etiology of AFM is unclear, but the most common link is viral. In 2014, the initial cluster of AFM was linked to enterovirus D68; a respiratory illness. Since 2014, "seasonal waves" of AFM have been cyclical, spiking about every two years. In 2016, links to enterovirus A71, adenovirus, rhinovirus, and herpesvirus were all detected.[2] Greater than 90% of the patients diagnosed with AFM all experienced a respiratory illness or fever consistent with a viral illness prior to becoming symptomatic with acute onset of limb weakness, and other symptoms.[3] The Centers for Disease Control and Prevention continues to investigate other causes like environmental toxins or a genetic link in making one person more susceptible than another.

SIGNS AND SYMPTOMS:

- Recent history of a respiratory illness or fever
- Neurological symptoms including sudden acute onset limb weakness, stiff neck, headache, and pain that rapidly develop and quickly progress over hours or days[4]
- Numbness or tingling in limbs
- Slurred speech
- Inability to pass urine
- Facial dropping
- Drooping eyelids
- Difficulty swallowing
- The most severe is respiratory failure[5]

MANAGEMENT/TREATMENT:

- Healthcare providers rely on careful examination as well as magnetic resonance imaging (MRI) and lab testing of the cerebrospinal fluid (CFS) for diagnosis.[6]
- Currently there is no specific therapy or intervention for the treatment of AFM, though an initial treatment phase that includes Intravenous immunoglobulin (IVIG) has been used, as well as steroids, and plasma exchange, but these treatments have yielded mix opinions.[7]
- Decrease the risk of exposure to viruses during cold and flu season, by instituting good hand washing with soap and water. (*Refer to HANDWASHING HANDOUTS in the APPENDIX).*
- Cover coughs and sneezes with tissue or sleeves. (*Refer to COUGH and COVER HANDOUT in the APPENDIX).*
- Stay home when sick.
- Clean and disinfect surfaces appropriately.
- Avoid touching hands or face.
- Ensure immunizations and influenza vaccine are current.

ACUTE FLACCID MYELITIS *(continued from previous page)*

MANAGEMENT/TREATMENT *(continued)*

- The treatment phase of AFM should include intensive rehabilitation therapy for speech, occupational and physical therapy to help restore function to the nervous system.[8]
- Activity–based Restorative Therapy (ABRT) uses high intensity, repetitive approach to drive the enteral nervous system's ability to spontaneously regenerate after spinal cord injury.[9]
- Nerve transfer surgery for upper extremities.[10]

SCHOOL NURSES ROLE/ SCHOOL RECOMMENDATIONS/FOLLOW-UP:

- The school nurse should gather any history of any recent respiratory, gastrointestinal or genitourinary symptoms when referring a student for further assessment if a student presents at school with weakness, pain in extremities, slurred speech, changes in bladder or bowel habits.[11]
- The school nurse should consult the state or local health department if he/she suspects a student may have AFM for surveillance purposes.[12]
- Educate school staff.
- Raise awareness to parents, guardians, students and community regarding AFM, stressing if a child experiences any signs of weakness, to take the child to the Emergency Room.[13]
- Develop a Section 504 plan for accommodations, if needed.
- Develop an Individualized Healthcare Plan (IHP), in partnership with the school-home team, as necessary.
- Review and revise Section 504 plan and IHP if complication/changes arise.
- Review and promote good handwashing.[14] *(Refer to HANDWASHING HANDOUTS in the APPENDIX).*
- Teach covering nose and mouth with a tissue or sleeve when coughing or sneezing, proper disposal of tissues; wash hands or use alcohol-based hand sanitizer after blowing nose or touching secretions.
- Collaborate with school staff regarding proper cleaning of tabletops, and surfaces in the school setting.[15]

POTENTIAL COMPLICATIONS:

- Paralysis of affected limb(s)
- Ventilator dependency due to respiratory muscle weakness
- Slurred speech
- Neurogenic bowel and bladder

ACUTE FLACCID MYELITIS *(continued from previous page)*

REFERENCES

[1] Levy, M., Giovannoni, G., Hawkes, C., Lechner-Scott, J., & Waubant, E. (2019, April). Acute flaccid myelitis in the 21st century: Reminiscence of poliomyelitis or a new emergent disease. Multiple Sclerosis and Related Disorders, 29, A1-A2 https://doi.org/10.1016/j.msard.2019.03.007

[2]American Academy of Pediatrics. (2019). *AFM in children*. https://www.healthychildren.org/English/health-issues/conditions/head-neck-nervous-system/Pages/AFM.aspx 1

[3]Centers for Disease Control and Prevention. (2019). *About acute flaccid myelitis*. https://www.cdc.gov/acute-flaccid-myelitis/about-afm.html

[4]American Academy of Pediatrics. (2019). *AFM in children*. https://www.healthychildren.org/English/health-issues/conditions/head-neck-nervous-system/Pages/AFM.aspx 1

[4] Ibid.

[5]The Transverse Myelitis Association. (2019). *Acute flaccid myelitis (AFM).* https://myelitis.org/wp-content/uploads/2019/03/2019_AFM.pdf

[6] Ibid.

[7] Centers for Disease Control and Prevention. (2019). *About acute flaccid myelitis*. https://www.cdc.gov/acute-flaccid-myelitis/about-afm.html

[7] American Academy of Pediatrics. (2019). *AFM in children*. https://www.healthychildren.org/English/health-issues/conditions/head-neck-nervous-system/Pages/AFM.aspx 1

[8] The Transverse Myelitis Association. (2019). Acute flaccid myelitis (AFM). https://myelitis.org/wp-content/uploads/2019/03/2019_AFM.pdf

[9] Ibid.

[10] Morens, D.M., Folkers, G.K., & Fauci, A.S. (2019). Acute flaccid myelitis: Something old and something new. mBio, 10(2), e00521-19. https://do.org/: 10.1128/mbio.00521-19

[11] Woldai, S. & Binnix, A. (2019). Acute flaccid myelitis: Nursing implications and public health. American Nurse Today, 14 (6), 25-27. https://www.americannursetoday.com/acute-flaccid-myelitis/

[12] The Transverse Myelitis Association. (2019). *Acute flaccid myelitis (AFM).* https://myelitis.org/wp-content/uploads/2019/03/2019_AFM.pdf

[13] Centers for Disease Control and Prevention. (2019). *About acute flaccid myelitis.* https://www.cdc.gov/acute-flaccid-myelitis/about-afm.html

[14] Ibid.

[15] Kilmer, M., Shreve, M., & Jarrett, A. (2019). *Clarifying the diagnosis of acute flaccid myelitis*. The Journal for Nurse Practitioners, 15(6), 444-448. https://doi.org/10.1016/j.nurpra.2019.01.007

OTHER REFERENCES CONSULTED

Betsy, T. (2019). Acute flaccid myelitis: An ongoing investigation. American Journal of Nursing, 119(2),60-62. https://doi.org/10.1097/01.NAJ.0000553207.44212.21

ADRENAL INSUFFICIENCY

OVERVIEW/DEFINITION:

Adrenal insufficiency is an endocrine disorder that occurs when the adrenal glands do not produce a sufficient amount of the hormone cortisol. Adrenal insufficiency can also affect the production of the hormone aldosterone. Cortisol and aldosterone are crucial for the body to regulate blood pressure, metabolism, heart contractibility and sodium balance. Cortisol also regulates the body's response to stress. Lack of cortisol production affects the body's ability to appropriately respond to physiological stressors. Onset of adrenal insufficiency is usually gradual.

There are a multitude of known causes for adrenal inefficiency. Adrenal insufficiency is classified as either primary or secondary.

Primary adrenal insufficiency[1] (commonly referred to as Addison's disease) occurs when the adrenal glands are compromised and do not produce the hormone cortisol. Addison's disease is caused by an autoimmune response in approximately 80-90% of cases.

Secondary adrenal insufficiency[2] occurs when the pituitary gland is diseased and unable to produce the hormone adrenocorticotropin (ACTH). ACTH stimulates the adrenal gland to produce the hormone cortisol. Impaired production of ACTH causes a decrease in the production of cortisol thereby triggering shrinkage of the adrenal glands. Secondary adrenal insufficiency is more common than primary adrenal insufficiency.

SIGNS AND SYMPTOMS:[3, 4, 5]

Symptoms are the same for primary and secondary adrenal insufficiency unless specifically noted.

- Muscle and joint pain
- Nausea and vomiting
- Diarrhea
- Hypotension
- Hypoglycemia (unexplained)
- Generalized weakness
- Growth delay
- Chronic fatigue
- Depression
- Irritability

Late Symptoms:

- Weight loss
- Bronze pigmentation to skin (occurs only with primary adrenal insufficiency)
- Salt cravings
- Severe weakness
- Confusion
- Pain in legs

ADRENAL INSUFFICIENCY *(continued from previous page)*

ANTICIPATED CONCERNS/PROBLEMS:[6, 7]

Adrenal Crisis is a serious complication of adrenal insufficiency. An adrenal crisis is a sudden, severe worsening of adrenal insufficiency symptoms. This can occur when an individual with adrenal insufficiency experiences a traumatic physical or emotional stressor.

An adrenal crisis is life-threatening. Symptoms of an adrenal crisis include:

- Dizziness/lightheaded
- Sudden, muscle pain (can be severe – often occurs in low back, abdomen or legs)
- Severe nausea and vomiting
- Severe abdominal pain
- Confusion
- Hypotension
- Neurological deficits (headache/confusion/seizure)
- Shock like symptoms
- Loss of consciousness
- Death (if left untreated)

Rapid physical deterioration can occur. **If a person with adrenal insufficiency exhibits these symptoms, act immediately!**

1. Administer prescribed Solu-Cortef IM
2. Call Emergency Medical Services (EMS).
3. Provide appropriate first aid care.
4. Notify parent/guardian.

MANAGEMENT/POTENTIAL INTERVENTIONS:[8]

Adrenal insufficiency results in a lack of essential hormones, and therefore treatment focuses on replacing these vital hormones. Individuals with adrenal insufficiency are glucocorticoid dependent and must take cortisol daily. Cortisol is taken orally once or twice a day. If necessary, aldosterone is replaced orally once a day. The student may also need to follow a high sodium diet and/or have salty snacks at school.

FOLLOW-UP:

1. Communicate and monitor, per healthcare provider instructions, necessary medication dosage changes. Medication dosages often need to be adjusted to meet a student's needs during times of stress. Once the stressor is over, the healthcare provider typically returns medication dosages to pre-illness (pre-injury) levels.
2. Encourage student to wear medical alert identification.

ADRENAL INSUFFICIENCY *(continued from previous page)*

NOTES:

- Develop an Emergency Care Plan (ECP) to accommodate an adrenal crisis and an Individualized Healthcare Plan (IHP) to address all other issues.
- Train appropriate staff involved with student.
- Children with adrenal insufficiency may experience short-term memory difficulties and/or learning disabilities
- Evaluate need for Section 504 accommodations or Special Education services.

REFERENCES

[1] Mayo Clinic. (2018). *Addison's disease.* http://www.mayoclinic.org/diseases-conditions/addisons-disease/basics/causes/con-20021340

[2] Merck Manual, Consumers Version. (2018). *Secondary adrenal insufficiency.* http://www.merckmanuals.com/professional/endocrine-and-metabolic-disorders/adrenal-disorders/secondary-adrenal-insufficiency

[3] American Academy of Pediatrics. (2019). *Addison disease.* https://familydoctor.org/condition/addisons-disease/?adfree=true

[4] Mayo Clinic. (2018). *Addison's disease.* http://www.mayoclinic.org/diseases-conditions/addisons-disease/basics/causes/con-20021340

[5] American Academy of Pediatrics. (2019). *Addison disease.* https://familydoctor.org/condition/addisons-disease/?adfree=true

[6] Merck Manual, Consumers Version. (2019). *Addison disease.* https://www.merckmanuals.com/home/hormonal-and-metabolic-disorders/adrenal-gland-disorders/addison-disease

[7] Mayo Clinic. (2018). *Addison's disease.* http://www.mayoclinic.org/diseases-conditions/addisons-disease/basics/causes/con-20021340

[8] Mayo Clinic. (2018). *Addison's disease.* http://www.mayoclinic.org/diseases-conditions/addisons-disease/basics/causes/con-20021340

OTHER REFERENCES CONSULTED

Medline Plus. (2019). *Addison disease.* https://medlineplus.gov/addisondisease.html

National Endocrine and Metabolic Diseases. (2018). *Adrenal insufficiency and Addison's disease.* https://www.niddk.nih.gov/health-information/endocrine-diseases/adrenal-insufficiency-addisons-disease/symptoms-causes

ALLERGIES

(Refer to ANAPHYLAXIS, FOOD ALLERGIES, LATEX ALLERGIES, STING ALLERGIES, POISON IVY/OAK, RASHES)

DEFINITION/ETIOLOGY:

The immune system reacts to a foreign substance that is not generally harmful (examples – certain foods, latex, pollen, insect stings/bites, medications or pet dander).[1]

SIGNS AND SYMPTOMS:[2]

Symptoms vary and depend on the persons' specific allergy. Allergy symptoms range from mild to life threatening, anaphylactic reactions.

Allergic Dermatitis	• Rash (papules/vesicles) at site of contact • Pruritus • May have areas of excoriation from scratching • Thickened dry skin that may ooze
Allergic Rhinitis	• Allergic shiners – bluish discoloration and edema below eyes • Clear nasal discharge • Sneezing • Itchy, watery and/or swollen eyes
Atopic Dermatitis (allergic type of eczema)	• Thickened, cracked, or scaly patches of skin • Patches red to brownish gray in color • Itchy skin • Extremely dry skin may ooze • Most commonly seen on arms, legs, but may appear anywhere on the body
Medication Allergy (penicillin, sulfa, anticonvulsants, iodine and insulin are the most common cause of medication allergies)	• Hives • Rash • Pruritus • Difficulty breathing/wheezing • Anaphylaxis

GENERAL MANAGEMENT/TREATMENT:[3]

General treatment

- Avoidance of allergen
- Medications (as prescribed) to reduce symptoms
- Immunotherapy (allergy shots)
- Emergency epinephrine

ALLERGIES *(continued from previous page)*

GENERAL MANAGEMENT/TREATMENT *(continued)*

Allergic Dermatitis

- Corticosteroids creams/ointments – to ease itching
- Corticosteroid (oral) – reduces inflammation, immune response and itching
- Antihistamines – to relieve severe itching
- Antibiotics – if lesions are infected from scratching

Allergic Rhinitis

- Antihistamines - relieves sneezing, runny nose, itching, and watery eyes
- Nasal corticosteroid sprays – start working quickly but may take several weeks to obtain the full effect of the medication
- Decongestants – reduce symptoms of nasal congestion
- Leukotriene inhibitor (i.e. Singulair®) - to relieve seasonal allergy symptoms
- Immunotherapy

Atopic Dermatitis

- **Oral corticosteroids – may be prescribed short-term to treat severe cases**. There is increased concern about the long-term use of oral corticosteroids.
- Corticosteroid creams or ointments - to ease scaling of skin and itching.
- Antihistamines-- to relieve severe itching.
- Antibiotics – if lesions are infected from scratching.
- Immunomodulators – reduces atopic dermatitis flare-ups**. These medications are approved for children over the age of two. The U.S. Food and Drug Administration (FDA) recommends that these medications be used only when other treatment options have failed**.

Medication Allergy

- **Discontinue medication that caused allergic response immediately.**
- Antihistamines - to relieve mild symptoms of rash/hives/itching.
- Bronchodilators - to relieve wheezing.
- Corticosteroids - reduce inflammation associated with allergic reaction.
- Epinephrine - for severe allergic reaction.

FOLLOW-UP:

- Refer to healthcare provider if symptoms do not respond to treatment.
- Educate as to the importance of avoiding known allergens.
- Develop an Individualized Healthcare Plan (IHP) for severe allergies – provide information regarding the importance of wearing a medical alert necklace/bracelet.
- Identify coexisting medical conditions such as asthma – commonly associated with allergic rhinitis and atopic dermatitis - anaphylactic reactions are more severe in students with asthma.
- Educate family and student on hand washing and keeping nails trimmed to prevent secondary infections from scratching.
- Instruct school staff to be aware of any bullying related to allergens.

ALLERGIES *(continued from previous page)*

POTENTIAL COMPLICATIONS:

General

- Skin infections from frequent scratching
- Another allergy
- Anaphylaxis (severe allergic reaction) (*Refer to ANAPHYLAXIS*)
- Death

Allergic rhinitis

- Sinusitis
- Otitis Media

NOTES:

- Appropriate school staff (including bus personnel and cafeteria and playground personnel) should receive in-service training to learn how to reduce exposures to allergens, respond to a student with a general allergic reaction and with child specific needs.
- Staff training in the use of injected epinephrine should be conducted according to state and district laws and policies.[4]
- All states (except HI) have adopted legislation that allows schools provide undesignated epinephrine auto injectors. Some states mandate stock emergency medication and some allow it – know your state's laws and regulations.

Allergy Resources for School Personnel

Allergy & Asthma Network
https://www.allergyasthmanetwork.org

Allergy & Anaphylaxis: A Practical Guide for Schools & Families
https://www.allergyasthmanetwork.org/outreach/publications/special-publications/allergy-anaphylaxis-practical-guide-for-schools-and-families/

American Academy of Allergy and Asthma and Immunology (AAAAI)
1-800-822-ASMA
https://www.aaaai.org/
Professional and patient education resources on the website

Asthma and Allergy Foundation of America
https://www.aafa.org/
Resources and free student Asthma Action Cards

Food Allergy and Anaphylaxis Network (FAAN)
U.S. Department of Health and Human Services
https://healthfinder.gov/FindServices/Organizations/Organization.aspx?code=HR2472
Specific School guidelines (including school bus and field trips) and teaching materials.

ALLERGIES *(continued from previous page)*

REFERENCES

[1] American Academy of Allergy, Asthma & Immunology. (2019). Allergies. https://www.aaaai.org/conditions-and-treatments/allergies

[2] Mayo Clinic. (2018). *Allergies.* https://www.mayoclinic.org/diseases- conditions/allergies/symptoms-causes/syc-20351497

[3] Mayo Clinic. (2018). *Allergies.* https://www.mayoclinic.org/diseases- conditions/allergies/symptoms-causes/syc-20351497

[4] Hogate, S., Giel, J., Selekman, J. (2019). Allergy. In J. Selekman, R. Adair Shannon, & C. F. Yonkaitis (Eds.), *School nursing: A comprehensive text* (3rd ed., pp. 500-522). F.A. Davis.

OTHER REFERENCES CONSULTED

Pham, M., Pistiner, M., & Wang, J. (2019). National school nurse survey of food allergy and anaphylaxis policies and education. Clinical communication. *The Journal of Allergy and Clinical Immunology: In Practice, 7*(7), pp. 2440–2442.e7. https://www.jaci-inpractice.org/article/S2213-2198(19)30277-6/abstract

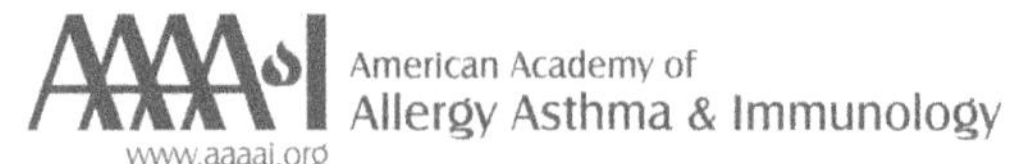

Anaphylaxis Emergency Action Plan

Patient Name: ______________________________ Age: __________

Allergies: ______________________________

Asthma ☐ Yes *(high risk for severe reaction)* ☐ No

Additional health problems besides anaphylaxis: ______________________________

____

Concurrent medications: ______________________________

____

	Symptoms of Anaphylaxis
MOUTH	itching, swelling of lips and/or tongue
THROAT*	itching, tightness/closure, hoarseness
SKIN	itching, hives, redness, swelling
GUT	vomiting, diarrhea, cramps
LUNG*	shortness of breath, cough, wheeze
HEART*	weak pulse, dizziness, passing out

Only a few symptoms may be present. Severity of symptoms can change quickly.
**Some symptoms can be life-threatening. ACT FAST!*

Emergency Action Steps - DO NOT HESITATE TO GIVE EPINEPHRINE!

1. Inject epinephrine in thigh using (check one): ☐ Adrenaclick (0.15 mg) ☐ Adrenaclick (0.3 mg)

☐ Auvi-Q (0.15 mg) ☐ Auvi-Q (0.3 mg)

☐ EpiPen Jr (0.15 mg) ☐ EpiPen (0.3 mg)

Epinephrine Injection, USP Auto-injector- authorized generic
☐ (0.15 mg) ☐ (0.3 mg)

☐ Other (0.15 mg) ☐ Other (0.3 mg)

Specify others: ______________________________

IMPORTANT: ASTHMA INHALERS AND/OR ANTIHISTAMINES CAN'T BE DEPENDED ON IN ANAPHYLAXIS.

2. Call 911 or rescue squad (before calling contact)

3. Emergency contact #1: home__________ work__________ cell__________

Emergency contact #2: home__________ work__________ cell__________

Emergency contact #3: home__________ work__________ cell__________

Comments: ______________________________

____

____

Doctor's Signature/Date/Phone Number

____

Parent's Signature (for individuals under age 18 yrs)/Date

FARE — FOOD ALLERGY & ANAPHYLAXIS EMERGENCY CARE PLAN

Food Allergy Research & Education

Name: ______________________ D.O.B.: ____________

Allergy to: ______________________

Weight: ________ lbs. Asthma: ☐ **Yes (higher risk for a severe reaction)** ☐ **No**

NOTE: Do not depend on antihistamines or inhalers (bronchodilators) to treat a severe reaction. USE EPINEPHRINE.

Extremely reactive to the following allergens: ______________________

THEREFORE:

☐ If checked, give epinephrine immediately if the allergen was LIKELY eaten, for ANY symptoms.

☐ If checked, give epinephrine immediately if the allergen was DEFINITELY eaten, even if no symptoms are apparent.

FOR **ANY** OF THE FOLLOWING:

SEVERE SYMPTOMS

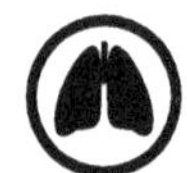

LUNG Shortness of breath, wheezing, repetitive cough

HEART Pale or bluish skin, faintness, weak pulse, dizziness

THROAT Tight or hoarse throat, trouble breathing or swallowing

MOUTH Significant swelling of the tongue or lips

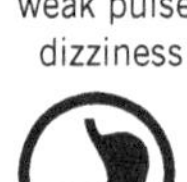

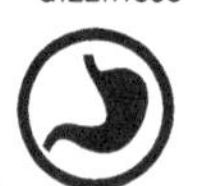

SKIN Many hives over body, widespread redness

GUT Repetitive vomiting, severe diarrhea

OTHER Feeling something bad is about to happen, anxiety, confusion

OR A COMBINATION of symptoms from different body areas.

1. **INJECT EPINEPHRINE IMMEDIATELY.**
2. **Call 911.** Tell emergency dispatcher the person is having anaphylaxis and may need epinephrine when emergency responders arrive.

- Consider giving additional medications following epinephrine:
  - » Antihistamine
  - » Inhaler (bronchodilator) if wheezing
- Lay the person flat, raise legs and keep warm. If breathing is difficult or they are vomiting, let them sit up or lie on their side.
- If symptoms do not improve, or symptoms return, more doses of epinephrine can be given about 5 minutes or more after the last dose.
- Alert emergency contacts.
- Transport patient to ER, even if symptoms resolve. Patient should remain in ER for at least 4 hours because symptoms may return.

MILD SYMPTOMS

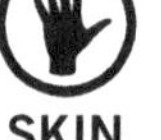

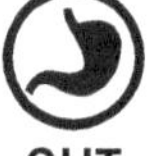

NOSE Itchy or runny nose, sneezing

MOUTH Itchy mouth

SKIN A few hives, mild itch

GUT Mild nausea or discomfort

FOR **MILD SYMPTOMS** FROM **MORE THAN ONE** SYSTEM AREA, GIVE EPINEPHRINE.

FOR **MILD SYMPTOMS** FROM **A SINGLE SYSTEM** AREA, FOLLOW THE DIRECTIONS BELOW:

1. Antihistamines may be given, if ordered by a healthcare provider.
2. Stay with the person; alert emergency contacts.
3. Watch closely for changes. If symptoms worsen, give epinephrine.

MEDICATIONS/DOSES

Epinephrine Brand or Generic: ______________

Epinephrine Dose: ☐ 0.1 mg IM ☐ 0.15 mg IM ☐ 0.3 mg IM

Antihistamine Brand or Generic: ______________

Antihistamine Dose: ______________

Other (e.g., inhaler-bronchodilator if wheezing): ______________

____

PATIENT OR PARENT/GUARDIAN AUTHORIZATION SIGNATURE　DATE　PHYSICIAN/HCP AUTHORIZATION SIGNATURE　DATE

FORM PROVIDED COURTESY OF FOOD ALLERGY RESEARCH & EDUCATION (FARE) (FOODALLERGY.ORG) 5/2018

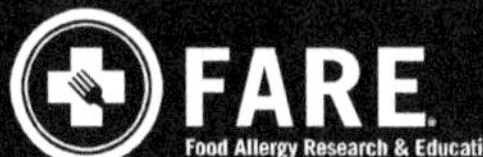

FOOD ALLERGY & ANAPHYLAXIS EMERGENCY CARE PLAN

HOW TO USE AUVI-Q® (EPINEPRHINE INJECTION, USP), KALEO

1. Remove Auvi-Q from the outer case.
2. Pull off red safety guard.
3. Place black end of Auvi-Q against the middle of the outer thigh.
4. Press firmly until you hear a click and hiss sound, and hold in place for 2 seconds.
5. Call 911 and get emergency medical help right away.

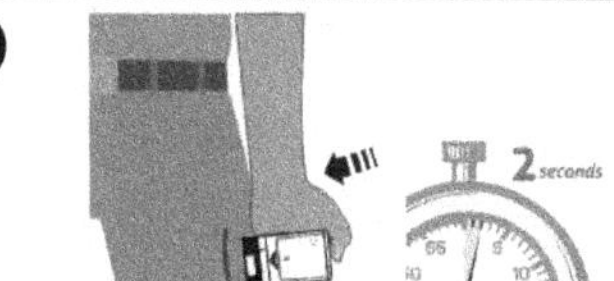

HOW TO USE EPIPEN® AND EPIPEN JR® (EPINEPHRINE) AUTO-INJECTOR AND EPINEPHRINE INJECTION (AUTHORIZED GENERIC OF EPIPEN®), USP AUTO-INJECTOR, MYLAN AUTO-INJECTOR, MYLAN

1. Remove the EpiPen® or EpiPen Jr® Auto-Injector from the clear carrier tube.
2. Grasp the auto-injector in your fist with the orange tip (needle end) pointing downward.
3. With your other hand, remove the blue safety release by pulling straight up.
4. Swing and push the auto-injector firmly into the middle of the outer thigh until it 'clicks'.
5. Hold firmly in place for 3 seconds (count slowly 1, 2, 3).
6. Remove and massage the injection area for 10 seconds.
7. Call 911 and get emergency medical help right away.

HOW TO USE IMPAX EPINEPHRINE INJECTION (AUTHORIZED GENERIC OF ADRENACLICK®), USP AUTO-INJECTOR, IMPAX LABORATORIES

1. Remove epinephrine auto-injector from its protective carrying case.
2. Pull off both blue end caps: you will now see a red tip.
3. Grasp the auto-injector in your fist with the red tip pointing downward.
4. Put the red tip against the middle of the outer thigh at a 90-degree angle, perpendicular to the thigh.
5. Press down hard and hold firmly against the thigh for approximately 10 seconds.
6. Remove and massage the area for 10 seconds.
7. Call 911 and get emergency medical help right away.

HOW TO USE TEVA'S GENERIC EPIPEN® (EPINEPHRINE INJECTION, USP) AUTO-INJECTOR, TEVA PHARMACEUTICAL INDUSTRIES

1. Quickly twist the yellow or green cap off of the auto-injector in the direction of the "twist arrow" to remove it.
2. Grasp the auto-injector in your fist with the orange tip (needle end) pointing downward.
3. With your other hand, pull off the blue safety release.
4. Place the orange tip against the middle of the outer thigh (upper leg) at a right angle (perpendicular) to the thigh.
5. Swing and push the auto-injector firmly into the middle of the outer thigh until it 'clicks'.
6. Hold firmly in place for 3 seconds (count slowly 1, 2, 3).
7. Remove and massage the injection area for 10 seconds.
8. Call 911 and get emergency medical help right away.

ADMINISTRATION AND SAFETY INFORMATION FOR ALL AUTO-INJECTORS:

1. Do not put your thumb, fingers or hand over the tip of the auto-injector or inject into any body part other than mid-outer thigh. In case of accidental injection, go immediately to the nearest emergency room.
2. If administering to a young child, hold their leg firmly in place before and during injection to prevent injuries.
3. Epinephrine can be injected through clothing if needed.
4. Call 911 immediately after injection.

OTHER DIRECTIONS/INFORMATION (may self-carry epinephrine, may self-administer epinephrine, etc.):

Treat the person before calling emergency contacts. The first signs of a reaction can be mild, but symptoms can worsen quickly.

EMERGENCY CONTACTS — CALL 911

RESCUE SQUAD: ____________________

DOCTOR: ____________________ PHONE: __________

PARENT/GUARDIAN: ____________________ PHONE: __________

OTHER EMERGENCY CONTACTS

NAME/RELATIONSHIP: ____________________ PHONE: __________

NAME/RELATIONSHIP: ____________________ PHONE: __________

NAME/RELATIONSHIP: ____________________ PHONE: __________

FORM PROVIDED COURTESY OF FOOD ALLERGY RESEARCH & EDUCATION (FARE) (FOODALLERGY.ORG) 1/2019

ALLERGY, LATEX

DEFINITION/ETIOLOGY (*Refer to ALLERGIES and ANAPHYLAXIS*):
Latex allergy is a reaction to certain proteins found in natural rubber latex (a product manufactured from a milky fluid that comes from the rubber tree). Natural rubber latex is different from synthetic rubber made from chemicals. Synthetic rubber products, including "latex" house paints, are not made with natural latex and do not trigger allergic reactions in people who are allergic to natural rubber latex products. The more frequently exposed a person is to latex either by direct contact or inhalation (e.g., staff administering daily care requiring use of gloves, persons with spina bifida who use latex catheters), the more likely they are to develop sensitivity.[1]

A latex allergy may cause allergic reactions ranging from sneezing or a runny nose to anaphylaxis, a potentially life-threatening condition. The severity of the reaction can get worse with repeated exposure to latex products. Almost half of people with a latex allergy have a history of an allergy to another substance.[2]

Delayed Reaction (due to chemicals used in processing latex):[3]

- Itchy, red, mildly swollen skin rash on sites which touched latex
- Typically appearing 12-36 hours after contact
- Blisters appear in severe cases

Immediate Allergic Reaction (due to proteins which are part of the natural latex):[4]

- Involves parts of the body that did not touch latex, or respiratory symptoms from airborne latex
- Hives on any part of the body
- "Hay fever-like" nasal stuffiness, sneezing, runny nose, itchy nose, eyes or roof of the mouth

Severe Reactions occur within minutes and involve multiple body systems.

- Wheezing, coughing, shortness of breath, and passing out - ***an emergency***
- **Anaphylaxis** - a life threatening blockage of the airway and shock

MANAGEMENT/TREATMENT:
Treatment is individualized but management essentially involves avoidance of the offending source that causes the reaction.

- *Delayed reactions*: short-term, over the counter, or prescribed antihistamines or steroid topical cream or ointment usually relieve rash.[5]

- *Hives or "hay fever"- like signs*: over-the-counter antihistamines provide relief. If no relief seek advice from healthcare provider.[6]

- *Wheezing, coughing or shortness of breath*: this may indicate severe reaction or anaphylaxis. **Seek medical advice immediately as this may become a medical emergency**. Anti-inflammatory and bronchodilator medications for reactive airway may be prescribed.[7]

ALLERGY, LATEX *(continued from previous page)*

MANAGEMENT/TREATMENT *(continued)*

- *Anaphylaxis*: epinephrine (e.g., Epi-Pen®, Auvi-Q®, AdrenaClick® and generic auto injectors) injected as quickly as possible, followed by immediate call to Emergency Medical Services (EMS) for transport to emergency facility.[8] (***Refer to ANAPHYLAXSIS).***

FOLLOW UP:

- Educate persons to avoid contact and exposure to items containing latex (such as gloves, condoms, bandages, balloons, rubber bands, erasers and toys). A list of common health care and daily items containing latex and alternative products is available through the Latex Allergy Toolbox at https://www.allergyasthmanetwork.org/education/allergies/latex-allergy/

- Persons with a latex allergy may need to avoid certain cross-reactive foods: avocado, banana, kiwi, chestnuts and tomato. There are other foods with a low degree of association to latex allergies.[9]

- Develop an Individualized Healthcare Plan (IHP) for a student with a latex allergy that includes specific actions to prevent exposure, staff training, and the Emergency Care Plan (ECP). Students at risk for a severe latex reaction should have auto-injectable epinephrine readily available.[10]

- Schools should provide latex free gloves for staff that use them in their daily job performance.

RESOURCES

- **NASN's Anaphylaxis Toolkit** at http://www.nasn.org/nasn/nasn-resources/practice-topics/allergies-anaphylaxis

- **FARE (Food Allery Research and Education)** at http://www.foodallergy.org/ Allergyhome.org. Specific information for schools at http://www.allergyhome.org/schools/

- **Allergy and Asthma Network** at https://www.allergyasthmanetwork.org/cms/wp-content/uploads/2018/11/Latex-Infographic-hoiz.pdf

- **Allergy & Asthma Network Latex Allergy Toolbox** at https://www.allergyasthmanetwork.org/education/allergies/latex-allergy/

ALLERGY, LATEX *(continued from previous page)*

REFERENCES

[1] Schoessler, S. & Selekman, J. (2019). Students with allergies. In J. Selekman, R. Adair Shannon, & C. F. Yonkaitis (Eds.), *School nursing: A comprehensive text* (3rd ed., pp. 500-522). F.A. Davis.

[2]American Academy of Allergy Asthma and Immunology. (2019). *Latex allergy*. https://www.aaaai.org/conditions-and-treatment/allergies/latex-allergy

[3] Ibid.

[4] Ibid.

[5] Mayo Clinic. (2019). *Latex allergy*. https://www.mayoclinic.org/diseases-conditions/latex-allergy/diagnosis-treatment/drc-20374291

[6] Ibid.

[7]American Academy of Allergy Asthma and Immunology. (2019). *Latex allergy*. https://www.aaaai.org/conditions-and-treatment/allergies/latex-allergy

[8] American College of Asthma, Allergy and Immunology. (2018). *Anaphylaxis.* https://acaai.org/allergies/anaphylaxis

[9] American Academy of Allergy Asthma and Immunology. (2019). *Latex allergy.* https://www.aaaai.org/conditions-and-treatment/allergies/latex-allergy

[10] National Association of School Nurses. (2019). *Allergies and anaphylaxis*. http://www.nasn.org/nasn/nasn-resources/practice-topics/allergies-anaphylaxis

OTHER REFERENCES CONSULTED

American College of Asthma, Allergy and Immunology. (2014). *Latex allergy*. http://acaai.org/allergies/types/skin-allergies/latex-allergy

Centers for Disease Control and Prevention. (2014). Latex allergy a prevention guide. http://www.cdc.gov/niosh/docs/98-113/

ALLERGY, STING

DEFINTION/ETIOLOGY:
An allergic reaction that occurs when the immune system overreacts to an insect sting/bite or hymenoptera sting (African bees, yellow jackets, wasps, hornets, fire ants). *Extreme hypersensitivity to a bee/insect sting is a potentially life-threatening condition.* *(Refer to ANAPHYLAXIS).*

SIGNS AND SYMPTOMS:[1]
Mild Reaction
- Erythema, warmth, tenderness
- Edema (swelling may extend as much as 10 cm)
- Hives (mild)
- Pain
- Pruritus (mild)

Severe Reaction
- Abdominal pain, nausea, vomiting, diarrhea
- Difficulty breathing/short of breath/wheezing
- Severe pruritis and hives over large areas of the body
- Difficulty swallowing/talking
- Swelling of the face, mouth or tongue
- Weakness/dizziness/fainting
- Hypotension/shock (rare)

MANAGEMENT/TREATMENT:[2, 3]
Students with known allergy should have a written emergency care plan including medication orders to receive their medication as soon as the sting is reported. Do not wait to observe a reaction.

Administer medication as ordered.

Mild Reaction [4]
1. Administer oral antihistamine medication as ordered (e.g. Benadryl®).
2. Remove stinger by scraping with hard edge (e.g. name badge) as soon as possible. The skin reaction will be worse the longer the stinger is left in the skin.
3. Wash area with soap and water.
4. Apply ice pack to reduce swelling and to slow the absorption of the venom.
5. Monitor for signs and symptoms of a severe reaction.

ALLERGY, STING *(continued from previous page)*

Severe reaction (*Refer to ANAPHYLAXIS*)

1. Administer epinephrine (EpiPen®, Adrenaclick®, Auvi-Q®, epinephrine injection, USP auto-injector [generic]) [5] in mid outer thigh.
    a. **CALL Emergency Medical Services (EMS) IMMEDIATELY!**
    b. Record time that medication was administered.
2. If student is able to swallow, administer oral antihistamine as prescribed.
3. Notify parent.
4. If possible, remove stinger as described above.

Be prepared to administer CPR.

FOLLOW-UP:

- Monitor for signs and symptoms of infection at sting/bite site.
- Replace used medication (Epipen®, Adrenaclick®, Auvi-Q®, epinephrine injection, USP auto-injector) for self-carry or health office.

POTENTIAL COMPLICATIONS:

- Infection at the site of the bee sting
- Anaphylaxis
- Death

NOTES:

- Educate staff on recognizing allergic reactions and action to take.
- Educate qualified staff (i.e., administrators, faculty, coaches) on administration of epinephrine (EpiPen© and others).
- Educate on the importance of wearing a medical identification necklace/bracelet.
- Educate student on how to avoid stings:
  — Avoid wearing heavy scents (perfumes, hygiene products).
  — Avoid wearing bright colored clothing.
  — Avoid swatting at bees (may incite the bee to sting).
  — Avoid drinking from open cans when the content of the can is not visible.
  — Avoid wearing sandals or walking barefoot in grass.

REFERENCES

[1] American Academy of Allergy Asthma and Immunology. (2019). *Stinging insect allergy.* https://www.aaaai.org/conditions-and-treatments/allergies/stinging-insect-allergy

[2] American College of Allergy, Asthma & Immunology. (2018). Insect Sting allergy. https://acaai.org/allergies/types/insect-sting-allergy

[3] American Academy of Pediatrics. (2019). *Allergy and anaphylaxis emergency plan.* https://www.aap.org/en-us/Documents/AAP_Allergy_and_Anaphylaxis_Emergency_Plan.pdf

[4] Mayo Clinic. (n.d.). Insect bites and stings: First aid. https://www.mayoclinic.org/first-aid/first-aid-insect-bites/basics/art-20056593

[5] Federal Drug Administration. (2018). *FDA approved first generic version of EpiPen.* https://www.fda.gov/news-events/press-announcements/fda-approves-first-generic-version-epipen

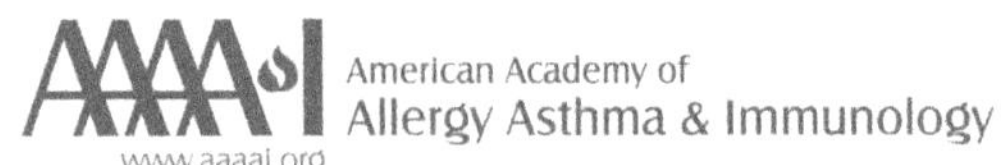

Anaphylaxis Emergency Action Plan

Patient Name: ______________________ Age: __________

Allergies: ______________________

Asthma ☐ Yes *(high risk for severe reaction)* ☐ No

Additional health problems besides anaphylaxis: ______________________

____

Concurrent medications: ______________________

____

Symptoms of Anaphylaxis

MOUTH	itching, swelling of lips and/or tongue
THROAT*	itching, tightness/closure, hoarseness
SKIN	itching, hives, redness, swelling
GUT	vomiting, diarrhea, cramps
LUNG*	shortness of breath, cough, wheeze
HEART*	weak pulse, dizziness, passing out

Only a few symptoms may be present. Severity of symptoms can change quickly.
**Some symptoms can be life-threatening. ACT FAST!*

Emergency Action Steps - DO NOT HESITATE TO GIVE EPINEPHRINE!

1. Inject epinephrine in thigh using (check one): ☐ Adrenaclick (0.15 mg) ☐ Adrenaclick (0.3 mg)

☐ Auvi-Q (0.15 mg) ☐ Auvi-Q (0.3 mg)

☐ EpiPen Jr (0.15 mg) ☐ EpiPen (0.3 mg)

Epinephrine Injection, USP Auto-injector- authorized generic
☐ (0.15 mg) ☐ (0.3 mg)

☐ Other (0.15 mg) ☐ Other (0.3 mg)

Specify others: ______________________

IMPORTANT: ASTHMA INHALERS AND/OR ANTIHISTAMINES CAN'T BE DEPENDED ON IN ANAPHYLAXIS.

2. Call 911 or rescue squad (before calling contact)

3. Emergency contact #1: home__________ work__________ cell__________

Emergency contact #2: home__________ work__________ cell__________

Emergency contact #3: home__________ work__________ cell__________

Comments: ______________________

____

____

Doctor's Signature/Date/Phone Number

____

Parent's Signature (for individuals under age 18 yrs)/Date

ANAPHYLAXIS

IMPORTANT:

- Students with a known life-threatening allergy should have an individualized healthcare plan (IHP) in place and all staff (including bus drivers) must be aware of the emergency plan and how to initiate it.
- Determine how epinephrine will be available to the student at all times (on person, in classroom(s)/cafeteria, when on bus or school sponsored event).
- Point to consider: Some schools have obtained *Standing Orders* or a specific *provider directed nursing protocol* for epinephrine from their school medical advisor or a local healthcare provider and non-specific epinephrine in the health room for unknown allergic reactions. Most states have laws which require schools to have stock epinephrine in schools.

OVERVIEW/DEFINITION:[1, 2]

Anaphylaxis is an acute systemic, potentially life-threatening allergic reaction that mimics other conditions and varies in its presentation. Disorders that present with similar symptoms are anxiety attacks, vasovagal episode, acute asthma, acute generalized urticaria, and aspiration of a foreign body.

- Every minute counts with anaphylaxis. Delay in treatment is associated with fatalities.
- Individuals considered to be at highest risk for anaphylaxis are those with allergies, asthma, or a history of anaphylactic reactions in the family.
- Most allergic reactions are not severe enough to cause anaphylaxis.
- It may occur in adults or children not previously known to be allergic or hypersensitive.
- Reactions range from mild, self-limited symptoms to rapid death.
- The reaction depends on sensitivity, amount ingested, and route of exposure. Each reaction can present very differently and vary in severity.

Clinical criteria for anaphylaxis:

Anaphylaxis is highly likely when any one of the following three criteria is occurs:[3]

- Acute onset of symptoms involving the skin, mucosal tissue, or both and **at least one** of the following:
  - respiratory compromise
  - reduced blood pressure
  - associated symptoms (hypotonia, syncope, incontinence)
- **Two or more** of the following that occur suddenly after exposure to a *likely* allergen:
  - involvement of the skin/mucosal tissue
  - respiratory compromise
  - reduced blood pressure
  - associated symptoms or persistent gastrointestinal symptoms
- Reduced blood pressure after exposure to a *known* allergen.

ANAPHYLAXIS *(continued from previous page)*

SIGNS AND SYMPTOMS:[4, 5]

- Symptoms of a reaction can occur within seconds to minutes but typically 15 minutes after exposure.[6]
- Symptoms do not always progress from mild to severe in all people.
- Symptoms may vary in multiple episodes in the same person.
- Anaphylaxis may only have one phase of symptoms but can also have a bi-phasic set of symptoms that occur hours after the initial phase of symptoms were resolved with treatment without an additional exposure.

All of the below can potentially lead to a life-threatening situation. Only a few symptoms may be present. CAUTION: The severity of the symptoms can change quickly:[7, 8]

Mouth	Itching, swelling of lips and or tongue, tingling (burning) sensation in mouth or around lips or drooling
Throat	Swelling of the tongue and throat, difficulty swallowing, itching, tightness/closure, hoarseness, changes in quality of voice*
Skin	Itching, hives, redness, swelling
Gut	Abdominal pain/cramping, nausea/vomiting, diarrhea
Lungs	Respiratory difficulty, shortness of breath, cough, shallow respirations, wheezing, stridor
Heart	Weak pulse, heart palpitations, drop in blood pressure, dizziness, light-headedness, loss of consciousness

**(See Anticipated Concerns below)*

Triggers:[9]

Extreme sensitivity to one or more of the following common triggers puts a student at risk for anaphylaxis:

- Food such as peanuts, tree nuts, shellfish, cow's milk or egg (most common triggers in children adolescents and young adults)
- Insect sting, usually bee, wasp or fire ants
- Latex rubber
- Medication or immunizations, usually by injection

ANTICIPATED CONCERNS:[10]

- Cardiac arrest
- Respiratory arrest
- Shock
- Coma
- Death

ANAPHYLAXIS *(continued from previous page)*

ANTICIPATED CONCERNS *(continued)*

- Respiratory difficulty and changes in quality of voice are symptoms of laryngeal edema and may signal closure of the airway. Laryngospasm (closure of the vocal cords blocking air intake) can occur as part of anaphylaxis or by itself without any of the above symptoms. **Call Emergency Medical Services (EMS) immediately.**
- Sudden standing or sitting after receiving the epinephrine injection can lead to empty ventricle syndrome, which can be fatal.[11] Keep the student lying on back with legs elevated, turn on side with risk of vomiting.
- Eighty to ninety percent of anaphylactic reactions include skin signs and when they are absent, anaphylaxis is harder to recognize.[12]
- Medications, age-related factors, and co-existent diseases may contribute to severe or fatal anaphylaxis. Co-factors such as infections, exercise, emotional stress, and may possibly amplify anaphylaxis.
- Side effects of epinephrine include anxiety, tachycardia, dizziness, sweating, headaches, tremors, nausea and vomiting.[13] Epinephrine has an impressive safety profile and should be given without delay.

MANAGEMENT/TREATMENT:[14]

- **Provide prompt medical attention.**
- **Epinephrine is the first line of treatment for anaphylaxis.**

Recommended Dosages:[15]

Immediate Injection of adrenalin 1:1000 SQ	Immediate administration of epinephrine
Age Infant-5 0.15cc	33-66 lbs. 0.15
Age 6-8 0.25cc	>66 lbs. 0.3
Age 9-18 0.3cc	

Follow student's individual Emergency Care Plan (ECP). Administer medication as ordered. The ECP should include medical orders and staff responsibilities for emergency care.

The following information should be sent with the EMS:

— Signs and symptoms of reaction.
— Emergency care measures instituted.
— Patient response to emergency care measures.
— Time of all activities, including administration of epinephrine.
— Epinephrine auto injector if given.
— Contact/emergency information.

ANAPHYLAXIS *(continued from previous page)*

Administration of non-specific stock epinephrine to an individual without an ECP:

1. Assess for signs and symptoms of anaphylaxis.
2. Remove from allergen if possible.
3. Secure leg and administer epinephrine into the outer thigh. May be administered through clothing. Avoid seams and check pockets.
4. Administer appropriate dose of epinephrine.
5. Do not leave person alone.
6. **Immediately call EMS**.
7. Lay flat, elevate feet, if vomiting or respiratory difficulty do not lay flat, if hypotensive lay on side.
8. Send information as mentioned above with EMS.
9. Dispose of used auto-injector according to OSHA guidelines.
10. Epinephrine can be repeated in five to 15-minute intervals one or two times.[16]

Epinephrine Auto Injectors

- Do not use epinephrine that is cloudy or discolored.
- Do not store injectable epinephrine devices in a frequently opened drawer as repeated motion may cause premature release and injury when handled.
- Do not store injectable epinephrine in car glove box/bus or where it can become overheated.
- Consider sending epinephrine home during school breaks depending on temperature of building when school is not in session.
- Do not store epinephrine in refrigerator. Normal **room temperature** is best (range is 59-86 Celsius.[17]
- Epinephrine auto injectors (EAI):
  - Should not be locked up during school or after school activities.
  - Shelf life is 12-18 months (see "Notes", bullet #5).
- Ask parents how they store EAI at home.

FOLLOW-UP:

- Review the student's ECP to make sure there are no changes required based on this incident.
- If this is the first known incident of an allergic reaction, ensure that an ECP (see sample below) Is developed and make sure all staff (including bus drivers) are aware of the ECP and how to initiate it.

ANAPHYLAXIS *(continued from previous page)*

FOLLOW-UP *(continued)*

- Provide health education with family, student, and school staff regarding further exposure to allergen.
- Emphasize wearing Medic Alert tag or bracelets (www.medicalert.org).
- Have parent/guardian replace epinephrine if expired or administered.
- Record as "Medical Alert" on student's record.

NOTES:

- Your district should have a written procedural guideline in place for anaphylaxis. Post this guideline in the health room.
- Create and maintain a healthy and safe educational environment.
- You may see anaphylaxis in an individual without a previously known life-threatening allergy.
- An emergency care plan should be in place and mock drills practiced regularly.
- Practice prevention as a school community – avoid known allergens.

REFERENCES

[1] Sicherer, H., & Simons, E. (2017). *Clinical guidelines regarding treatment with epinephrine in first aid of anaphylaxis.* https://pediatrics.aappublications.org/content/139/3/e20164006

[2] Campbell, R., & Kelso, J. (2018). *Anaphylaxis: Emergency treatment.* https://www.uptodate.com/contents/anaphylaxis-emergency-treatment

[3] Sicherer, H. & Simons, E. (2017). *Clinical guidelines regarding treatment with epinephrine in first aid of anaphylaxis.* https://pediatrics.aappublications.org/content/139/3/e20164006

[4] Mayo Clinic. (2018). *Anaphylaxis.* https://www.mayoclinic.org/diseases-conditions/anaphylaxis/symptoms-causes/syc-20351468

[5] Sicherer, H., & Simons, E. (2017). *Clinical guidelines regarding treatment with epinephrine in first aid of anaphylaxis.* : https://pediatrics.aappublications.org/content/139/3/e20164006

[6] Merck Manual, Professional Version. (2019). *Anaphylaxis.* https://www.merckmanuals.com/professional/immunology-allergic-disorders/allergic,-autoimmune,-and-other-hypersensitivity-disorders/anaphylaxis

[7] Mayo Clinic. (2018). *Anaphylaxis.* https://www.mayoclinic.org/diseases-conditions/anaphylaxis/symptoms-causes/syc-20351468

[8] American Academy of Allergy Asthma Immunology. (n.d.) *Anaphylaxis.* https://www.aaaai.org/conditions-and-treatments/library/allergy-library/anaphylaxis

[9] Ibid.

[10] Campbell, R., & Kelso, J. (2018). *Anaphylaxis: Emergency treatment.* https://www.uptodate.com/contents/anaphylaxis-emergency-treatment

ANAPHYLAXIS *(continued from previous page)*

[11] Simons, F.E.R., Ardussol, L.R.F., Bilo, M. B., El- Gamal, Y.M., Ledford, D.K., Ring, J., Sanchez-Borges, M., Gian Enrico Senna, G., Sheikh, A., Bernard Y., Thong, B.Y. for the World Health Organization. (2011). World allergy organization guidelines for the assessment and management of anaphylaxis. *The World Allergy Organization Journal*, *4*(2), pp.13-37. http://www.ncbi.nlm.nih.gov/pmc/articles/PMC3500036/

[12] Ibid.

[13] Pfizer Medical Information. (n.d.). *Health professional information.* https://www.pfizermedicalinformation.ca/en-ca/epipen

[14] Sicherer, H., & Simons, E. (2017). *Clinical guidelines regarding treatment with epinephrine in first aid of anaphylaxis.* https://pediatrics.aappublications.org/content/139/3/e20164006

[15] Schoessler, S., & Selekman, J. (2019). Students with allergies. In J. Selekman, R. A. Shanon, & C. F. Yonkaitus (Eds.), *School nursing: A comprehensive text* (3rd ed., pp. 500-522). F.A. Davis Company.

[16] Sicherer, H., & Simons, E. (2017). *Clinical guidelines regarding treatment with epinephrine in first aid of anaphylaxis.* https://pediatrics.aappublications.org/content/139/3/e20164006,

[17] Pfizer Medical Information. (n.d.). *Storage and stability.* https://www.pfizermedicalinformation.ca/en-ca/epipen/storage-and-stability

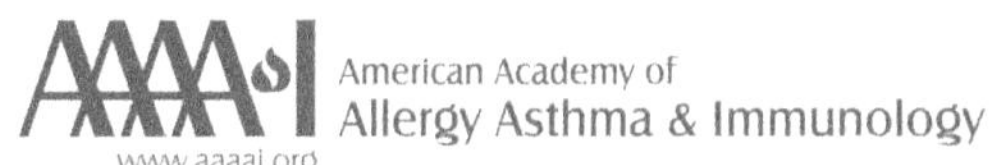

Anaphylaxis Emergency Action Plan

Patient Name: ______________________________ Age: __________

Allergies: ______________________________

Asthma ☐ Yes *(high risk for severe reaction)* ☐ No

Additional health problems besides anaphylaxis: ______________________________

____

Concurrent medications: ______________________________

____

	Symptoms of Anaphylaxis
MOUTH	itching, swelling of lips and/or tongue
THROAT*	itching, tightness/closure, hoarseness
SKIN	itching, hives, redness, swelling
GUT	vomiting, diarrhea, cramps
LUNG*	shortness of breath, cough, wheeze
HEART*	weak pulse, dizziness, passing out

Only a few symptoms may be present. Severity of symptoms can change quickly.
**Some symptoms can be life-threatening. ACT FAST!*

Emergency Action Steps - DO NOT HESITATE TO GIVE EPINEPHRINE!

1. Inject epinephrine in thigh using (check one):

☐ Adrenaclick (0.15 mg)	☐ Adrenaclick (0.3 mg)
☐ Auvi-Q (0.15 mg)	☐ Auvi-Q (0.3 mg)
☐ EpiPen Jr (0.15 mg)	☐ EpiPen (0.3 mg)

Epinephrine Injection, USP Auto-injector- authorized generic

☐ (0.15 mg)	☐ (0.3 mg)
☐ Other (0.15 mg)	☐ Other (0.3 mg)

Specify others: ______________________________

IMPORTANT: ASTHMA INHALERS AND/OR ANTIHISTAMINES CAN'T BE DEPENDED ON IN ANAPHYLAXIS.

2. Call 911 or rescue squad (before calling contact)

3. Emergency contact #1: home__________ work__________ cell__________

   Emergency contact #2: home__________ work__________ cell__________

   Emergency contact #3: home__________ work__________ cell__________

Comments: ______________________________

____

____

Doctor's Signature/Date/Phone Number

____

Parent's Signature (for individuals under age 18 yrs)/Date

FARE FOOD ALLERGY & ANAPHYLAXIS EMERGENCY CARE PLAN

Food Allergy Research & Education

Name:____ D.O.B.: ______________

Allergy to: ____

Weight: ______________lbs. Asthma: ☐ **Yes (higher risk for a severe reaction)** ☐ **No**

NOTE: Do not depend on antihistamines or inhalers (bronchodilators) to treat a severe reaction. USE EPINEPHRINE.

Extremely reactive to the following allergens: ______________________________

THEREFORE:

☐ If checked, give epinephrine immediately if the allergen was LIKELY eaten, for ANY symptoms.

☐ If checked, give epinephrine immediately if the allergen was DEFINITELY eaten, even if no symptoms are apparent.

FOR **ANY** OF THE FOLLOWING:

SEVERE SYMPTOMS

LUNG
Shortness of breath, wheezing, repetitive cough

HEART
Pale or bluish skin, faintness, weak pulse, dizziness

THROAT
Tight or hoarse throat, trouble breathing or swallowing

MOUTH
Significant swelling of the tongue or lips

SKIN
Many hives over body, widespread redness

GUT
Repetitive vomiting, severe diarrhea

OTHER
Feeling something bad is about to happen, anxiety, confusion

OR A COMBINATION of symptoms from different body areas.

1. **INJECT EPINEPHRINE IMMEDIATELY.**
2. **Call 911.** Tell emergency dispatcher the person is having anaphylaxis and may need epinephrine when emergency responders arrive.

- Consider giving additional medications following epinephrine:
  - » Antihistamine
  - » Inhaler (bronchodilator) if wheezing
- Lay the person flat, raise legs and keep warm. If breathing is difficult or they are vomiting, let them sit up or lie on their side.
- If symptoms do not improve, or symptoms return, more doses of epinephrine can be given about 5 minutes or more after the last dose.
- Alert emergency contacts.
- Transport patient to ER, even if symptoms resolve. Patient should remain in ER for at least 4 hours because symptoms may return.

MILD SYMPTOMS

NOSE
Itchy or runny nose, sneezing

MOUTH
Itchy mouth

SKIN
A few hives, mild itch

GUT
Mild nausea or discomfort

FOR **MILD SYMPTOMS** FROM **MORE THAN ONE** SYSTEM AREA, GIVE EPINEPHRINE.

FOR **MILD SYMPTOMS** FROM **A SINGLE SYSTEM** AREA, FOLLOW THE DIRECTIONS BELOW:

1. Antihistamines may be given, if ordered by a healthcare provider.
2. Stay with the person; alert emergency contacts.
3. Watch closely for changes. If symptoms worsen, give epinephrine.

MEDICATIONS/DOSES

Epinephrine Brand or Generic: ______________________

Epinephrine Dose: ☐ 0.1 mg IM ☐ 0.15 mg IM ☐ 0.3 mg IM

Antihistamine Brand or Generic: ______________________

Antihistamine Dose: ______________________

Other (e.g., inhaler-bronchodilator if wheezing): ______________

____

PATIENT OR PARENT/GUARDIAN AUTHORIZATION SIGNATURE DATE PHYSICIAN/HCP AUTHORIZATION SIGNATURE DATE

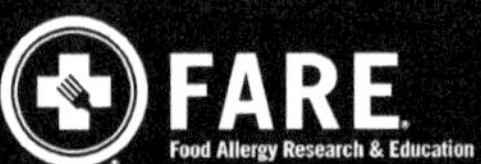

FOOD ALLERGY & ANAPHYLAXIS EMERGENCY CARE PLAN

HOW TO USE AUVI-Q® (EPINEPRHINE INJECTION, USP), KALEO

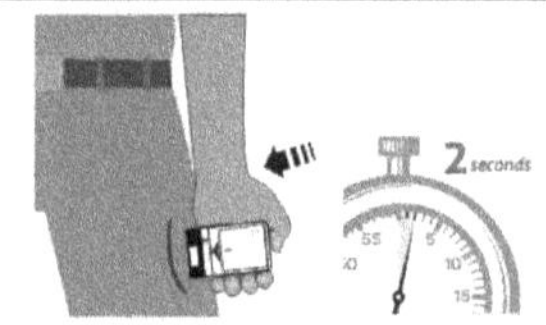

1. Remove Auvi-Q from the outer case.
2. Pull off red safety guard.
3. Place black end of Auvi-Q against the middle of the outer thigh.
4. Press firmly until you hear a click and hiss sound, and hold in place for 2 seconds.
5. Call 911 and get emergency medical help right away.

HOW TO USE EPIPEN® AND EPIPEN JR® (EPINEPHRINE) AUTO-INJECTOR AND EPINEPHRINE INJECTION (AUTHORIZED GENERIC OF EPIPEN®), USP AUTO-INJECTOR, MYLAN AUTO-INJECTOR, MYLAN

1. Remove the EpiPen® or EpiPen Jr® Auto-Injector from the clear carrier tube.
2. Grasp the auto-injector in your fist with the orange tip (needle end) pointing downward.
3. With your other hand, remove the blue safety release by pulling straight up.
4. Swing and push the auto-injector firmly into the middle of the outer thigh until it 'clicks'.
5. Hold firmly in place for 3 seconds (count slowly 1, 2, 3).
6. Remove and massage the injection area for 10 seconds.
7. Call 911 and get emergency medical help right away.

HOW TO USE IMPAX EPINEPHRINE INJECTION (AUTHORIZED GENERIC OF ADRENACLICK®), USP AUTO-INJECTOR, IMPAX LABORATORIES

1. Remove epinephrine auto-injector from its protective carrying case.
2. Pull off both blue end caps: you will now see a red tip.
3. Grasp the auto-injector in your fist with the red tip pointing downward.
4. Put the red tip against the middle of the outer thigh at a 90-degree angle, perpendicular to the thigh.
5. Press down hard and hold firmly against the thigh for approximately 10 seconds.
6. Remove and massage the area for 10 seconds.
7. Call 911 and get emergency medical help right away.

HOW TO USE TEVA'S GENERIC EPIPEN® (EPINEPHRINE INJECTION, USP) AUTO-INJECTOR, TEVA PHARMACEUTICAL INDUSTRIES

1. Quickly twist the yellow or green cap off of the auto-injector in the direction of the "twist arrow" to remove it.
2. Grasp the auto-injector in your fist with the orange tip (needle end) pointing downward.
3. With your other hand, pull off the blue safety release.
4. Place the orange tip against the middle of the outer thigh (upper leg) at a right angle (perpendicular) to the thigh.
5. Swing and push the auto-injector firmly into the middle of the outer thigh until it 'clicks'.
6. Hold firmly in place for 3 seconds (count slowly 1, 2, 3).
7. Remove and massage the injection area for 10 seconds.
8. Call 911 and get emergency medical help right away.

ADMINISTRATION AND SAFETY INFORMATION FOR ALL AUTO-INJECTORS:

1. Do not put your thumb, fingers or hand over the tip of the auto-injector or inject into any body part other than mid-outer thigh. In case of accidental injection, go immediately to the nearest emergency room.
2. If administering to a young child, hold their leg firmly in place before and during injection to prevent injuries.
3. Epinephrine can be injected through clothing if needed.
4. Call 911 immediately after injection.

OTHER DIRECTIONS/INFORMATION (may self-carry epinephrine, may self-administer epinephrine, etc.):

Treat the person before calling emergency contacts. The first signs of a reaction can be mild, but symptoms can worsen quickly.

EMERGENCY CONTACTS — CALL 911

RESCUE SQUAD: ____________________

DOCTOR: ____________________ PHONE: ____________

PARENT/GUARDIAN: ____________________ PHONE: ____________

OTHER EMERGENCY CONTACTS

NAME/RELATIONSHIP: ____________________ PHONE: ____________

NAME/RELATIONSHIP: ____________________ PHONE: ____________

NAME/RELATIONSHIP: ____________________ PHONE: ____________

ANXIETY DISORDER IN CHILDREN AND ADOLESCENTS

OVERVIEW/DEFINITION:

Feelings of anxiety can be a normal response to life's challenges, but sometimes a school aged children's fears and worry can develop into a behavioral health disorder. At some point anxiety affects 30% of children and adolescents, and in the past 10 years there has been a 17% increase in anxiety disorder diagnosis.[1]

According to the Centers for Disease Control and Prevention more than 7% of children aged three to 17 years have a diagnosed anxiety disorder.[2] Anxiety disorders include generalized anxiety disorder, social anxiety disorder, specific phobias, panic disorder, Post Traumatic Stress Disorder (PTSD), and separation anxiety disorder.

SIGNS AND SYMPTOMS:

Signs of anxiety[3]

- Physical complaints that seem to have no medical explanation such as recurring stomachaches, nausea, and headaches
- Excessive worries or fears about things like school failure, health issues, imagined dangers, or new situations
- Not participating in class, having few friends
- Other behavioral issues like seeming angry, irritable or acting out, overreacting
- Memory problems

Other signs include[4]

- School avoidance due to excessive anxiety about school
- Trouble falling or staying asleep
- Need for a great deal of emotional comfort from parents
- Lack of attention and focus, difficulty concentrating, and confusion
- Bad temper or low mood

Physiologic effects of anxiety[5]

- Anorexia
- Diarrhea
- Dry mouth
- Facial flushing
- Increased blood pressure, pulse, respirations
- Twitching
- Abdominal pain
- Faintness
- Fatigue
- Nausea

ANXIETY DISORDER IN CHILDREN AND ADOLESCENTS *(continued from previous page)*

MANAGEMENT/POTENTIAL INTERVENTIONS:

Because the nurse and the health office are seen by students as a place to get help and support, school nurses are in a unique position to help identify and manage anxiety; they are often the first point of entry for a student's behavioral health care.[6] It is estimated that 80% of children and adolescents do not get treatment for anxiety.[7] Identifying and treating anxiety early is essential for school success and long-term behavioral health prognosis.

- Be alert to students who visit the school nurse's office often with complaints of headache, stomachache, and fatigue, with no known medical cause, as possibly having anxiety.
- As part of the nursing assessment ask students about any feelings of worry, fear, or panic.
- Gather information about the child's attendance, get teacher feedback about behavior, and participation in class.
- Speak with the parent or guardian to gather information regarding any pertinent psychosocial or physical health history that may contribute to anxiety. Obtain an exchange of information to speak with medical provider to confirm there is no physical health cause for feelings of anxiety, like thyroid disease or diabetes.
- Do a HEADSS assessment on high school students. A HEADSS assessment [8] includes asking questions about:
    - Home & Environment
    - Education & Employment
    - Activities
    - Drugs
    - Sexuality
    - Suicide/Depression
- Use the OARS approach of therapeutic communication:[9]
    - Open ended questions
    - Affirmations
    - Reflective listening
    - Summaries
- Create a resource map of support in the school and community for students and their families that includes school psychologists, school counselors, school mental health providers, school social workers, community based organizations that can provide mental health services, university partners that have interns, mental health clinics, crisis response units, youth shelters, and private providers.
- Become trained in using anxiety screening tools after establishing referral resources for treatment.
- Create a quiet calm space in the health office with comfortable seating, soft lighting, a coloring book with pencils, story books about characters that feel anxious, and headphones with music.

ANXIETY DISORDER IN CHILDREN AND ADOLESCENTS *(continued from previous page)*

MANAGEMENT/POTENTIAL INTERVENTIONS *(continued)*

- Refer students suspected of having anxiety to the healthcare provider as medication management can be a helpful component of care.
- Offer activities that support the student to decrease their feelings of anxiety[10]
  - Make a calm down jar with water, glitter, and glitter glue that the child can shake and watch the glitter fall.
  - Offer them a stress ball to squeeze or a hairy tangle to twist.
  - Have "slime" in a container they can run through their hands.
  - Have the student make a worry box where they can write their worries and leave for later.
  - Encourage and teach them positive self-talk, help them make a positive mantra bracelet with beads.
- Other helpful tools include the 5-4-3-2-1 activity[11]
  - Before starting this exercise, have student pay attention to their breathing. Slow, deep, long breaths can help maintain a sense of calm and help them return to a calmer state. Once they settle their breath, go through the following steps:
  - 5: Acknowledge FIVE things they can see. It could be a picture, an item, a book.
  - 4: Acknowledge FOUR things they can touch. It could be their hair, their clothes, or the ground under their feet.
  - 3: Acknowledge THREE things they hear. This could be any external sound. If they can hear their stomach rumbling that counts! But have them focus on things they can hear outside of their body.
  - 2: Acknowledge TWO things they can smell.
  - 1: Acknowledge ONE thing they can taste or remember tasting.
- Use social emotional tools,[12] like the "feelings" thermometer, which helps youth develop strategies for their worries and concerns.
- Motivate students and parents to seek additional help and assist them in addressing barriers to seeking care.[13]
- Refer to the Section 504 team to evaluate under the Section 504 Rehabilitation Act to determine eligibility if you suspect the student has a disability such as anxiety. If eligible, by team determination, recommended accommodations that might be needed to help a child stay in school and learn in class include (but not limited to) seating as requested by student, help with directions, modified expectations for classroom participation and presentations, and extended time on tests in a quiet space.[14] WorryWiseKids.org provides these and other helpful suggestions to consider when developing a Section 504 plan.

ANXIETY DISORDER IN CHILDREN AND ADOLESCENTS *(continued from previous page)*

ANTICIPATED CONCERNS:

Potential complications:

- School failure or decreased academic success
- Not reaching full academic potential
- Truancy, school avoidance
- Loss of normal developmental experiences
- Loss of normal social experiences
- Substance abuse (alcohol, tobacco and other drugs)
- Self-injury
- Suicidal ideation
- Social isolation
- Illness falsification, somatization
- Later psychiatric disorders

Note: The earlier in life a child has symptoms that meet criteria for generalized anxiety disorder the more comorbidity they tend to have and the more impaired they are likely to be.[15]

FOLLOW UP:[16]

- Promote student success by developing and implementing Section 504 plans or Individualized Healthcare Plans (IHP).
- Provide behavioral health screening and basic behavioral health skills that include education about mental health disorders and cognitive behavioral skills.
- Recognize care coordination as a critical component of comprehensive behavioral health services and determine with the school mental health providers who is the most appropriate care coordinator.
- Make referrals and connect parents and children with school and community behavioral health resources.
- Have regular contact with students to provide ongoing assessment, and to monitor treatment compliance.
- Be aware of your own anxiety.
- Maintain confidentiality.

NOTES:

There is a free online course through the University of Maryland School of Medicine, Department of Behavioral Health- Mental Health Training Intervention for Health Providers in School Settings, (MH-TIPS).[17]

ANXIETY DISORDER IN CHILDREN AND ADOLESCENTS *(continued from previous page)*

REFERENCES

[1] Child Mind Institute. (2018). *Understanding anxiety in children and teens/2018 Children's Mental Health Report.* https://childmind.org/our-impact/childrens-mental-health-report/2018report/

[2] Centers for Disease and Prevention. (2019). *Data and statistics on children's mental health.* https://www.cdc.gov/childrensmentalhealth/data.html

[3] Dominion Hospital Blog. (2019). *How school nurses can help spot and manage anxiety in children and teens.* https://dominionhospital.com/blog/entry/how-school-nurses-can-help-spot-and-manage-anxiety-in-children-and-teens

[4] Children's National Health Center. (n.d.). *What is generalized anxiety disorder in children and teens?* https://childrensnational.org/visit/conditions-and-treatments/mental-health-behavioral-disorders/generalized-anxiety-disorder

[5] Wayne, G. (2016). *Anxiety: Nursing diagnosis and care plans.* https://nurseslabs.com/anxiety/

[6] Dominion Hospital Blog. (2019). *How school nurses can help spot and manage anxiety in children and teens.* https://dominionhospital.com/blog/entry/how-school-nurses-can-help-spot-and-manage-anxiety-in-children-and-teens

[7] Child Mind Institute. (2018). *Understanding anxiety in children and teens/2018 Children's Mental Health Report.* https://childmind.org/our-impact/childrens-mental-health-report/2018report/

[8] BC Children's Hospital. (n.d.). *H.E.A.D.S.S. a psychosocial interview for adolescents.* http://www.bcchildrens.ca/Youth-Health-Clinic-site/Documents/headss20assessment20guide1.pdf

[9] Oregon Health Authority, Center for Health Training. (2010). *The OARS model essential communication skills.* https://www.oregon.gov/oha/ph/HealthyPeopleFamilies/ReproductiveSexualHealth/Documents/edmat/OARSEssentialCommunicationTechniques.pdf

[10] O'Rourke, K. (2017). *10 therapist (and child)-approved activities to support kids with anxiety.* www.familytherapybasics.com/blog/2017/10/8/10-therapist-and-child-approved-activities-to-support-kids-with-anxiety

[11] Smith, S. & University of Rochester Medical Center Blog. (2018). *5-4-3-2-1-coping technique for anxiety.* www.urmc.rochester.edu/behavioral-health-partners/bhp-blog/April-2018/5-4-3-2-1-coping-technique-for-anxiety.aspx

[12] Driscoll, L. (2019). *A feelings thermometer.* www.socialemotionalworkshop.com/2019/03/feelings-thermometer

[13] Patterson, B.R., Bohnenkamp, J., Hoover, S., Bostic, J. & Selekman, J. (2019). Students with mental/behavioral health concerns and disorders. In J. Selekman, R. Adair Shannon, & C. F. Yonkaitis (Eds.), *School nursing: A comprehensive text* (3rd ed., pp. 756-789). F.A. Davis.

[14] Worrywisekids.org/The Children's and Adult Center for OCD and Anxiety. (2019). *Sample accommodations for anxious kids.* http://www.worrywisekids.org/node/40

[15] American Psychiatric Association. (2013). Anxiety disorders. In *Diagnostic and statistical manual of mental disorders* (5th ed., pp. 222-225). American Psychiatric Association Publishing.

[16] National Association of School Nurses. (2018). *The school nurse's role in behavioral/mental health of students* (Position Statement). Silver Spring, MD: Author. https://www.nasn.org/advocacy/professional-practice-documents/position-statements/ps-behavioral-health

[17] University of Maryland. (2019). *Mental health training for health professionals in schools.* https://mdbehavioralhealth.com/training

ASTHMA AND ASTHMA EMERGENCIES

OVERVIEW/DEFINITION:

Asthma is a chronic inflammatory disease of the airways. It is best understood as the clinical result of two linked processes, airway inflammation and bronchial hyper-reactivity. While bronchial hyper-reactivity is often genetically determined, it may be induced by viral infection. Airway inflammation is often triggered by allergies or viral illness. Environmental exposure to known allergens, indoor and outdoor air pollution, especially cigarette smoke at home, may aggravate symptoms and lead to more persistent and significant airways hyper-reactivity.

Asthma affects one in 10 children in the U.S.; therefore, in a typical classroom approximately two to three students are likely to have a diagnosis of asthma.[1] Asthma is a leading chronic illness among children and youth in the United States and a leading cause of school absenteeism.[2] The student with asthma may present with any of the following:

- Episodes of wheezing and shortness of breath related to exposure to an allergen, such as cats, dust, outdoor pollens or mold;
- Prolonged and often refractory cough and wheeze with shortness of breath related to acute respiratory viral illness; and
- Shortness of breath, cough or wheeze triggered by exercise or cold-air that takes more than just a minute or two from which to recover.

SIGNS AND SYMPTOMS:

Asthma symptoms vary from person to person. Symptoms range from minor wheezing to life-threatening asthma attacks. In most children without active symptoms, physical examination is normal. Common signs and symptoms are: [3]

- Shortness of breath
- Tightness (or pain) in chest
- Coughing
- Wheezing
- Difficulty sleeping due to cough, wheeze, shortness of breath, leading to daytime fatigue

Persistent cough or shortness of breath may be the only signs of active asthma. Wheezing is often but not always heard. Students with persistent cough and/or shortness of breath should be evaluated by their healthcare provider in order to distinguish between asthma from other conditions such as bronchitis or poor physical conditioning. The signs and symptoms may vary from student to student, are reversible with timely treatment, and typically are brought on by exposure to one or more triggers.[4]

Asthma may be classified as intermittent, mild persistent, moderate persistent, or severe persistent. These classifications are based on the frequency of symptoms, number of nighttime awakenings, frequency of rescue inhaler use, and interference with daily activities, along with lung function measurements.[5] However, children with any classification of asthma can experience a potentially life-threatening episode (exacerbation).

ASTHMA AND ASTHMA EMERGENCIES *(continued from previous page)*

SIGNS AND SYMPTOMS *(continued)*

Although the school nurse is not responsible for the diagnosis of asthma, the following chart is helpful in addressing the criteria associated with the asthma severity categories.

National Heart, Lung, and Blood Institute Asthma Severity Categories [6]					
Intermittent asthma	Symptoms < 2 days a week	Nighttime awakenings with symptoms < twice a month	Require short-acting medication < twice a week	Normal activities not interrupted	Symptom-free outside of rare episodes
Mild persistent asthma	Symptoms at least 2 times weekly but not daily	Nighttime episodes 1-4 times a month	Require short-acting medication at least 2 times weekly but not more than 2times in one day	Minor limitations in daily activities	Lung function 80% of normal or greater during episodes
Moderate persistent asthma	Daily symptoms	Nighttime awakenings > once per week but not nightly	Require daily use of short-acting medication	Some limitations in daily activities	Lung function 60-80% of normal without treatment
Severe persistent asthma	Symptoms several times daily	Frequent nighttime awakenings	Require use of short-acting medication several times daily	Significant limitation of activities	Lung function less than 60% of normal without treatment

Advanced asthma symptoms which require immediate action:

- Struggling to breath – may be hunched over in tripod position
- Abnormal breath sounds – absent/decreased/wheezing
- Retractions – intercostals, substernal, suprasternal
- Nasal flaring
- Using accessory muscles
- Bluish discoloration (cyanosis) around lips or nailbeds
- Inability to speak in full sentences without stopping to catch breath
- Tachycardia
- Tachypnea

ASTHMA AND ASTHMA EMERGENCIES *(continued from previous page)*

The presence of advanced signs or symptoms of a severe asthma attack in a student is considered a medical emergency, and prompt assessment and treatment are required. If student does not respond to treatment, Emergency Medica Services (EMS) should be contacted.

ANTICIPATED CONCERNS/PROBLEMS:

- Complications can range from secondary infections to more serious respiratory arrest.
- Permanent narrowing of the bronchial tubes.
- Unresponsiveness to medications.
- Side effects from long-term use of some asthma medications.
- Severe asthma attack resulting in increased emergency room visits and hospitalizations.

MANAGEMENT/INTERVENTIONS:

The goals of asthma management therapy are:[7]

- Few, if any, asthma symptoms
- Few, if any, awakenings during the night caused by asthma symptoms
- No need to take time off from school or work due to asthma
- Few or no limits on full participation in physical activities
- No emergency department visits
- No hospital stays
- Few or no side effects from asthma medicines

The school nurse is in a unique position to assess the student's asthma control and ability to administer inhaled medication, as well as to educate students and families about asthma control. The Asthma Control Test is a helpful tool that is often used to assist in this assessment. Students respond to five questions on a scale of one to five, with the lower scores indicating poor control.

1. In the past four weeks, how much of the time did your asthma keep you from getting as much done at work, school or at home?
2. During the past four weeks, how often have you had shortness of breath?
3. During the past four weeks, how often did your asthma symptoms (wheezing, coughing, shortness of breath, chest tightness or pain) wake you up at night or earlier than usual in the morning?
4. During the past four weeks, how often have you used your rescue inhaler or nebulizer medication (such as albuterol)?
5. How would you rate your asthma control during the past 4 weeks?

ASTHMA AND ASTHMA EMERGENCIES *(continued from previous page)*

MANAGEMENT/INTERVENTIONS *(continued)*

Asthma control currently relies on controlling acute episode and reducing inflammation, with the goal of normalizing lung function. When assessing control, the school nurse should consider the following components:

- Day and night symptoms
- Limitation of activities
- Frequency of use of Albuterol

Being proactive when a student is using albuterol more than twice a week is a key opportunity for the school nurse to play an active role in mitigating worsening asthma symptoms, even life-threatening exacerbations.

Treatment of acute symptoms of asthma with as-needed rescue is achieved with short-acting bronchodilators. Albuterol sulfate *(Proventil®, Ventolin®, Xopenex®, ProAir®)* is the most commonly prescribed metered dose inhaled rescue bronchodilator. It may also be given in tablet, extended release tablet, syrup, or nebulized with the means of an air compressor driven hand-held nebulizer.

Long-term controller medications are key to managing asthma. Anti-inflammatory therapy using an inhaled corticosteroid (such as Flovent® Diskus, QVAR® or Pulmicort®) or Flonase® steroid nasal spray should be added to as-needed bronchodilators. The use of long-term controller medication is especially important when evaluating the student with asthma who is taking only rescue medication for control. In low doses, inhaled corticosteroids have been shown to reduce mortality, hospitalizations, emergency asthma flares, exercise and allergen triggering, nighttime awakenings from asthma and total cost of care.

In order to receive the maximum benefit from inhaled medication, many healthcare providers will recommend spacers or valved holding chambers. These devices will help the medication to move past the mouth and throat and get deep into the lungs. They also help avoid breathing in the medication too fast.[8]

- A spacer is placed on the mouthpiece of the inhaler to create a "space" between the mouth and the medicine. The space helps break the medicine into smaller droplets which move more easily into the lungs.

- A valved holding chamber is a specific type of spacer that includes a one-way valve at the end of the mouthpiece, which traps and holds the medicine, giving the user time to take a slow deep breath. This stops the user from accidently breathing into the tube and allows all of the medicine to be inhaled.

ASTHMA AND ASTHMA EMERGENCIES *(continued from previous page)*

MANAGEMENT/INTERVENTIONS *(continued)*

Management should also include avoiding asthma triggers. Studies have shown that reducing exposure to specific allergens or irritants (such as cigarette smoke) improves asthma symptoms and reduces the amount of medication necessary for good control. Common triggers for asthmatic episodes include:[9]

- Cold, dry air
- Allergens (pets, dust, food)
- Respiratory illness
- Exercise
- Inhaled irritants (cigarette smoke, perfumes, strong scents)
- Poor indoor or outdoor air quality
- Emotion
- Aspirin and other nonsteroidal anti-inflammatory drugs (NSAIDs)
- Gastroesophageal reflux disease (GERD)

General guidelines for dealing with an asthma attack include:

- Implement student's Asthma Action Plan.
- Administer inhaled or nebulized bronchodilator (usually albuterol) as per Asthma Action Plan.
- Allow the student to assume a comfortable posture in a quiet setting.
- Measure peak flow, if possible, to document severity and response to therapy.
- Record pulse and respiratory rate.
- Monitor – do not leave student alone.
- Do not allow student to return to class until symptoms are resolved.
- If student does respond positively to treatment or condition worsens, contact EMS and transport
- Notify parent/guardian.

FOLLOW-UP:

- Monitor effectiveness of pharmacological therapy.
- Monitor student inhaler technique. Provide reinforcement as needed.
- Educate student/staff on asthma basics and how to manage an asthma emergency.
- Educate student/staff on how to properly care for inhaler.
- Consider need for Individualized Healthcare Plan (IHP) or Section 504 plan.

NOTES:

Every student identified with asthma should have a written **Asthma Action Plan**[10] approved by the student's healthcare provider and available in the school nurse's office. The Asthma Action Plan:

- Identifies the severity classification and known triggers
- Identifies whether the student should be taking daily control meds (especially inhaled steroids)

ASTHMA AND ASTHMA EMERGENCIES *(continued from previous page)*

NOTES *(continued)*

- Empowers the school nurse as a member of the student's asthma team and actively discussing with parent or healthcare provider when there are concerns about control or acute symptoms

The goal of asthma management is to optimize control of symptoms:

- Education regarding avoiding known triggers or irritants and the need to use medications as directed.
- Yearly influenza vaccine may be recommended.
- Students may be allowed to self-carry and self-administer short-acting rescue inhaled bronchodilators for use before exercise, when experiencing asthma symptoms, and during off-campus school sponsored activities. The decision to allow students to self-carry and self-administer should be made through collaboration between the healthcare provider, parent, and school nurse and in accordance with state law and district policy.
- Educate student/staff on the importance of avoiding extreme weather conditions. Student may need to stay indoors when:
  - It is extremely windy
  - Pollen count is high
  - Outdoor temperature is <32^0 F (including wind chill factor). Encourage student to cover mouth and nose with a scarf or mask during cold weather!
  - Outdoor temperature is > 90^{0}F (including heat index)
- Support *CDC's Controlling Asthma in Schools* strategies which includes five main components: education, having student action plans, allowing self-carry when appropriate, improving indoor air quality and reducing triggers, and developing an asthma friendly school.[11]

Note on inhalers:

Albuterol inhalers should have a dose counter. You **cannot** get an accurate estimate of how much active ingredient is in a canister by floating it in water (and you risk damaging the valve). Counters also help indicate if a person is overusing the inhaler and needs a different controller medication plan.

Spacers or valved holding chambers should be used for children who are not yet able to master the metered-dose inhaler technique.

REFERENCES

---

[1] Barrett, M. & Murphy Moore, C. (2019). Students with common health chronic respiratory conditions: Asthma and cystic fibrosis. In J. Selekman, R. Shannon, & C. Yonkaitis (Eds.), *School nursing: A comprehensive text* (3rd ed., pp. 523-540). F.A. Davis.

[2] Centers for Disease Control and Prevention. (2018). *Asthma*. https://www.cdc.gov/healthyschools/asthma/index.htm

[3] Merck Manual. (2019). *Asthma*. https://www.merckmanuals.com/professional/pulmonary-disorders/asthma-and-related-disorders/asthma#v31726177

[4] Ibid.

ASTHMA AND ASTHMA EMERGENCIES *(continued from previous page)*

[5] Ibid.

[6] National Heart, Lung, and Blood Institute, U.S. Department of Health and Human Services. (2012). *Asthma care quick reference: Diagnosing and managing asthma.* https://www.nhlbi.nih.gov/files/docs/guidelines/asthma_qrg.pdf

[7] National Heart, Lung, and Blood Institute, U.S. Department of Health and Human Services. (2011). *Asthma guidelines.* https://www.nhlbi.nih.gov/health-pro/resources/lung/naci/asthma-info/asthma-guidelines.htm

[8] American Lung Association. (2018). *Valved holding chambers and spacers.* https://www.lung.org/lung-health-and-diseases/lung-disease-lookup/asthma/living-with-asthma/managing-asthma/valved-holding-chambers-and.html

[7] MedlinePlus. U.S. National Library of Medicine. (2018). *Signs of an asthma attack.* www.nlm.nih.gov/medlineplus/asthma.html

[10] American Lung Association. (2019.) *Asthma action plan for home and school.* https://www.lung.org/assets/documents/asthma/asthma-action-plan-for-home.pdf

[11] Centers for Disease Control and Prevention. (2018). *Controlling asthma in schools.* https://www.cdc.gov/asthma/controlling_asthma_factsheet.html

OTHER REFERENCES CONSULTED

American Lung Association. https://www.lung.org/lung-health-and-diseases/lung-disease-lookup/asthma/

American Academy of Asthma, Allergy, and Immunology (AAAAI). https://www.aaaai.org/conditions-and-treatments/asthma

Allergy and Asthma Network. https://www.allergyasthmanetwork.org/

Centers for Disease Control and Prevention: Asthma – School and Childcare Providers. (2018). https://www.cdc.gov/asthma/schools.html

National Association of School Nurses Asthma Resources. https://www.nasn.org/nasn/nasn-resources/practice-topics/asthma

National Heart, Lung, and Blood Institute, U.S. Department of Health and Human Services. https://www.nhlbi.nih.gov/files/docs/resources/lung/asth_sch.pdf

ATTENTION DEFICIT HYPERACTIVITY DISORDER

DEFINITION/ETIOLOGY:

The American Psychiatric Association defines attention deficit hyperactivity disorder (ADHD) as "characterized by a pattern of behavior, present in multiple settings e.g., school and home),[1] that can result in performance issues in social, educational, or work settings." It is one of the most commonly diagnosed disorders in childhood and is considered a chronic condition often persisting in individuals into adolescence or adulthood.[2] ADHD is a neurobehavioral disorder that is characterized by inattention, hyperactivity and/or impulsive behaviors that may include behaviors like failure to pay close attention to details, difficulty organizing tasks, and activities, excessive talking, fidgeting, or an inability to remain seated in appropriate situations.[3] The behaviors affect cognitive, educational, behavioral, emotional, and social functioning. Children with ADHD differ in their symptoms, causes, prognosis, and responses to treatment. Some children are thought to have attention deficit without hyperactivity. These students may perform poorly in school despite normal intellect because they cannot sit still, attend, or complete a task. They are often rejected by their peers. Boys are affected more than girls. Symptoms may appear by age three years but often the condition is not medically diagnosed until school age.[4]

SIGNS AND SYMPTOMS:

Diagnostic criteria

The DSM-5 (2013) sets diagnostic criteria for ADHD. Children must have at least six symptoms from either (or both) the inattention group of criteria and the hyperactivity and impulsivity criteria, while older adolescents and adults (over age 17 years) must present with five. Using DSM-5, several of the individual's ADHD symptoms must be present prior to age 12 years.[5]

The DSM-5 lists the following symptoms of inattention. The symptoms must have persisted for at least six months to a degree that is maladaptive and inconsistent with developmental level.

Inattention

- Often fails to give close attention to details or makes careless mistakes in schoolwork, work, or other activities.
- Often has difficulty sustaining attention in tasks or play activities.
- Often does not seem to listen when spoken to directly.
- Often does not follow through on instructions and fails to finish schoolwork or chores (not due to oppositional behavior or failure to understand instructions).
- Often has difficulty organizing tasks and activities.
- Often avoids, dislikes, or is reluctant to engage in tasks that require sustained mental effort (such as schoolwork or homework).
- Often loses things necessary for tasks or activities (e.g., toys, school assignments, pencils, books, or tools).[6]
- Is often easily distracted by extraneous stimuli.
- Is often forgetful in daily activities.

The following symptoms of hyperactivity-impulsivity are listed by the DSM-5 and must have persisted for at least six months to a degree that is maladaptive and inconsistent with developmental level.

ATTENTION DEFICIT HYPERACTIVITY DISORDER *(continued from previous page)*

SIGNS AND SYMPTOMS *(continued)*

Hyperactivity
- Often fidgets with hands or feet or squirms in seat.
- Often leaves seat in classroom or in other situations in which remaining seated is expected.
- Often runs about or climbs excessively in situations in which it is inappropriate. (adolescents or adults may only feel restless).
- Often has difficulty playing or engaging in leisure activities quietly.
- Is often "on the go" or often acts as if "driven by a motor".
- Often talks excessively.[7]

Impulsivity
- Often blurts out answers.
- Often has difficulty waiting for a turn.
- Often interrupts or intrudes on others.
- Some hyperactive-impulsive or inattentive symptoms that caused impairment were present before age 12 years.
- Some impairment from the symptoms is present in two or more structured settings (e.g., at school and at home).
- There must be clear evidence of clinically significant impairment in social, academic, OR occupational functioning.[8]

DIAGNOSTIC PROCEDURES:
- Observations may be conducted:
  - At home, in several locations and circumstances (e.g. mealtime, outdoor play, performance of homework and household chores)
  - At healthcare provider's office
  - At school - classroom, cafeteria, and playground
  - At church, restaurants and family gatherings
- Information from standardized ADHD rating scales or other pertinent evaluations such as school testing
- Interview of parent/child/teachers/others including developmental history
- History and physical examination

MANAGEMENT/TREATMENT:
While there is no cure for ADHD, it can be successfully managed. Treatment management may include medication and educational and behavioral interventions.
- **Educational:** The student may benefit from an Individualized Educational Plan (IEP) or a Section 504 plan that addresses the child's learning or behavior through individualized accommodations or modification of lesson plans, teacher instruction, special class placement.
- **Family Support:** routines, rules and relationships, support and advocacy groups.

ATTENTION DEFICIT HYPERACTIVITY DISORDER *(continued from previous page)*

MANAGEMENT/TREATMENT *(continued)*

- **Psychological/behavioral:** counseling, (group, individual and family), behavior modification, social skills training.
- **Medication:** Stimulants are the first line medication prescribed for uncomplicated ADHD. Dosage is not based on body weight; rather dosages are calculated on achieving desired effect with minimal side effects. Non-stimulant and Alpha-Agonists can also be used.[9]

Types of Medication
Methylphenidate (Ritalin®)
Methylphenidate (sustained release or once daily forms)
Concerta® ER (extended release)
Metadate CD
Metadate ER (extended release)
Methylin
Ritalin SR (sustained release)
Daytrana® transdermal patch
DextroAmphetamines
Dexedrine®
Dexedrine® spansules
DextroStat®
Adderall® (mixture)
Methamphetamine (Desoxyn®)
Dexmethylphenidate (Focalin®)
Lisdexamfetamine dimesylate (Vyvanse®)
Atomoxetine (Strattera®) which works on norepinephrine
Pemoline (Cylert®)

High blood pressure medication for ADD/ADHD — Certain blood pressure medications can be used to treat ADD/ADHD. Options include clonidine (Catapres®) and guanfacine (Tenex®). They are especially beneficial for those with tics or Tourette's Syndrome. While these medications can be effective for hyperactivity, impulsivity, and aggression, they are less helpful when it comes to attention problems.[10]

FOLLOW-UP:

Stimulants (Methylphenidate [Ritalin®], etc.) can cause loss of appetite: control by taking medication with or after meal. Monitor growth; height and weight three times each school year (e.g. September, January, and May).

In an adolescent it is important to screen for substance abuse as stimulants may be abused or sold to others. Alternatively, one of the non-stimulant medications can be chosen.[11]

ATTENTION DEFICIT HYPERACTIVITY DISORDER *(continued from previous page)*

POTENTIAL COMPLICATIONS:
Monitor for adverse effects of medications. The following are the most common adverse effects. For a complete list, see Physician's Desk Reference® or other drug resource.

- Risk of liver toxicity
- Abdominal pain, stomach-ache, headache
- Jitteriness, nervousness, anxiety, irritability
- Sleeplessness if taken after 4-5 p.m.
- New onset tic
- Decreased appetite, weight loss[12]

NOTES:
Families require support and education regarding the diagnosis and management of this condition.

Medication Reminder
A healthcare provider must individualize dose for each child.

- All have side effects and must be monitored closely, especially early in therapy.
- Do not insist that child be put on medication.
- If child is prescribed medication, try to obtain child's assent. All psychoactive medications work better if they are taken willingly by child with parental cooperation.
- It may be necessary to continue medication into adolescence and adult years.
- Children and teens should not take medication without supervision.

Associated Disorders (Co-morbid conditions)
While ADHD does not cause psychological problems, children with ADHD are more likely to have co-morbid conditions. The most common associated disorders seen with ADHD include oppositional defiant disorder, conduct disorder and learning disabilities.

Conduct Disorder
A repetitive and persistent pattern of behavior in which the basic rights of others or major age-appropriate societal norms or rules are violated, as manifested by the presence of three or more of the following criteria in the past 12 months, with at least one criterion present in the past six months:

- Aggression to people and animals
- Destruction of property
- Deceitfulness or theft
- Serious violations of rules

Oppositional Defiant Disorder (ODD)
A pattern of negativistic, hostile, and defiant behavior lasting at least six months, during which four or more of the components are present.

Note: Consider a criterion met only if the behavior occurs more frequently than is typically observed in individuals of comparable age and development level. The disturbance in behavior causes clinically significant impairment in social, academic, or occupational functioning. ODD may start during preschool years. Conduct disorder usually appears in older children.[13]

ATTENTION DEFICIT HYPERACTIVITY DISORDER *(continued from previous page)*

REFERENCES

[1]American Psychiatric Association. (2013). Neurodevelopmental disorders in *Diagnostic and statistical manual of mental disorders* (5th ed., pp. 59-66). American Psychiatric Association.

[2] Star, N., & Bowman-Harvey, C. (2017). Cognitive-perceptual disorders. *Pediatrics primary care* (6th ed., pp. 393-403). Elsevier, Inc.

[3] Ibid.

[4] American Psychiatric Association. (2013). Diagnostic and statistical manual of mental disorders (5th ed., pp. 59-66. American Psychiatric Association.

[5] Ibid.

[6] Ibid.

[7] Ibid.

[8] Ibid.

[9] Star, N., & Bowman-Harvey, C. (2017). Cognitive-perceptual disorders. *Pediatrics primary care* (6th ed., pp. 393-403) Elsevier, Inc.

[10] Ibid.

[11] Ibid.

[12] Ibid.

[13] American Psychiatric Association. (2013). Diagnostic and statistical manual of mental disorders (5th ed., pp. 59-66). American Psychiatric Association.

OTHER REFERENCES CONSULTED

American Academy of Pediatrics, Subcommittee on Attention-Deficit/Hyperactivity Disorder, Steering Committee on Quality Improvement and Management. (2011). ADHD: Clinical practice guideline for the diagnosis, evaluation, and treatment of Attention-Deficit/Hyperactivity Disorder in children and adolescents. *Pediatrics, 123*(5). Published online October 16, 2011. https://pediatrics.aappublications.org/content/pediatrics/early/2011/10/14/peds.2011-2654.full.pdf

American Psychiatric Association. (2019). *Attention deficit hyperactivity disorder.* http://www.dsm5.org/Documents/ADHD%20Fact%20Sheet.pdf

Foley, M. (2019). Students with attention deficit- hyperactivity disorder and specific learning disabilities. In J. Selekman, R. Adair Shannon, & C. F. Yonkaitis (Eds.), *School nursing: A comprehensive text* (3rd ed., pp. 549-574). F.A. Davis.

Goldson, E., & Reynolds, A. (2018). Child development and behavior. In W. Hay, M. Levin, R. Deterding, & M. Abzug (Eds.), *Current diagnosis and treatment pediatrics* (24th edition, pp. 105-107). McGraw Hill Education, Inc.

Mayo Clinic. (2017). *Attention-deficit/hyperactivity disorder (ADHD) in children*. http://www.mayoclinic.com/helth/adhd/DS00275

National Institutes of Health. (2016). *Attention deficit hyperactivity disorder.* http://www.nimh.nih.gov/health/publications/attention-deficit-hyperactivity-disorder/index.shtml

AUTISM SPECTRUM DISORDER

DEFINITION/ETIOLOGY:

Autism Spectrum Disorder (ASD) falls under a group of complex neurodevelopmental disorders. According to the fifth edition of the Diagnostic and Statistical Manual of Mental Disorders (DSM)[1], Asperger's Syndrome, Pervasive Developmental Disorder – Not Otherwise Specified, and Childhood Disintegrative Disorder are no longer separate diagnoses. All these subcategories of autism are now incorporated into a single category - the Autistic Spectrum Disorder (ASD) diagnosis, with severity specified for each individual. While most children maintained their diagnoses in spite of this change, it is important to note that some children who have social deficits but lack other characteristics such as repetitive behaviors who may have previously been diagnosed with PDD-NOS may be instead carry a diagnosis of *social communication disorder*.[2]

Prevalence varies according to race, gender, and ethnic group[2]. Recent reports indicate that one in 59 children are diagnosed with an ASD.[3]

The exact etiology of autism is unknown. Given the varied severity and symptoms of autism, the etiology is most likely multifactorial. Potential contributing factors include:

- Children with medical conditions such as congenital rubella syndrome, phenylketonuria, tuberous sclerosis, Tourette syndrome, RETT syndrome, epilepsy, tuberous sclerosis, or fragile X syndrome have a higher risk of being diagnosed with ASD.[4] There are a few case reports that suggest children with mitochondrial disorders may have a higher rate of autism than the general population, though more research is needed on this topic. Children with these conditions may display some autistic features even if they do not meet full diagnostic criteria.
- Genetic predisposition – based on sibling research studies, there is also a genetic tendency; families that have one child diagnosed with ASD have a higher occurrence of autism in subsequent children.
- Brain structure abnormalities – some children diagnosed with ASD have enlarged ventricles, abnormalities of the cerebellar vermis and of the brain stem nuclei.
- Gender – males are approximately four times more likely to be diagnosed with autism than females.[5, 6]
- Environmental – while suspected, and supported by some correlational and observational studies, there remains no high-level evidence supporting an environmental connection to ASD.[7]

SIGNS AND SYMPTOMS:

Autism symptoms appear within the first three years of life.[8] Symptoms vary from person to person, and diagnostic evaluation involves a multidisciplinary approach. Potential team members include trained healthcare providers (developmental pediatrician/neurologist) and psychiatrists/psychologists who administer specific autistic behavioral testing/evaluations. Diagnostic criteria are based on social communication/interaction and restricted/repetitive behaviors that interfere with functional abilities.

AUTISM SPECTRUM DISORDER *(continued from previous page)*

SIGNS AND SYMPTOMS *(continued)*

Social communication/interaction symptoms (deficits must be met in each of the two categories)

- Impaired social interaction/emotional interaction
  - Difficulty reciprocating social and emotion interactions with others
  - Difficulty making friends
  - Does not display physical affection
  - May reject physical affection
  - Prefer not to be held or touched by others
  - Absence of social play
  - Difficulty verbalizing needs
  - Difficulty with nonverbal communication
  - Tend to avoid eye contact (poor eye contact)
  - Inability to understand facial expressions, gestures and tone of voice
- Unable to maintain relationships
  - Lack empathy for others
  - Difficulty playing with others

Restrictive/repetitive movements (two of the four symptoms must be met)

- Repetitive speech (ECHOLALIA) / motor movements (rocking back and forth, hand flapping)
- Strict adherence to routines/rituals – resistant to change
- Highly restricted interest – these interests are often obsessive and may be limited to specific topics/activities (lining up cars, etc.)
- Hypo/hyper reactive to sensory input
- Self-abusive behaviors (head banging) [9, 10]

MANAGEMENT/TREATMENT:

There is no cure for autism. ASD can be diagnosed by experienced professionals in children as young as two years of age. Refer children with suspected autism diagnosis for evaluation. Early detection and interventions improve quality of life and overall outcomes. Interventions should be based on student need, and may include:

- Speech therapy
- Physical therapy
- Occupational therapy
- Behavioral therapy – social work services
- Family therapy – to promote social interaction
- Special education services
- Pharmacological therapy – antipsychotic medication for aggressive and harmful behaviors, ADHD medications to help treat impulsive and hyperactive behaviors, antidepressant for anxiety, etc.

AUTISM SPECTRUM DISORDER *(continued from previous page)*

MANAGEMENT/TREATMENT *(continued)*

- Nutritional therapy – Many children with autism often experience nutritional deficits or feeding difficulties due to restrictive interests or other biological factors such as poor digestion leading to pain and discomfort. Some research suggests that children with ASD have a higher rate of digestive difficulties than the general population. [11] Preliminary anecdotal evidence from parents and clinicians supports nutritional intervention for autism as a potential strategy for improving health and potentially associated problematic behaviors.

FOLLOW-UP:

- Tend to lose skills that they once possessed.
- Ongoing evaluation of interventions to determine effectiveness is necessary.
- Monitor for potential medication side effects. Some medications can interact, causing dangerous side effects. Report suspected side effects to parent/prescriber.

POTENTIAL COMPLICATIONS:

Comorbidities may include:

- ADHD
- Pica
- Seizure disorder – more than 20 % of individuals with autism develop seizure disorder by adulthood[12]
- Sleep disorders
- Gastrointestinal issues

NOTES:

Controversy remains on whether a link exists between autism and certain childhood vaccines, especially the measles, mumps and rubella vaccine (MMR). Educate parent/guardian that no reliable, high-quality study has shown a link between autism and any particular vaccine; however, some vaccine injuries (rare but serious adverse effects from vaccination), including but not limited to encephalopathy or encephalitis, may present with autistic-like symptoms and/or regression. [13, 14, 15, 16, 17] Educate parent on the potential complications of contracting a vaccine preventable disease such as rubeola, mumps, rubella, and/or pertussis versus the risk of a serious adverse event from a vaccination. Encourage parents to report any adverse events of vaccination to the Vaccine Adverse Event Reporting System (VAERS) in conjunction with their healthcare provider.

Some parents/guardians seek alternative therapy in the treatment of autism including chelation therapy. Chelation therapy is thought to remove mercury and heavy metals from the body and is considered dangerous, as it also removes beneficial elements and minerals. There have been deaths associated with chelation therapy as an alternative therapy for autism. As needed, educate parents/guardians on the dangers of chelation therapy vs. any potential benefit.

AUTISM SPECTRUM DISORDER *(continued from previous page)*

NOTES *(continued)*

Dietary interventions – parents/guardians may choose vitamin supplements, and special diets such as the gluten-free and casein-free diet, FODMAPS diet, or ketogenic diet in the treatment of ASD. More research is needed regarding how effective dietary interventions are in addressing ASD; however, these diets are generally not harmful to generally healthy individuals and should be supported within the school environment if this is parental preference. Refer parents/guardians with questions related to dietary interventions to a registered dietician or nutritionist with an expertise in ASD.

RESOURCES

- **Autism Research Institute**
  https://www.autism.org/

- **Autism Society of America**
  http://www.autism-society.org/
  1(800) 328-8476

- **Autism Speaks**
  http://www.autismspeaks.org/what-autism/symptoms

- **Centers for Disease Control and Prevention (CDC)**
  http://www.cdc.gov/ncbddd/autism/facts.html
  1(800) 232-4636

- **Early Childhood Technical Assistance Center (ECTA)**
  http://www.ectacenter.org/contact/ptccoord.asp
  919-962-2001

- **National Institute of Neurological Disorders and Stroke**
  http://www.ninds.nih.gov/disorders/autism/detail_autism.htm

AUTISM SPECTRUM DISORDER *(continued from previous page)*

REFERENCES

[1] American Academy of Pediatrics. (2018). *CDC: Autism rates increase slightly to 1 in 59 children.* https://www.aappublications.org/news/2018/04/26/autism042618

[2] Ibid.

[3] Ibid.

[4] Rossignol, D.A., Genuis, S.J., & Frye, R.E. (2014). Environmental toxicants and autism spectrum disorders: A systematic review. *Translational Psychiatry*, *4*, e360. https://www.nature.com/articles/tp20144

[5] Ibid.

[6] Centers for Disease Control and Prevention (CDC). (2018). *Autism spectrum disorders.* http://www.cdc.gov/ncbddd/autism/facts.html

[7] Rossignol, D.A., Genuis, S.J., & Frye, R.E. (2014). Environmental toxicants and autism spectrum disorders: A systematic review. *Translational Psychiatry*, *4*, e360. https://www.nature.com/articles/tp20144

[8] Centers for Disease control and Prevention. (2017). *Signs and symptoms of autism spectrum disorders. https://www.cdc.gov/ncbddd/autism/signs.html*

[9] American Psychiatric Association. (2013). *Diagnostic and statistical manual of mental disorders* (5th ed.). American Psychiatric Publishing.

[10] Centers for Disease Control and Prevention (CDC). (2018). *Autism spectrum disorders.* http://www.cdc.gov/ncbddd/autism/facts.html

[11] Chaidez, V., Hansen, R. L., & Hertz-Picciotto, I. (2014). Gastrointestinal problems in children with autism, developmental delays or typical development. *Journal of Autism and Developmental Disorders, 44*(5), 1117–1127.https://doi.org/10.1007/s10803-013-1973-x

[12] National Institute of Neurological Disorders and Stroke. (2019). *Autism spectrum disorder fact sheet.* https://www.ninds.nih.gov/Disorders/Patient-Caregiver-Education/Fact-Sheets/Autism-Spectrum-Disorder-Fact-Sheet

[13] Centers for Disease Control and Prevention (CDC). (2018). *Frequently asked questions on mitochondrial disease.* https://www.cdc.gov/ncbddd/autism/mitochondrial-faq.html

[14] Shoffner, J., Hyams, L., Langley, G. N., Cossette, S., Mylacraine, L., Dale, J., Ollis, L., Kuoch, S., Bennett, K., Aliberti, A., & Hyland, K. (2010). Fever plus mitochondrial disease could be risk factors for autistic regression. *Journal of Child Neurology*, *25*(4), 429–434. https://doi.org/10.1177/0883073809342128

[15] Qudah, Z.A., Abukwaik, W., Patel, H., & Souayah, N. (2012). Encephalitis after vaccination in United States: A Report from the CDC/FDA Vaccine Adverse Event Reporting System [1990-2010]. *Neurology* Apr 2012, *78* (1 Supplement) P03.151. https://n.neurology.org/content/78/1_Supplement/P03.151

[16] Srivastava, S., & Sahin, M. (2017). Autism spectrum disorder and epileptic encephalopathy: Common causes, many questions. *Journal of neurodevelopmental disorders*, *9*(23). https://doi.org/10.1186/s11689-017-9202-0

[17] Weibel, R.E., Caserta, B., Benor, D. E., & Evans, G. (1999). acute encephalopathy followed by permanent brain injury or death associated with further attenuated measles vaccines: A review of claims submitted to the National Vaccine Injury Compensation Program. *Pediatrics, 101*(3). https://pediatrics.aappublications.org/content/101/3/383

BACK AND NECK INJURY

DEFINITION/ETIOLOGY:
The etiology of back and neck injury is multifactorial. Severe injuries may occur from a traumatic blow to the back or neck that fractures, dislocates, or compresses a vertebra. Most injuries are sprains and strains.[1] Back and neck injuries may result from motor vehicle accidents and playground injuries. Youth are at increased risk of injury because they often participate in higher-risk behaviors and physical activities/sports. Severe injuries may occur to athletes (such as football, soccer, gymnastics, etc.) trampoline jumpers, horseback riders, divers who hit bottom, etc. Neck injuries can occur when the neck is forcefully flexed, and the chin strikes the chest.

SIGNS AND SYMPTOMS:[2]
Symptoms depend on the location of the injury. Symptoms can affect the neck, arms, legs, back and shoulders. Symptoms may include:

- Pain made worse by pressure or movement
- Pain may radiate into arm or leg
- Nerve involvement: weakness, tingling, numbness, or inability to move arm or leg

Signs of a serious injury include: [3]

- Extreme pain in neck or back
- Abnormal positioning of neck or back
- Loss of sensation
- Loss of bowel and bladder function
- Difficulty walking
- Lacks control over extremities
- Paralysis
- Difficulty breathing
- Shock
- Loss of consciousness

When damage to the spinal cord is suspected, DO NOT MOVE STUDENT until assessment is done.

MANAGEMENT/TREATMENT:[4]
Treatment depends on the extent of the injury.

1. If you suspect a neck injury or back injury do not move, bend, or rotate neck or spinal column of student. Permanent complications such as paralysis could result. If severe injury is suspected and the student is wearing a helmet with shoulder pads (typical of American football), the helmet should remain in place unless its presence presents a compromise to the student airway or facial access.[5,6]. Helmets with no attached padding (baseball, biking, etc.) should be removed to allow spinal neutrality.
2. ***Assess airway, breathing, and circulation – if airway is compromised, and Cardiopulmonary Resuscitation (CPR) is necessary, use jaw thrust maneuver instead of head tilt. Call Emergency Medical Services (EMS) immediately.[7]***
3. Perform comprehensive neurological assessment. If you suspect a serious injury, immobilize student until assessment is completed.

BACK AND NECK INJURY *(continued from previous page)*

MANAGEMENT/TREATMENT *(continued)*

4. Assess student's ability to move extremities slowly, and only move a small amount. Test response to stimuli, such as a finger touch or pin prick. Determine strength by checking hand grasp.
5. If severe neck or back injury is suspected or if pain, sensory impairment, or weakness persists, have student remain in current position and **call EMS for additional evaluation.** Moving the student may cause further injury or damage. Keep child warm and calm until help arrives.
6. If sensation is intact, pain is minimal to absent, and student is able to move all extremities normally, allow student to slowly sit up and then walk.
7. If all neurological signs are normal and student is able to move all extremities freely, ice may be applied to relieve pain if allowed per school district protocol. Some states require orders to apply ice.
8. Notify parent/guardian for any degree of injury.
9. Refer to healthcare provider for further follow-up and treatment if necessary.
10. If prescribed, administer pain/anti-inflammatory medications as ordered. Monitor for medication side effects.
11. Student may return to play/activity when they are symptom free and have a normal examination by a healthcare provider including no neck or back pain, sensory deficits, or limitations to spinal range of motion.[8, 9]
12. Complete injury/incident report.

FOLLOW UP:

- Student with minor injuries who remains at school should be observed several times during school day.
- Notify physical education teacher and coaches of injury and potential accommodations.

POTENTIAL COMPLICATIONS (serious injuries):[10]

- Chronic pain
- Fecal and bladder incontinence
- Permanent paralysis

BACK AND NECK INJURY *(continued from previous page)*

NOTES:

BACK PACKS AND BACK PAIN

The amount of weight carried by children in their backpacks is an important issue that deserves serious consideration. Loading of the spine is a risk factor for low back pain not only in adults but also in children; the load that children most commonly carry is their school backpack. **A backpack limit of 5-10% of ideal body weight for students is recommended**[11] (obese children already carry an additional built-in burden which should not be used in calculating 15% of body weight). The backpack should have two wide (at least 2") shoulder straps and a waist or chest strap to distribute the load with the backpack never hanging more than 4 inches past the student's waist.[12] Although back pain in children is likely to be multifactorial, heavy backpacks are probably an important contributing cause. Some schools have policies on the use of backpacks and rolling cases.

While increasing numbers of children are developing back pain, it is difficult to assign the cause of this increase to heavy backpack use alone. Students may also have back or neck pain due to postural lordosis, spondylolysis, and/or Scheuermann's kyphosis. Back pain in the absence of injury requires evaluation to rule out potentially serious causes such as malignancy or spinal meningitis.[13]

REFERENCES

---

[1] MedlinePlus. U.S. National Library of Health. (2019). *Back injuries.* http://www.nlm.nih.gov/medlineplus/backinjuries.html

[2] Mayo Clinic. (2017). *Spinal cord injuries.* http://www.mayoclinic.org/diseases-conditions/spinal-cord-injury/basics/symptoms/con-20023837

[3] Ibid.

[4] Merck Manual. (2018). *Evaluation of neck and back pain.* http://www.merckmanuals.com/professional/musculoskeletal-and-connective-tissue-disorders/neck-and-back-pain/evaluation-of-neck-and-back-pain

[5] Kleiner, D.M. & Cantu, R.C. (2016). *The spine-injured football player and helmet removal.* https://www.acsm.org/docs/default-source/files-for-resource-library/basics_player-helmet-removal.pdf?sfvrsn=1276d818_2

[6] Ghiselli, G., Schaadt, G., & McAllister, D. R. (2003). On-the-field evaluation of an athlete with a head or neck injury. *Clinics in Sports Medicine*, *22*(3), 445-465. https://doi.org/10.1016/S0278-5919(02)00109-6

[7] Mayo Clinic. (2019). *Spinal injuries: First aid.* https://www.mayoclinic.org/first-aid/first-aid-spinal-injury/basics/art-20056677

[8] Anderson, C., & Johnson, R. J. (1993). Neck injuries: Backboard, bench, or return to play? *The Physician and Sports Medicine*, *21*(8), 23-34. https://doi.org/10.1080/00913847.1993.11947585

[9] Cantu, R. C.; Li, Y.; Abdulhamid, M.; Chin, L. (2013). Return to play after cervical spine injury in sports. *Current Sports Medicine Reports,* 12(1),14–17. https://doi.org/10.1249/JSR.0b013e31827dc1fb

[10] Nigrovic, P. (2018). *Back pain in children and adolescents: Causes.* https://www.uptodate.com/contents/back-pain-in-children-and-adolescents-causes

BACK AND NECK INJURY *(continued from previous page)*

[11] American Academy of Pediatrics. (2019). *Backpack safety.* https://www.healthychildren.org/English/safety-prevention/at-play/Pages/Backpack-Safety.aspx

[12] Ibid.

[13] Anderson, C., & Johnson, R. J. (2017). Neck injuries: backboard, bench, or return to play? *The Physician and Sports Medicine*, *21*(8), 23-34. https://doi.org/10.1080/00913847.1993.11947585

BED BUGS

OVERVIEW/DEFINITION:[1, 2]

Bed bugs (*Cimex lectularius*) are small, reddish brown, wingless, flat, parasitic insects that bite humans and animals while they sleep. They feed for five to 10 minutes exclusively on human blood typically between 2:00 – 5:00 am. They can go without feeding for up to six months. Bite marks may take up to two weeks to develop. They are not known to transmit or spread disease and should not be considered a medical or public health hazard.

Bedbugs were eradicated at one time in most developed countries because of the use of DDT, a pesticide that is no longer used and is banned because of its toxicity. The discontinuation of DDT use and the increase of international travel are thought to have led to bedbugs becoming a problem again.[3]

Bed bug infestations usually occur in areas where people sleep, e.g. beds, bed frames, mattress seams, box springs, behind wallpaper, or any other clutter or objects around a bed.[4] The insects can travel anywhere from eight to 15 feet but are found to live usually within eight feet of where people sleep. Bedbugs hide in luggage and clothing, crawl and hitchhike so they can be transported easily. They may be brought to school in book bags and clothing.

SIGNS AND SYMPTOMS BITES:[5, 6]

- Bites may take up to two weeks to appear
- Itchy bites, sometimes in a row
- Bites usually found on face, arms, legs, neck
- Bites may have a red dot in the middle of a raised bump
- Some people have no reaction to bedbug bites
- Some people may experience an allergic reaction that results in severe itching, blisters or hives
- Difficult to distinguish bed bug bites from other insect bites

ANTICIPATED CONCERNS/PROBLEMS:[7]

- Scratching may lead to secondary infection
- Boils
- Cellulitis
- Allergic symptoms (e.g. swelling/pain at the bite site)
- Anaphylaxis (on rare occasions)

MANAGEMENT/POTENTIAL INTERVENTIONS:

- **No exclusion is necessary** [8]
- Avoid scratching
- Relief for itching may include:[9]
    - antiseptic creams or lotions
    - prescribed steroid creams
    - antihistamines (such as Benadryl®)

BED BUGS *(continued from previous page)*

FOLLOW-UP:
For School Buildings[10]

- Limit items that travel back and forth between home and school.
- Avoid clutter.
- Clean cubbies/lockers routinely (seasonally).
- Vacuum rugs frequently. Dispose of vacuum cleaner bags/filters in tightly sealed plastic bag.
- Avoid fabric-covered furniture, pillows in schools.
- Provide space between coat hooks and backpacks.
- Keep "Lost and Found" clothing, backpacks, etc. in closeable plastic storage bins.
- Involve facilities maintenance and pest management staff to address any bed bug infestation in schools.

Families may need to contact their landlord or contact a professional exterminator to eliminate any home infestation. Exterminators may use a combination of pesticides and nonchemical treatments. Nonchemical treatments may include: [11]

- **Vacuuming** - dispose of vacuum filter and bags in a tightly sealed plastic bag.
- **Washing clothes -** and other items in water at least 120°F (49° C) can kill bedbugs.
- **Using clothes dryer -** placing wet or dry items in a clothes dryer set at high heat for 30–60 minutes will kill bedbugs and their eggs.
- **Freeze –** leave articles outside when temperatures are below 32°F or place small articles in a sealed bag and put in the freezer.

NOTES:
SIGNS OF A BED BUG INFESTATION

- Tiny black specks seen in mattress seams are typically bed bug feces.
- Pale yellow empty exoskeletons are left after a bedbug molts.
- Small smears red or rusty stains on bed sheets may be blood of a crushed a bedbug.

PREVENTION:

- Bed bugs are not inclined to burrow through clothing. Cover as much skin as possible when sleeping.
- Keep nails short to prevent infection from scratching.

The school nurse can be extremely helpful in helping families and staff from overreacting to this nuisance condition. Education is very important, reminding people that bed bugs do not discriminate, and infestations is not a reflection of cleanliness. Bed bugs do not infest the person; they infest the living area and require extermination.[12]

Having a plan/guideline that includes how the school will physically address prevention and elimination of bed bugs and how families will be notified is helpful.

BED BUGS *(continued from previous page)*

REFERENCES

[1] American Academy of Pediatrics. (2020). Bedbugs. In S. Aronson, & T. Shope (Eds.), *Managing infectious diseases in child care and schools* (5th ed., pp. 63-64). American Academy of Pediatrics.

[2] Merck Manual. (2018). *Bed bugs.* https://www.merckmanuals.com/professional/dermatologic-disorders/parasitic-skin-infections/bedbugs

[3] Plumer, B. (2016). *Why bed bugs have made a horrifying comeback. Vox.* https://www.vox.com/2015/4/27/8502491/bed-bugs-kill-increase

[4] Mayo Clinic. (2018). *Bed bugs.* https://www.mayoclinic.org/diseases-conditions/bedbugs/symptoms-causes/syc-20370001

[5] Center for Disease Control and Prevention. (2017). *Bed bugs FAQs.* http://www.cdc.gov/parasites/bedbugs/faqs.html

[6] Mayo Clinic. (2018). *Bed bugs.* https://www.mayoclinic.org/diseases-conditions/bedbugs/symptoms-causes/syc-20370001

[7] Center for Disease Control and Prevention. (2017). *Bed bugs FAQs.* http://www.cdc.gov/parasites/bedbugs/faqs.html

[8] Mayo Clinic. (2018). *Bed bugs.* https://www.mayoclinic.org/diseases-conditions/bedbugs/symptoms-causes/syc-20370001

[9] American Academy of Dermatologists Inc. (2018). *Bed bugs: Overview.* https://www.aad.org/public/diseases/itchy-skin/bed-bugs#overview

[10] Mayo Clinic. (2018). *Bed bugs.* https://www.mayoclinic.org/diseases-conditions/bedbugs/symptoms-causes/syc-20370001

[11] American Academy of Pediatrics. (2020). Bedbugs. In S. Aronson, & T. Shope (Eds.), *Managing infectious diseases in child care and schools* (5th ed., pp. 63-64). American Academy of Pediatrics.

[12] Ibid.

OTHER REFERENCES CONSULTED

Environmental Protection Agency. (2019). *Bed bugs: Get them out and keep them out.* www.epa.gov/bedbugs

IdentifyUs. (2017). *Bed bugs.* https://identify.us.com/idmybug/bed-bugs/

Quirós, G. (2019, July 9). *How best to snag and destroy bedbugs?* National Public Radio (NPR). https://www.npr.org/sections/health-shots/2019/07/09/739473492/how-best-to-snag-and-destroy-bedbugs?utm_source=dlvr.it&utm_medium=twitter

EPA

EPA 730-F-15-001
June 2016

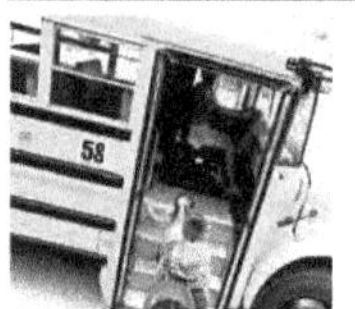

Bed Bugs in Schools

Guidance for School Nurses

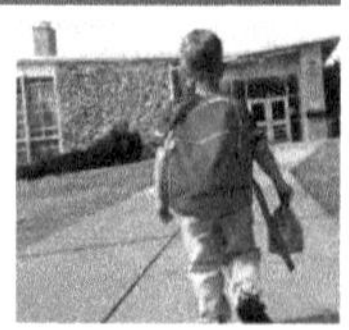

Managing bed bugs can be a major challenge for any school. School nurses are often called upon to provide vital information to students, parents, teachers, and administrators. These tips on identifying, managing and preventing bed bugs will help you to effectively respond if bed bugs appear in your school.

If You Think You Have Spotted a Bed Bug

- Collect and keep it intact for proper identification.
- Discretely remove the student from class but do not send him/her home or exclude them from school.
- Check the student's clothing and belongings for possible bed bugs.
- Inspect the area around where the bug was found.

Have a Positive Bed Bug ID?

- Oversee the case until the problem is resolved.
- Tell the child's parents about the bed bug sighting.
- Provide the student and parents with information on bed bug control.

What to Tell Parents

- Having a bed bug infestation does not mean their home isn't clean.
- A true bed bug infestation is unlikely in the school.
- It is not necessary for the school to close because of bed bugs.
- Students should limit the items they bring to school.
- Students should store school supplies in protective boxes at home and not under or near beds or couches.

Finding a confirmed bed bug on a student or their belongings may not mean their home or school is infested.

Successful Bed Bug Management

- Uses a combination of strategies such as prevention, inspection, vacuuming, steam/heat treatment, and, if needed, pesticides.
- Recognizes that pesticides alone may not eliminate bed bugs.
- Involves placing clothes in a dryer on high heat for at least 30 minutes to kill any bed bugs.
- May include professional steam or radiant heat treatments.

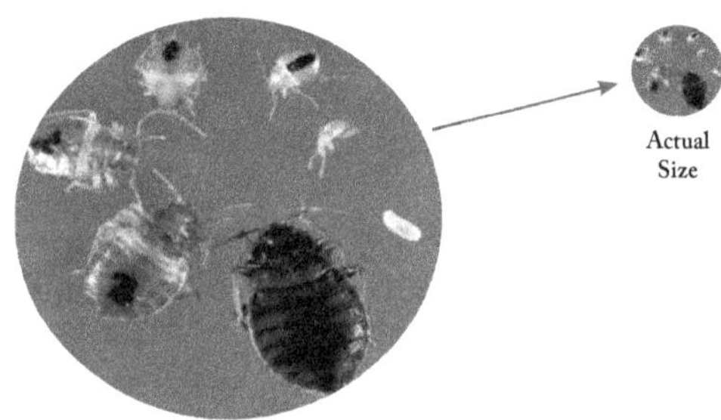

Bed Bug Hot Spots in Schools

- Student and staff closets, lockers, coats and backpacks.
- Faculty lounges, classrooms or other areas with upholstered furniture or cots.
- Dormitories or other sleeping areas.

Learn more at epa.gov/bedbugs

Bed Bugs: School Response Flowchart

School Responsibility:
Providing a healthy, pest-free environment in which students can excel
Parent/Caregiver Responsibility:
Providing a safe and healthy living environment for the student

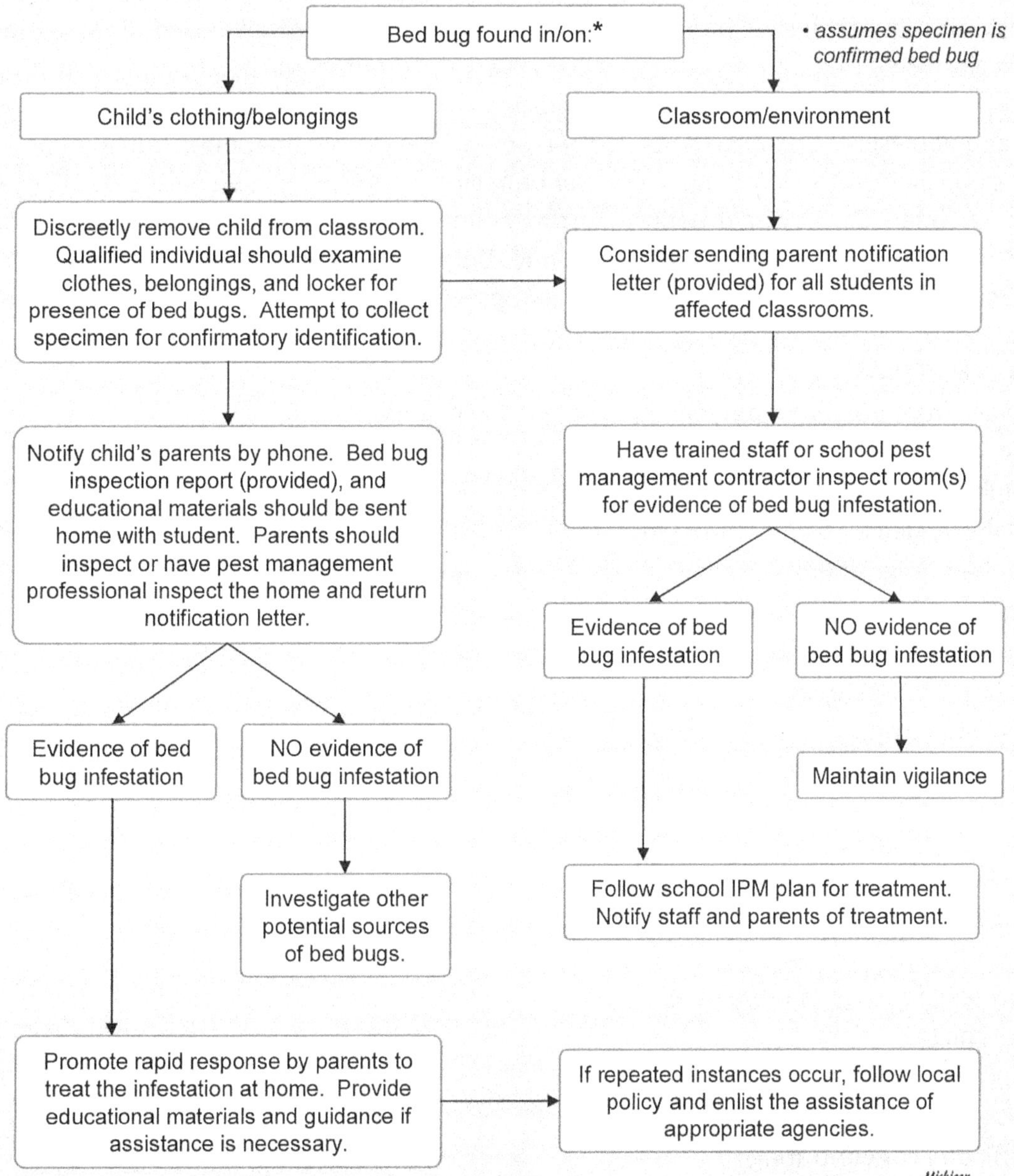

Bed bug found in/on:*

* *assumes specimen is confirmed bed bug*

Child's clothing/belongings

Discreetly remove child from classroom. Qualified individual should examine clothes, belongings, and locker for presence of bed bugs. Attempt to collect specimen for confirmatory identification.

Notify child's parents by phone. Bed bug inspection report (provided), and educational materials should be sent home with student. Parents should inspect or have pest management professional inspect the home and return notification letter.

- Evidence of bed bug infestation → Promote rapid response by parents to treat the infestation at home. Provide educational materials and guidance if assistance is necessary. → If repeated instances occur, follow local policy and enlist the assistance of appropriate agencies.
- NO evidence of bed bug infestation → Investigate other potential sources of bed bugs.

Classroom/environment

Consider sending parent notification letter (provided) for all students in affected classrooms.

Have trained staff or school pest management contractor inspect room(s) for evidence of bed bug infestation.

- Evidence of bed bug infestation → Follow school IPM plan for treatment. Notify staff and parents of treatment.
- NO evidence of bed bug infestation → Maintain vigilance

See the Schools and Daycares section of Michigan's Bed Bug Prevention and Control Manual for detailed instructions.
Michigan Bed Bug Working Group (May 2010)

Michigan Department of Education | Michigan Department of Community Health MDCH | Michigan Department of Agriculture

BIPOLAR DISORDER

DEFINITION/ETIOLOGY:[1]
Bipolar disorder (previously called manic-depressive disorder) is a behavioral health disorder characterized by extreme changes in energy and affect, mood swings, periods of unusual highs (mania) and lows (depression). The exact etiology is unknown. However, genetics and environment have been linked to bipolar disorder. Onset usually occurs in mid-to-late adolescence, though there are cases in children. Children and adolescents diagnosed as bipolar are typically unpredictably explosive, moody, and aggressive toward themselves and others. Their mood cycles are mixed and unpredictable, which is very different from the adult presentation of bipolar disorder which has cycles of mania (euphoric behavior) followed by periods of depression. In children and adolescents mania is not usually a period of extreme happiness but seen as aggressive, explosive, and a violent episode. The behavioral outburst can be very dangerous (e.g. hitting, kicking, biting, destroying property, hurting animals, using weapons, etc.) and can last until the child or adolescent is too exhausted to continue. Bipolar disorder is a life-long illness but in most cases, can be controlled with medications and psychological counseling.

SIGNS AND SYMPTOMS:
Symptoms vary from person to person. Symptoms may include:[2]
Manic stage

- Euphoria
- Flight of ideas
- Feelings of grandiose
- Agitation/irritation
- Aggressive behaviors
- Inflated self-esteem
- Risky behaviors
- Substance/alcohol abuse
- Talking fast
- Decreased need for sleep

Depressive stage:

- Withdrawn
- Sadness/feelings of hopelessness
- Irritability
- Anxiety
- Fatigue
- Difficulty concentrating
- Chronic pain with unknown cause
- Suicidal thoughts

Children and adolescents may demonstrate symptoms of intense rage, aggressive and impulsive behaviors. These symptoms can be misdiagnosed as Obsessive-Compulsive Disorder or Attention Deficit/Hyperactive Disorder (ADHD).

BIPOLAR DISORDER *(continued from previous page)*

MANAGEMENT/TREATMENT:[3]

- Primary treatment includes daily medication and psychotherapy.
- If indicated, administer medication during the school day per the healthcare provider's orders.
- Potential medication treatment includes:

Drug	Purpose/Examples of medications	Comments
Lithium®	Prevents extreme highs and lows, stabilizes mood; may need to take lithium for several weeks before feeling better; provider will order regular blood test to monitor lithium levels	• Monitor for side effects – dry mouth, gastrointestinal issues; **beware of lithium toxicity** – gastrointestinal issues, dizziness, weakness, slurred speech, seizures, nystagmus, coma; follow up with healthcare provider immediately if lithium toxicity is suspected • Risk of lithium toxicity increases with dehydration; therefore, maintain hydration
Antipsychotics	Used to treat acute mania. Examples include risperidone, olanzapine, ziprasidone, chlorpromazine, aripiprazole, paliperidone, and quetiapine.	• Monitor for side effects which may include weight gain, sedation and neurological symptoms
Anticonvulsants	Used to stabilize mood. Examples include carbamazepine, divalproex and lamotrigine	• Monitor for potential side effects – weight gain, dizziness, drowsiness

- Develop an individualized healthcare plan (IHP) to manage in school care along with a behavioral health care if indicated.

FOLLOW UP:[4]

- Be aware that some adolescents are non-adherent to drug regimens (often due to side effects such as weight gain)
- Educate parent/guardian and student that bipolar disorder is a lifelong illness that requires lifelong treatment
- Monitor for medication side effects and communicate regularly with healthcare provider and parents/guardian

BIPOLAR DISORDER *(continued from previous page)*

POTENTIAL COMPLICATIONS:

- Poor school attendance/performance
- Difficulty maintaining relationships
- Suicide

REFERENCES

[1] American Academy of Child Adolescent Psychiatry (AACAP). (2018*). Bipolar disorder resource center.* https://www.aacap.org/AACAP/Families_and_Youth/Resource_Centers/Bipolar_Disorder_Resource_Center/Home.aspx

[2] American Psychiatric Association (APA). (2013). *Diagnostic and statistical manual of mental disorders (DSM-V)* (5th ed.) https://doi.org/10.1176/appi.books.9780890425596

[3] Ibid.

[4] Patterson, B.R., Bohnenkamp, J., hoover, S., Bostie, J. & Selekman, J. (2019). Students with mental / behavioral health concerns and disorders. In J. Selekman, R.A. Shannon, & C. F. Younkaitis (Eds.), *School Nursing: A comprehensive text* (3rd ed., pp. 756-790). F. A. Davis.

OTHER REFERENCES CONSULTED

American Psychiatric Association. (2019). *Help with* bipolar *disease.* http://www.psychiatry.org/bipolar-disorder

Halter, M.J. (2018). Bipolar and related disorders. In M. J. Halter (Ed.), *Varcarolis' foundations of psychiatric-mental health nursing: A clinical approach* (8th ed., pp.223-239). Elsevier.

Mayo Clinic. (2019). *Bipolar disorder.* https://www.mayoclinic.org/search/search-results?q=bipolar%20disorder

Merck Manual. (2019). *Bipolar disorders in children and adolescents.* http://www.merckmanuals.com/professional/pediatrics/mental_disorders_in_children_and_adolescents/bipolar_disorder_in_children_and_adolescents.html?qt=bipolar disorder&alt=sh

Walton, K., & Kersey, S.J. (2020). Mental health disorders. In B. Richardson (Ed.*), Pediatric primary care: Practice guideline for nurses* (4th ed., pp. 673-689). Jones and Bartlett.

BITES: Animal and Human **(if skin is broken)**

DEFINITION/ETIOLOGY:

Soft tissue injuries resulting from animal or human bites that include a puncture wound or crushing injury combined with lacerations. Commonly, such injuries are to the arm/hand and to the head, face, and neck.

SIGNS AND SYMPTOMS:

- Pain and bleeding
- Punctures and/or lacerations are usually jagged; pieces of tissue may be torn away in severe bites.

ANTICIPATED COMPLICATIONS/PROBLEMS:

Animal bites[1]

- Early cellulitis - *Pasteurella multocida*
- Secondary infection – *Staphylococcus aureus*
- Rabies

Human bites[2]

- Cellulitis
- Hepatitis B or Hepatitis C
- Herpes Simplex Virus
- Tetanus
- Human Immunodeficiency Virus (low risk)
- Other infections

MANAGEMENT/TREATMENT:

1. Stop bleeding by applying firm pressure with clean, dry gauze or cloth.
2. Wash and irrigate with copious amounts of soap and water.
3. Apply loose dressing.
4. Topical antibiotics may be applied if prescribed.
5. Refer bites with broken skin to a healthcare provider.
6. Check immunization records for last tetanus, and Hepatitis vaccines (if appropriate), and record.

FOLLOW-UP:[3, 4]

Human bites: Notify parents of both the student that was bitten and the student that inflicted the bite. School policy may also require notification to administration of any bite incident.

Prevention of Infection

- Dog bites are likely to be open, jagged lacerations that can be thoroughly irrigated, have a low infection rate, and usually require no prophylactic antibiotics.
- Cat bites are usually deep puncture wounds and have a high infection rate. They often require prophylactic antibiotics.

BITES: Animal and Human *(continued from previous page)*

FOLLOW-UP *(continued)*

- **Human bites *that break the skin* have the greatest potential for infection. Also, consider transmission of Hepatitis B to both parties** (consult current AAP Redbook for guidance or follow school district policy).[5]

<u>**Prevention of Tetanus**[6]</u>

- If no previous active immunization with tetanus toxoid, encourage tetanus immune globulin and begin series of tetanus toxoid.
- If active immunization is 10 years ago or longer: Booster of tetanus toxoid (adult Td).
- If active immunization within the past five years:
    - Mild bite—no booster.
    - Severe bite—booster adult Td.
- Severe, neglected, old (over 24 hours) or dirty bites—Adult Td, unless person has had one in the previous 12 months.

NOTES:[7, 8, 9]

- Follow procedure for notifying animal control agency of animal bites.
- When there is a bite on a hand, there is an increased risk of infection due to the structure, thin skin and circulation of the hand.
- While it is theoretically possible for any mammal to develop rabies, rodents have not been implicated in transmitting the disease; therefore, a child bitten by a squirrel, rat, mouse, gerbil, hamster or rabbit is not considered to be in danger, but a healthcare provider should be consulted.
- Common carriers of rabies are dogs, cats, foxes, skunks and raccoons. Bats carry rabies but only bite if handled. Children who touch a dead or sick bat are at small risk, but a healthcare provider and public health department should be notified (airborne infection from bat guano is only a theoretical possibility).
- Unprovoked bites (especially from a dog) raise greater suspicion than if animal is provoked or teased. The biting animal must be confined and observed 10 days—notify the health department or police. If the animal cannot be apprehended, then a series of rabies vaccine injections may need to be given.[10]
- Isolate all students from area where bite occurred (if on school property) until animal control/police arrive.
- Bites on fingers and face are more dangerous.

BITES: Animal and Human *(continued from previous page)*

REFERENCES

[1] Garth, A. P., Harris, N. S., & Spanierman, C.S. (2018). *Animal bites in emergency medicine*. http://emedicine.medscape.com/article/768875-overview

[2] Barrett, J., & Revis, D.R. (201). *Human bites*. http://emedicine.medscape.com/article/768978-overview

[3] Ibid.

[4] Ball, J., Binder, R., & Cowen, K. (Eds.). (2017). Alterations in skin integrity. *Principles of pediatric nursing: caring for children* (7th ed., pp.936-937). Pearson Education, Inc.

[5] American Academy of Pediatrics, Committee on Infectious Diseases. (2018). Infections spread by blood and body fluids. In D.W. Kimberlin, M.T. Brady, M.T., M.A. Jackson, & S.S. Long (Eds.), *Red Book, (2018-2021): Report of the Committee on Infectious Diseases* (31st ed., pp. 143-146). American Academy of Pediatrics.

[6] Mayo Clinic. (2016). *Rabies, overview*. https://www.mayoclinic.org/diseases-conditions/rabies/symptoms-causes/syc-20351821

[7] American Academy of Pediatrics. (2016). Bites (human and animal). In S.S. Aronson & T.R. Shope (Eds.), *Managing infectious diseases in child care and schools, a quick reference guide* (5th ed., pp. 65-66). American Academy of Pediatrics.

[8] Garth, A. P., Harris, N. S., & Spanierman, C.S. (2018). *Animal bites in emergency medicine*. http://emedicine.medscape.com/article/768875-overview

[9] Mayo Clinic. (2016). *Rabies, overview*. https://www.mayoclinic.org/diseases- conditions/rabies/symptoms-causes/syc-20351821

[10] Centers for Disease Control and Prevention. (2019). *What is rabies?* https://www.cdc.gov/rabies/about.html

OTHER REFERENCES CONSULTED

Medline Plus, U.S. National Library of Medicine. (2016). *Rabies*. https://medlineplus.gov/rabies.html#cat11

Merch Manual, Professional Version. (2018). *Human and mammal bites*. https://www.merckmanuals.com/professional/injuries-poisoning/bites-and-stings/human-and-mammal-bites?query=animal%20bites

BLISTERS

DEFINITION/ETIOLOGY:

A blister is a round or oval bubble of fluid under the skin,[1] that may or may not be painful or itchy depending on the cause. The cause is varied:

- Irritation (friction/shoes; repetitive activity/rowing, shoveling)
- Burns from intense heat (sunburn, hot liquids or appliances, etc.)
- Exposure to cold (frostbite)
- Skin diseases — Numerous skin diseases can cause blisters (contact dermatitis such as poison ivy, oak and sumac). There also are inherited forms of blistering skin conditions, such as epidermolysis bullosa (in which pressure or trauma commonly leads to blisters) and porphyria cutanea tarda (in which sun exposure provokes blisters).[2]
- Medications — Many medications, such as nalidixic acid (NegGram®) and furosemide (Lasix®), can cause mild, blistering skin reactions. Others, such as the doxycycline (Vibramycin®), can increase the risk of blistering sunburn by increasing the skin's sensitivity to sunlight. In rare and extreme cases, medications can trigger a life-threatening, blistering disorders called erythema multiforme or toxic epidermal necrolysis, also known as TEN, which typically involves 30% or more of the body's surface and causes severe skin damage.[3]
- Infection (impetigo, eczema, ringworm, herpes, varicella [chicken pox])

SIGNS AND SYMPTOMS:

- Blisters from irritation and burns are red and often painful, particularly if the blister is on a weight bearing part of the body (foot) or in an area that is frequently used (hand).
- Contact dermatitis and allergic skin responses have redness and are itchy.
- Blisters or vesicles (a small fluid-filled irritation up to five mm wide) may be present with some infections.[4]
- Depending on the source of the infection, these vesicles can be red, itchy, and/or painful. A vesicle larger than five mm wide is referred to as a bulla.[5]

MANAGEMENT/TREATMENT:

- Treatment is largely symptomatic.
- Leave skin covering the blister intact. If the blister is broken, skin integrity is compromised leaving an entry for bacteria. Unbroken skin over a blister may provide a natural barrier to bacteria and decreases the risk of infection.[6]
- Cover the broken blister with a sterile dressing and attempt to avoid activity that requires further friction or pressure on the affected area.
- If a blister breaks, wash the area with soap and water, then apply a sterile dressing.[7]
- Monitor for signs of infection.

BLISTERS *(continued from previous page)*

POTENTIAL COMPLICATIONS:

- Infection after blister skins over or blister ruptures.
- Signs of infection include increasing redness, edema, the area is warm to touch, area becomes increasingly more painful, or purulent drainage is present.

FOLLOW UP:

Monitor for signs of infection and refer to healthcare provider if redness increases, edema present, area warm to touch, area becomes increasingly more painful, or purulent drainage is present.

NOTES:

Prevention

- Proper fitting shoes, socks, clothing, and equipment for walking, running and participation in athletic/sports activities.
- If an area of redness appears, stop the activity.
- Observe sun-safety cautions and use sunscreen.[8]
- Dress appropriately for winter weather and know the signs of frostbite.
- Be able to identify poison ivy, oak, and sumac.
- To prevent blisters caused by infections, wash hands often and never touch skin sores, cuts or any open or broken areas of skin on other people.[9]

REFERENCES

[1] Harvard Health Publishing. (2019). *Blisters (overview).* https://www.health.harvard.edu/a_to_z/blisters-overview-a-to-z

[2] Ibid.

[3] Ibid.

[4] Medline Plus, US National Library of Medicine. (2019). *Vesicles.* https://medlineplus.gov/ency/article/003939.htm

[5] Ibid.

[6] Mayo Clinic. (2018). *Blisters: First aid.* https://www.mayoclinic.org/first-aid/first-aid-blisters/basics/art-20056691

[7] Harvard Health Publishing. (2019). *Blisters (overview).* https://www.health.harvard.edu/a_to_z/blisters-overview-a-to-z

[8] The Merck Manual. (2019). *Sunburn.* https://www.merckmanuals.com/professional/dermatologic-disorders/reactions-to-sunlight/sunburn

[9] Mayo Clinic. (2018). *Blisters: First aid.* https://www.mayoclinic.org/first-aid/first-aid-blisters/basics/art-20056691

OTHER REFERENCES CONSULTED

American Academy of Dermatology. (2018). How to prevent and treat blisters. https://www.aad.org/public/skin-hair-nails/injured-skin/blisters

BURNS

DEFINITION/ETIOLOGY:

Lesions caused by extreme heat or other cauterizing agents. Burns are classified by depth of injury, percentage of body surface area (BSA) involved, location of the burn, and association with other injuries.[1]

First-degree or superficial burns: Only involves the top layer of skin (epidermis).

Second degree or partial-thickness burns: Involves the epidermis and extends into the dermis.

Third degree or full-thickness burns: Full thickness of skin is destroyed and involves the epidermis, dermis, and fat layer. Usually destroys the sweat glands, hair follicles, and nerve endings as well.

Fourth degree burns: Full thickness through all layers of skin into the muscle and bone.

Minor burns: Less than 10% of the body surface area (BSA) for partial thickness burns or less than 2% for full thickness burns. Partial or full thickness burns of the hands, feet, face, eyes, ears and perineum are considered major.[2] The Rule of Nine is a tool that can be used and adapted for children to calculate the percentage of body surface area.[3]

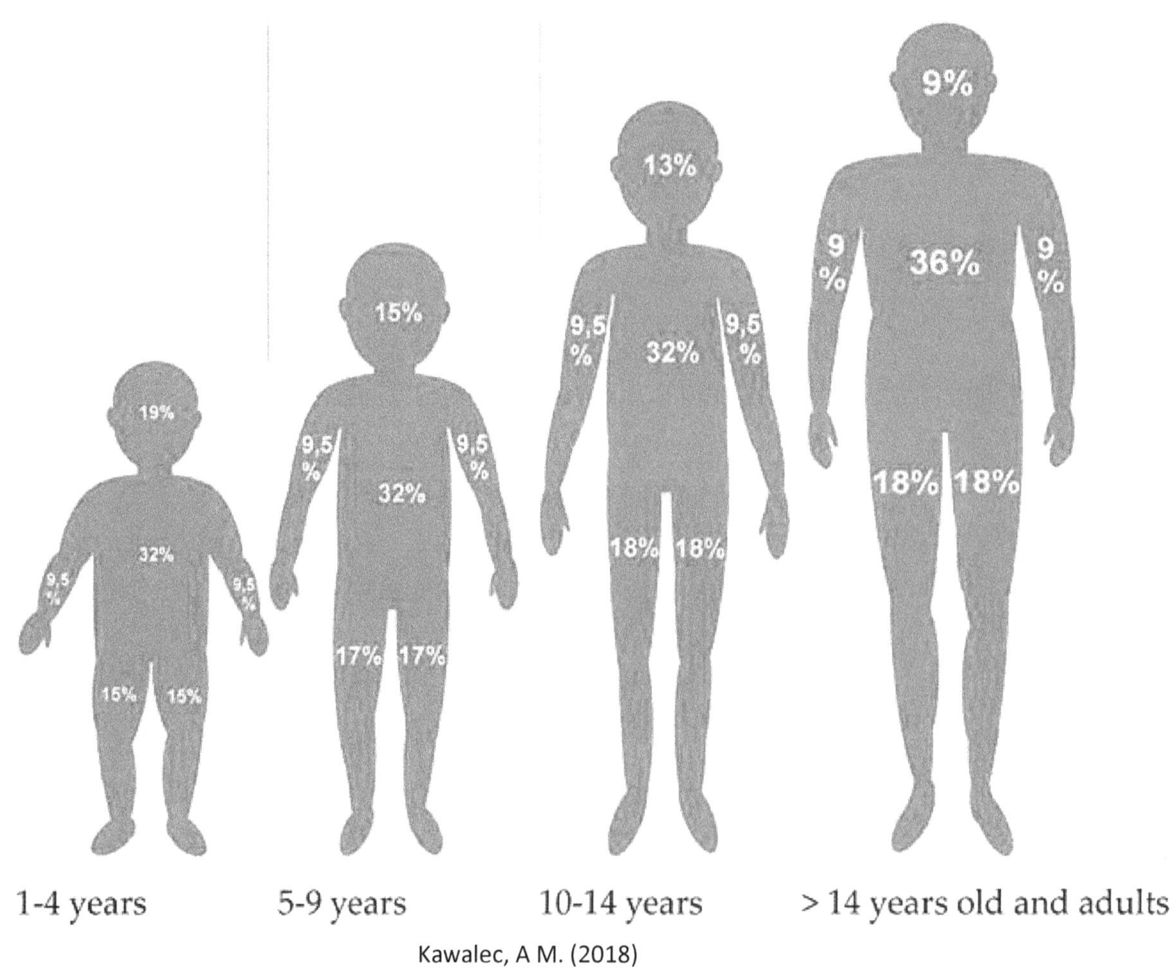

Kawalec, A M. (2018)

BURNS *(continued from previous page)*

SIGNS AND SYMPTOMS:

- **Superficial burns**
  - Begins with pain and redness as in minimal sunburn without blisters.
  - Later, slight to no peeling of skin.
- **Partial-thickness burns**
  - Begins with pain, redness, and blisters as in moderate to severe sunburn.
  - Later, skin peels in large pieces, scarring only if secondary infection ensues.
- **Full thickness burns**
  - Begins with little or no pain (nerves are gone), with red, black, pale, yellow or white discoloration.
  - Some unbroken blisters may be present.
  - Third degree burns always scar and often need a skin graft.[4]

MANAGEMENT/TREATMENT:

General

1. For superficial and partial-thickness burns: Rapidly immerse burn in cool water. This not only helps stop the pain, but it also stops destruction of tissue.
2. Wash gently but thoroughly with antiseptic soap, pat dry with sterile pad.
3. Avoid Vaseline®, butter, antibiotic or other greasy ointments.
4. Avoid tight, air-excluding bandages.
5. Check date of latest tetanus booster and receive booster if needed.
6. Complete injury report if burn occurred in school/school program.

Superficial burns

1. Cool compress or submerge in cool water (not ice).
2. Wash gently with soap and dry.
3. No further treatment necessary.

Partial-thickness burns

1. Cool compress.
2. Wash gently with antiseptic soap and dry.
3. DO NOT break blisters.
4. Apply non-sticking dressing that does not exclude air.
5. Notify parent.
6. Monitor daily for infection.

Full-thickness burns

1. Cover with clean or sterile dressing or sheet.
2. Evacuate to emergency room or healthcare provider's office.

BURNS *(continued from previous page)*

MANAGEMENT/TREATMENT *(continued)*

<u>Chemical burn</u>

1. Flush with copious amounts of cool water for 15 minutes.
2. **Refer in all cases for further medical treatment.**

<u>Electrical burns</u>

Refer in all cases for further medical treatment.

FOLLOW-UP:

- Change dressing daily (if this is not done at home) until danger of infection has passed.
- Observe for signs of secondary infection such as drainage, change in color of the wound, pain and or swelling.
- Teach student and parent/guardian to clean the affected area gently twice a day with soap and water and keep the area clean.
- Teach student and parent/guardian signs and symptoms of infection and the need to see the healthcare provider if they occur.
- Refer to healthcare provider for any developing signs of infection or if no improvement after FIRST day of treatment.
- Observe for scarring, especially on flexor areas of arms, legs, and neck and refer to healthcare provider as indicated.
- Children with facial scarring need emotional support on return to school. Prepare classmates/peers.

POTENTIAL COMPLICATIONS:

- Minor burns are typically superficial and do not cause complications.
- Moderate to severe burns can cause serious complications due to tissue damage and extensive fluid loss. Complications include dehydration, infection, shock, muscle and tissue damage, chemical imbalances, etc.

NOTES:

- Facial burns, hands and feet burns, genitalia burns: refer to healthcare provider in all cases.
- Send date of last tetanus booster with all healthcare provider referrals.
- Be alert to possible child abuse, self-tattoo, or deliberate injury.
- Record shape/size of burns as well as document history of event.
- Do not use ice on burns as it can cause further damage.
- Children with burns greater than 10% of body surface area should be admitted to the hospital.[5] It would be helpful to include a tool & diagram such as the Rule of 9's (different for adults and children) used to calculate percentage of body surface area.

Teach children safety rules such as **stop, drop, and roll** if their clothing catches on fire so they can help extinguish the flame and prevent getting burned more extensively.

BURNS *(continued from previous page)*

NOTES *(continued)*

Burns are a common cause of accidental death in children. It also may be associated with child abuse. Areas of prevention include:

- Hot liquids should be placed away from counter and stove edges with the handles facing backwards.
- Water heater thermostats should be kept less than 120 degrees F (49 degrees C).
- Irons and electrical cords should be kept out of reach of children.
- Barriers should be used around fireplaces.[6]

REFERENCES

[1] Degolier, S. & Garzon, D. (2017). Common injuries. In C. E. Burns, A.M. Dunn, M. H. Brady, N.B. Starr. C.G. Blosser, & D.L. Farzon (Eds.). *Pediatric primary care* (6th ed., pp. 1131-1135). Elsevier.

[2] Ibid.

[3] Kawalec, A. M. (2018). Problem of burns in children: Opportunities for health improvement. *Essentials of Accident and Emergency Medicine.* https://www.intechopen.com/books/essentials-of-accident-and-emergency-medicine/problem-of-burns-in-children-opportunities-for-health-improvement

[4] Ibid.

[4] Carney, K. P., & Roswell, K. (2018). Emergencies and injuries. In W. Hay, M. Levin, R. Deterding, & M. Abzug (Eds.), *Current diagnosis and treatment pediatrics* (24th ed., pp.309-331). McGraw Hill Education, Inc.

[6] Ibid.

OTHER REFERENCES CONSULTED

Mayo Clinic. (2018). *Burns: First aid.* https://www.mayoclinic.org/diseases-conditions/burns/symptoms-causes/syc-20370539

Cosby, M. F., Lyons, E., & Prestidge, L. (2019). Students with acute illness and injury. In J. Selekman, R. Adair Shannon, & C. F. Yonkaitis (Eds.), *School nursing: A comprehensive text* (3rd ed., pp. 449-453). F.A. Davis.

CARDIAC CONDITIONS, LIFE THREATENING

DEFINITION/ETIOLOGY:
Sudden death in children and adolescents is rare. About 25% of cases occur during sports. Most children/adolescents with sudden cardiac death (SCD) have underlying heart disease, with hypertrophic cardiomyopathy and long QT syndrome (LQTS) being among the most common life-threatening cardiac conditions. Other conditions that may contribute to sudden cardiac death include congenital aortic stenosis, myocarditis, abnormal development of cardiac arterial vessels, and aortic dissection.[1]

HYPERTROPHIC CARDIOMYOPATHY (HCM)

HCM is the most common cause of SCD in the United States in people under 30 years of age. HCM often presents itself in mid to late adolescence, and usually presents without warning clinical signs or symptoms. Diagnosis is confirmed echocardiography; however, an electrocardiogram may show left ventricular hypertrophy or T-wave abnormalities.[2]

HCM is an autosomal dominant congenital disorder typically characterized by asymmetric septal hypertrophy and marked disarray of ventricular muscle fibers, which contribute to the risk of arrhythmias even in patients with minimal hypertrophy and no evident left ventricular outflow tract obstruction.[3]

Risk factors:
- septal thickness ≥30 mm
- family history of sudden cardiac death

SIGNS AND SYMPTOMS:
- non-sustained ventricular tachycardia [VT] (i.e., VT that lasts <30 seconds)
- syncope
- hypotensive response to exercise

MANAGEMENT/TREATMENT:[4]
Call Emergency Medical Services (EMS) or your local emergency number if the student experience any of the following symptoms for more than a few minutes:
- Rapid or irregular heartbeat
- Difficulty breathing
- Chest pain

CARDIAC CONDITIONS, LIFE THREATENING *(continued from previous page)*

LONG QT INTERVAL (LQTS)[5]

Long QT syndrome (LQTS) is a rare inherited cardiac disorder that occurs in about one in 2500–3500 individuals. LQTS results from a delay in repolarization of the heart muscle following a ventricular contraction leading to a ventricular arrhythmia (ventricular tachycardia and/or fibrillation). Diagnosis is difficult because only in a percentage of cases a prolonged QT interval is noted on during an electrocardiogram (ECG/EKG). These episodes may lead to palpitations, fainting, and sudden death due to ventricular fibrillation. For symptomatic patients, the presenting symptom is usually syncope, which is due to the type of ventricular tachycardia. The syncope may occur with specific triggers, such as stress, swimming, and loud auditory stimuli, or it may occur when the child is relatively bradycardic, as during rest or sleep.

Risk factors:

- female predominance
- family history of congenital long QT syndrome
- pre-existing cardiovascular disease
- electrolyte imbalance
- concurrent administration of interacting drugs
- anorexia nervosa

SIGNS AND SYMPTOMS:

Not all people with long QT syndrome experience signs and symptoms. Yet some may experience the following signs and symptoms:

- fainting
- dizziness
- seizures
- sudden death

MANAGEMENT/TREATMENT:

Diagnosing LQTS is not an easy diagnosis to make because the majority of people with LQTS have no signs or symptoms. Patients diagnosed with LQTS are advised to avoid drugs that would further prolong the QT interval. Some of the more common medication to avoid include:[6]

- certain antibiotics, i.e. macrolides, fluoroquinolones, trimethoprim-sulfa
- some azole antifungals
- antiemetic's and promotility agents such as ondansetron, phenergen, and cisapride
- cough/cold medications, i.e. pseudoephedrine
- stimulant medications, i.e. methylphenidate
- pain and sedatives such as chloral hydrate, oxycodone, and methadone
- anti-depressants including tricyclic antidepressants and some selective serotonin reuptake inhibitors including citalopram and fluoxetine.
- other groups include antiarrhythmic drugs, antineoplastic drugs, diuretics (because of electrolyte abnormalities), other psychotropic medications and even some herbs.

CARDIAC CONDITIONS, LIFE THREATENING *(continued from previous page)*

MANAGEMENT/TREATMENT *(continued)*

Treatment is usually the administration of arrhythmia medications (such as beta blockers) which prevents severe symptoms and sudden death in most cases. In severe cases, an implantable cardioverter-defibrillator (ICD) may be indicated.

All signs and symptoms need to be taken seriously. Children/adolescents need to be referred to the healthcare provider for follow up and possible cardiologist referral. The school nurse should request a healthcare provider note to ensure that student has been appropriately followed by a healthcare provider along with recommendations/restrictions for school activities.

IMPLICATIONS FOR SCHOOL NURSES:

- It is critical that the school nurse has clear orders from the student's healthcare provider and guidance from their parent or guardian regarding the plan of care for the student with any life-threatening cardiac conditions.[7]
- An Individualized Healthcare Plan (IHP) should be created and include medications, signs and symptoms to watch for, physical activity or any other restrictions, and any plans that need to be implemented in the event of an emergency.
- All sports activities need to be stopped until the student has been cleared to participate by their healthcare provider.
- Emergency preparedness is essential with trained staff in cardiopulmonary resuscitation and automatic external defibrillators.
- School physicals, especially sports physical examination polices, need to be adhered to prior to participation.

POTENTIAL COMPLICATIONS:

- Sudden Death

REFERENCES

[1] McKelvie, R.S. (2019). *Sudden cardiac death in athletes. Merck Manual Professional Version.* https://www.merckmanuals.com/professional/cardiovascular-disorders/sports-and-the-heart/sudden-cardiac-death-in-athletes?query=Sudden%20cardiac%20death%20in%20children%20and%20adolescents

[2] Martchenke, J., & Rummell, M. (2017). Cardiovascular disorders. In C. Burns, A. Dunn, M. Brady, N. Starr, C. Blosser, & D. Garzon Maaks (Eds.), *Pediatric primary care: a clinical approach* (6th ed., pp. 756-794). Elsevier.

[3] Ibid.

[4] O'Brian, P., & Evangelista, J. (2019). Heart and vascular assessment. In K.G. Duderstadt (Ed.), *Pediatric physical exam* (3rd. ed., pp. 110-132). Elsevier.

[5] Ibid.

[6] Martchenke, J., & Rummell, M. (2017). Cardiovascular disorders. In C. Burns, A. Dunn, M. Brady, N. Starr, C. Blosser, & D. Garzon Maaks (Eds.), *Pediatric primary care: a clinical approach* (6th ed., pp. 756-794). Elsevier.

[7] Cosby, M., Lyons, E., & Prestige, L. (2019). Students with acute illness and injury. In J. Selekman, R.A. Shannon, & C. F. Younkaitis (Eds.), *School Nursing: A comprehensive text* (3rd ed., pp. 417-456). F.A. Davis.

CELIAC DISEASE

DEFINITION/ETIOLOGY:

Celiac disease is an autoimmune response to eating gluten. Gluten is a protein found in wheat, barley, rye and other grains. When a person with celiac disease eats gluten the body's immune system reacts by causing inflammation of the intestinal villa in the small colon. The small villa absorbs nutrients from food in the gastrointestinal (GI) system. Damage to the villa prevents absorption of necessary nutrients leading to malnutrition.

Celiac disease is more common in Caucasian, females. It is estimated to affect one in 100 people worldwide. Celiac disease also has genetic tendencies with about 50% of individuals with celiac disease reporting that they have a family member who also has the disorder.[1]

SIGNS AND SYMPTOMS:

Signs and symptoms vary from person to person. Some individuals with Celiac disease are asymptomatic – leading to undiagnosed cases of Celiac disease. Other individuals with Celiac disease may present with gastrointestinal symptoms including:[2]

- chronic diarrhea (30% persons with celiac disease);
- bloating;
- flatulence;
- constipation (20% persons with celiac disease);
- abdominal pain and distention;
- nutritional deficiency;
- nausea, vomiting;
- foul-smelling (pale) stool;
- poor appetite, lack of energy, muscle wasting; and
- weight loss (after eating gluten-containing products).

It is important to note that not everyone with Celiac disease experience GI symptoms. Other symptoms may include:

- irritability;
- iron deficiency anemia;
- osteopenia/osteoporosis; and
- itching/blistering dermatitis (called dermatitis herpetiformis – rash usually appears elbows, knees, buttocks and back).

Symptoms also vary depending on age. School age children may experience growth and development delays secondary to poor nutritional absorption, delayed puberty, and damage to dental enamel of secondary teeth.

CELIAC DISEASE *(continued from previous page)*

MANAGEMENT/TREATMENT:
There is no cure for Celiac disease. It is a lifelong disorder. Management includes strict avoidance to gluten (wheat, barley, rye and other grains). Typically, once gluten is removed from the diet, symptoms start to improve within a few days. It can take several months to years for complete healing of the intestinal villa to occur. The healthcare provider may recommend daily vitamin supplements due to poor nutrient absorption (Vitamin B12, folic acid, calcium, and iron).[3]

If no improvement in symptoms after starting gluten-free diet, look for hidden sources of gluten.

- Gluten can be found in products such as lip balm, cosmetics, hair and oral hygiene products.
- Check with pharmacist to see if gluten is in prescribed prescription and/or over the counter medications, vitamins and nutritional supplements that student may be taking to manage condition.

Foods made from corn and rice products, soy and potato flour, and fresh fruits are usually tolerated well.[4]

FOLLOW-UP:

- Educate students/parent/staff on necessity of strict gluten avoidance, including reading food labels for "hidden" gluten such as flour as a filler or thickener.
- Consult with school's Registered Dietician to ensure necessary dietary accommodations are made in school meals.
- Only use non-food items for manipulatives in classroom projects.
- Avoid using modeling dough (Play-Doh®) for art or classroom projects.
- To facilitate the avoidance of accidental exposure, include information to teachers and staff on student's medical condition in accordance with the school district's policies and procedures on sharing confidential information.
- Develop an Individualized Healthcare Plan (IHP) or Section 504 Plan, as appropriate, to assure plans are in place to accommodate student's needs.

POTENTIAL COMPLICATIONS:

- Malnutrition
- Osteoporosis
- Liver disease
- Neurological conditions
- Infertility
- Lactose intolerance
- Intestinal cancers (intestinal lymphoma and bowel cancer)

NOTES:
Monitor for other autoimmune disorders such as autoimmune thyroid disease, Type 1 diabetes, Addison's disease, Sjogren's syndrome, multiple sclerosis and rheumatoid arthritis.

CELIAC DISEASE *(continued from previous page)*

REFERENCES

[1] Celiac Disease Foundation. (2015). *Celiac disease foundation.* Retrieved from https://celiac.org/celiac-disease/what-is-celiac-disease/

[2] Mayo Clinic. (2013). *Celiac disease.* Retrieved from http://www.mayoclinic.org/diseases-conditions/celiac-disease/basics/definition/con-20030410

[3] Ball, J., Binder, R., Cowen, K. & Shaw, M. (Eds.). (2017). Infant, child, and adolescent nutrition. *Principles of pediatric nursing: Caring for children* (7th ed., pp. 297-298). Pearson Education, Inc.

[4] John, T. (2019). Students with other chronic conditions. In J. Selekman, R. Shannon, & C. Yonkaitis (Eds.), *School nursing: A comprehensive text* (3rd ed., pp. 710- 712). F.A. Davis.

OTHER REFERENCES CONSULTED

Merck Manual. (2018). *Celiac disease*. Retrieved from http://www.merckmanuals.com/professional/SearchResults?query=celiac+disease

National Institute of Diabetes and Digestive and Kidney Diseases. (2016). *Celiac disease.* Retrieved from https://www.niddk.nih.gov/health-information/digestive-diseases/celiac-disease/definition-facts

CHEST PAIN

DEFINITION/ETIOLOGY:
Chest pain is a common complaint in the health office and accounts for six in 1000 visits to urban emergency departments and urgent care clinics.[1] Pediatric chest pain can be classified as cardiac or non-cardiac. Non-cardiac is the most prevalent cause of chest pain in school-aged children and adolescents. Chest pain can originate from any structure in the chest - lungs, ribs, chest wall, diaphragm, joints between sternum and ribs, and heart. It can be caused from injury, infection, respiratory conditions, referred pain from the abdomen, or irritation. The pain may also be the result of stress or anxiety.

Although chest pain is common in children and adolescents, it is very rare that this pain is related in any way to their heart (unless child is known to have heart defect or disease). Often the source of the pain cannot be determined.[2] While the pain may be a symptom of serious disease, most chest pain is benign or self-limiting. Several factors influence the pain perceived by the child, including maturation of the nervous system, the child's developmental stage, and previous pain experiences.[3]

SIGNS AND SYMPTOMS:
Signs and symptoms will vary widely with cause and the person's age and personality. For many people, the heart is the most identifiable organ in the chest, so they describe discomfort by saying their "heart hurts". It is important to remember this may be a figure of speech and not to overreact. The determination of the cause of pain is a diagnostic decision and the term "heart pain" should be assessed similarly to other types of pain, focusing on associated signs and symptoms and severity and conveying that information to a healthcare provider. Children complaining of chest pain should be assessed for associated symptoms, such as syncope, palpitations, nausea/vomiting, shortness of breath, cough, or wheezing.[4]

MANAGEMENT/TREATMENT:

1. Conduct an assessment[5]
    - It is important to take a careful history; make close observation as person describes symptoms. Determine if history of recent injury, presence of underlying health condition (asthma, heart defect or cardiovascular history, recent illness, sickle cell disease, history of genetic disorder).
    - Determine onset of symptoms (acute, gradual, growing worse).
    - Length of time with symptoms?
    - Has this pain occurred before?
    - Any association with activity (including at rest, only after activity, on inspiration, after coughing, etc.)?
    - What makes it better?
    - What makes it worse?
    - Determine type of pain - constant, intermittent, sharp, dull, radiating, etc.
    - Are there associated respiratory symptoms?
    - Assess skin condition (indicative of oxygen exchange).
    - Assess psychological demeanor (calm, anxious, dramatic), history of increased stress.
    - History of huffing, smoking, vaping, or other drug use.
    - Perform a general physical assessment including vital signs and note any irregularities.

CHEST PAIN *(continued from previous page)*

MANAGEMENT/TREATMENT *(continued)*

2. The person who has pain of acute onset that:
    a. interferes with breathing and/or sleep,
    b. is precipitated by exercise, or
    c. is associated with alteration of vital signs and dizziness, palpitations, syncope, or fever,

   should be evaluated by their healthcare provider. Symptomatic individuals should not be allowed to drive alone.

3. Emergency Medical Services (EMS) should be contacted if an individual is more seriously compromised, particularly with symptoms of cyanosis, difficulty breathing, and decreased level of consciousness. Activate EMS if open chest wound or signs and symptoms of pneumothorax (rapid/shallow respiration, painful respiration, cyanosis, and hypotension). (*Refer to SPONTANEOUS PNEUMOTHORAX*).

COMMON ILLNESSES THAT CAUSE CHEST PAIN [6]

Costochondritis
A condition where there is inflammation in the cartilage between the sternum and ribs. It may be caused by a viral illness or by frequent coughing. The pain will occur with inhalation. Most people will have tenderness over the costochondral joint (depression on side of sternum where rib joins sternum). May be treated with OTC anti-inflammatories.

Musculoskeletal Injury/Pain
The most common cause of pediatric chest pain. Children frequently strain chest wall muscles while wrestling, carrying heavy books, or exercising. Direct trauma to the chest may result in a mild contusion of the chest wall or, with more significant force, a rib fracture, hemothorax, or pneumothorax. If pain can be reproduced through direct palpation of the chest wall, it is almost always musculoskeletal in nature. In most cases, there is a straightforward history of trauma and the diagnosis is clear.

Respiratory Conditions
Children who have severe, persistent cough, asthma, bronchitis, pleurisy or pneumonia may complain of chest pain due to overuse of chest wall muscles. Some children may complain of chest pain with exercise due to exercise-induced asthma. Pulmonary embolism should be considered in adolescent girls taking oral contraceptives.

Psychogenic Disturbances
Stress or anxiety can precipitate chest pain in both boys and girls. Often the stress that results in somatic complaints is not readily apparent and not all these children present with hyperventilation or an anxious appearance. However, if the child has had a recent major stressful event, such as separation from friends, divorce in the family, or school failure that correlates temporally with the onset of the chest pain, it is reasonable to conclude that the symptoms are related to the event.

CHEST PAIN *(continued from previous page)*

COMMON ILLNESSES THAT CAUSE CHEST PAIN *(continued)*

Gastrointestinal Disorders
Conditions such as reflux esophagitis often cause chest pain in young children and adolescents. The pain is described classically as burning, substernal in location, and worsened by reclining or eating spicy foods. Be aware that students with eating disorders such as purging may have pain secondary to esophageal trauma related to the purging. The timing of the pain in relation to eating may suggest a gastrointestinal cause.

Miscellaneous Causes
Some young children will complain of chest pain following ingestion of a coin or other foreign body that lodges in the esophagus. Generally, the child or parent/guardian gives a clear history of recent foreign body ingestion.

Some instances of chest pain are related to an underlying disease. A careful history and physical exam will often sort these out and assist in determining level of intervention needed. For instance, sickle cell disease may lead to vaso-occlusive crises or acute chest syndrome. Marfan syndrome may result in chest pain and fatal dissection of an abdominal aortic aneurysm. Collagen vascular disorders may lead to pleural effusions. Shingles may result in severe chest pain that precedes or occurs simultaneously with the classic rash.

REFERENCES

[1] Schreiner T.L., Yang, M. L., Martin, J.A. Messer, R., Demarest, S., & Walleigh, D. (2018). Cardiovascular diseases. In W.W. Hay, M. J. Levin, R.R. Deterding, R.R., & Abzug, M.J. (Eds.*), Current diagnosis and treatment: Pediatrics* (24nd ed., pp.610-611). McGraw Hill Education.

[2] American Heart Association. (2019). *Commonly asked questions about children and heart disease*. http://www.heart.org/HEARTORG/Conditions/More/CardiovascularConditionsofChildhood/Commonly-Asked-Questions-About-Children-and-Heart-Disease_UCM_311917_Article.jsp

[3] Ball, J., Binder, R., & Cowen, K. (Eds.). (2017). Pain assessment and management in children. *Principles of pediatric nursing: caring for children* (7th ed., pp. 310-332). Pearson Education, Inc.

[4] Schreiner T.L., Yang, M. L., Martin, J.A. Messer, R., Demarest, S., & Walleigh, D. (2018). Cardiovascular diseases. In W.W. Hay, M. J. Levin, R.R. Deterding, R.R., & Abzug, M.J. (Eds.*), Current diagnosis and treatment: Pediatrics* (24nd ed., pp.610-611). McGraw Hill Education.

[5] Jakubowski, T. & Perron, T. (2019). Students with Common Health Complaints. In J. Selekman, R. Shannon, & C. Yonkaitis (Eds.), *School nursing: A comprehensive text* (3rd ed., pp. 350-351). F.A. Davis.

[6] Ibid.

CHILDHOOD CANCER

Childhood cancer is the second leading cause of death in children.[1] On a positive note, it is still a rare disease, and has a survival rate of 80% (defined as surviving five [5] years after diagnosis).[2] Because children are growing, childhood cancer is unlike cancer seen in adults. Adult cancers tend to be slow in growth, but childhood cancers grow quickly, and a child may become ill in a short period of time. Childhood cancers predominate in the areas of the body that exhibit rapid growth such as the blood, lymphatic system, central nervous system, and bones.[3]

DEFINITION/ETIOLOGY:

Cancer results when cells divide without controls or so quickly that they divide before they mature. The rapid growth results in immature, abnormal cells that invade surrounding tissue and quickly metastasize to other areas. The etiology of childhood cancer varies from adult cancers and is often unknown, although some genetic and environmental exposures may place children at risk.[4]

Numerous types of cancers are seen in children. Following is a brief overview of the most common cancers seen in children.[5]

Leukemia	Leukemia is the most commonly diagnosed childhood cancer. Leukemia is characterized by an abnormal amount of white blood cells (WBC) in the body. It is considered a cancer of the bone marrow and blood. As the WBC's proliferate, the cells they produce are immature. The increasing production of WBC's affects normal production of red blood cells and platelets. Abnormal WBC's are called blast cells. The common types of leukemia in children are acute lymphoblastic leukemia (ALL) and acute myeloid leukemia (AML). Typical symptoms include lethargy, bruising and other abnormal bleeding, bone and joint pain, weakness and weight loss. (*Refer to Leukemia for further information, if needed*).
Brain tumor	Second most common cancer in children. The overall prognosis is dependent on the size, type, and location of the tumor. Neurological symptoms such as headache, blurred vision, dizziness, change in gait or fine motor skills, nausea, and vomiting are often seen. School staff may note a change in school performance and/or concentration. Typically, occurring tumors include astrocytoma, glioma, medulloblastoma, and ependymoma.
Neuroblastoma	Tumors that form along the sympathetic nervous system chain. They are often found above the kidneys in the adrenal glands but can start anywhere.
Bone tumors	Tend to occur in older children and in the teenage years. **Osteosarcoma-** usually affects the large bones of the arms and legs. **Ewing's sarcoma-** can occur anywhere but most likely found in spine, ribs or pelvis.
Lymphoma	These malignant diseases affect the lymph system and tissues. The two main types of lymphoma are Hodgkin lymphoma (also known as Hodgkin disease) and Non-Hodgkin lymphoma.
Retinoblastoma	Originates in the retina of the eye. Dependent on the size of the tumor, it may be necessary to remove the entire eye. This tumor is often discovered during well child exams and is rarely seen in children over the age of six.
Wilm's tumor	Also known as nephroblastoma. Wilm's tumor is the most common kidney cancer. Symptoms include swelling or lump in the abdomen. Other symptoms such as poor appetite, fever, pain, or nausea may be present. **Nursing alert: DO NOT** palpate the abdomen if this tumor is suspected.

CHILDHOOD CANCER *(continued from previous page)*

SIGNS AND SYMPTOMS (General):[6]

Note: Keep in mind that symptoms may have a relatively fast onset, secondary to the rapidly growing cells in children

- Pain in one area of the body
- Loss of appetite
- Weight loss
- Anemia, loss of energy, paleness
- Increased susceptibility to infection
- Easy bruising
- Prolonged bleeding
- Sudden vision changes
- An unusual lump or swelling
- Neurological disturbances: change in behavior, change in gait, headache, dizziness, blurred or double vision
- Symptoms are related to the location of the cancer
- Unexplained fever or illness
- Limping
- Sudden eye or vision changes

MANAGEMENT/TREATMENT: [7]

- Treatment is based on the type of cancer and may include surgery, radiation, targeted drug therapy, immunotherapy and/or chemotherapy.
- In some cases, a bone marrow transplant may be indicated for treatment.
- In addition to treating the cancer, the effects of the tumor on the body (i.e. pain) and any side effects from treatment must be managed.
- Be aware that 80% of patients use some type of complementary treatment such as acupuncture, exercise, aromatherapy or hypnosis in addition to conventional care.
- Cancer therapy is complex and is usually managed by a pediatric oncologist but may also include radiation oncologists, pediatric surgeons and pediatric oncology nurses.
- In most cases, the oncology team develops an individualized treatment plan for the child that may be followed for several years.
- Side effects from treatment include increased susceptibility to infection, bleeding/bruising, hair loss, loss of appetite, nausea, vomiting.
- Students may need an Individualized Healthcare Plan (IHP) to help address any medical or other needs while attending school when receiving treatment.

CHILDHOOD CANCER *(continued from previous page)*

FOLLOW-UP:

1. Potential for infection
   a. Monitor for signs and symptoms of infection
   b. Notify parent/guardian if temperature > 99.9
   c. Notify parent/guardian of any exposure to communicable diseases
   d. Educate student, staff and class on handwashing techniques
   e. Provide health promotion information

2. Bleeding
   a. Educate staff regarding potential for abnormal bleeding and situations to report to the school nurse.
   b. Monitor for petechiae, nosebleeds, bleeding gums or prolonged bleeding.
   c. Contact parent/guardian for nosebleeds lasting longer than 10 minutes.

3. Pain
   a. Contact parent/guardian with any new complaints of pain or severe pain.
   b. Partner with oncology team for chronic pain management.
   c. Administer analgesics only if ordered specifically for the student, even if standing orders available.

4. Gastro-intestinal (GI) side effects (nausea, vomiting, constipation, diarrhea)
   a. Educate staff on potential GI side effects and importance of notifying school nurse.
   b. Maintain adequate hydration.
   c. Accommodate for frequent, small meals throughout the day if necessary.
   d. Provide opportunities for rest as needed.
   e. Notify parent/guardian if vomiting persists.

5. Alteration in coping
   a. Assess for stress and coping abilities.
   b. Provide resource information to families.
   c. Monitor for body image disturbances through observation, discussion, and collaboration with parents and school staff. Hair loss, surgical scars, and effects of long-term corticosteroids can contribute to altered body image.
   d. Offer therapeutic forms of expression and stress management for the child, such as art.
   e. Provide support to siblings and make appropriate referrals as needed.

POTENTIAL COMPLICATIONS:

It is important for the school nurse to be aware of late effects of treatment in survivors of childhood cancers. Potential adverse outcomes include decreased growth and development, developmental delays, cognitive disorders, heart or lung disease, infertility and development of secondary cancers.

CHILDHOOD CANCER *(continued from previous page)*

INTERVENTIONS FOR THE SCHOOL NURSE:

- Monitor growth.
- Monitor development and refer student for Individualized Educational Plan or Section 504 plan if regression is noted.
- Provide psycho-social support and referrals as needed.
- Educate staff on potential complications.
- Plan for school re-entry following extended absences.
- Refer for social skills training, vocational rehabilitation, cognitive remediation therapy as needed.
- Be knowledgeable of complementary treatments that these children and families may be using in addition to conventional cancer treatments.

SCHOOL RE-ENTRY:

It is often recommended that the student remain in school as much as possible to maintain a sense of normalcy and to continue with established peer relationships. Homebound or hospital-based instruction should be instituted when the student is unable to attend school. Prior to the student returning to school:

- Schedule a meeting with the parent/ guardian and appropriate school staff which may also include the counselor, teacher, school psychologist, principal, healthcare provider.
- Establish guidelines for care while the child is at school, along with a plan for any potential emergencies.
- Create an IHP.
- Update parent/guardian emergency contact numbers.
- With parent/guardian permission, consider a presentation to the class prior to student returning to school. Often a provider from the child's cancer treatment team is willing to assist with transitioning the student back to school.
- Continue to monitor the student after the child returns to school, re-evaluate and revise the plan as needed.

CHILDHOOD CANCER *(continued from previous page)*

IMPLICATIONS FOR LEARNING:

- Treatment and follow-up appointments will affect attendance.
- Side effects from cancer and treatment impacts learning and performance.
- Learning problems may emerge years after treatment is completed.
- Common problems seen after treatment:
    - Attention disorders
    - Cognitive deficits
    - Difficulty remembering and processing information
    - Difficulty "keeping up"
    - Delayed processing
    - Difficulty with reading
    - Difficulty with handwriting
    - Difficulty with new material
    - Lower grades than before treatment
    - Alterations in executive functioning
    - Behavioral disorders
    - Trouble reading social cues

It may be necessary to institute an Individualized Education Plan (IEP) or Section 504 Plan to provide the necessary academic accommodations and supports.

NOTE: There may be cases when not all treatment options have been successful. The shift in care will become palliative. Often these students wish to continue to attend school. Accommodations can be made to make the child comfortable and have optimal quality of life while at school.

*Refer to **Do Not Attempt Resuscitation (DNAR)** for further information, if needed.*

REFERENCES

[1] American Cancer Society. (2019). *Cancer in children/ Key statistics for childhood cancers.* https://www.cancer.org/cancer/cancer-in-children/key-statistics.html

[2] Ibid.

[3] John, T. (2019). Students with other chronic conditions. Alterations in cellar health: cancer. In J. Selekman, R. Adair Shannon, & C. F. Yonkaitis (Eds.), *School nursing: A comprehensive text* (3rd ed., pp. 680-684). F.A. Davis.

[4] Ibid.

[5] Ibid.

[6] American Cancer Society. (2019). *Finding cancer in children.* https://www.cancer.org/cancer/cancer-in-children/finding-childhood-cancers-early.html

[7] American Cancer Society. (2016). *Treating children with cancer.* https://www.cancer.org/cancer/cancer-in-children/how-are-childhood-cancers-treated.html

CONCUSSION/HEAD INJURY *(Refer to LACERATIONS)*

OVERVIEW/DEFINITION:

A **concussion** is a type of traumatic brain injury (TBI) that affects children, adolescents and young adults. Children and teens take longer to recover than adults. It is caused by a blow, bump or jolt to the head. The impact generally causes the brain to move back and forth in the head. Approximately 3.8 million sports/recreation related concussions happen each year and over 50% are not reported.[1] Most concussions occur without loss of consciousness. All concussions are serious and recognition and proper response when they first occur can help aid recovery and prevent further injury. Subsequent or repeated concussions can have lifelong complications or even death. Although 90% of concussions resolve within 2 weeks, students who experience a concussion may exhibit cognitive and emotional issues that can impact the learning process and requires a collaborative approach in which the school nurse plays a vital role in supporting the student and educating the school team on potential implications in the school setting.[2]

Other head injuries include:

- **Trauma to scalp:** laceration, bruise, abrasion
- **Trauma to bony skull:** fracture
- **Trauma to brain:** contusion, laceration, hematoma

SIGNS AND SYMPTOMS:[3, 4]

Concussion

a. **Physical**
   - Headache
   - Nausea or vomiting
   - Dizziness
   - Fatigue, feeling "foggy"
   - Blurry or double vision
   - Sensitivity to light
   - Vomiting
   - Unequal size of pupils
   - Unusually rapid or slow pulse rate

b. **Cognitive**
   - Difficulty concentrating
   - Difficulty remembering
   - Feeling slowed down
   - Difficulty thinking clearly

c. **Emotional**
   - Irritable
   - Sad
   - Nervous

CONCUSSION/HEAD INJURY *(continued from previous page)*

SIGNS AND SYMPTOMS *(continued)*

1. **Scalp injury:**[5]
   - Abrasion.
   - Laceration: more bleeding than similar cut on other parts of the body because the skin over the scalp has a larger blood supply.
   - Bruise: causes mildly painful swelling (synonyms: pump-knot, goose-egg). Edges may feel depressed, but it is not to be mistaken for the depressed skull fracture described below.
   - In all these conditions, there is no disturbance of consciousness unless there is accompanying injury to the brain.

2. **Skull fracture:**[6]
   - Non-displaced linear fracture: no symptoms except pain unless the base (bottom) of the skull is fractured (X-ray required for diagnosis).
   - Basal skull fracture: usually associated with severe injury which almost always produces disturbance of consciousness or leakage of blood or spinal fluid from the mouth, nose, or ear.
   - Depressed skull fracture: due to a fragment or larger piece of bone pressing down on the brain as a result of trauma. Usually it cannot be felt by palpation and requires an X-ray for diagnosis.

Red Flags:[7] Students should seek guidance from their healthcare provider or be sent to the emergency room if they suddenly experience any of the following:

Pupils are different in size	Headache that does not go away	Restless/Agitated
Seizures	Slurred speech	Weakness or numbness
Neck Pain	Increasing confusion	Unusual behavior change
Extreme drowsiness	Repeated vomiting	Loss of consciousness

ANTICIPATED SERIOUS CONCERNS:[8]
- Epidural/subdural hematoma
- Intracranial hemorrhage
- Cervical spinal injury
- Skull fracture
- Cerebrospinal fluid leak

CONCUSSION/HEAD INJURY *(continued from previous page)*

MANAGEMENT/POTENTIAL INTERVENTIONS:[9, 10, 11]

Concussion:

- Assess concussion ABC's. (**A**ssess situation, **B**e alert for signs and symptoms, **C**ontact healthcare provider).
- Observe student for 30 minutes.
- Complete the Concussion Signs and Symptoms Checklist.[12] (*At end of chapter.*)
- Contact parent/guardian.
- Any student expected of having a concussion or serious head injury should be removed from play immediately and sent for a healthcare provider evaluation.
- A student should be admitted to the hospital for observation if he/she has been unconscious for more than 5 minutes or has amnesia.[13]
- Students should not participate in any high-risk activity such as contact sports, bike riding and physical education (PE) class while experiencing the symptoms of a concussion.
- Students should return to their normal activities gradually. Only when student's symptoms have reduced significantly, in consultation with their healthcare provider, should they gradually return to activities. If symptoms worsen or return, activities should be lessened, and students/family should be encouraged to contact their healthcare provider.
- Students should get plenty of rest and avoid high risk, high intensity activities until symptoms resolve.
- When returning to school students may need accommodations such as a shortened school day, less testing, rest periods during the day, reduced computer use and classroom screen time (e.g. use of SMART boards and tablets), restrictions on physical education and/or recess or moderations to the workload.
- Prior to returning to sports students should take part in a "return to play" protocol that gradually allows the student to increase activities while monitoring for symptoms. The Centers for Disease Control and Prevention (CDC) recommends a six-step return to play progression plan.[14]

Scalp injury:

- Abrasion: wash with plain soap. Apply pressure with 4x4 gauze or other clean cloth until bleeding stops. Dressing is usually not necessary.
- Laceration: same as abrasion but apply pressure longer to make sure bleeding stops. (*Refer to LACERATIONS*).
- Bruise: apply cold pack to relieve pain. DO NOT apply pressure. Prognosis excellent if no sign of brain injury.

Skull fracture:[15]

- If skull fracture suspected, refer to healthcare provider or Emergency medical Services (EMS).
- Linear fracture: Limitation of activity as directed by the healthcare provider.
- Basal fracture: refer to medical facility.
- Depressed skull: if fragment is significantly depressed to encroach on brain, surgery may be required to elevate bony segment.
- Depending on the severity of the skull fracture, a student may need accommodations for return to school based on symptoms similar as those with a concussion.

CONCUSSION/HEAD INJURY *(continued from previous page)*

FOLLOW-UP:

- Students and parents/guardians should be educated on the signs and symptoms of a concussion and be instructed on the importance of not hiding their injury.
- Online concussion training is available on the CDC website.[16]

NOTES:[17, 18]

- Check to see if your state/district has a return to play/learn protocol. School nurses should be involved in the development of return to play/return to learn protocols.
- Students with chronic conditions such as migraines or ADHD may take longer to recover from a concussion.
- Students with depression and/or anxiety may also have trouble dealing with the complications of a concussion.
- Neurocognitive testing to assess concentration, memory and processing speed may be done to help assess the impact of the concussion.
- Children and adolescents should avoid computer use (at home and at school), texting and video games while symptoms persist.
- After a concussion a collaborative approach to the student's needs in school will support the student's successful recovery.
- Guidance counselors, teachers, nurses and support staff must be educated on the complications of concussions and the impact on learning.
- Students who have experienced concussion symptoms over a longer period of time that is expected may benefit from an Individualized Health Care Plan (IHP) or Section 504 accommodation plan.

REFERENCES

---

[1] Harmon, K., Clugston, J., Dec, K. Hainline, B., Herring, S., Kane, S., Kontos, A.P., Leddy, J.J., McCrea, M., Poddar, S.K., Putukian, M., Wilson, J.C., & Roberts, W.O. (2018). American Medical Society for Sports Medicine position statement on concussion in sport. *British Journal of Sports Medicine.* https://bjsm.bmj.com/content/53/4/213

[2] Ibid.

[3] Centers for Disease Control and Prevention. (2019). *Heads up to school nurses, A fact sheet for school nurses.* https://www.cdc.gov/headsup/pdfs/schools/TBI_factsheet_NURSE-508-a.pdf

[4] Ball, J., Binder, R., & Cowen, K. (Eds.). (2017). Alterations in Neurologic Function. In *Principles of pediatric nursing: Caring for children* (7th ed., pp. 782-83). Pearson Education, Inc.

[5] Ibid.

[6] Ibid.

[7] Centers for Disease Control and Prevention. (2019). *Heads up to school nurses, A fact sheet for school nurses.* https://www.cdc.gov/headsup/pdfs/schools/TBI_factsheet_NURSE-508-a.pdf

[8] Centers for Disease Control and Prevention. (2019). *HEADS up to healthcare providers.* https://www.cdc.gov/headsup/providers/index.html

[9] Centers for Disease Control and Prevention. (2019). *Heads up to school nurses, A fact sheet for school nurses.* https://www.cdc.gov/headsup/pdfs/schools/TBI_factsheet_NURSE-508-a.pdf

[10] Mayo Clinic. (2019). *Concussion.* http://www.mayoclinic.com/health/concussion/DS00320

CONCUSSION/HEAD INJURY *(continued from previous page)*

[11] Harmon, K., Clugston, J., Dec, K. Hainline, B., Herring, S., Kane, S., Kontos, A.P., Leddy, J.J., McCrea, M., Poddar, S.K., Putukian, M., Wilson, J.C., & Roberts, W.O. (2018). American Medical Society for Sports Medicine position statement on concussion in sport. *British Journal of Sports Medicine.* https://bjsm.bmj.com/content/53/4/213

[12] Centers for Disease Control and Prevention. (2019). *Concussion signs and symptoms checklist.* https://www.cdc.gov/headsup/pdfs/schools/TBI_schools_checklist_508-a.pdf

[13] Ball, J., Binder, R., & Cowen, K. (Eds.). (2017). Alterations in Neurologic Function. In *Principles of pediatric nursing: Caring for children* (7th ed., pp. 782-83). Pearson Education, Inc.

[14] Centers for Disease Control and Prevention. (2019) *Returning to sports and activities.* https://www.cdc.gov/headsup/basics/return_to_sports.html

[15] Merck Manual, Consumer Version. (2017). *Skull fracture.* https://www.merckmanuals.com/home/injuries -and-poisoning/head-injuries/skull-fracture?query=Traumatic%20Brain%20Injury%20(TBI)

[16] Centers for Disease Control and Prevention. (2019). *HEADS up to healthcare providers.* https://www.cdc.gov/headsup/providers/index.html

[17] Centers for Disease Control and Prevention. (2019). *Returning to school.* https://www.cdc.gov/headsup/basics/return_to_school.html

[18] Harmon, K., Clugston, J., Dec, K. Hainline, B., Herring, S., Kane, S., Kontos, A.P., Leddy, J.J., McCrea, M., Poddar, S.K., Putukian, M., Wilson, J.C., & Roberts, W.O. (2018). American Medical Society for Sports Medicine position statement on concussion in sport. *British Journal of Sports Medicine.* https://bjsm.bmj.com/content/53/4/213

OTHER REFERENCES CONSULTED

National Association of School Nurses. (2016). *Concussions –the role of the school nurse* (Position Statement). Author. https://www.nasn.org/advocacy/professional-practice-documents/position-statements/ps-concussions?CLK=64d6f38e-d04e-4c10-b245-75bf53c3e4d6

Concussion Signs and Symptoms

Checklist

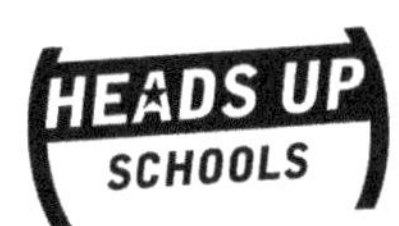

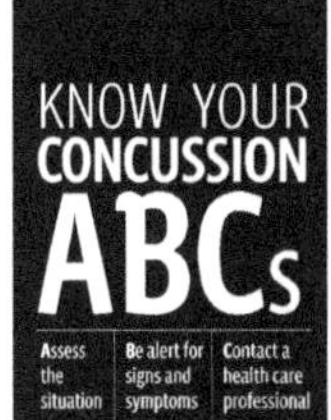

Student's Name: ________________________ **Student's Grade:** ______ **Date/Time of Injury:** ____________

Where and How Injury Occurred: *(Be sure to include cause and force of the hit or blow to the head.)* ________________________

____

Description of Injury: *(Be sure to include information about any loss of consciousness and for how long, memory loss, or seizures following the injury, or previous concussions, if any. See the section on Danger Signs on the back of this form.)* ________________________

____

____

DIRECTIONS:

Use this checklist to monitor students who come to your office with a head injury. Students should be monitored for a minimum of 30 minutes. Check for signs or symptoms when the student first arrives at your office, fifteen minutes later, and at the end of 30 minutes.

Students who experience *one or more* of the signs or symptoms of concussion after a bump, blow, or jolt to the head should be referred to a health care professional with experience in evaluating for concussion. For those instances when a parent is coming to take the student to a health care professional, observe the student for any new or worsening symptoms right before the student leaves. Send a copy of this checklist with the student for the health care professional to review.

OBSERVED SIGNS	0 MINUTES	15 MINUTES	30 MINUTES	☐ MINUTES Just prior to leaving
Appears dazed or stunned				
Is confused about events				
Repeats questions				
Answers questions slowly				
Can't recall events *prior* to the hit, bump, or fall				
Can't recall events *after* the hit, bump, or fall				
Loses consciousness (even briefly)				
Shows behavior or personality changes				
Forgets class schedule or assignments				
PHYSICAL SYMPTOMS				
Headache or "pressure" in head				
Nausea or vomiting				
Balance problems or dizziness				
Fatigue or feeling tired				
Blurry or double vision				
Sensitivity to light				
Sensitivity to noise				
Numbness or tingling				
Does not "feel right"				
COGNITIVE SYMPTOMS				
Difficulty thinking clearly				
Difficulty concentrating				
Difficulty remembering				
Feeling more slowed down				
Feeling sluggish, hazy, foggy, or groggy				
EMOTIONAL SYMPTOMS				
Irritable				
Sad				
More emotional than usual				
Nervous				

To download this checklist in Spanish, please visit: www.cdc.gov/Concussion. Para obtener una copia electrónica de esta lista de síntomas en español, por favor visite: www.cdc.gov/Concussion.

May 2010

→More

Danger Signs:

Be alert for symptoms that worsen over time. The student should be seen in an emergency department right away if s/he has:

- ❒ One pupil (the black part in the middle of the eye) larger than the other
- ❒ Drowsiness or cannot be awakened
- ❒ A headache that gets worse and does not go away
- ❒ Weakness, numbness, or decreased coordination
- ❒ Repeated vomiting or nausea
- ❒ Slurred speech
- ❒ Convulsions or seizures
- ❒ Difficulty recognizing people or places
- ❒ Increasing confusion, restlessness, or agitation
- ❒ Unusual behavior
- ❒ Loss of consciousness (even a brief loss of consciousness should be taken seriously)

Additional Information About This Checklist:

This checklist is also useful if a student appears to have sustained a head injury outside of school or on a previous school day. In such cases, be sure to ask the student about possible sleep symptoms. Drowsiness, sleeping more or less than usual, or difficulty falling asleep may indicate a concussion.

To maintain confidentiality and ensure privacy, this checklist is intended only for use by appropriate school professionals, health care professionals, and the student's parent(s) or guardian(s).

For a free tear-off pad with additional copies of this form, or for more information on concussion, visit: www.cdc.gov/Concussion.

Resolution of Injury:

__ Student returned to class
__ Student sent home
__ Student referred to health care professional with experience in evaluating for concussion

SIGNATURE OF SCHOOL PROFESSIONAL COMPLETING THIS FORM: ______________________

TITLE: ______________________

COMMENTS:

For more information on concussion and to order additional materials for school professionals **FREE-OF-CHARGE**, visit: www.cdc.gov/Concussion.

U.S. Department of Health and Human Services
Centers for Disease Control and Prevention

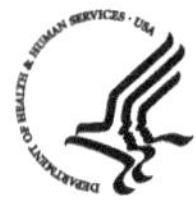

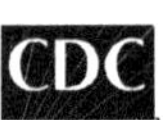

CONJUNCTIVITIS (Pink Eye)

DEFINITION/ETIOLOGY:

Inflammation, swelling, and/or infection of the conjunctiva (thin transparent layer of tissue that lines the inner surface of the eyelid and covers the white part of the eye), caused by allergens, irritants (e.g., foreign object, dust, smoke), bacterial (staphylococcal, streptococcal, haemophilus) or viral (usually adenovirus, but also herpes simplex) infections. Both bacterial and viral conjunctivitis are contagious.[1, 2]

SIGNS AND SYMPTOMS:[3]

- Redness of sclera
- Discharge: purulent or watery
  - Purulent drainage may cause blurred vision
- Itching or burning in one or both eyes
- Eyelids may be red and/or swollen
- Crusts in inner corner of eyes, especially on waking from sleep
- Gritty feeling in eyes
- Increased sensitivity to light

Physical Findings That Help Differentiate Etiology:[4, 5]

Allergic	• Red, itchy, tearing eyes. Eyes may feel gritty. • Puffy eyelids. • Occurs in response to agent causing allergic reaction. • Discharge remains watery/stringy; bilateral. • Runny nose, sneezing. • No contagious period.
Bacterial	• The common meaning of "pink eye": purulent drainage (thick, yellow to green-yellow) and more crusting during sleep causing matting of the eyelashes. • Often beginning unilaterally and progressing to bilateral. Is spread to others by hand, contaminated eye mascara, etc. • Contagious until start of antibiotic treatment. • Contagious period ends when medication begins. Approximately 50% of cases resolve without treatment in one to two weeks.
Viral	• Usually less severe, watery discharge but may be thick and white to pale yellow. • Photophobia. • Self-limiting. Lasts three to five days. • Most often bilateral. • Highly contagious but does not require antibiotics. • May occur with the common cold. • Contagious period continues while symptoms are present.
Chemical	• Usually appears shortly after contact with irritating substance. • No contagious period.

CONJUNCTIVITIS (Pink Eye) *(continued from previous page)*

MANAGEMENT/TREATMENT:

- Focus is on alleviating symptoms and based on the cause of the condition:
    - Bacterial conjunctivitis
        - treated with ophthalmic antibiotic therapy
        - student may return to school once treatment initiated (no longer necessary to wait 24 hours after initiation of treatment)[6]
    - Viral conjunctivitis
        - no antibiotic treatment required
    - Allergic conjunctivitis
        - topical antihistamine ophthalmic drops or artificial tears may provide some relief
- Conjunctivitis without fever and behavioral change does not necessitate exclusion from school.[7]
- Most children get better after five to six days without antibiotics.
- Students who wear contacts should remove contacts at the onset of symptoms of conjunctivitis and seek evaluation by ophthalmologist if symptoms don't improve in 24-48 hours.[8]
- Hands become contaminated by direct contact with discharge from infected eye, or by touching other surfaces contaminated by respiratory secretions.
- Review handwashing and other measures to prevent an spread of infection.
- Over-the-counter drops may be used for comfort of mild allergic or viral conjunctivitis.
- Cool compress for temporary relief.
- Check visual acuity; it should be normal or unchanged from the student's usual acuity.
- Refer any case with subconjunctival hemorrhage.
- Discourage home treatment with cold ointment or steroid drops.

FOLLOW UP:

- If healthcare provider orders medication, instruct student and parent/guardian to take for the entire prescribed time.
- Educate about handwashing and keeping fingers/hands away from eyes. Instruct the student to not share face washcloths and eye makeup. (*Refer to HANDWASHING APPENDIX*).
- Discard unused eye makeup.

POTENTIAL COMPLICATIONS:

Conjunctivitis can cause inflammation in the cornea that can affect vision. Students who experience eye pain, foreign body sensation, blurred vision or light sensitivity should seek prompt evaluation by a healthcare provider.[9]

CONJUNCTIVITIS (Pink Eye) *(continued from previous page)*

REFERENCES

[1] American Optometric Association (AOA). (n.d.). *Conjunctivitis*. http://www.aoa.org/patients-and-public/eye-and-vision-problems/glossary-of-eye-and-vision-conditions/conjunctivitis

[2] Merck Manual. (2018). *Overview of conjunctivitis.* http://www.merckmanuals.com/professional/eye-disorders/conjunctival-and-scleral-disorders/overview-of-conjunctivitis

[3] American Optometric Association (AOA). (n.d.). *Conjunctivitis*. Retrieved from http://www.aoa.org/patients-and-public/eye-and-vision-problems/glossary-of-eye-and-vision-conditions/conjunctivitis

[4] Ball, J., Bindler, R., Cowen, K. & Shaw, M. (Eds.). (2017). Alterations in the eye, nose, ear and throat function. *Principles of Pediatric Nursing: Caring for Children* (7th ed., p. 444). Pearson Education, Inc.

[5] Jakubowski, T. & Perron, T. (2019). Students with common health complaints. In J. Selekman, R. Adair Shannon, & C. F. Yonkaitis (Eds.), *School nursing: A comprehensive text* (3rd ed., pp. 340-341). F.A. Davis.

[6] Ibid.

[7] American Academy of Pediatrics. (2020). Recognizing the ill child: Inclusion/exclusion criteria. In S. Aronson, & T. Shope (Eds.), *Managing infectious diseases in child care and schools* (5th ed., pp. 45-50). American Academy of Pediatrics.

[8] Mayo Clinic. (2019). *Pink eye (conjunctivitis).* http://www.mayoclinic.com/health/pink-eye/DS00258

[9] Ibid.

ADDIONAL REFERENCE CONSULTED

American Academy of Pediatrics. (2020). Pinkeye (conjuctivitis). In S. Aronson, & T. Shope (Eds.), *Managing infectious diseases in child care and schools* (5th ed., pp. 141-142). American Academy of Pediatrics.

SUGGESTED RESOURCES

Centers for Disease Control and Prevention. (2019). *Conjunctivitis (Pink Eye).* https://www.cdc.gov/conjunctivitis/about/treatment.html

CONJUNCTIVITIS (Pink Eye) *(continued from previous page)*

HELP PROTECT YOURSELF FROM GETTING & SPREADING PINK EYE (CONJUNCTIVITIS)

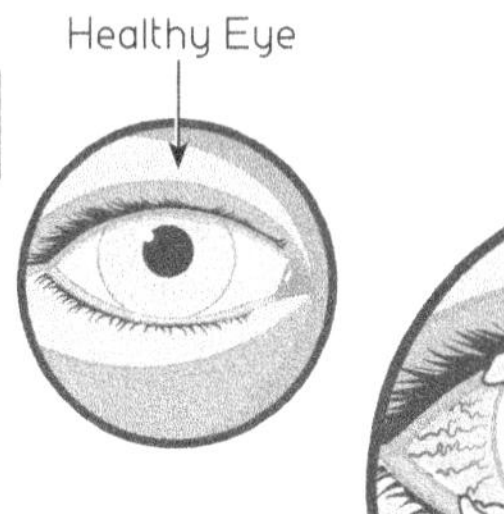

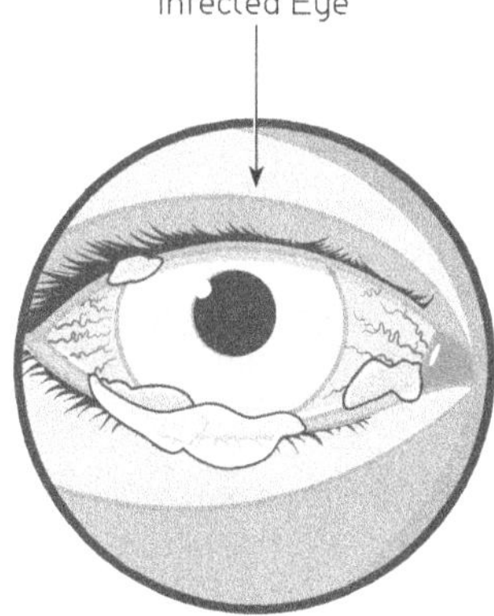

PINK EYE IS OFTEN HIGHLY CONTAGIOUS.

IT CAN BE CAUSED BY

- Viruses (very contagious)
- Bacteria (very contagious)
- Allergens, like pollen (not contagious)
- Irritants, like smoke or dust (not contagious)

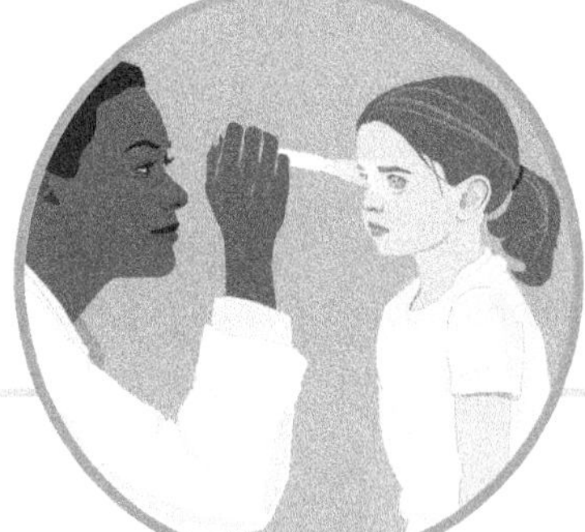

SYMPTOMS USUALLY INCLUDE:

- Redness or swelling
- Watery eyes
- A gritty feel
- Itchiness, irritation, or burning
- Discharge
- Crusting of the eyelids or eyelashes

SEE A DOCTOR IF YOU HAVE PINK EYE ALONG WITH ANY OF THE FOLLOWING:

- Eye pain
- Sensitivity to light or blurred vision
- Intense eye redness
- Symptoms that get worse or don't improve
- A weakened immune system, for example from HIV or cancer treatment
- Pre-existing eye conditions

 Newborns with symptoms of pink eye should see a doctor right away.

A doctor can usually diagnose the cause of pink eye based on symptoms and patient history.

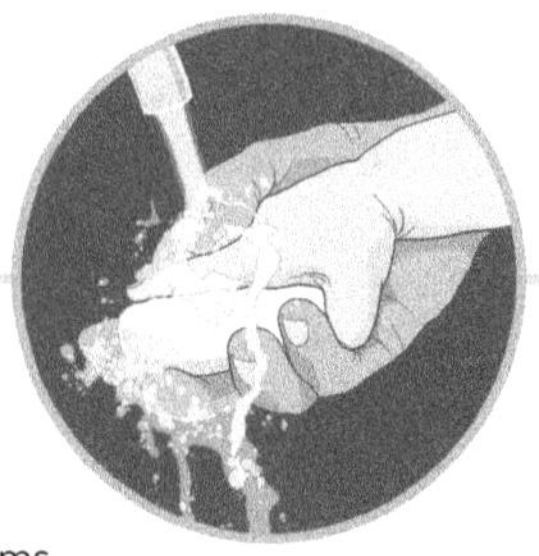

PROTECT YOURSELF AND OTHERS FROM PINK EYE

- Wash your hands often with soap and water, and help young children do the same. Wash hands especially well after touching someone with pink eye or their personal items.
- Avoid touching or rubbing your eyes. This can worsen the condition or spread it to your other eye.
- Avoid sharing personal items, such as makeup, eye drops, towels, bedding, contact lenses and containers, and eyeglasses.
- Do not use the same eye products for your infected and non-infected eyes.
- Stop wearing contact lenses until your eye doctor says it's okay.
- Clean, store, and replace your contact lenses as instructed by your eye doctor.

WWW.CDC.GOV/PINKEYE

CS284341-C

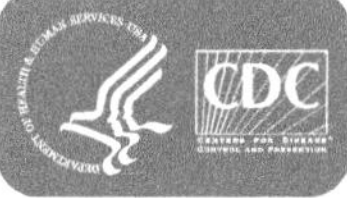

CONSTIPATION (Idiopathic or Functional)

DEFINITION/ETIOLOGY:

Constipation is a common gastrointestinal disorder in children. It results in abnormal bowel patterns with stools that are hard, dry and painful or difficult to pass.[1] Constipation is termed idiopathic or functional if it cannot be explained by any anatomical, physiological, radiological or histological abnormalities.

Factors that may contribute to and should also be included in school nurse assessments for constipation in children are: [2]

- impaired mobility
- lack of exercise
- withholding bowel movements due to pain or busy schedules
- discomfort with using public restrooms
- dehydration
- dietary and fluid intake
- fever
- toilet training
- medications
- family history of constipation and/or other medical conditions

Excessive use of laxatives and enemas can also stop regular bowel movements, as the body may begin to rely on them for defecation.

SIGNS AND SYMPTOMS:

- Infrequent bowel activity that deviates from individual bowel activity
- Excessive and foul-smelling flatulence
- Foul smelling stools
- Irregular stool texture
- Passing occasional enormous stools or frequent small pellets
- Intentionally withholding or straining to stop passage of stools (retentive posturing or changing positions)
- Soiling or overflow
- Abdominal pains, which go away after a large bowel movement[3]
- Abdominal distension or discomfort
- Lack of energy, general malaise
- Urinary incontinence
- Improved appetite with the passage of stool
- Anal pain and bleeding associated with hard stools
- History of painful or hard bowel movements or constipation
- History of large diameter stools which may obstruct the toilet

CONSTIPATION *(continued from previous page)*

SIGNS AND SYMPTOMS *(continued)*

- Passing ribbon stools
- Failure to thrive
- Abdominal distension with vomiting
- History of constipation symptoms since birth

MANAGEMENT/TREATMENT:

- Provide developmentally appropriate behavioral interventions that are negotiated and non-punitive, including:
    - Scheduling toileting to establish a regular bowel habit.
    - Discuss the use of a bowel diary that records information on bowel regimen.
- Provide education to students and families about:
    - How the bowels work
    - Symptoms that might indicate a serious underlying problem
    - How to take medication to treat constipation
    - What to expect when taking laxatives
    - Strategies to enhance production of bowel movement:
        - Drink lots of water and other liquids to help relieve and prevent constipation.[4]
        - Increase high-fiber foods like vegetables, fruits and whole grains in diet, while decreasing high-fat meats, dairy products and eggs, rich deserts and sugary sweets.[5]
        - Increase physical activity and stay active.
        - Establish regular bowel habits.
- Administer medications according to the healthcare provider's orders.
- Provide developmentally appropriate education and guidance regarding toilet training in children.
- Use a combination of history and physical examination when assessing for fecal impaction.
- Disimpaction treatment/therapy - Be sure to inform families that disimpaction treatment/therapy can initially increase symptoms of soiling and abdominal pain.
- Seek medical attention if symptoms persist for more than two weeks or do not resolve with over the counter or home remedies.[6]
- Children should be taken to their healthcare provider right away if they have constipation and are experiencing any of the following symptoms:
    - bleeding from his or her rectum
    - blood in his or her stool
    - bloating
    - constant pain in his or her abdomen
    - vomiting
    - weight loss

CONSTIPATION *(continued from previous page)*

FOLLOW-UP:

- Support the family and student during the prescribed treatment plan by following the treatment plan and documenting bowel activities, including accidents at school.
- Follow up by the healthcare provider for acute constipation and to assess for chronic constipation.
- The frequency of assessment by the healthcare provider should be tailored to the individual needs of the child and their families. This may be based on the child or young person's response to treatment, measured by frequency, amount and consistency of stools.

POTENTIAL COMPLICATIONS:[7]

- Fecal impaction
- Long-lasting constipation
- Painful bowel movements
- Bladder control problems
- Hemorrhoids
- Anal fissures
- Rectal prolapse
- Possible fecal incontinence
- Increase in abdominal pain

NOTES:

Develop a Section 504 plan and Individualized Healthcare Plan for chronic or ongoing constipation as needed.

REFERENCES

---

[1] Healthychildren.org. (2017). *Constipation in children.* https://www.healthychildren.org/English/health-issues/conditions/abdominal/Pages/Constipation.aspx

[2] American Academy of Pediatrics, healthychildren.og. (2019). *Constipation in children.* https://www.healthychildren.org/English/health-issues/conditions/abdominal/Pages/Constipation.aspx

[3] American Academy of Pediatrics. (2019). *Constipation.* https://www.aap.org/en-us/about-the-aap/aap-press-room/aap-press-room-media-center/Pages/Constipation.aspx

[4] MedlinePlus. (2019). *Constipation.* https://medlineplus.gov/constipation.html

[5] National Institute on Aging. (2013). *Concerned about constipation?* https://www.nia.nih.gov/health/concerned-about-constipation

[6] National Institute of Diabetes and Digestive and Kidney Diseases. (2019). Symptoms & causes of constipation in children. https://www.niddk.nih.gov/health-information/digestive-diseases/constipation-children/symptoms-causes

[7] National Institute of Diabetes and Digestive and Kidney Diseases. (2019*). Definition & facts for constipation in children.* https://www.niddk.nih.gov/health-information/digestive-diseases/constipation-children/definition-facts

CONTACT LENS PROBLEMS

OVERVIEW/DEFINITION:

Contact lenses are used as a substitute for glasses in most situations. They may also be used to treat myopia, hyperopia, astigmatism, presbyopia or for cosmetic purposes to change eye color. Contacts are generally prescribed for children beginning at 12-13 years old.[1] Children less than ages of eight to nine are prescribed contact lenses for medical reasons only.[2]

Lens types include soft lenses, rigid gas permeable lenses, extended wear lenses, disposable lenses, and specialty lenses. Decorative lenses are illegally sold in beauty salons, novelty stores and online. These lenses are non-fitted lenses and cover a larger part of the eye, putting the wearer at a higher risk for a severe complication. Decorative lenses, if desired should be prescribed by an eye care professional.[3]

Most problems encountered from wearing contact lenses are from inexperienced wearers, improper wear or care, or delay in follow-up with the eye healthcare provider. These problems range from a lens being out of position, eye irritations such as dryness, a foreign body on or under lens, to more serious complications such as pink eye, corneal abrasion, infection, corneal ulcer, and permanent vision loss.[4]

ANTICIPATED CONCERNS/PROBLEMS: [5]

- Unable to wear due to dry eyes
- Unable to wear due to work or home environment (dusty)
- Severe allergies
- Contact lenses that do not fit properly can scratch eyes

As a new contact lens wearer, it is not uncommon to have:

- Tearing upon insertion
- Scratchy feeling or like there is something in the eye
- Mild light sensitivity
- Slight headache especially if stronger prescription
- Distorted vision that may be caused from:
  - Lens that is not centered
  - Soft lens inside out
  - Wearing disposable lenses beyond the suggested time
  - Not wearing lenses for several days (cornea may lose adaptation)
  - Dirty lens

SIGNS AND SYMTPOMS OF AN EYE IRRITATION, INFECTION, OR SERIOUS COMPLICATION INCLUDE:[6]

- Persistent pain
- Burning and tearing
- Redness that will not clear
- Hazy vision that continues an hour or more after lens removal
- Continued sensitivity to light
- Swelling of eye

CONTACT LENS PROBLEMS *(continued from previous page)*

MANAGEMENT/POTENTIAL INTERVENTIONS:
Seek care from eye healthcare professional if symptoms of an eye irritation or infection (above) occur.

Removing Displaced Lenses[7]

- Blink several times to make sure lens is in the eye. Blinking may center the lens.
- Wash hands before touching the eye or lens.
- Use your finger to feel the lens through the eyelid.
- Look in the opposite direction of the lens (downward, upward, to the right or left) to visualize the lens.
- When the lens is visualized, use your finger to move the lens back on the cornea.
- Massaging the lens through eyelid may help move it back in place.
- If unable to move back in correct position, remove and re-insert a cleaned or new contact
- If you are unable to remove the lens, seek care from an eye healthcare professional.

FOLLOW-UP:

- Annual eye exams
- Extended wear lenses require exams every three to six months.[8]

Teaching Tips:[9, 10]

- Wash your hands before touching your eye or handling lenses.
- Don't wear lenses longer than prescribed.
- Don't sleep in your lenses unless specifically fitted for that purpose.
- Don't use saliva or water as a cleaning agent. The risk of bacterial contamination is great.
- Do not use homemade solutions that are not sterile. Do not use distilled or tap water for any part of the cleaning regimen.
- Use only solutions recommended by fitter – some are not compatible with other lenses and/or may be allergenic to wearer.
- Experts consider the "rub and rinse" method to be the superior cleaning method.[11]
- Don't get cosmetics, sprays, etc. on lenses.
- Finish with makeup before handling lenses.
- Remove contacts before shower or swimming or hot tub.
- Don't reuse the solution in your lens case. Throw away and use a new case every three months or if you get an eye infection.
- Do not rinse lenses in hot water or store in a hot or unusually cold place; lens may warp.
- Used lenses stored for 30 days should not be worn without re-disinfecting.
- Frequent blinking is essential for all contacts to maintain moisture and a constant supply of oxygen to the corneas.
- Wearing non-prescription decorative lenses or circle lenses purchased online or in novelty shops can result in permanent eye damage.
- Smokers have a higher incidence of problems wearing contact lenses than non-smokers.

CONTACT LENS PROBLEMS *(continued from previous page)*

FOLLOW-UP *(continued)*

Tips for new contact users:

- Avoid dry eyes by drinking water and using rewetting drops if necessary.
- Keep your fingernails short to avoid tearing the lens or scratching your eye.
- Put the lens in the same eye first to avoid mixing lenses up.

NOTES:[12]

- Contact lenses are recommended for children based on their age and maturity.
- Extended wear lenses are generally not recommended for children and teens.
- Children with seasonal allergies are not good candidates for contact lenses.

REFERENCES

[1] American Academy of Ophthalmology, Eye Smart. (2019). *Contact lenses for vision correction.* https://www.aao.org/eye-health/glasses-contacts/contact-lens-102

[2] Weinstock, F., Rhee, M., Stoppler, M. (2017). *Contact Lenses.* www.emedicinehealth.com/contact_lenses/article_em.htm

[3] American Academy of Ophthalmology, Eye Smart. (2019). *Contact lenses for vision correction.* https://www.aao.org/eye-health/glasses-contacts/contact-lens-102

[4] Ibid.

[5] Ibid.

[6] United States Food and Drug and Administration, Medical Devices. (2018). *Contact lenses.* https://www.fda.gov/medical-devices/consumer-products/contact-lenses

[7]American Academy of Ophthalmology. (2012). *Eye smart: How do I get a contact lens out of the top of my eye?* https://www.aao.org/eye-health/ask-ophthalmologist-q/stuck-contact-lens

[8] Weinstock, F., Rhee, M., Stoppler, M. (2017). *Contact Lenses.* www.emedicinehealth.com/contact_lenses/article_em.htm

[9] American Academy of Ophthalmology, Eye Smart. (2019). *Contact lenses for vision correction.* https://www.aao.org/eye-health/glasses-contacts/contact-lens-102

[10] United States Food and Drug and Administration, Medical Devices. (2018). *Contact lenses.* https://www.fda.gov/medical-devices/consumer-products/contact-lenses

[11] 1800 contact CONNECT. (2017). *Contact* lenses *for beginners*. https://www.1800contacts.com/connect/how-to-clean-contacts

[12] United States Food and Drug and Administration, Medical Devices. (2018). *Contact lenses.* https://www.fda.gov/medical-devices/consumer-products/contact-lenses

OTHER REFERENCES CONSULTED

Merck Manual. (2018). *Contact lenses.* https://www.merckmanuals.com/professional/eye-disorders/refractive-error/contact-lenses?query=contact%20lenses

CROHN'S DISEASE

DEFINITION/ETIOLOGY:

Crohn's disease is a debilitating, chronic inflammatory bowel disease (IBD) that causes intermittent inflammation in the lining of the digestive tract. Inflammation commonly occurs in the ileum of the small intestines and colon but can occur in any area in the gastrointestinal tract. This frequently causes fissures and fistulas. There can also be segments of intestinal tract that are disease free. The exact cause of Crohn's disease is unknown but may be caused by environmental exposure of a genetically susceptible person. It peaks in late adolescence and early adulthood with 25 to 40% of cases diagnosed in childhood and adolescence.[1] There is no known cure for Crohn's disease. It is characterized by periods of flare-ups and periods of remission that may last weeks to years. A person has a higher incidence of developing Crohn's disease if they have a relative with the disease.[2] Diagnosis is generally made by a pediatric gastroenterologist through the use of colonoscopy and endoscopy.

SIGNS AND SYMPTOMS:[3]

Symptoms range from mild to severe and differ from person to person. Symptoms may include:

- Abdominal pain/intestinal cramping
- Diarrhea (can be severe)
- Fatigue, low grade fever, often of unknown etiology
- Anorexia
- Low grade fever – secondary to inflammation and/or infection
- Weight loss
- Malnutrition
- Impaired growth and development including sexual development
- Rectal bleeding

MANAGEMENT/TREATMENT:

The overall goal of treatment is to reduce inflammation in the intestines, obtain remission and allow for continued growth and development to help foster a normal lifestyle. Students with abdominal cramps and diarrhea may be prescribed anti-diarrheal and anti-spasmodic medications to relieve acute symptoms.

Other treatment options may include anti-inflammatory medications (such as 5 aminosalicyclic acid) and/or antibiotics for acute infection. Individuals with severe symptoms may be prescribed corticosteroids to reduce symptoms. These medications help to induce and maintain remission by decreasing the acute symptoms. The use of immunomodulators and biologics have also been utilized for those who do not respond to traditional medications.[4]

Surgical intervention may be necessary if an individual does not respond to medications. Up to 15 to 20% of children require surgery within two years of the diagnosis and most patients eventually require surgery.[5] Surgery before puberty may improve the growth rate. Surgery does not cure the disease. Surgery removes the area of intestine that is severely inflamed, symptomatic and is not responding to medications.[6]

CROHN'S DISEASE *(continued from previous page)*

Nutritional support is an important component of management. Students should be supported in selecting foods that are nutritionally dense and avoid triggering foods. Oral supplemental nutrition through the use of nasogastric, gastrostomy or parental hyperalimentation may be needed. The use of amino acids as exclusive elemental nutrition may also be utilized to induce remission.[7]

POTENTIAL COMPLICATIONS:

- Malnutrition/ growth failure (poor intestinal absorption)
- Anemia
- Fistula (may become infected and form an abscess)
- Intestinal obstruction with scarring
- Anal fissures
- Ulcers (mouth, genital and/or anal)
- Pancreatitis
- Osteoporosis (poor intestinal absorption/corticosteroids also increase the risk of developing osteoporosis)
- Increased risk of colon cancer
- Pericarditis/arthritis
- Uveitis or other ophthalmological manifestations
- Risk for opportunistic infections due to use of corticosteroids[8]

FOLLOW UP:

- Monitor for medication side effects.
- Monitor height, weight and body mass index (BMI).
- Diet may aggravate Crohn's disease. Dietary needs/restrictions should be provided to the school nutrition services for potential school-based dietary accommodations. Individual may be on a low fat, low fiber diet (fiber may make symptoms worse). May also need to limit dairy products and avoid spicy foods and caffeine.
- Monitor for potential need of school-based social work services.
- Smoking aggravates symptoms. Educate students and families on the need to avoid cigarette/cigar smoke.
- Homebound school services may be necessary for extended absences Educate teachers and other school staff with legitimate educational interest on the student's condition and its impact on the educational process.
- Complete and Individualized Healthcare Plan (IHP) to address the student's individual needs.
- The student may require multiple medications during the school day. It would be important to develop a medication administration plan that limits missed educational time.

CROHN'S DISEASE *(continued from previous page)*

(continued from previous page)

NOTES:

Evaluate to determine eligibility for possible Section 504 accommodations. Possible accommodations may include:

- Free access to bathroom
- Self-paced activity at school
- Provide rest as needed throughout the academic day
- Access to snacks/water throughout the school day
- School-based dietary/meal accommodations
- Extra change of clothes at school
- Allow for excessive tardiness or absenteeism due to medical condition
- Academic accommodations during periods of flare-ups (extended test taking time, extended time to turn in assignments, second set of books for home use, etc.)

REFERENCES

[1] Ball, J.W., Binder, R. C., Cowen, K. J., & Shaw, M.R. (Eds.). (2017). Gastrointestinal disorders. *Principles of pediatric nursing: Caring for children, (7th ed., p.869).* Pearson Education.

[2] Willer, E., Peterson, B., Smith, A. (2017). Gastrointestinal disorders. In C. Burns, A.M. Dunn, M.A. Brady, N.B. Starr, C.G. Blosser, & D.L. Garzon (Eds.), *Pediatric primary care* (6th ed., pp. 868-871). Elsevier.

[3] John, T. (2019). Students with other chronic conditions. In J. Selekman, R. Adair Shannon, &C. F. Yonkaitis (Eds.), *School nursing: A comprehensive text* (3rd ed., pp. 709-711). F.A. Davis.

[4] Ibid.

[5] Willer, E., Peterson, B., Smith, A. (2017). Gastrointestinal disorders. In C. Burns, A.M. Dunn, M.A. Brady, N.B. Starr, C.G. Blosser, & D.L. Garzon (Eds.), *Pediatric primary care* (6th ed., pp. 868-871). Elsevier.

[6] Ibid.

[7] John, T. (2019). Students with other chronic conditions. In J. Selekman, R. Adair Shannon, & C. F. Yonkaitis (Eds.), *School nursing: A comprehensive text* (3rd ed., pp. 709-711). F.A. Davis.

[8] Willer, E., Peterson, B., Smith, A. (2017). Gastrointestinal disorders. In C. Burns, A.M. Dunn, M.A. Brady, N.B. Starr, C.G. Blosser, & D.L. Garzon (Eds.), Pediatric *primary care* (6th ed., pp. 868-871). Elsevier.

OTHER REFERENCES CONSULTED

Centers for Disease Control and Prevention (CDC). (2018). *What is inflammatory bowel disease?* http://www.cdc.gov/ibd/what-is-ibd.htm

Mayo Clinic. (2019). *Crohn's disease.* http://www.mayoclinic.org/diseases-conditions/crohns-disease/basics/definition/CON-20032061

National Institute of Diabetes and Digestive and Kidney Diseases. (2017). *What I need to know about Crohn's disease?* http://www.niddk.nih.gov/health-information/health-topics/digestive-diseases/crohns-disease/Pages/ez.aspx

CYSTIC FIBROSIS

DEFINITION/ETIOLOGY:[1]

Cystic fibrosis (CF) is an autosomal recessive genetic disease caused by a mutation of the **Cystic Fibrosis Transmembrane Regulator** (CFTR) gene, altering the salt balance in body secretions. Cystic fibrosis affects mainly the exocrine glands, resulting in a thick, sticky mucous that compromises the organs, primarily the lungs and pancreas. The exocrine glands produce sweat, saliva, pancreatic digestive juice and respiratory tract mucous. In children with cystic fibrosis, air becomes trapped in the small airways, leading to hyperventilation, atelectasis, and secondary respiratory infections. Obstructions in the pancreatic ducts impede natural enzyme flow that enables the body to digest fats, fat soluble vitamins, and proteins.

SIGNS AND SYMPTOMS:[2]

Vary with the severity of the disease.

- Salty taste to the skin – increased amount of sodium and chloride in sweat
- Weight loss despite voracious appetite
- Frequent, foul-smelling, greasy stools
- Stools may be gray or clay colored
- Flatulence
- Abdominal pain
- Delayed growth
- Thick, sticky sputum
- Productive coughing
- Wheezing
- Frequent respiratory infections

MANAGEMENT/TREATMENT:

There is no cure for cystic fibrosis. Treatment is aimed at preventing and controlling infections that occur in the lungs, removing and loosening mucus from the lungs, treating and preventing intestinal blockage, and providing adequate nutrition.[3]

1. Develop an Individualized Healthcare Plan (IHP) and a Section 504 Plan, if indicated.
    a. Identify signs of airway distress and appropriate responses.
    b. **Allow student time during school day to go to nurse's office for administration of pancreatic enzymes prior to snacks and meals and/or chest physical therapy.**
    c. **Allow unlimited access to bathroom and water.**
    d. **Develop plan to get homework or tutor during absences and hospitalizations.**

2. Chest physical therapy to loosen thick mucus secretions
    a. Postural drainage
    b. Chest percussion
    c. Positive expiratory pressure therapy
    d. Mechanical devices such as Flutter/Vest devices

CYSTIC FIBROSIS *(continued from previous page)*

MANAGEMENT/TREATMENT *(continued)*

3. Medications
    a. Pancreatic enzymes to aid in digestion with each meal/snack
    b. Aerosolize drugs thins mucus making it easier to cough up
    c. Bronchodilators to open airways
    d. Vitamin supplements (secretions prevent body from absorbing fat-soluble vitamins A, D, E and K)
    e. Antibiotics to treat respiratory infections, may need longer duration of treatment than normal
4. Maintain adequate nutrition
    a. High calorie/diet high in protein and fat
    b. May need nutritional supplements
    c. May need supplemental feedings per nasogastric tube, or Total Parenteral Nutrition (TPN)
    d. For long term nutritional support, a gastrostomy or jejunostomy tube may be placed
5. Physical activity as tolerated
    a. Allow student to set his or her own pace, accommodate for rest periods as needed.
    b. Encourage adequate hydration (especially during hot weather or after exercise; due to increased salt in sweat, may need supplement salt).
    c. Physical activity loosens lung secretions.
    d. Improves overall physical condition of heart and lungs.
6. Psychosocial assessment
    a. May feel different from peers
    b. Need for special diet, medications, respiratory management
    c. Potential for bullying from others

FOLLOW-UP:

- Assist student with administration of pancreatic enzymes.
- Act as a liaison with CF care centers to coordinate care for school.
- Monitor nutritional status – measure height/weight a minimum of two times per year.
- Educate staff regarding chronic cough:
    - Not contagious
    - Should not suppress cough – clears secretions
    - Allow student to keep water bottle on desk
    - Preferential seating near door so student may leave classroom as needed for heavy coughing
- Allow bathroom privileges as needed for digestive problems
- Tissues/plastic bag at desk for productive cough. Students with CF may have frequent complications that require hospitalization. The school nurse serves as the liaison between the school and healthcare providers to foster continuity of care during return to school transitions.[4]

CYSTIC FIBROSIS *(continued from previous page)*

POTENTIAL COMPLICATIONS:

- Asthma can result from chronic inflammation of the bronchial tubes
- Chronic respiratory infections (pneumonia, bronchitis, chronic sinusitis)
- Liver damage due to blocked bile duct
- Cystic fibrosis-related diabetes (CFRD)– features similar to Type 1 and Type 2 diabetes but considered a separate condition
- Depressed growth rate
- Osteoporosis and/or osteopenia secondary to compromised absorption of calcium and vitamin D
- Infertility – 98% in males
- Death – typically as a result of lung complications

NOTES:

As noted, children with CF are more likely to suffer complications from an illness. Educate students and families regarding the importance of healthy lifestyle behaviors to help mitigate these complications:

- Practice appropriate handwashing. (*Refer to HANDWASHING APPENDIX).*
- Obtain immunizations, especially pneumococcal and influenza.
- Avoid cigarette smoke.
- Promote healthy eating habits.
- If there is more than one student with CF in a school building, avoid assigning both students to the same classroom [5] or seated at least six feet apart.
- Multiple students with CF within a school should be assigned separate bathrooms, lunch tables, drinking fountains, and lockers. [6]

RESOURCES

- **Cystic Fibrosis Foundation** http://www.cff.org/AboutCF/
- **Cystic Fibrosis Foundation, specific for school**: http://www.cff.org/LivingWithCF/AtSchool/
- **National Lung Heart and Blood Institute** http://www.nhlbi.nih.gov/health/health-topics/topics/cf/
- **Merck Manual.** (2019). *Cystic fibrosis.* http://www.merckmanuals.com/professional/pediatrics/cystic-fibrosis-cf/cystic-fibrosis#SymptomsAndSigns
- **National Lung, Heart Blood Institute.** (n.d.). https://www.nhlbi.nih.gov/health-topics/cystic-fibrosis

CYSTIC FIBROSIS *(continued from previous page)*

REFERENCES

[1] Ball, J., Bindler, R., Cowen, K., & Shaw, M. (Eds.). (2017). Alterations in respiratory function. *Principles of Pediatric Nursing: Caring for Children* (5th ed., p. 506). Pearson Education, Inc.

[2] Cystic Fibrosis Foundation. (n.d.). *About cystic fibrosis.* http://www.cff.org/AboutCF/

[3] Mayo Clinic. (n.d.). *Cystic fibrosis.* http://www.mayoclinic.com/health/cystic-fibrosis/DS00287

[4] Barrett, M. & Murphy Moore, C. (2019). Students with chronic respiratory conditions: Asthma and cystic fibrosis. In J. Selekman, R. Adair Shannon, & C. F. Yonkaitis (Eds.), *School nursing: A comprehensive text* (3rd ed., pp. 540-546). F.A. Davis Company.

[5] Cystic Fibrosis Foundation. (n.d.). *Living with CF at school.* http://www.cff.org/LivingWithCF/AtSchool/

[6] Barrett, M. & Murphy Moore, C. (2019). Students with chronic respiratory conditions: Asthma and cystic fibrosis. In J. Selekman, R. Adair Shannon, & C. F. Yonkaitis (Eds.), *School nursing: A comprehensive text* (3rd ed., pp. 540-546). F.A. Davis Company.

CYTOMEGALOVIRUS (CMV)

DEFINITION/ETIOLOGY:
Cytomegalovirus (CMV) is one of a group of highly host-specific herpes viruses (herpes 1 & 2, Epstein Barr and varicella/shingles). The virus cycles between stages of an active infection and dormancy and an infected person can "shed" the virus at any time. Depending upon the age and the immune status of the host, CMV can cause a variety of clinical syndromes, collectively known as cytomegalic inclusion disease, although the majority of infections are very mild or subclinical. [1] Young children are often infected from the saliva of playmates and older people by sexual partners. CMV can be transmitted through body fluids including urine, blood, saliva, secretions (e.g. breast milk, tears, semen, and vaginal fluids), blood transfusion products, transplanted organs and during the birthing process.[2]

<u>CLINICAL MANIFESTATIONS</u>:[3, 4]

Congenital CMV *(*Fetus/Newborn): may cause intrauterine death or severely affect newborn. These negative outcomes may include microcephaly, poor temperature control, hearing loss, vision impairment, *c*hronic liver disease, developmental disabilities, intellectual disabilities, pneumonia, seizures, and other conditions. Symptoms may develop months after birth. Approximately 10% of babies with Congenital CMV are symptomatic.

Acquired CMV (Infant/Toddler*)* occurs postnatally: milder infections may be asymptomatic with excretion of virus in the urine.

Older Children/Adults: CMV is present in the environment; about half of adults have antibodies against the organism; blood transfusions and organ transplants can convey infection; immunosuppressed and pregnant individuals are at particular risk.

SIGNS AND SYMPTOMS:[5, 6]

- Generally, none except in the severely affected newborn; those who survive will usually be served under Individuals with Disabilities Education Act (i.e., special education) due to cognitive impairment and other developmental disabilities.
- An infectious mononucleosis-like syndrome can occur in older children and young adults (fever, sore throat, fatigue, jaundice, and swollen glands).
- More serious symptoms may be seen in people with compromised immunity affecting the liver, stomach, eyes, and lungs.
- Diagnosis is made by rising antibody titer in blood, or isolation of virus from the urine.

MANAGEMENT/TREATMENT:[7, 8, 9]

- Acute disease is rarely diagnosed in school-age children.
- Special education staff and other school personnel who handle diapers should always use "universal/standard precautions". *(Refer to Standard Precautions Appendix*).
- Quarantine is unnecessary but pregnant teachers should not change diapers of known children shedding CMV.
- No vaccine is available. Recent clinical trials show that vaccines help prevent CMV or decrease symptoms.

CYTOMEGALOVIRUS (CMV) *(continued from previous page)*

MANAGEMENT/TREATMENT *(continued)*

- Specific treatment with intravenous antiviral drugs is generally reserved for individuals who are immunosuppressed.
- CMV has a predilection for the retina with the possible development of retinitis.

FOLLOW UP:

- Some children will have serial urine cultures to determine when they stop shedding the virus.
- Educate staff that **pregnant women and immunosuppressed individuals are the only ones at significant risk.**[10]

POTENTIAL COMPLICATIONS:

Most babies born with CMV never develop symptoms or disabilities. However, 1 in 5 babies do have symptoms or long-term complications from congenital CMV.[11] Some resolve while others can be permanent. Examples of potential complications of CMV include:[12]

Temporary Symptoms	Permanent Symptoms or Disabilities
• Liver problems	• Hearing loss
• Spleen problems	• Vision loss
• Jaundice (yellow skin and eyes)	• Mental disability
• Purple skin splotches	• Small head (microcephaly)
• Lung problems	• Lack of coordination
• Small size at birth	• Seizures
• Seizures	• Death
• Pneumonia	
• Intestinal complications	
• Mononucleosis	

Children with compromised immunity may present with an illness similar to infectious mononucleosis and other organs may be affected. Symptoms may include:[13, 14, 15]

- Fever
- Pneumonia
- Diarrhea
- Ulcers in the digestive tract, possible causing bleeding
- Hepatitis
- Encephalitis
- Behavioral changes
- Seizures
- Coma
- Visual impairment and blindness

CYTOMEGALOVIRUS (CMV) *(continued from previous page)*

POTENTIAL COMPLICATIONS *(continued)*

Most people infected with CMV experience few if any symptoms. Some adults may also present with symptoms similar to mononucleosis (fatigue, fever and muscle aches).

PREVENTION:[16, 17]

- Use Universal/Standard Precautions (for infection). (*Refer to STANDARD PRECAUTIONS APPENDIX*).
- Encourage childbearing staff to consult a healthcare provider and inform them of the risk of CMV exposure. Once informed of the risk and referred to their healthcare provider, childbearing staff should sign a document that they are aware of the risk to an unborn child. The document should be stored in the personnel file in the Human Resource Office.[18] (See NOTES, bullet 2).
- Practice good handwashing. (*Refer to HANDWASHING APPENDIX*).
- Avoid contact with infectious body fluids (drool, other oral secretions, and diapers).
- Avoid contact with tears and saliva of infected child.
- Avoid sharing food, eating utensils and drinking from the same glass.
- Do not put a child's pacifier in your mouth.
- Do not use someone else's toothbrush.
- Do not touch inside of mouth, nose or eye after contact with body fluids of an infection person.
- Clean surface and toys.

NOTES:[19, 20, 21, 22,23]

- In settings for children <three years old, exclusion or screening children for CMV does not have any benefit since it is so prevalent.
- In 2015, there was successful litigation against a childcare facility because they did not provide information about the risk of CMV exposure during pregnancy and did not encourage consultation with a healthcare provider.
- After neonatal infection, virus may be excreted for five to six years (children aged seven and older rarely pose a threat); CMV is excreted (urine, saliva) by a large number of children in day care centers, which may represent a community reservoir.
- If the mother has a primary CMV infection during pregnancy, the risk of transmitting the disease is high. However, if CMV is reactivated during pregnancy the risk of transmission to the fetus is low.
- If congenital CMV is suspected, it is important to test the infant within three weeks otherwise it is considered acquired CMV.
- CMV should be considered if an infant becomes severely ill shortly after birth.
- If CMV is found in breast milk, breast-feeding is not discouraged as usually no signs, symptoms or disease occur.
- Approximately 60 percent to 90 percent of adults have had a CMV infection resulting in lifelong latent infection.

CYTOMEGALOVIRUS (CMV) *(continued from previous page)*

NOTES *(continued)*

- Once CMV is in the body, it remains present for life. If healthy, CMV is often dormant and goes undiagnosed.
- CMV does not reactivate unless an individual is immunosuppressed.
- No cure is available for CMV, but antiviral medication is available to slow down the infection for those at risk.

REFERENCES

[1] American Academy of Pediatrics, Committee on Infectious Diseases. (2018). Cytomegalovirus infection. In D.W. Kimberlin, M.T. Brady, M.T., M.A. Jackson, & S.S. Long (Eds.), *Red Book, (2018-2021): Report of the Committee on Infectious Diseases* (31st ed., pp. 310-317). American Academy of Pediatrics.

[2] Centers for Disease Control. (2018). *Cytomegalovirus (CMV) and congenital CMV infection.* http://www.cdc.gov/cmv/overview.html

[3] Merck Manual Professional Version. (2018). *Cytomegalovirus Infections.* https://www.merckmanuals.com/professional/infectious-diseases/herpesviruses/cytomegalovirus-cmv-infection?query=CMV

[4] Schleiss, M., Windle, M., & Steele, R. (2018). Pediatric cytomegalovirus infection clinical presentation._*Medscape.* https://emedicine.medscape.com/article/963090-clinical

[5] Centers for Disease Control. (2018). *Cytomegalovirus (CMV) and congenital CMV infection.* http://www.cdc.gov/cmv/overview.html

[6] American Academy of Pediatrics, Committee on Infectious Diseases. (2018). Cytomegalovirus infection. In D.W. Kimberlin, M.T. Brady, M.T., M.A. Jackson, & S.S. Long (Eds.), *Red Book, (2018-2021): Report of the Committee on Infectious Diseases* (31st ed., pp. 310-317). American Academy of Pediatrics.

[7] Centers for Disease Control. (2018). *Cytomegalovirus (CMV) and congenital CMV infection.* http://www.cdc.gov/cmv/overview.html

[8] American Academy of Pediatrics. (2020). Cytomegalovirus. In S. Aronson, & T. Shope, (Eds.), *Managing infectious diseases in child care and schools* (5th ed., p.81-82). American Academy of Pediatrics.

[9] National Institute of Neurological Disorders and Stroke. (2019). *NINDS neurological consequences of cytomegalovirus infection information page.* https://www.ninds.nih.gov/Disorders/All-Disorders/Neurological-Consequences-Cytomegalovirus-Infection-Information-Page

[10] American Academy of Pediatrics, Committee on Infectious Diseases. (2018). Cytomegalovirus infection. In D.W. Kimberlin, M.T. Brady, M.T., M.A. Jackson, & S.S. Long (Eds.), *Red Book, (2018-2021): Report of the Committee on Infectious Diseases* (31st ed., pp. 310-317). American Academy of Pediatrics.

[11] Centers for Disease Control. (2018). *Cytomegalovirus (CMV) and congenital CMV infection.* http://www.cdc.gov/cmv/overview.html

[12] Merck Manual Professional Version. (2018). *Cytomegalovirus Infections.* https://www.merckmanuals.com/professional/infectious-diseases/herpesviruses/cytomegalovirus-cmv-infection?query=CMV

[13] Centers for Disease Control. (2018). *Cytomegalovirus (CMV) and congenital CMV infection.* http://www.cdc.gov/cmv/overview.html

CYTOMEGALOVIRUS (CMV) *(continued from previous page)*

[14] Merck Manual Professional Version. (2018). *Cytomegalovirus Infections.* https://www.merckmanuals.com/professional/infectious-diseases/herpesviruses/cytomegalovirus-cmv-infection?query=CMV

[15] Schleiss, M., Windle, M., & Steele, R. (2018). Pediatric cytomegalovirus infection clinical presentation._*Medscape.* https://emedicine.medscape.com/article/963090-clinical

[16] American Academy of Pediatrics. (2020). Cytomegalovirus. In S. Aronson, & T. Shope, (Eds.), *Managing infectious diseases in child care and schools* (5th ed., pp.81-82). American Academy of Pediatrics.

[17] Centers for Disease Control. (2018). *Cytomegalovirus (CMV) and congenital CMV infection.* http://www.cdc.gov/cmv/overview.html

[18] American Academy of Pediatrics. (2020). Cytomegalovirus. In S. Aronson, & T. Shope, (Eds.), *Managing infectious diseases in child care and schools* (5th ed., pp.81-82). American Academy of Pediatrics.

[19] National Institute of Neurological Disorders and Stroke. (2019). *NINDS neurological consequences of cytomegalovirus infection information page.* https://www.ninds.nih.gov/Disorders/All-Disorders/Neurological-Consequences-Cytomegalovirus-Infection-Information-Page

[20] American Academy of Pediatrics, Committee on Infectious Diseases. (2018). Cytomegalovirus infection. In D.W. Kimberlin, M.T. Brady, M.T., M.A. Jackson, & S.S. Long (Eds.), *Red Book, (2018-2021): Report of the Committee on Infectious Diseases* (31st ed., pp. 310-317). American Academy of Pediatrics.

[21] Mayo Clinic. (2017). *Cytomegalovirus infection.* https://www.mayoclinic.org/diseases-conditions/cmv/symptoms-causes/syc-20355358

[22] American Academy of Pediatrics. (2020). Cytomegalovirus. In S. Aronson, & T. Shope, (Eds.), *Managing infectious diseases in child care and schools* (5th ed., pp.81-82). American Academy of Pediatrics.

[23] Merck Manual Professional Version. (2018). *Cytomegalovirus Infections.* https://www.merckmanuals.com/professional/infectious-diseases/herpesviruses/cytomegalovirus-cmv-infection?query=CMV

DENTAL EMERGENCIES

DEFINITION/ETIOLOGY:

Nearly one half of children have a dental injury to a tooth during their childhood.[1] Tooth and mouth injuries are generally not considered life threatening but may require immediate dental or medical attention. Falls, sports-related injuries, and fights are the most common causes of tooth injury in children. Mouth injuries can also occur when a child trips or is pushed with an object in the mouth.[2] Frequently, injury to a tooth or the oral cavity can be prevented or lessened by use of appropriate equipment or a mouth guard.

Mouth guards are one of the least expensive pieces of protective gear available. They can help prevent or minimize tooth and jaw injuries. The American Association of Orthodontists recommends mouth guards be worn any time the teeth could be hit by a ball, a hard object, another player or the pavement. The recommendation applies to organized sports and leisure activities like bicycling.[3]

Tooth decay (cavities) while not an emergency, is one of the most common chronic conditions of childhood in the United States. About 1 in 5 (20%) children aged five to 11 years have at least one untreated decayed tooth,[4] and about 1 in 7 (13%) adolescents aged 12–19 years have at least one untreated decayed tooth.[5] The percentage of children and adolescents aged five to 19 years with untreated tooth decay is twice as high for those from low-income families (25%) compared with children from higher-income households (11%).[6] Untreated decay can result in pain and emergent conditions including dental abscess which will impede a students ability to learn. (*Refer to ORAL HEALTH).*

Prevention education is critical as injuries to permanent teeth are costly financially, physiologically, and emotionally having a lasting impact on a person's dentition, self-esteem and confidence.

SIGNS AND SYMPTOMS:

A healthcare provider should be contacted for the following.[7] Depending upon the circumstances, this contact may be done over the phone, at the pediatrician's or dentist's office, or in an emergency department:

- If there is pain, tenderness, or sensitivity (to hot/cold or pressure) in a tooth
- If there is an avulsed tooth (knocked out due to trauma) or luxated/dislocated tooth
- If there is a broken, loose, or missing tooth after trauma (the tooth could have been inhaled or swallowed)
- If there is bleeding that does not stop after applying pressure for 10 minutes
- If there is pain in the jaw when opening or closing the mouth
- If there is difficulty swallowing or breathing
- If there is an object stuck in the roof of the mouth, cheek, tongue, or throat (do NOT remove the object)
- If there is a large or gaping cut inside the mouth or on the face
- If the child could have a puncture in the back of the throat

DENTAL EMERGENCIES *(continued from previous page)*

SIGNS AND SYMPTOMS *(continued)*

- If there is a cut on the lip that extends through the lip's border into the surrounding skin
- If after a mouth or tooth injury, the child is weak, numb, or has blurred vision or slurred speech
- If the parent is concerned about the child's condition
- If the child develops a fever (temperature ≥100.4ºF/38ºC) or other signs of infection after a mouth or tooth injury (localized redness, pus, increasing pain); signs of more serious infection may include neck pain or stiffness, inability to open the mouth completely, drooling, or chest pain.

MANAGEMENT/TREATMENT:

AVULSED TOOTH*[8]

If a knocked out tooth is handled correctly, there is a good possibility the dentist will be able to put the tooth placed back into the socket if the child is seen within 30 minutes. Approximately 85% of avulsed teeth placed in the socket within 5 minutes survive.

1. **Activate Emergency Medical Services (EMS) or contact parent/guardian for transport immediately to the dentist.**
2. **Do not touch the root of the tooth.**
3. Do not change the tooth's protective coating by trying to clean it. At most, gently rinse off debris with cool water.
4. Gently place the tooth back into its socket (do not use force) **only** if the student is alert and cooperative. Instruct student to keep pressure on tooth by biting gently on clean gauze.
5. If unable to replace tooth in socket, place the tooth in a protective container filled with pH balanced solution for transport with the student to the Emergency Department or dental specialist. If this solution is not available, use saline solution or cold milk or the child's saliva. **Do not store in tap water**.
6. Do not attempt to reinsert a **primary** tooth back in the socket. This might cause damage to the developing permanent tooth. Instead, the tooth should be taken to the dentist so that he or she can be sure the tooth was lost in its entirety and the root not broken.

**Maxillary central incisor is most frequently avulsed.*

FRACTURED TOOTH

1. Rinse the mouth with warm water.
2. Call parent. Refer to dentist for follow-up treatment.
3. Save fragment/large chip.
4. Place tooth fragment in water and send with the child to the dentist.
5. Apply cool compress to reduce facial swelling.
6. If possible, call dentist and describe extent of chip.
7. Cover jagged edge of tooth with gauze.
8. Apply cold compress or a washcloth with ice to the cheek to reduce pain and swelling.

DENTAL EMERGENCIES *(continued from previous page)*

MANAGEMENT/TREATMENT *(continued)*

LUXATED/DISLOCATED TOOTH

1. For permanent tooth, **time is of the essence**.
2. Reposition tooth gently.
3. Call parent and dentist for emergency visit.
4. Put gauze around tooth and have student hold it there during transportation to dentist.

FRACTURED JAW [9]

1. Immobilize jaw placing a scarf, tie or towel under the chin. Tie the ends on top of the head. Avoid pressure on the neck.
2. Apply cold packs to reduce pain/edema.
3. Notify parent/guardian and dentist.

PUNCTURE WOUNDS

1. Do not remove the embedded object in any part of the mouth.
2. Seek immediate medical care.
3. This injury may require referral to surgeon.

FOLLOW-UP:

- Monitor hygiene and diet: After a tooth or mouth injury, continue keeping the teeth clean. Encourage brushing twice per day with a soft bristled toothbrush. Occasionally, a mouthwash will be prescribed to prevent swelling and infection.
- If a child's tooth is loose or the mouth is sore, a soft diet is recommended for several days. Children who have stitches in the mouth should avoid spicy or salty food, popcorn, and straws for approximately one week.
- Monitor for persistent pain, sensitivity to hot and cold, discoloration of tooth.
- Possible tetanus booster if less than 12 years old.
- Monitor for persistent bleeding - prolonged or recurrent, after dental injury or extraction of tooth:
    1. Place a sterile gauze pad on the extraction site and have the student gently bite on it for 30 minutes.
    2. Replace soaked gauze pads as necessary.
    3. Consult a dentist if bleeding persists over 1 hour; sooner if bleeding appears excessive. If bleeding is spontaneous without trauma, refer to healthcare provider.

DENTAL EMERGENCIES *(continued from previous page)*

POTENTIAL COMPLICATIONS:

- Dental pulp fracture
- Displaced tooth
- Embedded tooth fragments
- Discoloration of tooth
- Loss of tooth
- Possible root canal or crown in the future
- Wounds may heal with a scar that may affect swallowing and speech

NOTES:

- When a facial or dental injury occurs at school, the school nurse, rather than a dentist, may be the first one contacted.
- Taking a quick, complete, injury specific history is essential.
- If the child has no life-threatening symptoms (airway compromise, change in mental status or level of consciousness, or excessive bleeding), briefly obtain any additional history that would influence advice, such as past medical history, whether the child has any special healthcare needs, or significant social information.
- Next, it becomes important to determine if the injury requires a medical or dental referral. The head, neck, and oral cavity have a tremendous vascular supply; therefore, blood may obscure a significant injury, or it may make a mild injury appear much worse that it is. If it is clear the injury is primarily dental, help the parent/guardian to access a child's dentist immediately.

Other considerations include:

1. Education on prevention of dental injuries
    a. Types and use of mouth guards
    b. Do not put anything but food in the mouth
    c. Sit while eating
    d. Do not chew hard candy, popcorn kernels, ice, etc.
2. Special hygiene and diet instructions following an injury.

DENTAL EMERGENCIES *(continued from previous page)*

REFERENCES

[1] McTigue, D. J., & Thompson, A. (2015). *Patient information: Mouth and dental injuries in children.* http://www.uptodate.com/contents/mouth-and-dental-injuries-in-children-beyond-the-basics?view=print

[2] Ibid.

[3] American Association of Orthodontists. (2017*). Preventing accidents.* https://www.aaoinfo.org/system/files/media/documents/Prevent_Accidents_flyer-13-l.pdf

[4] Centers for Disease Control and Prevention. (2017). *Oral health in schools.* https://www.cdc.gov/healthyschools/npao/oralhealth.htm

[5] Ibid.

[6] Ibid.

[7] McTigue, D. J., & Thompson, A. (2015). *Patient information: Mouth and dental injuries in children.* http://www.uptodate.com/contents/mouth-and-dental-injuries-in-children-beyond-the-basics?view=print

[8] Illinois Emergency Medical Services. (2017). *Guidelines for the nurse in the school setting (3rd ed.).* https://www.luriechildrens.org/globalassets/documents/emsc/resourcesguidelines/guidelines-tool-and-other-resources/practice-guidelinestools/guidelinesfornurseinschoolsetting3rdeditionapril2017.pdf

[9] Ibid.

DEPRESSION

DEFINITION/ETIOLOGY:
Depression is an affective illness or mood disorder characterized by dysphoric moods (emotions such as sadness, irritability, mood swings, and hopelessness) and affect (sad facies) and self-devaluation (e.g., feeling worthless). Clinical depression is characterized by a combination of specific symptoms that persist *more than three weeks* and *cause functional problems* at home, school or in social relationships.[1] Depression is a leading cause of school failure, especially in students with learning difficulties, and suicidal ideation.[2]

CAUSES:
Primary or familial-genetic depression. About a third of depressed children have a biological parent who is affectively ill.[3] Research suggests that the right parietotemporal cortex of the brain plays a role in depression. In depressed states, there is a relatively low level of the neurotransmitters serotonin and norepinephrine.

Secondary or symptomatic depression is a response to problems such as early childhood traumas, chronic health conditions, learned patterns of helpless thinking, learning disabilities, peer pressure, significant losses or having a family member commit suicide.

Comorbidity with other mental health disorders (anxiety, disruptive disorders, Attention Deficit/Hyperactivity Disorder [ADHD], substance abuse) is common in adolescents.

SIGNS AND SYMPTOMS:
Depression is expressed differently among age groups. Developmentally, preschoolers may have difficulty expressing feelings and emotions. Symptoms in preschool age children include regression of developmental milestones and nonorganic failure to thrive.

Children are more likely to have:
- Somatic complaints
- Separation anxiety
- Insomnia at night and fears (i.e. being alone, of the dark, something bad happening)
- Irritability

Adolescents exhibit both emotional and behavioral symptoms:
<u>Emotional:</u>
- Crying spells for no apparent reason
- Irritability
- Difficulty focusing or concentrating – decline in school performance
- Fatigue
- Feelings of helplessness, worthlessness, isolation
- Feeling sad or down
- Tremendous sensitivity to failure or rejection
- Loss of interest and pleasure in developmentally appropriate activities
- Socially withdrawn from friends and family
- Recurrent suicidal ideations

DEPRESSION *(continued from previous page)*

SIGNS AND SYMPTOMS *(continued)*

Behavioral:

- Appetite changes associated with weight gain or weight loss
- Agitation, disruptive behavior
- Decrease in school performance
- Insomnia or hypersomnia
- Somatic complaints – headaches, stomachaches, etc.
- Disheveled appearance
- Self-mutilation (cutting, burning, excessive piercing/tattooing)
- Extreme risk taking

MANAGEMENT/TREATMENT:

1. **If immediate danger is suspected, student must not be left alone while Emergency Medical Services (EMS) or local emergency crisis number is called.**

2. **Therapy**:
   Young children may benefit the most from play therapy. Comprehensive treatment including both individual (cognitive behavioral therapy/interpersonal psychotherapy) and family therapy has been shown to be effective in treating depression in older children and adolescents.[4] The focus is not on emotions, but on behaviors that influence feelings, e.g., "feels sad but act positive to help you feel better."

3. **Medication:**
   Treatment may also include the use of antidepressant medication. These drugs affect neurotransmitters such as serotonin and norepinephrine in the brain. The choice of drug is related to age, weight, family history of illness and response to medication, and the nature of depression or its related conditions, e.g., bipolar disorder. Selective serotonin reuptake inhibitors (SSRI's) such as Prozac, Zoloft and Paxil have fewer side effects than older antidepressants. Other classes of drugs include tricyclics and MAOI's (monoamine oxidase inhibitors).

Antidepressants may increase the risk that a child/teen may have suicidal ideations. Closely monitor children/teens who take antidepressants. Educate staff and parents/guardians regarding the warning signs of suicide (talking, writing, or drawing about death, giving belongings away, withdrawing from family and friends, etc.). ***(Refer to Suicide Ideation/Threats).***

DEPRESSION *(continued from previous page)*

MANAGEMENT/TREATMENT *(continued)*

4. **Electroconvulsive therapy (ECT)** may be used in adolescents when there is no improvement in symptoms with other therapies.[5]

5. **School-home Communication**
   A team approach with consistent messages from adults at home and school that reassure the child/youth and do not allow him/her to drop routines and social interactions.

FOLLOW UP:
- Collaborate with community-based providers.
- Monitor for adverse effects from pharmacotherapy.
- Participate in the Section 504 planning for accommodations.
- Develop an Emergency Care Plan for students who exhibit behaviors that are safety concerns.
- Develop an Individualized Healthcare Plan (IHP) as necessary.
- Encourage exercise: clinical evidence links physical activity with mood improvement [6]

POTENTIAL COMPLICATIONS:
- Alcohol/Substance Abuse
- Anxiety
- Family/relationship conflicts
- Involvement with the court system
- School problems
- Social isolation
- Self-mutilation
- Suicide

NOTES:
The school nurse may suspect depression with:
- Teacher referrals for inattention, falling asleep in class (due to inadequate sleep at night).
- Frequent student visits for tiredness, headache, stomachache, panic attack, and muscle aches.
- Vague vision problems.
- Referrals for school avoidance (school "phobia") or declining school performance.
- Informal observation of weight change, disheveled appearance, irritability with friends, dropping out of extracurricular activities.
- Consider depression as a significant factor in students with learning failures or discipline infractions, e.g., fights, especially among males.
- Anticipate depression as a response to chronic illness, significant losses or stress, abuse, neglect or exposure to violence.

DEPRESSION *(continued from previous page)*

NOTES *(continued)*

The school nurse is the key school professional to:

- Report responses to medication and communicate any concerns for missed or excessive doses with the parent and prescribing healthcare provider.
- Inform teachers of anticipated side effects as needed.
- Develop an IHP, in partnership with the school-home team, to respond constructively to somatic complaints (without minimizing significant illnesses or injuries) and reinforce positive behaviors, e.g., good attendance, engaging in school activities.
- Educate the student about the need for consistent medication use and to not take anyone else's medication.
- Educate staff and students (health education) to recognize that children of any age can experience and exhibit signs of depression.

Other:

- Screening in 12-18-year olds for major depression is recommended by the U.S. Prevention Task Force if support systems are in place for diagnosis, therapy and follow up.[7]
- Some diseases such as hypothyroidism or anemia can cause symptoms that look like depression. The healthcare provider may order diagnostic tests to rule out these physical conditions.

RESOURCES

- **Families for Depression Awareness**. (2019). http://familyaware.org
- **National Association of School Nurses.** (2019). https://www.nasn.org/nasn/nasn-resources/practice-topics/mental-health. Helpful handouts including interventions and screening.
- **U.S. Department of Health and Human Services**. (2019). Substance Abuse and Mental Health Services (SAMHSA). Evidenced Based Practice Resource Center. https://www.samhsa.gov/ebp-resource-center

REFERENCES

---

[1] American Psychiatric Association. (2013). Diagnostic and statistical manual of mental disorders (DSM-V) (5th ed.) American Psychiatric Association.

[2] American Academy of Child and Adolescent Psychiatry. (2019). *Depression in children and teens.* https://www.aacap.org/AACAP/Families_and_Youth/Facts_for_Families/FFF-Guide/The-Depressed-Child-004.aspx

[3] CASA of Arizona. (2020). *Childhood depression*. https://www.azcourts.gov/casa/Training/Training-Courses/Childhood-Depression

[4] Centers for Disease Control and Prevention. (2019). *Children's mental health: Anxiety and depression in children.* https://www.cdc.gov/childrensmentalhealth/depression.html

[5] American Psychiatric Association. (2013). Diagnostic and statistical manual of mental disorders (DSM-V) (5th ed.) American Psychiatric Association.

DEPRESSION *(continued from previous page)*

[6] National Institute of Mental Health. (2019). *Depression basics*.
https://www.nimh.nih.gov/health/publications/depression/index.shtml

[7] Centers for Disease Control and Prevention. (2019). *Children's mental health: Anxiety and depression in children.*
https://www.cdc.gov/childrensmentalhealth/depression.html

DIABETES EMERGENCIES *(Refer to DIABETES TYPE I)*

DEFINITION/ETIOLOGY:

A diabetic emergency is a life-threatening condition. Diabetic emergencies occur when there is a severe imbalance between blood glucose, physical activity and insulin. There are two types of diabetic emergencies: hypoglycemia and hyperglycemia.

HYPOGLYCEMIA

Hypoglycemia is low blood glucose and is the greatest immediate danger to the student with diabetes. Causes include:

- Too much insulin
- Not enough food or student eats less than insulin dose calculated
- Delayed snack or missed meal
- Too much exercise without snack before
- Prescribed or over-the-counter medication

SIGNS AND SYMPTOMS: HYPOGLYCEMIA[1]

- Vary from person to person
- Symptoms develop rapidly without warning
- Children may not always demonstrate outward symptoms
- Some students (especially young or nonverbal children) may not recognize or communicate symptoms of hypoglycemia (hypoglycemia unaware)

Mild	Moderate	Severe
○ Hunger ○ Difficulty concentrating or inattention ○ Headache ○ Irritability ○ Shakiness, ○ Sweaty and/or pale ○ Weakness ○ Anxious ○ Dizziness ○ Not feeling well ○ Heart Racing ○ Tingling in extremities	○ Sleepiness ○ Erratic behavior including mood changes (aggression, crying, bizarre behavior) ○ Disorientation ○ Confusion ○ Poor coordination ○ Restlessness ○ Slurred speech ○ Slow thinking ○ Numbness	○ Inability to swallow ○ Unresponsiveness ○ Unconscious ○ Seizures

DIABETES EMERGENCIES *(continued from previous page)*

MANAGEMENT/TREATMENT: <u>HYPOGLYCEMIA</u>
Treatment for hypoglycemia is individualized and is based on the student's blood glucose target ranges and history.[2]

Mild-Moderate Hypoglycemia blood glucose below the level indicated in the student's Emergency Care Plan (ECP) (for most students <70 -80mg/dl or > 70 mg/dL with symptoms)[3]

Note: Continuous glucose monitoring and alternate testing sites that test interstitial fluid may lag behind fingerstick blood glucose results. If there is any concern as to the accuracy of the sensor reading, a fingerstick should be done to confirm the glucose reading, especially if there are arrows indicating that the glucose is changing quickly, or it is within the first 24 hours of a sensor.[4]

- Follow student's ECP. Note student specific blood glucose targets.
- If possible*, perform a fingerstick blood glucose check and follow ECP.
- Follow the *"Rule of 15"*[5] immediately give 15 gram fast-acting carbohydrate such as one of the following:
  - Three to four glucose tablets
  - Four oz. fruit juice or regular soft drink (not diet)
  - One to two tablespoons of honey or glucose
  - One tube glucose gel

Recheck blood glucose level 15 minutes after treatment

- If blood glucose level is still below target range, repeat treatment, contact parent/guardian.
- Suspend basal insulin infusion if indicated in ECP.
- Follow with protein snack plus if it is more than a one hour until meal.

Once the student's blood glucose returns to target range. Check the blood glucose one hour later.

***Note do not delay treatment if a low blood glucose is suspected. If monitoring supplies are unavailable treat with 15-gram carbohydrates.**

Severe hypoglycemic reaction:

- **Position student on side** Position student on side as vomiting is a potential side effect of glucagon.[6]
  - **Do not attempt to give anything by mouth**
  - **Suspend insulin pump if in use**
- If student becomes unconscious, has a seizure or is unable to swallow, administer glucagon IM or SQ or intranasally per licensed healthcare provider's order.
- While treating, have another staff member, activate Emergency Medical Services (EMS) if glucagon is administered.
- Notify parent/guardian.
- Monitor student until EMS arrives.
- Notify student's healthcare provider per ECP.

DIABETES EMERGENCIES *(continued from previous page)*

HYPERGLYCEMIA

Hyperglycemia is a blood glucose level above target range and is **not** considered a medical emergency in the acute stage.[7] Untreated hyperglycemia can progress to ketoacidosis, which **is** a medical emergency.

Causes are:

- Late, missed or too little insulin
- Illness, infection, stress, hormonal response (e.g., menses)
- Expired or heat damaged insulin
- Problem with insulin pump site or pump malfunction
- Excess food intake (for amount of insulin or binge eating)
- Insufficient exercise

SIGNS AND SYMPTOMS: HYPERGLYCEMIA[8]

- Usually develops slowly

Mild	Moderate (mild symptoms plus)	Severe (DKA)
○ Increased thirst ○ Increased urination ○ Change in appetite and nausea ○ Blurry vision ○ Fatigue ○ Hunger, headache ○ Weight loss ○ Lack of concentration	○ Inability to concentrate ○ Abdominal cramps ○ Nausea and vomiting ○ Dry Mouth ○ Lightheaded	○ Nausea and/or vomiting ○ Abdominal cramps ○ Lethargic ○ Breath that smells fruity ○ Respiratory problems, Shortness of breath ○ Weakness ○ Confusion ○ Moderate to Large ketones

MANAGEMENT/TREATMENT: HYPERGLYCEMIA (Blood glucose above target or > 250)[9]

- Follow student's ECP - refer to Diabetes Medical Management Plan (DMMP) for specific instructions.
- Check blood or urine for ketones and report findings to family and/or healthcare provider per DMMP.
- Supplemental insulin may be ordered by licensed healthcare provider. Calculate the Insulin Correction Dose needed and administer supplemental insulin dose in accordance with the student's ECP or DMMP for Hyperglycemia.
- For students using insulin infusion pumps, the lack of rapid-acting insulin increases their risks of developing DKA more rapidly.[10]

DIABETES EMERGENCIES *(continued from previous page)*

MANAGEMENT/TREATMENT: HYPERGLYCEMIA *(continued)*

- For students using an insulin pump:
  - If student uses a pump, check to see if pump is connected properly and functioning by giving a correction bolus through the pump and checking blood glucose level one hour later.
  - If moderate or large ketones are present, change pump site and treat ketones with an injection of insulin by syringe or insulin pen per DMMP.
  - For infusion site failure: Insert new infusion set and/or replace reservoir or give insulin by syringe or insulin pen.
  - For suspected pump failure: Suspend or remove pump and give insulin by syringe or insulin pen per DMMP.[11]
- Encourage the student to drink extra water or non-caloric beverages.
- If asymptomatic and no ketones are present, the student may return to the classroom with access to fluids and unrestricted bathroom privileges.
- Restrict participation in physical activity as specified in the DMMP, note moderate exercise only if ketones are negative and the student is not nauseous or vomiting.
- Repeat ketone testing in one to two hours or next void.
- Recheck blood glucose every two hours or as indicated by the ECP.
- Notify parents/guardians and/or healthcare provider as specified in the DMMP.

ROLE OF THE SCHOOL NURSE:

- Develop and implement an Individualized Healthcare Plan (IHP) and an ECP from student's DMMP[12] which includes:
  - Specific detailed procedures and responsibilities performed by school staff
  - Glucagon administration and storage
  - Section 504 Plan
  - Disaster Plan
  - Plan for field trips and after school activities

- Provide diabetes training ***(Refer to DIABETES TYPE 1)*** Level I, II or III to teachers, cafeteria manager, bus driver and sports coaches.
- Manage and monitor trained staff - delegate diabetes care tasks as permitted by local guidelines, state laws and nurse practice act.
- Distribute and review of ECP with appropriate classrooms and staff.
- Obtain materials and medical supplies necessary for performing diabetes care tasks from parents/guardians.
- Arrange for insulin pump training for nurse and staff for students using insulin pump therapy. Students with insulin pumps require the nurse and staff (as appropriate) to be oriented to the specific unit.

DIABETES EMERGENCIES *(continued from previous page)*

FOLLOW UP:

- Monitor student for continued signs or symptoms of hypoglycemia or hyperglycemia.
- Report incidence to parents/guardians/healthcare provider as required by ECP.
- Inventory supplies used to treat hypoglycemia or hyperglycemia.

PREVENTION:

- Obtain history and review signs and symptoms of hypoglycemia and hyperglycemia experienced with individual student (if known).
- Encourage consistent routine (mealtimes, carbohydrate intake and physical activity).
- Notify parents/guardians in advance of schedule changes and special events.
- Provide a snack if physical activity occurs just before lunch period or in the late afternoon.
- Keep a fast-acting carbohydrate accessible during exercise.
- Keep emergency glucose/glucose in key places, especially in large schools (physical education area, nurse's office, locker, main office).

NOTES:

- Check state laws, nurse practice act and school district policy to determine what tasks of diabetes care can be delegated to unlicensed school personnel.
- Glucagon usually works within 10 minutes.
- Student should wear Medic Alert identification.

RESOURCES:

- **American Diabetes Association**. Provides staff training tools and sample diabetes management and Section 504 plans. www.diabetes.org

- **Diabetes Care Tasks at School** the American Diabetes Association's *Diabetes Care Tasks at School: What Key Personnel Need to Know* is an 18-module training curriculum. Each module has a PowerPoint presentation and some a corresponding video segment. https://www.diabetes.org/resources/know-your-rights/safe-at-school-state-laws/training-resources-school-staff/diabetes-care-tasks-school

- **NDEP GUIDE National Diabetes Education Program**. (2016). *Helping the student with diabetes succeed: A guide for school personnel.* https://www.niddk.nih.gov/health-information/communication-programs/ndep/health-professionals/helping-student-diabetes-succeed-guide-school-personnel

DIABETES EMERGENCIES *(continued from previous page)*

REFERENCES

[1] National Diabetes Education Program. (2016). *Helping the student with diabetes succeed: A guide for school personnel.* https://www.niddk.nih.gov/health-information/communication-programs/ndep/health-professionals/helping-student-diabetes-succeed-guide-school-personnel

[2] Wyckoff, L. (2019). Students with diabetes. In J. Selekman, R.A. Shannon, & C.F. Younkaitis (Eds.), *School Nursing: A comprehensive text* (3rd ed., pp. 575-602). F.A. Davis.

[3] National Diabetes Education Program. (2016). *Helping the student with diabetes succeed: A guide for school personnel.* https://www.niddk.nih.gov/health-information/communication-programs/ndep/health-professionals/helping-student-diabetes-succeed-guide-school-personnel

[4] Wood, J., & Peters, A. (2018*). The Type 1 diabetes self-care manual: A complete guide to diabetes across the lifespan for people with diabetes, parents and caregivers.* American Diabetes Association.

[5] MedlinePlus [Internet]. Bethesda (MD): National Library of Medicine (US); [updated 2018 February]. 15/15 Rule. https://medlineplus.gov/ency/imagepages/19815.htm

[6] National Diabetes Education Program. (2016). *Helping the student with diabetes succeed: A guide for school personnel.* https://www.niddk.nih.gov/health-information/communication-programs/ndep/health-professionals/helping-student-diabetes-succeed-guide-school-personnel

[7] Ibid.

[8] National Diabetes Education Program. (2016). *Helping the student with diabetes succeed: A guide for school personnel.* https://www.niddk.nih.gov/health-information/communication-programs/ndep/health-professionals/helping-student-diabetes-succeed-guide-school-personnel

[9] Joslin Diabetes Center. (2019). *High blood glucose, what it means and how to treat it.* https://www.joslin.org/info/high_blood_glucose_what_it_means_and_how_to_treat_it.html

[10] Brown, C. (2016). 21st-century diabetes: Technology leads the way. *NASN School Nurse, 31* (5), 254-256. https://doi.org/10.1177/1942602X16661198

[11] National Diabetes Education Program. (2016). *Helping the student with diabetes succeed: A guide for school personnel.* https://www.niddk.nih.gov/health-information/communication-programs/ndep/health-professionals/helping-student-diabetes-succeed-guide-school-personnel

[12] Ibid.

DIABETES INSIPIDUS

DEFINITION/ETIOLOGY:

Nephrogenic Diabetes Insipidus (NDI) is a disorder caused by hypofunction of the posterior pituitary gland. The normal storage and release of the antidiuretic hormone (ADH) vasopressin results in a person's kidneys passing an abnormally large volume of urine that is insipid—dilute and odorless. In most people, the kidneys pass about one to two quarts of urine a day. In people with diabetes insipidus, the kidneys can pass 3 to 20 quarts of urine a day. As a result, a person with diabetes insipidus may need to drink large amounts of liquids.[1] NDI can be inherited or occur secondary to conditions that impair renal concentrating ability.[2]

Inherited NDI

- Most commonly X-linked inherited trait
- In rare cases, caused by an autosomal recessive or autosomal dominant mutation that affects both males and females[3]

Acquired NDI can occur when disorders or drugs disrupt the medulla or distal nephrons and impair urine concentrating ability, making the kidneys appear insensitive to vasopressin.

- Among these disorders are polycystic kidney disease, sickle cell nephropathy, pyelonephritis, and certain cancers.
- Many drugs, especially lithium, but also others (e.g. demeclocycline, amphotericin B, dexamethasone, dopamine, ifosfamide, ofloxacin, orlistat)[4] may contribute to the development of NDI.

SIGNS AND SYMPTOMS:

Signs and symptoms are related to dehydration and hypernatremia including:

- Polyuria (Increased urination) may result in nocturia or daytime incontinence
- Polydipsia (Increased thirst)
- Dehydration - thirst, dry skin, fatigue, sluggishness, dizziness, nausea
- Hypernatremia may cause neurologic symptoms such as confusion, seizures or coma

MANAGEMENT/TREATMENT:

- The primary treatment for diabetes insipidus involves drinking enough liquid to prevent dehydration. In addition, medical management may include thiazide diuretics, NSAIDS and a low-salt, low protein diet.
- Contact the parent/guardian for immediate medical evaluation if the student exhibits uncontrolled polyuria and dehydration.[5]

FOLLOW-UP:

- Educate school staff.
- Participate in Section 504 meetings to make sure the student always has unrestricted access to water and unrestricted bathroom privileges.
- Monitor for ongoing signs of dehydration.

POTENTIAL COMPLICATIONS:

Severe dehydration leading to coma and even death can result if fluid loss is greater than liquid intake.

DIABETES INSIPIDUS *(continued from previous page)*

REFERENCES

[1] Young, B., & Verbalis, J. (2015). *Diabetes insipidus*. https://www.niddk.nih.gov/health-information/kidney-disease/diabetes-insipidus

[2] Hechanova, L. A. (2019). *Nephrogenic diabetes insipidus - Genitourinary disorders*. Merck Manuals Professional Edition. https://www.merckmanuals.com/professional/genitourinary-disorders/renal-transport-abnormalities/nephrogenic-diabetes-insipidus

[3] Ibid.

[4] Ibid.

[5] John, T. (2019). Students with other chronic health conditions. In J. Selekman, R.A. Shannon, & C. F. Younkaitis (Eds.), *School Nursing: A comprehensive text* (3rd ed., p. 409). F.A. Davis.

DIABETES -TYPE 1

DEFINITION/ETIOLOGY:

Type 1 diabetes, previously called juvenile or insulin-dependent diabetes, is an autoimmune disease in which there is destruction of the beta cells (insulin producing cells) of the pancreas leading to an absolute insulin deficiency and the subsequent need for exogenous insulin.[1] Insulin is a hormone (chemical messenger) necessary to convert food into energy for normal cell functioning. Without insulin, food is converted into glucose but is unable to move into the cell resulting in high levels in the blood stream and depriving the brain and muscles of the glucose needed to function. Diabetes is the third most common chronic health condition affecting an estimated 2.22/1,000 children and adolescents.[2] It occurs one in 350 children by age 18. Although type 1 can occur at any age, it typically manifests between age four and seven or between 10 and 14 years.[3] The incidences of both type 1 and type 2 diabetes among youths is increasing, particularly type 2 among youths of minority racial and ethnic groups and type 1 in children younger than 5 years old.[4]

Type 1 diabetes was once thought to be of sudden onset, but research suggests that the autoimmune process progresses over time and presents rather suddenly with hyperglycemia when the declining number of beta-cells can no longer compensate. At the point when 80% of the beta cells are no longer producing insulin, hyperglycemia occurs and the possibility for ketosis increases.[5] According to a new staging classification system, type 1 diabetes develops in three stages:

- Stage 1 is defined as the presence of β-cell autoimmunity as evidenced by two or more islet autoantibodies with normoglycemia and is presymptomatic.
- Stage 2 is the presence of β-cell autoimmunity with dysglycemia and is presymptomatic.
- Onset of symptomatic disease resulting from insulin deficiency in children with type 1 diabetes occurs at stage 3.[6]

Type 1 diabetes is most often diagnosed during childhood and requires lifelong insulin replacement, by multiple daily injections with syringe/vial or pen/needle or continuous subcutaneous insulin infusion via an insulin pump.

Normal fasting blood glucose is 70-100 mg/dl. An A1c target of <7.5% should be considered in children and adolescents with type 1 diabetes but should also be individualized based on the needs and situation of the patient and family.[7] A lower goal (<7.0%) is reasonable if it can be achieved without excessive hypoglycemia.[8] With increasing use of continuous glucose monitoring devices (CGM), outcomes other than A1c, such as time with glucose in target range and frequency of hypoglycemia, may be considered in the overall assessment of glycemic control.[9] High blood sugar levels (hyperglycemia) without adequate insulin can lead to Diabetic Ketoacidosis (DKA), in which the body breaks down stored fat and proteins, resulting in production of ketone (acid) bodies, dehydration, cerebral edema, and potentially death. Low blood sugar levels (hypoglycemia) can lead to loss of consciousness, brain damage, and potentially death. The management strategies used to achieve and maintain target blood sugar levels are individualized for each child. Advances in technology have provided more options for treatment than ever before.[10]

COMORBID CONDITIONS:

- Thyroid dysfunction
- Celiac Disease and other autoimmune disorders including Addison's disease

DIABETES -TYPE 1 *(continued from previous page)*

SIGNS AND SYMPTOMS:

Hyperglycemia:

- Polydipsia (Increased thirst)
- Polyuria (Increased urination) may result in nocturia or daytime incontinence
- Polyphagia (Increased hunger)
- Unexplained weight loss
- Impaired growth
- Fatigue
- Vision changes
- Nausea and vomiting

Hypoglycemia: *

- Shakiness
- Dizziness
- Pale skin
- Weakness
- Confusion
- Behavior change/irritability/emotional
- Loss of consciousness
- Seizure

***Symptoms of hypoglycemia vary from person to person. Some children do not demonstrate any outward symptoms of hypoglycemia and young children may be unable to communicate the symptoms that they are experiencing. Hypoglycemic unawareness (inability to recognize symptoms of low blood glucose) also known as Impaired Awareness of Hypoglycemia (IAH) is a syndrome in which the ability to detect the onset of hypoglycemia is diminished or absent. This is believed to be caused by changes in hormonal counter regulation system, especially a decrease in the hormonal response of epinephrine.[11]**

MANAGEMENT/TREATMENT:

- Monitor blood glucose levels with glucometer or CGM per healthcare provider orders. Often testing is before snack, meals, physical education/sports, before dismissal and as needed for symptoms of hypoglycemia and hyperglycemia.

- Insulin - injection via pen/syringe or continuous subcutaneous (pump) vary among children and dosages are individualized with each administration. Basal/Bolus regimen most mimics the normal pancreatic function. Basal insulin may be injected using a long acting insulin or administered continuously via a pump. Dosing determined by the Diabetes Medical Management Plan (DMMP) may be based on a sliding scale, carb to insulin ratio and sensitivity factors.

- Physical activity is important in maintaining stable blood glucose levels. Exercise is also a risk factor for hypoglycemia that can occur during the activity, immediately following and up to 48 hours after activity. Exercise may help lower blood glucose levels in the absence of ketones. However, exercise is **NOT** recommended when the blood glucose is elevated, **and** ketones are present in the blood or urine due to increased risk of DKA;[12] follow the DMMP.

DIABETES -TYPE 1 *(continued from previous page)*

MANAGEMENT/TREATMENT *(continued)*

- Medical nutrition therapy is important in diabetes prevention, managing existing diabetes and slowing the rate of development of diabetes related complications.[13] A well-balanced diet is recommended for all children. Insulin dosing may be determined by calculating the total carbohydrate to be consumed divided by the insulin to carbohydrate ratio (I:C ratio) and correcting (adding or subtracting insulin) for the current blood sugar level divided by the sensitivity (Grams of carbohydrate divided by I:C ratio) + (Blood sugar - target blood sugar divided by sensitivity factor). Accurate nutritional information including the carbohydrate count is critical to avoid underdosing or overdosing of insulin.[14]

- Treatment of hypoglycemia follows "The Rule of 15"- 15 grams of carbohydrate and recheck the blood glucose in 15 minutes for mild hypoglycemia. Episodes of moderate hypoglycemia may require the use of glucose gel if alert, but unable to follow directions. Emergency glucagon administration is indicated for episodes of severe hypoglycemia resulting in loss of consciousness and/or seizures.[15] *(**Refer to Diabetes Emergencies**).*

- Treatment of hyperglycemia per the child's emergency plan. Encourage drinking water. Urine or blood ketone testing as ordered by healthcare provider during episodes of hyperglycemia and illness. *(**Refer to Diabetes Emergencies**).*

General Management

Diabetes requires an individualized care and lifestyle plan balancing daily dietary intake, physical activity, medication (if ordered) and self-monitored blood glucose.[16] Children can learn to use glucometers and, in time, to self-administer insulin as ordered. A lab test called hemoglobin A1c or simply "A1c" measures the past three to four months' fasting and post meal blood glucose levels. A1C should be measured in all children and adolescents with type 1 diabetes at three-month intervals to assess their overall glycemic control.[17]

A team approach including students, families, healthcare providers, and school staff (food services, physical education, counseling staff, teachers, bus drivers and administration) led by the school nurse, can assist with risk reduction as well as condition management. The school nurse is the coordinator of care in school, but all staff that have responsibility for the student should have basic training to understand diabetes and the needs of these students.

Training for school personnel is recommended to follow three levels of training.[18]

- Level One training should be provided as basic information to all personnel.
- Level Two training is more in depth for those who have direct contact with the child during the school day.
- Level Three training is in-depth training for a small group of unlicensed personnel who will assist with specific diabetes management for the student, for those states that allow the registered nurse to delegate tasks (see your state Nurse Practice Act).

DIABETES -TYPE 1 *(continued from previous page)*

General Management *(continued)*

The **Diabetes Medical Management Plan (DMMP)** prepared by the student's personal diabetes healthcare team, contains the medical orders prescribed for the student. It provides the basis for all the health care and education plans designed to help the student manage diabetes effectively in the school setting.[19] From the DMMP, the school nurse develops an Individualized Healthcare Plan (IHP) to guide management throughout the school day.

An **emergency care plan (ECP)** is developed by the school nurse to help guide diabetes management during episodes of hypo/hyperglycemia. These documents are necessary attachments to Section 504 accommodation plans or an Individualized Education Plan (IEP). The school IHP should be adapted to the student's developmental level. As appropriate, the plan includes immediate access to diabetes supplies and permission to self-manage tasks in the classroom or least restrictive setting. The plan also addresses emergency evacuation/school lock-down instructions, before and after school activities, field trips and transportation needs.

FOLLOW-UP:

- Routine blood glucose monitoring, if ordered
- Monitor height, weight, and blood pressure
- Dietary goals – reinforce need for healthy eating habits
- Review carbohydrate counting/plate method for healthy nutrition
- Encourage routine exercise - at least 60 minutes of moderate to vigorous activity daily

POTENTIAL COMPLICATIONS:

Short term

- Hypoglycemia
- Hyperglycemia

Long term

- Cardiovascular disease
- Nephropathy
- Neuropathy
- Retinopathy
- Susceptible to skin infections
- Gastroparesis

DIABETES -TYPE 1 *(continued from previous page)*

REFERENCES

[1] American Diabetes Association. (2017). Classification and diagnosis of diabetes. In Standards of Medical Care in Diabetes 2017. *Diabetes Care, 40*(Suppl. 1), S11–S24. https://doi.org/10.2337/dc17-S005

[2] Pettitt D.J., Talton, J., Dabelea, D., Divers, J., Imperatore, G., Lawrence, J.M., Liese, A.D., Linder, B., Mayer-Davis, E.J., Pihoker, C., Saydah, S.H., Standiford, D.A., Hamman, R.F. & SEARCH for Diabetes in Youth Study Group. (2014). Prevalence of diabetes in U.S. youth in 2009: The SEARCH for diabetes in youth study. *Diabetes Care, 37*(2),402-8. http://care.diabetesjournals.org/content/37/2/402.abstract?ijkey=53ec8c3e487408c90ded10ff545e010c3cc4c52e&keytype2=tf_ipsecsha

[3] Merck Manual Professional Version. (2018). *Diabetes mellitus in children and adolescents.* https://www.merckmanuals.com/professional/pediatrics/endocrine-disorders-in-children/diabetes-mellitus-in-children-and-adolescents

[4] Mayer-Davis, E.J., Lawrence, J. M., Dabelea, D., Divers, J., Isom, S., Dolan, L., Imperatore, G., Linder, B., Marcovina, S., Pettitt, D.J., Pihoker, C., Saydah, S.,& Wagenknecht, L., for the SEARCH for Diabetes in Youth Study. (2017). Incidence trends of Type 1 and Type 2 diabetes among youths, 2002-2012. *New England Journal of Medicine* 2017, *376* (15),1419–1429. https://www.nejm.org/doi/full/10.1056/NEJMoa1610187

[5] Genuth, M., Palmer, J., & Nathan, D. (2016). Classification and diagnosis of diabetes. In C. C. Cowie, S. S. Casagrande, A. Menke, M. A. Cissell, M. S. Eberhardt, J. B. Meigs, ... J. E. Fradkin (Eds.), *Diabetes in America* (3rd ed., pp. 1–39). National Institutes of Health. https://www.ncbi.nlm.nih.gov/pmc/articles/PMC3006051/

[6] Chiang, J.L., Maahs, D.M., Garvey, K.C., Hood, K.C., Laffel, L.M., Weinzimer, S.A., Wolfsdorf, J.I., & Schatz, D. (2018). Type 1 diabetes in children and adolescents: A position statement by the American Diabetes Association. *Diabetes Care 2018, 41*, 2648-2668. https://doi.org/10.2337/dci18-0023

[7] Ibid.

[8] Ibid.

[9] Ibid.

[10] Brown, C. (2016). 21st-century diabetes: Technology leads the way. *NASN School Nurse, 31* (5), 254-256. https://doi.org/ 10.1177/1942602X16661198

[11] International Society for Pediatric and Adolescent Diabetes (ISPAD). (2018). ISPAD clinical practice consensus guidelines 2018. *Pediatric Diabetes, 19*(27), 287–301. https://www.ispad.org/page/ISPADGuidelines2018 doI: 10.1111/pedi.12698

[12]Chiang, J.L., Maahs, D.M., Garvey, K.C., Hood, K.C., Laffel, L.M., Weinzimer, S.A., Wolfsdorf, J.I., & Schatz, D. (2018). Type 1 diabetes in children and adolescents: A position statement by the American Diabetes Association. *Diabetes Care 2018, 41*, 2648-2668. https://doi.org/10.2337/dci18-0023

[13] Wyckoff, L. (2019). Students with diabetes. In J. Selekman, R.A. Shannon, & C. F. Younkaitis (Eds.), *School Nursing: A comprehensive text* (3rd ed.) (pp. 575-602). Philadelphia, PA: F.A. Davis.

[14] Chiang, J.L., Maahs, D.M., Garvey, K.C., Hood, K.C., Laffel, L.M., Weinzimer, S.A., Wolfsdorf, J.I., & Schatz, D. (2018). Type 1 diabetes in children and adolescents: A position statement by the American Diabetes Association. *Diabetes Care 2018, 41*, 2648-2668. https://doi.org/10.2337/dci18-0023

[15] International Society for Pediatric and Adolescent Diabetes (ISPAD). (2018). ISPAD clinical practice consensus guidelines 2018. *Pediatric Diabetes, 19*(27), 287–301. https://www.ispad.org/page/ISPADGuidelines2018 doI: 10.1111/pedi.12698

[16] Chiang, J.L., Maahs, D.M., Garvey, K.C., Hood, K.C., Laffel, L.M., Weinzimer, S.A., Wolfsdorf, J.I., & Schatz, D. (2018). Type 1 diabetes in children and adolescents: A position statement by the American Diabetes Association. *Diabetes Care 2018, 41*, 2648-2668. https://doi.org/10.2337/dci18-0023

DIABETES -TYPE 1 *(continued from previous page)*

[17] Chiang, J.L., Maahs, D.M., Garvey, K.C., Hood, K.C., Laffel, L.M., Weinzimer, S.A., Wolfsdorf, J.I., & Schatz, D. (2018). Type 1 diabetes in children and adolescents: A position statement by the American Diabetes Association. *Diabetes Care 2018, 41*, 2648-2668. https://doi.org/10.2337/dci18-0023

[18] National Institute of Diabetes and Digestive and Kidney Diseases. (2016). *Helping the student with diabetes succeed: A guide for school personnel.* https://www.niddk.nih.gov/health-information/communication-programs/ndep/health-professionals/helping-student-diabetes-succeed-guide-school-personnel?dkrd=hispt1099

[19] Ibid.

DIABETES READING RESOURCES

1. American Association of Diabetes Educators. *Management of children with diabetes in the school setting: AADE position statement.* (2016). https://www.diabeteseducator.org/docs/default-source/practice/practice-resources/position-statements/diabetes-in-the-school-setting-position-statement_final.pdf
2. American Diabetes Association. *State laws, regulations and policies for school diabetes care. Safe at School.* https://www.diabetes.org/resources/know-your-rights/safe-at-school-state-laws
3. Individuals with Disabilities Education Act, 20 U.S.C. 1400 et seq.; 34 CFR Part 300. http://idea.ed.gov/uploads/finalregulations.pdf
4. Jackson, C.C., Albanese-O'Neill, A., Butler, K.L., Chiang, J.L., Deeb, L.C., Hathaway, K., Kraus, E.,Weissberg-Benchell, J.,Yatvin, A.L.,& Siminerio, L.M. (2015). Diabetes care in the school setting: A position statement of the American Diabetes Association. *Diabetes Care,38*(10),1958-63. http://care.diabetesjournals.org/content/38/10/1958.full?patientinform-links=yes&legid=diacare;38/10/1958%20-%20xref-ref-1-1
5. Section 504 of the Rehabilitation Act of 1973, 29 U.S.C. 794; 35 CFR Part 104. http://www2.ed.gov/policy/rights/reg/ocr/edlite-34cfr104.html
6. Siminerio, L.M., Albanese-O'Neill, A., Chiang, J.L., Hathaway, K., Jackson, C.C., Weissberg-Benchell, J., Wright, J.L., Yatvin, A.L. & Deeb, L.C. (2014). Care of young children with diabetes in the child care setting: A position statement of the American Diabetes Association. *Diabetes Care,37*(10),2834-42. http://care.diabetesjournals.org/content/37/10/2834.full?ijkey=ce6766e4e9245b58a32155afd8fe9fbd39c2c690&keytype2=tf_ipsecsha
7. The Diabetes Control and Complications Trial Research Group. (1993). The effect of intensive treatment of diabetes on the development and progression of long-term complications in insulin-dependent diabetes mellitus. *New England Journal of Medicine, 329*(14),977-86. https://www.ncbi.nlm.nih.gov/pubmed/8366922?dopt=Abstract

DIABETES - TYPE 2

DEFINITION/ETIOLOGY:

Type 2 diabetes, formerly called adult-onset or non-insulin dependent diabetes, was once an adulthood disease. However, Type 2 diabetes in youth (under 20 years of age) has increased over the past 20 years, and recent estimates suggest an incidence of ~5,000 new cases per year in the U.S.[1] About one-third of American youth are overweight, a problem closely related to the increase in children with type 2 diabetes, some as young as 10 years old.[2] The Centers for Disease Control and Prevention (CDC) projections based on the SEARCH database, indicate that over the next 40 years, the prevalence of type 2 diabetes in youth will quadruple.[3,4] Type 2 diabetes in youth differs from Type 2 in adults in that there is a more quickly progressing decline in beta cell function and complications develop sooner.[5,6] Type 2 diabetes is defined by impaired secretion of the hormone insulin from the beta cells of the pancreas, insulin-resistance, or a combination of both processes.[7] This is unlike Type 1 diabetes where there is an absolute insulin deficiency due to destruction of the islet of langerhan (the insulin producing cells in the pancreas). Insulin is a hormone that is necessary to convert food into energy for normal body functioning. Without adequate insulin, food converted into glucose remains in the blood stream and is unable to enter the cells, depriving the brain and muscles of glucose. The accumulation of glucose within the blood stream damages tissues and blood vessels, leading to nephropathy/kidney disease, retinopathy/eye disease, neuropathy/nervous system, gastroparesis (slowing of the digestive system), heart disease, risk of stroke, poor wound healing and amputations.[8]

Type 2 diabetes results from a physiological resistance to rising levels of insulin and usually has a relative (not absolute) insulin deficiency. Insulin resistance occurs when the pancreas produces elevated amounts of insulin in response to large amounts of glucose in the blood stream.[9] Over time, cells stop responding to all that insulin—they've become insulin resistant. The pancreas keeps making more insulin to try to make cells respond. Eventually, the pancreas can't keep up, and glucose keeps rising. While there is a genetic predisposition for type 2 diabetes, it requires an "environment" to develop - usually being overweight (especially with a body type that stores excess fat around the waist more than the hips) due to high calorie diet and too little activity.

Metabolic syndrome is a cluster of conditions that occur together, increasing the risk of heart disease, stroke and type 2 diabetes. These conditions include increased blood pressure, high blood sugar, excess body fat around the waist, and abnormal cholesterol or triglyceride levels. Type 2 diabetes disproportionately impacts youth of ethnic and racial minorities and can occur in complex psychosocial and cultural environments, which may make it difficult to sustain health lifestyle changes and self-management behaviors.[10,11] Detected early, type 2 diabetes can be managed by changes in diet and daily activity but may require oral medication and, at times, insulin injections.

COMORBID CONDITIONS:

- Polycystic Ovarian Syndrome (PCOS)
- Hypertension
- Dyslipidemia
- Fatty liver
- Obstructive sleep apnea

DIABETES - TYPE 2 *(continued from previous page)*

RISK FACTORS[12]

- Obesity- body mass index (BMI) 85th-94th and >95th percentile for age and gender
- Family history of Type 2 diabetes
- Ethnicity - Hispanic, Non-Hispanic white, African American, Asian/Pacific Islander
- Sedentary lifestyle
- Low socioeconomic status
- Small-for-gestational age birthweight
- Maternal history of gestational diabetes during pregnancy during the child's gestation

Type 2 diabetes risk factor identification is an important aspect of prevention and control. Because Type 2 diabetes develops gradually over time often patients do not recognize the signs and symptoms. Risk-based screening for prediabetes and/or type 2 diabetes should be considered in children and adolescents after the onset of puberty or over 10 years, who are overweight (over 85%) and who have one or more additional risk factors for diabetes.[13]

SIGNS AND SYMPTOMS:

Hyperglycemia:

- Increased thirst (polydipsia)
- Increased urination (polyuria)
- Increased hunger (polyphagia)
- Unexplained weight loss/no weight change
- Vaginal yeast infections
- Fatigue
- Slow healing wounds
- Vision changes
- High blood pressure
- Elevated blood lipids
- Acanthosis Nigricans (later sign of insulin resistance) - dark, velvety textured skin primarily noted in the axillary, inner elbow, posterior neck and groin areas that signify insulin resistance that may or may not be present with Type 2 diabetes. Often this condition is mistaken for poor hygiene.

Hypoglycemia: *

- Shakiness
- Dizziness
- Pale skin
- Weakness
- Confusion
- Behavior change/irritability/emotional
- Loss of consciousness**
- Seizure**

***Some children do not demonstrate any outward symptoms of hypoglycemia or may have hypoglycemic unawareness (inability to recognize symptoms of low blood glucose).**

DIABETES - TYPE 2 *(continued from previous page)*

MANAGEMENT/TREATMENT:[14]

- Monitor blood glucose levels with glucometer if ordered (may also have a continuous glucose monitoring system [CGM]) per healthcare provider orders. Testing recommendations are for those who are taking insulin or oral medications with a risk of hypoglycemia, who may be initiating or changing treatment regimens or have concurrent illnesses.
- Metformin (only oral medication approved for children with Type 2 diabetes), may be ordered. Metformin is recommended as a first-line therapy, unless initial diagnosis included DKA. If there is significant hyperglycemia, insulin may be initiated to reverse glucose toxicity. Insulin delivery systems and dosages vary. There is potential to discontinue insulin, begin oral therapy and progress to management with diet, and exercise only (unlike Type 1 Diabetes where insulin is the only option for treatment).[15]
- Lifestyle management including eating a balanced diet, achieving and maintaining a healthy weight and exercising regularly.[16] Nutrition recommendations are based on requirements for all healthy youth, as there is no research on optimal nutrient requirements for children and adolescents with diabetes. Exercise improves blood glucose control because of decreased insulin resistance. Activity recommendations are for 60 minutes of exercise daily.
- If child or youth is being treated with insulin, dosing is usually related to total carbohydrate count of each meal along with blood glucose level.
- Treatment of hypoglycemia follows "The Rule of 15" [17] - 15 grams of carbohydrate and recheck in 15 minutes for mild hypoglycemia. Moderate episodes of hypoglycemia may require the use of glucose gel if alert, but unable to follow directions. Emergency glucagon administration for episodes of severe hypoglycemia and the child is unconscious or has a seizure. (*Refer to DIABETES EMERGENCIES*). ** While glucagon may not be prescribed for the child with Type 2 diabetes, it should be considered if the child is treated with insulin.
- Treatment of hyperglycemia per the child's emergency plan.[18] Encourage drinking water. Urine or blood ketone testing as ordered by healthcare provider during episodes of hyperglycemia and illness. (See Diabetes Emergencies Guidelines). **Often ketone testing is NOT ordered for children with Type 2 diabetes due to decreased risk for DKA.

****Severe hypoglycemia is not as common with Type 2 diabetes but should be considered when on insulin management.**

DIABETES - TYPE 2 *(continued from previous page)*

MANAGEMENT/TREATMENT *(continued)*

General Management

Diabetes requires an individualized care and lifestyle plan balancing daily dietary intake, physical activity, medication (if ordered) and self-monitored blood glucose. If ordered, children can learn to use glucometers and, in time, to self-administer insulin as ordered. A lab test called hemoglobin A1c or simply "A1c" measures the past three to four months' fasting and post meal blood glucose levels to indicate the effectiveness of blood glucose control. While a non-diabetic A1c ranges from 4-6%, the goal for the child with type 2 diabetes is <7%.[19]

A team approach including students, families, healthcare providers, and school staff (food services, physical education, counseling staff, teachers, bus drivers and administration) led by the school nurse, can assist with risk reduction as well as disease management. The school nurse is the coordinator of care in school, but all staff that have responsibility for the student should have basic training to understand Type 2 diabetes and the needs of these students.

Training for school personnel is recommended to follow three levels of training.[20]

- Level One training should be provided as basic information to all personnel.
- Level Two training is more in depth for those who have direct contact with the child during the school day.
- Level Three training is in-depth training for a small group of unlicensed personnel who will assist with specific diabetes management for the student, for those states that allow the registered nurse to delegate tasks (see your state Nurse Practice Act).

The Diabetes Medical Management Plan (DMMP) prepared by the student's personal diabetes healthcare team, contains the medical orders prescribed for the student. It provides the basis for all the health care and education plans designed to help the student manage diabetes effectively in the school setting.[21] From the DMMP, the school nurse develops an Individualized Healthcare Plan (IHP) to guide management throughout the school day. An Emergency Care Plan (ECP) is developed by the school nurse to help guide the management during episodes of hypo/hyperglycemia. These documents are necessary attachments to a Section 504 Plan or an Individualized Education Plan (IEP). The school healthcare plan should be adapted to the student's developmental level. As appropriate, the plan includes immediate access to diabetes supplies and permission to self-manage tasks in the classroom or least restrictive setting. The plan also addresses emergency evacuation/school lock-down instructions.

DIABETES - TYPE 2 *(continued from previous page)*

FOLLOW-UP:

- Routine blood glucose monitoring, if ordered.
- Monitor height, weight, and blood pressure.
- Dietary goals – reinforce need for healthy eating habits.
- Review carbohydrate counting method prescribed (May use basic carbohydrate counting based on "carbohydrate choices." One choice contains about 15 grams of carb. Others use what's called the "plate method" to eat a reasonable portion of carbohydrate-containing foods at each meal by limiting grains and starchy vegetables to a quarter of the plate.[22]
- Encourage routine exercise - at least 60 minutes of moderate to vigorous activity daily.[23]

POTENTIAL COMPLICATIONS:

Short term

- Hypoglycemia
- Hyperglycemia

Long term microvascular and macrovascular changes resulting in:[24]

- Cardiovascular disease including hypertension and stroke
- Nephropathy
- Neuropathy
- Retinopathy
- Susceptible to skin infections
- Gastroparesis

REFERENCES

---

[1] Pettitt, D.J., Talton, J., Dabelea, D., Divers, J., Imperatore, G., Lawrence, J.M., Liese, A.D., Linder, B., Mayer-Davis, E.J., Pihoker, C., Saydah, S.H.,S tandiford, D.A., & & Hamman, B.S. for the SEARCH for Diabetes in Youth Study Group. (2014). Prevalence of diabetes in U.S. youth in 2009: the SEARCH for diabetes in youth study. *Diabetes Care*. *37*(2),402-8. http://care.diabetesjournals.org/content/37/2/402.abstract?ijkey=53ec8c3e487408c90ded10ff545e010c3cc4c52e&keytype2=tf_ipsecsha

[2] Centers for Disease Control and Prevention. (2019). *Prevent Type 2 diabetes in kids.* https://www.cdc.gov/diabetes/prevent-type-2/type-2-kids.html?CDC_AA_refVal=https%3A%2F%2Fwww.cdc.gov%2Fdiabetes%2Flibrary%2Ffeatures%2Ftype-2-_kids.html

[3] Imperatore, G., Boyle, J.P., Thompson, T.J., Case, D., Dabelea, D., Hamman, R.F., Lawrence, J.M., Liese, A.D., Liu, L.L., Mayer-Davis, E.J., Rodriguez, B.L., & Standiford, D., for the SEARCH for Diabetes in Youth Study Group. (2012). Projections of type 1 and type 2 diabetes burden in the U.S. population aged <20 years through 2050: dynamic modeling of incidence, mortality, and population growth. *Diabetes Care,* 35(12),2515-20. https://doi.org/10.2337/dc12-0669

[4] Pettitt, D.J., Talton, J., Dabelea, D., Divers, J., Imperatore, G., Lawrence, J.M., Liese, A.D., Linder, B., Mayer-Davis, E.J., Pihoker, C., Saydah, S.H.,S tandiford, D.A., & & Hamman, B.S. for the SEARCH for Diabetes in Youth Study Group. (2014). Prevalence of diabetes in U.S. youth in 2009: the SEARCH for diabetes in youth study. *Diabetes Care*. *37*(2),402-8. http://care.diabetesjournals.org/content/37/2/402.abstract?ijkey=53ec8c3e487408c90ded10ff545e010c3cc4c52e&keytype2=tf_ipsecsha

DIABETES - TYPE 2 *(continued from previous page)*

[5] Arslanian, S., Bacha, F., Grey, M., Marcus, M.D., White, N.H., & Zeitler P. (2018). Evaluation and management of youth-onset type 2 diabetes: A position statement by the American Diabetes Association. *Diabetes Care, 41*,2648–2668. https://doi.org/10.2337/dci18-0052

[6] Copeland, K.C., Zeitler, P., Geffner, M., Guandalini, C., Higgins, J., Hirst, K., ... TODAY Study Group. (2011). Characteristics of adolescents and youth with recent-onset type 2 diabetes: the TODAY cohort at baseline. *Journal of Clinical Endocrinology Metabolism, 96*(1),159–67. https://doi.org/10.1210/jc.2010-1642

[7] American Diabetes Association. (2019). *Standards of* medical care in diabetes—*2019 abridged for primary care providers clinical diabetes*, *37*(1), 11-34. https://doi.org/10.2337/cd18-0105

[8] Centers for Disease Control and Prevention. (2019). *Prevent diabetes*. https://www.cdc.gov/diabetes/prevention/lifestyle-program/about-prediabetes.html

[9] Centers for Disease Control and Prevention. (2019). *Diabetes: What's insulin resistance got to do with It?* https://www.cdc.gov/diabetes/library/spotlights/diabetes-insulin-resistance.html

[10] Liu, L.L., Lawrence, J.M., Davis, C., Liese, A.D., Pettitt, D.J., Pihoker, C., Dabelea, D., Hamman, R., Waitzfelder, B., & Kahn, H.S. for SEARCH for Diabetes in Youth Study Group. (2010). Prevalence of overweight and obesity in youth with diabetes in USA: the SEARCH for diabetes in youth study. *Pediatric Diabetes*,*11*(1),4-11. https://doi.org/10.1111/j.1399-5448.2009.00519.x

[11] Whalen, D.J., Belden, A.C., Tillman, R., Barch, D.M., & Luby, J.L. (2016). Early adversity, psychopathology, and latent class profiles of global physical health from preschool through early adolescence. *Psychosomatic Medicine,* 78, 1008–1018. https://doi.org/10.1097/PSY.0000000000000398

[12] Copeland, K.C., Zeitler, P., Geffner, M., Guandalini, C., Higgins, J., Hirst, K., ... TODAY Study Group. (2011). Characteristics of adolescents and youth with recent-onset type 2 diabetes: the TODAY cohort at baseline. *Journal of Clinical Endocrinology Metabolism, 96*(1),159–67. https://doi.org/10.1210/jc.2010-1642

[13] American Diabetes Association. (2019). Children and adolescents: Standards of medical care in diabetes—2019. *Diabetes Care,* 42 (Supplement 1). https://doi.org/10.2337/dc19-s013

[14] American Diabetes Association. (2019). *Standards of* medical care in diabetes—*2019 abridged for primary care providers clinical diabetes*, *37*(1), 11-34. https://doi.org/10.2337/cd18-0105

[15] Arslanian, S., Bacha, F., Grey, M., Marcus, M.D., White, N.H., & Zeitler P. (2018). Evaluation and management of youth-onset type 2 diabetes: A position statement by the American Diabetes Association. *Diabetes Care, 41*,2648–2668. https://doi.org/10.2337/dci18-0052

[16] American Diabetes Association. (2019). Introduction: Standards of medical care in diabetes—2019. *Diabetes Care, 42* (Supplement 1), S1-S2. https://doi.org/10.2337/dc19-Sint01

[17] MedlinePlus. (2019). 15/15 rule. Bethesda (MD): National Library of Medicine. https://medlineplus.gov/ency/imagepages/19815.htm

[18] National Diabetes Education Program. (2016). *Helping the student with diabetes succeed: A guide for school personnel.* https://www.niddk.nih.gov/health-information/communication-programs/ndep/health-professionals/helping-student-diabetes-succeed-guide-school-personnel

[19] Ibid.

[20] National Institute of Diabetes and Digestive and Kidney Diseases. (2016). H*elping the student with diabetes succeed: a guide for school personnel.* https://www.niddk.nih.gov/health-information/communication-programs/ndep/health-professionals/helping-student-diabetes-succeed-guide-school-personnel?dkrd=hispt1099

[21] Centers for Disease Control and Prevention. (2017). *Prevent type 2 diabetes in kids*. https://www.cdc.gov/diabetes/prevent-type-2/type-2-kids.html?CDC_AA_refVal=https://www.cdc.gov/diabetes/library/features/type-2-kids.html

DIABETES - TYPE 2 *(continued from previous page)*

[22] Tsai, A., & American Diabetes Association. (2015). The basics of carbohydrate counting. In *Diabetes Forecast.* *http://www.diabetesforecast.org/2015/may-jun/the-basics-of-carb-counting.html*

[23] Centers for Disease Control and Prevention. (2017). *Prevent type 2 diabetes in kids.* https://www.cdc.gov/diabetes/prevent-type-2/type-2-kids.html?CDC_AA_refVal=https://www.cdc.gov/diabetes/library/features/type-2-kids.html

[24] The National Institute of Diabetes and Digestive and Kidney Diseases Health Information Center. (n.d.), *Preventing diabetes complications.* https://www.niddk.nih.gov/health-information/diabetes/overview/preventing-problems

DIABETES READING RESOURCES

1. American Association of Diabetes Educators. Management of children with diabetes in the school setting: AADE position statement. 2016. Available from: https://www.diabeteseducator.org/docs/default-source/practice/practice-resources/position-statements/diabetes-in-the-school-setting-position-statement_final.pdf
2. American Diabetes Association. State laws, regulations and policies for school diabetes care. Safe at School. https://www.diabetes.org/resources/know-your-rights/safe-at-school-state-laws
3. Individuals with Disabilities Education Act, 20 U.S.C. 1400 et seq.; 34 CFR Part 300. http://idea.ed.gov/uploads/finalregulations.pdf
4. Jackson, C.C., Albanese-O'Neill, A., Butler, K.L., Chiang, J.L., Deeb, L.C., Hathaway, K., ...Siminerio, L.M. (2015). Diabetes care in the school setting: A position statement of the American Diabetes Association. *Diabetes Care,38*(10),1958-63. http://care.diabetesjournals.org/content/38/10/1958.full?patientinform-links=yes&legid=diacare;38/10/1958%20-%20xref-ref-1-1
5. Section 504 of the Rehabilitation Act of 1973, 29 U.S.C. 794; 35 CFR Part 104. http://www2.ed.gov/policy/rights/reg/ocr/edlite-34cfr104.html
6. Siminerio, L.M., Albanese-O'Neill, A., Chiang, J.L., Hathaway, K., Jackson, C.C., Weissberg-Benchell, J., Wright, J.L., Yatvin, A.L., Deeb, L.C. & American Diabetes Association. (2014). Care of young children with diabetes in the child care setting: A position statement of the American Diabetes Association. *Diabetes Care,37*(10),2834-42. http://care.diabetesjournals.org/content/37/10/2834.full?ijkey=ce6766e4e9245b58a32155afd8fe9fbd39c2c690&keytype2=tf_ipsecsha
7. The Diabetes Control and Complications Trial Research Group. (1993). The effect of intensive treatment of diabetes on the development and progression of long-term complications in insulin-dependent diabetes mellitus. *New England Journal of Medicine, 329*(14),977-86. https://www.ncbi.nlm.nih.gov/pubmed/8366922?dopt=Abstract

DIARRHEA

DEFINITION/ETIOLOGY:

Diarrhea is a common pediatric concern. Diarrhea is an increase in the number of stools (three [3] or more per day) and consists of loose, watery and more frequent bowel movements deviating from the normal stooling pattern. Severe diarrheal stools are watery, may be green and/or contain mucous or blood. Diarrhea can be acute, chronic or persistent. Acute diarrhea is typically caused by parasites, bacterial or viral infections and is the most common. Diarrhea is considered chronic if it lasts at least 4 weeks.[1] There are many causes of diarrhea. The most common causes of diarrhea are viruses, bacteria, parasites, and medications.[2]

Below is a partial list of common causes of diarrhea.

Infections [3]

- Acute gastroenteritis (viral) – norovirus: often referred to as "stomach flu". It causes diarrhea and sometimes nausea/vomiting and stomach pain. It is highly contagious.
- Rotavirus: most common in young children and infants. Usually seen in the winter and early spring months. The rotavirus vaccine is available for this population and can protect children from this viral illness.
- Bacterial diarrhea – salmonella, shigella, E. Coli, campylobacter, C. difficile
- Parasites (Giardia, cryptosporidium)

Diseases of the colon[4]

- Celiac disease
- Crohn's disease
- Ulcerative colitis
- Irritable Bowel Syndrome (IBS)

Psychogenic diarrhea[5]

- Fear/anxiety
- Encopresis

Other[6]

- Food allergy/Food intolerance/Lactose intolerance
- Medications such as antibiotics
- Artificial sweeteners or high sugar diet
- Constipation with fecal retention

SIGNS AND SYMPTOMS:

- Abdominal pain, abdominal cramps, or bloating[7]
- Viral gastroenteritis – vomiting and frequent watery diarrhea stools
- May have signs of dehydration (decreased urine output, thickening of saliva, thirst, feeling dizzy when standing up, etc.)[8]
- Vital signs—may have increased pulse and lower blood pressure if dehydrated[9]
- Fever is sometimes present, but usually not a high temperature
- Weight loss

DIARRHEA *(continued from previous page)*

MANAGEMENT/TREATMENT:

- Treatment is dependent on etiology. Treat underlying cause.
- Monitor for signs and symptoms of dehydration (tachycardia, hypotension, lethargy).
- If signs of dehydration are present, refer to healthcare provider immediately.[10]
- If well hydrated but acutely ill, notify parent/guardian.
- If all symptoms are mild, observe in school health office/clinic and offer preferably oral rehydrating solution. Notify parent/guardian.[11]
- Reinforce the practice of good handwashing to remove germs and prevent the spread of illness.[12]
- Although many cases of diarrhea are not caused by an infectious disease, public health guidelines may call for the exclusion of the child from school or childcare if the feces are not able to be contained in a diaper or in a toilet.[13]
- Very young children who attend school, significantly developmentally delayed children of any age, or children whose physical disabilities include lack of bowel control, are the children who may need to be excluded for diarrhea, even if the cause is known to be non-infectious.[14]
- **Diarrhea from suspected or known food borne illnesses is reportable to the health department, in most states[15]**
- Instruct parent/guardian to notify the healthcare provider immediately if no urine output for 12 hours, temperature 102° F or greater, blood or mucous noted in stool, severe abdominal pain, no tears when crying, irritability or lethargy.[16]
- Review handwashing with child. (*Refer to HANDWASHING APPENDIX*).

FOLLOW UP:

- Obtain diagnosis and assess the risk to other students in the school.
- Examine child on re-entry to school (temperature and hydration status).
- Give medication as prescribed.
- Report any relapse.

POTENTIAL COMPLICATIONS:[17]

Dehydration is a complication of intense diarrhea due to the loss of excess fluids and electrolytes. Dehydration limits the body's ability to carry out normal functions due to the lack of water/fluid intake. **Serious consequences can result if lost fluids are not replenished.**

NOTES:[18]

Prevention

- Proper handwashing prevents the spread of viral diarrhea.
- Guard against contaminated food.
- Wash fruits and vegetables before eating them.
- Clean kitchen counters well after contact with raw meat, especially poultry.
- Follow Centers for Disease Control and Prevention's food and water safety habits when traveling to developing countries (https://wwwnc.cdc.gov/travel/page/food-water-safety).
- Educate parent/guardian(s) on vaccine preventable diarrhea (rotavirus).

Refer to HANDWASHING APPENDIX

DIARRHEA *(continued from previous page)*

REFERENCES

[1] Mayo Clinic. (2019). *Diarrhea.* http://www.mayoclinic.org/symptoms/diarrhea/basics/definition/sym20050926

[2] National Digestive Diseases Information Clearinghouse (NDDIC). (2016). *Diarrhea.* http://www.niddk.nih.gov/health-information/health-topics/digestive-diseases/diarrhea

[3] American Academy of Pediatrics. (2019). *Diarrhea.* http://kidshealth.org/parent/infections/common/diarrhea.html#

[4] Mayo Clinic. (2019). *Diarrhea.* http://www.mayoclinic.org/symptoms/diarrhea/basics/definition/sym20050926

[5] Jakubowski, T. & Perron, T. (2019). Students with common health complaints: Diarrhea. In J. Selekman, R. Adair Shannon, & C. F. Yonkaitis (Eds.), *School nursing: A comprehensive text* (3rd ed., pp. 354-355). F.A. Davis Company.

[6] Ibid.

[7] Merck Manual. (2019). *Diarrhea.* https://www.merckmanuals.com/professional/pediatrics/symptoms-in-infants-and-children/diarrhea-in-children#v1083520

[8] National Digestive Diseases Information Clearinghouse (NDDIC). (2016). *Diarrhea.* http://www.niddk.nih.gov/health-information/health-topics/digestive-diseases/diarrhea

[9] Ibid.

[10] Ibid.

[11] Centers for Disease Control and Prevention (CDC). (2018). *Norovirus.* http://www.cdc.gov/norovirus/about/index.html

[12] Centers for Disease Control and Prevention (CDC). (2019). *Handwashing: Clean Hands Save Lives.* https://www.cdc.gov/handwashing/

[13] Centers for Disease Control and Prevention (CDC). (2018). *Norovirus.* http://www.cdc.gov/norovirus/about/index.html

[14] Ibid.

[15] Ibid.

[16] WebMD. (2017). D*iarrhea: Why it happens and how to treat it.* http://www.webmd.com/digestive-disorders/digestive-diseas diarrhea#1

[17] National Digestive Diseases Information Clearinghouse (NDDIC). (2016). *Diarrhea.* http://www.niddk.nih.gov/health-information/health-topics/digestive-diseases/diarrhea

[18] American Academy of Pediatrics. (2019). *Diarrhea.* http://kidshealth.org/parent/infections/common/diarrhea.html#

OTHER REFERENCES CONSULTED

Merck Manual. (2019). *Diarrhea in children.* https://www.merckmanuals.com/professional/pediatrics/symptoms-in-infants-and-children/diarrhea-in children?query=diarrhea

DIPHTHERIA

DEFINITION/ETIOLOGY:

Diphtheria is an acute, highly contagious, potentially life-threatening infection caused by *Corynebacterium diphtheriae* that can either invade sites along the respiratory tract, present as a cutaneous infection, or manifest in an asymptomatic carrier state. In the respiratory system the bacteria produces a toxin.[1] It is transmitted from person-to-person through respiratory droplets (coughing or sneezing). Persons can also become infected by coming in contact fomites, an object (telephone, keyboard, doorknobs, toys, and dish) that has been contaminated by an infected person. Contact with infected skin lesions can also spread the infection. Humans are the only known reservoir for *C. diphtheria.* Today, diphtheria is rare in the United States and other developed countries due to widespread vaccination programs.[2, 3]

SIGNS AND SYMPTOMS:[4]

Pharyngeal/Respiratory Diphtheria

- Weakness
- Sore throat
- Fever and chills
- Swollen glands (neck)
- Difficulty swallowing
- Loss of appetite
- Within two to three days, a thick coating (pseudomembrane) can build up in the throat or nose; may cause difficulty breathing

The normal incubation period is two to five days, although it could range one to 10 days from the time of exposure to onset of symptoms. Symptoms may vary depending on the primary site of infection. Diagnosis is determined by symptoms most notably the hallmark gray colored pseudomembrane covering the nose/throat. Definite diagnosis is made by laboratory results of throat or lesion swabs – confirming the presence of toxin in the body. Treatment begins when a diagnosis of diphtheria is suspected.

MANAGEMENT/TREATMENT:

- Hospitalization
- Diphtheria Antitoxin (DAT) to counteract toxin in severe cases
- Antibiotics (penicillin or erythromycin) to kill and eliminate bacteria
- If experiencing respiratory difficulties – healthcare provider may remove pseudomembrane covering nose and/or throat
- Isolation until two consecutive cultures taken 24 hours apart are negative[5]
- Untreated person who is infected may be contagious for up to four weeks. If the person is treated appropriately, the contagious period can be limited to less than four days.

DIPHTHERIA *(continued from previous page)*

POTENTIAL COMPLICATIONS:

- Obstructed airway
- Myocarditis, endocarditis
- Polyneuropathy
- Paralysis
- Pneumonia
- Respiratory failure
- Septic arthritis
- Case fatality is 5-10% with higher deaths rates in persons under five years old[6]

FOLLOW-UP:

- Recovery from diphtheria is not always followed by life-time immunity; therefore post recovery vaccination is needed.
- Follow-up cultures should be performed at 24 to 48 hours and two weeks following infection to document clearance.[7]

NOTES:

<u>General Considerations</u>

- Diphtheria is a reportable disease (local health department).
- Follow local and state health department guidelines regarding potential outbreak control and management.

<u>Cutaneous Diphtheria</u>

- It is rare in the U.S.
- Persons with poor hygiene or living in crowded conditions are those most often seen with diphtheria. Those at risk include the homeless and IV drug users.[8]
- Cutaneous infection manifests as non-healing sores or ulcers with a gray membrane [9]
- The toxin may be absorbed into the heart, kidneys, and nerves.
- The infection is treated by thoroughly cleaning the skin with soap and water and with antibiotics.

<u>Prevention</u> [10]

- Vaccine (primary and post-exposure).
- Post exposure cultural and antibiotics for close contacts.
- Diphtheria is a vaccine preventable disease (VPD) when diphtheria vaccine is appropriately given to infants and children, to pre-teens and teens, and to adults.
- Follow Centers for Disease Control and Prevention (CDC), American Academy of Pediatrics (AAP), and /or State Departments of Health recommendations for immunization schedules.

DIPHTHERIA *(continued from previous page)*

REFERENCES

[1] Naiditch, M. J., & Bower, A. G. (1954). Diphtheria: A study of 1,433 cases observed during a ten-year period at the Los Angeles County Hospital. *The American Journal of Medicine*, *17*(2), 229-245. https://doi.org/10.1016/0002-9343(54)90261-2

[2] Centers for Disease Control and Prevention. (2019). *Diphtheria.* http://www.cdc.gov/diphtheria/index.html

[3] Center for Disease Control and Prevention (CDC). (2015). Diphtheria. In J. Hamborsky, A.Kroger, & S. Wolfe (Eds.), *Epidemiology and prevention of vaccine-preventable diseases, the pink book: Course textbook (13th ed.).* Washington D.C. Public Health Foundation. http://www.cdc.gov/vaccines/pubs/pinkbook/dip.html

[4] Centers for Disease Control and Prevention. (2019). *Diphtheria.* http://www.cdc.gov/diphtheria/index.html

[5] American Academy of Pediatrics, Committee on Infectious Diseases. (2018). Diphtheria. In D.W. Kimberlin, M.T. Brady, M.T., M.A. Jackson, & S.S. Long (Eds.), *Red Book, (2018-2021): Report of the Committee on Infectious Diseases* (31st ed., pp. 319-323). American Academy of Pediatrics.

[6] Ibid.

[7] Centers for Disease Control and Prevention. (2019). *Diphtheria: For clinicians.* http://www.cdc.gov/diphtheria/index.html

[8] Lowe, C. F., Bernard, K. A., & Romney, M. G. (2011). Cutaneous diphtheria in the urban poor population of Vancouver, British Columbia, Canada: a 10-year review. *Journal of Clinical Microbiology*, *49*(7), 2664-2666. https://jcm.asm.org/content/jcm/49/7/2664.full.pdf

[9] Höfler, W. (1991). Cutaneous diphtheria. *International Journal of Dermatology*, *30*(12), 845-847. https://doi.org/10.1111/j.1365-4362.1991.tb04348.x

[10] Centers for Disease Control and Prevention. (2019). *Diphtheria.* http://www.cdc.gov/diphtheria/index.html

DYSPHAGIA (SWALLOWING DISORDERS)

DEFINITION/ETIOLOGY:[1]

Swallowing disorders, also known as dysphagia, causes difficulty swallowing. The swallowing process is very complex. Breakdown in the oral phase, pharyngeal phase or esophageal phase can cause swallowing disorders. Swallowing issues in school age children may be evident with the following diagnoses: cerebral palsy, severe developmental disabilities, meningitis, encephalopathy, gastrointestinal conditions, prematurity or low birth rate, cognitive impairment, head/neck cancer treated with radiation/chemotherapy, brain injury, spinal cord injury, muscular dystrophy, heart disease, cleft lip and/or palate, autism, head and neck abnormalities, muscle weakness in the face and neck respiratory difficulties or medications that cause lethargy or decreased appetite.[2]

Students with autism (this may be secondary to sensory difficulties with different textures), cognitive impairments, cerebral palsy and other nervous system disorders (this may be secondary to neurological dysfunction affecting motor skills and loss of function in the nerves in the spinal cord and brain) may experience swallowing difficulties.

SIGNS AND SYMPTOMS:[3]

- Coughing after eating/drinking
- Shortness of breath after eating/drinking
- Loss of pigmentation in the face after eating/drinking
- Wheezing and/or gasping during feeding
- Wet vocal quality after eating/drinking
- Feeling of food items sticking in the oral or pharyngeal phase of the swallow
- Pocketing food in oral cavity
- Residue in oral cavity after swallowing
- Choking after eating/drinking
- Anterior loss of food/drink from the oral cavity and/or drooling
- Over-filling oral cavity with food or drink
- Student feeling of "drowning"
- Reoccurring pneumonia
- Absent swallow
- Swallow delay
- Weight loss
- Difficulty chewing or initiating swallow
- Regurgitation
- Dehydration

DYSPHAGIA (SWALLOWING DISORDERS) *(continued from previous page)*

MANAGEMENT/TREATMENT:

- If any of the above signs and symptoms are present during feeding, follow up is needed. In cases of extreme choking/respiratory symptoms, oral feeding should stop at school until student is evaluated.
- Collaborate with school speech language pathologist on any swallowing concerns.
- Notify parent/guardian of symptoms and need for follow up with healthcare provider. Videofluoroscopic swallow study, sometimes known as a Modified Barium Swallow Study or a Fiberoptic Endoscopic Evaluation of Swallowing (FEES) is often indicated.
- After a complete swallow study has been completed, the student may have a change in diet level or may need to implement compensatory strategies. The nurse should request a copy of the swallow summary and the swallow/feeding management plan from the healthcare provider.

Diet Levels:[4]

Levels of Solids:

- Level 7 – Regular: normal foods.
- Level 6 – Soft and Bite-Sized: tender and moist throughout with no thin liquid leaking or dripping from the food. Chewing ability needed.
- Level 5 – Minced and Moist: very soft, small moist lumps, minimal chewing ability needed.
- Level 4 – Pureed: smooth, no lumps, not sticky, no chewing ability needed.
- Level 3 – Liquidized: eaten from a spoon or drunk from a cup, cannot be eaten with a fork as it slowly drips through, effort needed to drink through wide straw.

Levels of Liquids:

- Level 4 – Extremely Thick: sits in a mound on top of fork, does not drip through fork, holds shape on spoon, falls easily off spoon if tilted, must not be firm or sticky.
- Level 3 – Moderately Thick: eaten from a spoon or drunk from a cup, cannot be eaten with a fork as it slowly drips through, effort needed to drink through wide straw.
- Level 2 – Mildly Thick: "Sippable" from a cup but effort needed to drink this from a standard straw/nipple.
- Level 1 – Slightly Thick: thicker than water, can flow through a standard straw/nipple.
- Level 0 – Thin: Flows like water, flows easily through straw/nipple.

Compensatory Strategies:

- Avoid straws
- Small bites
- Chin tuck
- Turn head left or right
- Alternate liquids and solids
- Dry swallows after each bite of food or sip of drink
- Slow rate while eating or drinking
- Sit upright when eating and drinking
- Crush medications
- Pills in puree
- Extra swallows with each bite of food or drink
- Present food/drink on spoon

DYSPHAGIA (SWALLOWING DISORDERS) *(continued from previous page)*

MANAGEMENT/TREATMENT *(continued)*

Considerations for the Educational Setting[5]

- Safety
- Promote health to maximize attendance
- Develop a plan for adequate nutrition/hydration during the school day
- Skill development
- Access to Free Appropriate Public Education (FAPE): students must receive proper nutrition to access their learning environment

FOLLOW-UP:

- Educate staff and students on the signs and symptoms of swallowing disorders.
- Educate staff on chocking alleviation as indicated.
- Consider swallowing disorders as a significant factor in students with learning difficulties.
- Develop and implement an Individualized Healthcare Plan (IHP).
- Re-assess per the Feeding/Swallowing Plan.

POTENTIAL COMPLICATIONS:

- Silent aspiration
- Aspiration[6]
- Pneumonia[7]
- Weight loss
- Decreased enjoyment of eating or drinking orally

In some cases, nasogastric feedings are initiated until signs and symptoms are resolved
Placement of gastronomy feeding tube (G-tube or button) if oral feeding will be limited or nothing by mouth (NPO) for extended period of time.

NOTES:[8]

- Although only a small percentage, one per cent, of adolescents, ages three to 17, present with a swallowing disorder, it is important to be aware of swallowing disorders as they can be life threatening.

DYSPHAGIA (SWALLOWING DISORDERS) *(continued from previous page)*

The school nurse is the key professional to:

- Report signs and symptoms of swallowing difficulty to parents and speech language pathologist.
- Educate teachers on diet levels and monitor that students are consistently receiving their solid and liquid diet levels as ordered.
- Initiate individualized staff training for feeding as needed.
- Monitor medications, weight, temperature, lung sounds in at risk students.
- Develop and implement IHP and swallowing/diet plan based on healthcare provider orders.
- Educate student on importance of following their liquid and solid diet orders.
- Participate in dysphagia management team with the speech-language pathologist, occupational therapist, physical therapist, nutritionist, and parent.

REFERENCES

[1]American Speech-Language-Hearing Association. (2015). *Pediatric dysphagia: Considerations for evaluation in the school setting.* http://www.asha.org/PRPSpecificTopic.aspx?folderid=8589934965§ion=Assessment#Considerations_for_Evaluation_in_the_School_Setting

[2]Langmore, S. E. & Krisciunas, G. P. (2010). Dysphagia after radiotherapy for head and neck cancer: Etiology, clinical presentation, and efficacy of current treatments. *Perspectives on Swallowing and Swallowing Disorders (Dysphagia)*19(2), 32-38. https://doi.org/10.1044/sasd19.2.32

[3]Mayo Clinic. (2014). *Dysphagia.* https://www.mayoclinic.org/diseases-conditions/dysphagia/symptoms-_causes/syc-20372028

[4]International Dysphagia Diet Standardization Initiative. (2019). *Food & drinks classification and testing adult & pediatric.* https://iddsi.org/Documents/IDDSIFramework-CompleteFramework.pdf

[5] Homer, E. M. (2018). *"Demystifying swallowing and feeding in the school setting."* Live Webinar, American Speech and Hearing Association, January 18, 2018.

[6] Mayo Clinic. (2014). *Dysphagia.* https://www.mayoclinic.org/diseases-conditions/dysphagia/symptoms-_causes/syc-20372028

[7] Ibid.

[8] Homer, E. M. (2018). *"Demystifying swallowing and feeding in the school setting."* Live Webinar, American Speech and Hearing Association, January 18, 2018.

OTHER REFERENCES CONSULTED

American Speech-Language-Hearing Association. (2015). *Swallowing disorders (dysphasia) in adults.* http://www.asha.org/public/speech/swallowing/Swallowing-Disorders-in-Adults/

Groher, M.E. & Cary, M.A. (2010). *Dysphagia: Clinician Management in Adults and Children.* Mosby Elsevier Inc.

EAR PAIN

DEFINITION/ETIOLOGY:[1]
Otalgia or earache/pain can be caused by external or middle ear conditions or by referred pain from other sources. Infections of the ear are one of the most common diseases of childhood. The incidence of middle ear infection increases in winter and spring. Conditions of the ear can be responsible for transient or permanent hearing loss in students and therefore can have a great impact in the educational setting.

Causes of Specific Ear Pain:[2]

External ear including external auditory canal

- Infection/inflammation (otitis externa, cellulitis, furuncle or abscess, perichondritis of the pinna)
- Cerumen (wax) impaction
- Trauma
- Foreign object
- Tumor or growth

Middle ear [3, 4] - Eustachian tube and Mastoid

- Eustachian tube dysfunction
- Infection/inflammation (otitis media, middle ear effusion, mastoiditis)
- Trauma
- Tumor or growth
- Allergies
- Enlarged adenoids
- Extended pacifier use

Referred ear pain

- Pharyngeal lesions (peritonsillar abscess, retropharyngeal abscess, nasopharyngeal fibroma)
- Mouth lesions (acute stomatitis or glossitis, dental problem)
- Laryngeal and esophageal sources, e.g., laryngeal ulceration, esophageal foreign body, esophageal reflux (acid reflux)

Other

- Temporomandibular joint (TMJ) dysfunction

SIGNS AND SYMPTOMS:

- **Otitis externa**[5] or inflammation of the external ear canal, is also called “swimmer’s ear”. It is commonly seen after frequent exposure to moisture or swimming. *Pseudomonas aeruginosa* and *staphylococcus aureus* is the most common pathogen responsible for otitis externa, fungal infections are less common. The student has pain which may begin gradually or suddenly and is increased with pressure on the tragus or when the pinna is moved.
    - Otorrhea (discharge coming from the external canal) is common
    - Erythema (redness) of the ear canal
    - Itching and irritation

EAR PAIN *(continued from previous page)*

SIGNS AND SYMPTOMS *(continued)*

    - Pressure and fullness in the ear may be reported
    - Possibility of hearing loss if there is enough swelling to occlude the canal

- **Otitis Media (OM)**[6] is an acute inflammation of the middle ear. It is the most common cause of ear pain, and may accompany a simple "cold". The tympanic membrane is dull, often bulging and sometimes erythematous (red). The most common cause is Moraxella catarrhalis, Streptococcus pneumoniae, and Haemophilus influenzae.[7] OM often resolves spontaneously.
    - Ear pain, fever
    - Inability to sleep
    - Lethargy
    - Diarrhea and vomiting may be present
    - Sudden hearing loss may occur

  Otitis media may also be classified as Acute Otitis Media (AOM) referring to a sudden onset and the presence of a middle ear effusion. Three or more episodes of AOM in six months or four or more episodes in 12 months is considered Recurrent AOM.[8]

- **Middle Ear Effusion** (MEE) may complicate an upper respiratory infection. A collection of watery fluid fills the middle ear canal and can interfere with hearing. In most cases, the fluid is absorbed spontaneously within 2-3 weeks, but If it persists for 1-3 months it can lead to a hearing loss and a myringotomy may be indicated.[9] The child is often asymptomatic and afebrile but may have:
    - Mild or intermittent ear pain
    - Fullness, or "popping" in the ear
    - Dizziness
    - Loss of balance

- **Otitis Media with Effusion (OME)** is an accumulation of serous fluid in the middle ear without signs and symptoms of acute infection. Many children develop OME after a course of antibiotics for AOM. Bubbles or fluid levels may be seen behind the tympanic membrane. Chronic OME is associated with hearing loss and a speech assessment may be needed.

- **Impacted Cerumen** may cause ear pain if the cerumen hardens and touches the tympanic membrane. Although cerumen is a naturally forming lubricant and protector of the ear canal, excessive production may block the ear canal causing hearing loss until removed.

- **Foreign Objects** may be placed in the ear canal by small children or those with special needs. If present for more than a few days it is likely there will be foul smelling discharge or pain from abrasions to the auditory canal. ***(Refer to FOREIGN OBJECTS).***

EAR PAIN *(continued from previous page)*

SIGNS AND SYMPTOMS *(continued)*

Mastoiditis is a severe condition caused by extension of a middle ear infection into the periosteum of the skull. Symptoms would include displacement of the pinna away from the skull, erythema, edema and tenderness on palpation. This would require prompt evaluation from a healthcare provider.

Severe ear pain may be a sign of a ruptured eardrum or foreign body, especially if the onset is sudden.

ANTICIPATED CONCERNS/PROBLEMS:

- Ruptured ear drum
- Hearing loss
- Delayed speech and language

MANAGEMENT/POTENTIAL INTERVENTIONS:

- School nurses should feel confident in carrying out an otoscopic examination of the ear and should update otoscope skills if it is not a common practice.[10]

- A complete assessment (ear diagram)[11] of the ear is critical in addition to evaluation of respiratory status, signs of illness, possible sources of referred pain, balance, and dizziness.[12]

- The student with severe pain should be evaluated promptly. If a live insect is the cause of pain, inspection by otoscope may be difficult because the light may aggravate an insect and cause additional pain. Notify parents/guardians and advise taking the child to his/her healthcare provider.

- For otitis externa,[13] the parents/guardians should be advised to take the student to a healthcare provider. Clean any drainage gently from pinna of the ear using clean technique/standard precautions and apply a warm dry compress to the affected ear to relieve pain. Topical antibiotic treatment (eardrops) may be prescribed, but only after confirming that the eardrum is intact. If the eardrum has been perforated a nontoxic topical medication will be ordered. Swimming should be discouraged during antibiotic treatment. The parent/guardian should be advised to have the child use ear plugs to avoid moisture to the ear when swimming. Prevent recurrence (which is common) by instilling two to three drops of isopropyl alcohol in the ear canals after swimming, showering or during hot humid weather if prescribed by the healthcare provider with an order for the school nurse.[14]

- For healthy school- aged children with OM, guidelines recommend observation and pain management for 48 to 72 hours as the majority of OM will resolve spontaneously.[15]

- Removal of cerumen should be done in the office of the healthcare provider and may be done using a curette or irrigation.

EAR PAIN *(continued from previous page)*

MANAGEMENT/POTENTIAL INTERVENTIONS *(continued)*

- When administering ear drops to a child or adult pull up and back on the affected ear. If necessary, have the person lie on their side with the infected ear up to facilitate the medication moving into the ear canal.[16]

- To decrease ear pain, have the child sit up and/or blow a pinwheel to relieve pain.[17]

FOLLOW-UP:[18]

- Screening hearing acuity and comparing the result with a previous screen can be helpful after the student recovers from an acute ear infection.
- If mild hearing loss is found on screening in the absence of any other signs or discomfort, consider a re-check after a few weeks.
- Most OME will resolve without treatment, but if OME becomes chronic, there is a language delay, learning problems, or a significant hearing loss is suspected, a healthcare referral is indicated.

PREVENTION:

Educate parents and children about preventive measures for recurrent ear pain:[19]

- Avoid exposure to second hand smoke.
- Avoid wood burning stoves.
- Using a pacifier several hours a day may increase the occurrence of OM.
- Avoid allergy triggers.
- Avoid putting things in the ear.
- Dry ears well after swimming and bathing.
- Encourage breast feeding to increase immunity.
- Encourage childhood immunizations of Haemophilus influenzae and Pneumococcus pneumonia.

NOTES:

- As child ages ear infections may decease or stop.
- School nurse should be knowledgeable about current treatment guidelines for ear pain.[20]

REFERENCES

[1] Ball, J., Bindler, R., Cowen, K., & Shaw, M. (Eds.). (2017). *Alterations in eye, ear, nose, and throat function. Principles of Pediatric Nursing: Caring for Children* (7th ed., pp. 440-473). Pearson Education, Inc.

[2] Merck Manual, Professional Version. (2019). *External ear obstructions.* https://www.merckmanuals.com/professional/ear,-nose,-and-throat-disorders/external-ear-disorders/external-ear-obstructions?query=referred%20ear%20pain

[3] Ball, J., Bindler, R., Cowen, K., & Shaw, M. (Eds.). (2017). Alterations in eye, ear, nose, and throat function. *Principles of Pediatric Nursing: Caring for Children* (7th ed., pp. 440-473). Pearson Education, Inc.

EAR PAIN *(continued from previous page)*

[4] Jakubowski, T. & Perron, T. (2019). Students with common health complaints: Ear problems. In J. Selekman, R. Adair Shannon, & C. F. Yonkaitis (Eds.), *School nursing: A comprehensive text* (3rd ed., pp. 342-344). F.A. Davis Company.

[5] Merck Manual, Professional Version. (2019). *Otitis media (secretory).* https://www.merckmanuals.com/professional/ear,-nose,-and-throat-disorders/middle-ear-and-tympanic-membrane-disorders/otitis-media-secretory?query=otitis%20media

[6] Mayo Clinic. (2019). *Ear infection (middle ear).* https://www.mayoclinic.org/diseases-conditions/ear-infections/diagnosis-treatment/drc-20351622

[7] Ball, J., Bindler, R., Cowen, K., & Shaw, M. (Eds.). (2017). Alterations in eye, ear, nose, and throat function. *Principles of Pediatric Nursing: Caring for Children* (7th ed., pp. 440-473). Pearson Education, Inc.

[8] Ibid.

[9] Merck Manual, Professional Version. (2019). *Otitis media (secretory).* https://www.merckmanuals.com/professional/ear,-nose,-and-throat-disorders/middle-ear-and-tympanic-membrane-disorders/otitis-media-secretory?query=otitis%20media

[10] Jakubowski, T. & Perron, T. (2019). Students with common health complaints: Ear problems. In J. Selekman, R. Adair Shannon, & C. F. Yonkaitis (Eds.), *School nursing: A comprehensive text* (3rd ed., pp. 342-344). F.A. Davis Company.

[11] Medline Plus, U.S. National Library of Medicine. (2019). *Earache.* https://medlineplus.gov/ency/article/003046.htm

[12] Ibid.

[13] Mayo Clinic. (2019). *Swimmer's ear.* https://www.mayoclinic.org/diseases-conditions/swimmers-ear/diagnosis-treatment/drc-20351688

[14] Merck Manual, Professional Version. (2019). *Acute otitis externa (acute).* https://www.merckmanuals.com/professional/ear,-nose,-and-throat-disorders/external-ear-disorders/external-otitis-acute?query=otitis%20externa

[15] Merck Manual, Professional Version. (2019). *Antibiotics for otitis.* https://www.merckmanuals.com/professional/SearchResults?query=otitis+media

[16] Mayo Clinic. (2019). *Swimmer's ear.* https://www.mayoclinic.org/diseases-conditions/swimmers-ear/diagnosis-treatment/drc-20351688

[17] Ball, J., Bindler, R., Cowen, K., & Shaw, M. (Eds.). (2017). Alterations in eye, ear, nose, and throat function. *Principles of Pediatric Nursing: Caring for Children* (7th ed., pp. 440-473). Pearson Education, Inc.

[18] Ibid.

[19] Ibid.

[20] Lieberthal, A., Carroll, A., Chonlaitree, T., Ganiats, T., Hoberman, A., Jackson, M., Joffe, M.D., Miller, D.T., Rosenfeld, R.M., Sevilla, X.D., Schwartz, R.H., Thomas, P.A., & Tunkel, D.E. (2013). *Clinical practice guideline: The diagnosis and treatment of acute otitis media.* https://pediatrics.aappublications.org/content/131/3/e964.full

OTHER REFERENCES CONSULTED

Academy of Pediatrics. (2016). *Signs and symptoms chart*. In S. Aronson, (Ed.), *Managing infectious diseases in child care and schools* (4th ed., pp. 53). American Academy of Pediatrics.

Roa, S. (2018). Travel medicine. In W.W. Hay, M.J. Levin, R. R. Deterding, & M. J. Abzug (Eds.), *Current diagnosis and treatment: Pediatrics* (24th ed., pp. 1373-74). McGraw Hill Education.

Yoon, P.J., Scholes, M.A., & Friedman, N.R. (2018). Ear, Nose, and throat. In W.W. Hay, M.J. Levin, R. R. Deterding, & M. J. Abzug (Eds.), *Current diagnosis and treatment: Pediatrics* (24th ed., pp. 478- 508). McGraw Hill Education.

EATING DISORDERS

OVERVIEW:
An eating disorder is a medical and psychiatric illness that is marked by persistent disturbances in eating behavior, such as extreme reduction of food intake or extreme overeating, that results in altered consumption or absorption of foods and ultimately in impaired physical health or psychological functioning.[1] There are often feelings of significant concern about body weight or shape. Eating disorders have complicated genetic, biological, behavioral, and social causes. It is more common for women to develop eating disorders but the rate among men is increasing.[2] Although eating disorders may include disorders such as pica, rumination disorder and binge eating disorder the two most commonly seen types are anorexia nervosa (AN) and bulimia nervosa (BN). Eating disorders will often surface during adolescence but can occur at any age. People with eating disorders frequently have co-occurring disorders such as depression, anxiety and substance use disorder.[3] In addition to many short-term problems, they also can develop serious physical complications such as cardiac or kidney disorders that can be fatal.

ANOREXIA NERVOSA

DEFINITION/ETIOLOGY:
Anorexia is characterized by induced and sustained weight loss that is less than minimally normal or expected, intense fear of gaining weight or becoming fat and disturbances in the way the body is viewed with a persistent lack of perception of the seriousness of the low body weight.[4] Speculation on traits that may lead to this disorder are low self-esteem, rigid self-control, fear of maturation, obsession with appearance, and perfectionism.

There are two subtypes of AN:[5]

Restrictive which puts a severe restriction on the type and amount of food that is absorbed or ingested.

Binge eating/purge which, in addition to restriction, also includes binge eating with episodes of purging (vomiting) in an effort to eliminate the food they have eaten.

SIGNS/SYMPTOMS:[6]
- Refusal to maintain body weight at minimal normal weight for age and height or failure to make expected weight gain during period of growth.
- Obsessed with weight. Intense fear of gaining weight or becoming fat, even though underweight.
- Disturbance in the way in which one's body weight, size, or shape is experienced, e.g., the person claims to "feel fat" even if emaciated, believes that one area of the body is "too fat" even when obviously underweight.
- Weight loss accomplished by reduction in total food intake, often with extensive exercising.
- Frequently there is self-induced vomiting, use of laxatives, enemas or diuretics (in such cases Bulimia Nervosa may also be present).

EATING DISORDERS *(continued from previous page)*

SIGNS AND SYMPTOMS *(continued)*

- Often undiagnosed until weight loss is marked. By the time the person is profoundly underweight, there are other signs, such as hypothermia, bradycardia, hypotension, edema, lanugo (fine hair), and a variety of metabolic changes.
- Other symptoms may include abnormal laboratory tests (CBC, electrolytes, liver, kidney, etc.), fatigue, insomnia, thinning of hair, brittle nails, dizziness, anemia, lowering of body temperature and/or constipation.
- Amenorrhea - in most cases, amenorrhea follows weight loss, but may appear before noticeable weight loss has occurred.

MANAGEMENT/TREATMENT:[7]

- **Initial diagnosis** is most important.
  - Often eating disorder is not suspected at home because child is not seen unclothed.
- Refer to healthcare provider if condition is suspected.
- Engage the family in the process.
- Cognitive behavioral therapy may be effective.
- The use of Selective Serotonin Reuptake Inhibitor (SSRIs) is often used to address anxiety and depression.
- Effective treatment is often long term and may require hospitalization to restore weight and address medical complications.
- Establish liaison with parents/guardians, healthcare provider, and therapists – develop multidisciplinary approach in health plan in consultation with healthcare provider and therapist along with school mental health staff.

FOLLOW UP:

- Provide a confidential and welcoming clinic where the student can freely discuss problems.
- Monitor for secondary physical effects of under-nutrition.
- Relapse is common.
- **Significant mortality if not treated:** involuntary commitment may be considered if refusal to seek psychiatric care.

COMPLICATIONS:

- Under-nutrition can become severe enough to affect secondary endocrine, metabolic, and electrolyte disturbances of bodily functions, including osteoporosis.
- Prolonged anorexia may lead to alcohol and substance addiction, fertility problems and death due to cardiac arrhythmia, congestive heart failure, or suicide.
- Suicide risk is also elevated in AN with rates reported as 12 per 100,000 per year.[8]
- AN has a mortality rate of 5-6% which is the highest mortality rate of any psychiatric disorder.[9]

EATING DISORDERS *(continued from previous page)*

BULIMIA NERVOSA

DEFINITION/ETIOLOGY:
Recurrent episodes of binge eating with compensatory behaviors such as vomiting, laxative use or excessive exercise. Episodes occur at least once weekly for three months. Risk factors may include temperament, environment and genetic predispositions. Dieting is often precursor to disordered eating.[10]

SIGNS/SYMPTOMS:[11]

- Recurrent episodes of binge eating
- Normal weight or overweight, although some may be slightly under weight
- Rapid consumption of a large amount of food in a discrete period of time, usually done in secrecy
- A feeling of lack of control over eating behavior during the eating binges
- Self-induced vomiting, use of laxatives or diuretics, strict dieting or fasting
- Vigorous exercise in order to prevent weight gain
- Persistent over concern with body shape and weight
- Chapped, cracked, irritated, or sore fingers or knuckles called "Russell's sign" from self-induced vomiting
- If person purges by vomiting, may have tooth enamel damage and sore throats
- Frequent trips to bathroom following meals
- A depressed mood that may be part of a depressive disorder is commonly observed

MANAGEMENT / TREATMENT:[12]

- Refer to healthcare provider if condition is suspected.
- Engage the family in the process.
- Refer for nutritional counseling and family therapy if appropriate.
- Cognitive behavioral therapy may be effective in changing behaviors and attitudes towards eating and binging through cognitive restructuring and problem-solving skills.
- The use of SSRIs is often used to address anxiety and depression.
- Establish a liaison with parents/guardians, healthcare provider, and therapists – develop a multidisciplinary approach in health plan in consultation with healthcare provider and therapist along with school mental health staff.

FOLLOW UP:

- Monitor behavior and compliance to mental health and eating plan.
- Monitor for physical effects.
- Provide a confidential and welcoming clinic where the student can freely discuss problems.

EATING DISORDERS *(continued from previous page)*

COMPLICATIONS: [13]

- Negative self-esteem and problems with social functioning
- Dehydration-may lead to kidney failure
- Repeated vomiting causing inflammation or tears in the lining of the esophagus and erosion of tooth enamel
- Electrolyte imbalance -may lead to cardiac arrhythmia
- Absence of menstrual periods
- Anxiety and depression
- Under-nutrition- can become severe enough to affect secondary endocrine, metabolic, and electrolyte disturbances of bodily functions, including osteoporosis
- Prolonged bulimia- may lead to alcohol and substance addiction, mental health issues, fertility problems and death due to cardiac arrhythmia, congestive heart failure, or suicide

NOTE: Anorexia and bulimia are two serious life-threatening conditions that are curable if identified early, treated by trained therapists, and supplemented by support groups.

REFERENCES

---

[1] American Psychiatric Association. (2013). Trauma and stress related disorders. In *Diagnostic and statistical manual of mental disorders* (5th ed., pp. 349-347). American Psychiatric Association.

[2] Patterson, B, Bohnenkamp, J., Hoover, S., Bostic, J. Selekman, J. (2019). Students mental and behavioral health. In J. Selekman, R. Adair Shannon, & C. F. Yonkaitis (Eds.), *School nursing: A comprehensive text* (3rd ed., pp. 780-781). F.A. Davis.

[3] Ibid.

[4] American Psychiatric Association. (2013). Trauma and stress related disorders. In *Diagnostic and statistical manual of mental disorders* (5th ed., pp. 349-347). American Psychiatric Association.

[5] National Institute of Mental Health. (2018). *Eating disorders.* http://www.nimh.nih.gov/health/publications/eating-disorders/complete-index.shtml

[6] Ibid.

[7] Patterson, B, Bohnenkamp, J., Hoover, S., Bostic, J. Selekman, J. (2019). Students mental and behavioral health. In J. Selekman, R. Adair Shannon, & C. F. Yonkaitis (Eds.), *School nursing: A comprehensive text* (3rd ed., pp. 780-781). F.A. Davis.

[8] American Psychiatric Association. (2013). Trauma and stress related disorders. In *Diagnostic and statistical manual of mental disorders* (5th ed., pp. 349-347) American Psychiatric Association.

[9] Campbell, K., & Peebles, R. (2014). Eating disorders in children and adolescents; State of art review. *Pediatrics, 1*(34) (pp. 582-592). https://doi.org/10.1542/peds.2014-0194

[10] American Psychiatric Association. (2013). Trauma and stress related disorders. In *Diagnostic and statistical manual of mental disorders* (5th ed., pp. 349-347). American Psychiatric Association.

[11] Patterson, B, Bohnenkamp, J., Hoover, S., Bostic, J. Selekman, J. (2019). Students mental and behavioral health. In J. Selekman, R. Adair Shannon, & C. F. Yonkaitis (Eds.), *School nursing: A comprehensive text* (3rd ed., pp. 780-781). F.A. Davis.

[12] Ibid.

EATING DISORDERS *(continued from previous page)*

[13] Mayo Clinic. (2018). *Bulimia nervosa.* http://www.mayoclinic.org/diseases-conditions/bulimia/basics/definition/con-20033050

OTHER REFERENCES CONSULTED

National Eating Disorders Association. (2018.). *Get the facts on eating disorders.* https://www.nationaleatingdisorders.org/get-facts-eating-disorders

Kids Health from Nemours. (2019). *Eating disorders.* https://kidshealth.org/en/parents/eating-disorders.html

The Heathly Teen Project. (2015). *Adolescent eating disorders such as anorexia, bulimia and binge eating disorders are treatable.* http://www.healthyteenproject.com/adolescent-eating-disorders-ca

ECZEMA (Atopic Dermatitis)

DEFINITION/ETIOLOGY:
Eczema is a form of noncontagious dermatitis or inflamed skin. It presents as itchy, scaly patches that is often in the creases of the elbows or behind the knees. Other common places are neck, wrist or ankles.[1] The exact cause is unknown, but researchers believe people develop eczema from a combination of inherited genes and environmental factors.[2] Atopic (allergic nature) dermatitis is a common type of eczema characterized by acute or chronic skin eruptions.[3] Eczema affects about 1 in 10 children.[4] Symptoms almost always develop before age five.[5] More than half of these children will outgrow eczema before they are teenagers, but almost half will eventually develop hay fever or asthma.[6]

SIGNS AND SYMPTOMS:

- **Chronic or atopic:** Areas of involvement are antecubital and popliteal area, face and neck but can appear anywhere on the body. Usually dry, scaly, easily irritated. May be red or depigmented. Usually seen in school age children. Crusting may be present. Atopic eczema is chronic and characterized by remissions and exacerbations. Be aware of the Allergy Triad: Allergies-Eczema-Asthma either with the child or with positive family history.[7]
- **"Itch-scratch cycle":** Scratching or rubbing itchy skin causes further irritation and traumatizes sensitive tissue that increases the risk of secondary infection. Itching can also cause skin damage that eventually leads to thickened brownish areas on the skin (lichenification).
- Symptoms range from a small patch to a painful rash affecting large areas of the body.[8]

DIFFERENTIAL DIAGNOSES: There is no definitive test available to diagnose eczema[9]

- Seborrheic dermatitis (severe dandruff)[10]
- Contact dermatitis, e.g. poison ivy[11]
- Psoriasis[12]
- Herpes virus[13]
- Molluscum[14]

MANAGEMENT/TREATMENT:

Eczema tends to come and go; periods of mild or no symptoms and then times of severe symptoms or "flare ups".

- Keep skin hydrated:
  - Keep hydrated by drinking water which will increase moisture to the skin.[15]
  - Keep baths brief. Pat dry.[16]
  - Avoid excessive soap exposure; use mild soap. Avoid using scented soap.[17]
  - Apply an emollient (moisturizer) or a cool washcloth to itchy areas.[18]
- Topical corticosteroids and non-steroid creams or ointments may also be beneficial.[19]
- Antibiotic ointment for secondary infection may be prescribed by the healthcare provider.[20]
- Oral antihistamine to relieve itching may be used at bedtime, watch for drowsiness.[21]

ECZEMA (Atopic Dermatitis) *(continued from previous page)*

MANAGEMENT/TREATMENT *(continued)*

- Use soft cotton clothing and bedding. Avoid wool or rough fabrics. Do not rub skin with washcloth.[22]
- Keep fingernails short to minimize skin damage and potential secondary infection from scratching.[23]
- Control temperature and humidity extremes (high or low); gently pat sweaty skin dry.[24]
- Treatment is aimed at avoiding triggers that may cause flare-ups and breaking the "itch-scratch cycle".[25]

Flare-ups may be seasonal, due to factors like irritants, allergens, or stress however may not be able to identify cause. Skin that gets too dry, exposed to certain harsh soaps or detergents, tobacco smoke, excessive heat or sweating may be more susceptible to eczema.[26]

FOLLOW UP:[27]

- Secondary infection is common, especially due to scratching. Resembles impetigo at the edges of eczematous skin; may show as isolated circular crusts with moist or dry pus underneath.
- Observe for fever, flu-like symptoms, pain or swollen lymph nodes.
- Identify trends in flare-ups for possible allergies to chemicals, foods, or environmental factors, e.g., dust mites. This will help to develop a plan to avoid triggers at school. In severe cases a Section 504 plan may be needed.
- Advise others that eczema is not contagious.[28]
- Children are subject to teasing and social distancing which exacerbates stress and low self-esteem. Stress is a common eczema trigger during tween and teen years. Managing stress can reduce flares.
- Sleep disturbances are common, particularly during flare-ups. If the child is tired or irritable, ask the parent/guardian about night symptoms and management.
- Involve children in their care by asking about their experiences and giving them choices and some control over treatment, such as who applies the topical product, and privacy.
- Follow an eczema treatment plan for home and school.[29]

REFERENCES

---

[1] American Academy of Dermatology/Association. (2018). *Eczema resource center.* https://www.aad.org/public/diseases/eczema/eczema-resource-center

[2] National Eczema Association. (2017). *Atopic dermatitis 101 for parents.* https://nationaleczema.org/wp-content/uploads/2018/03/FactSheetAD_101_PEDS_FINAL_edited.pdf

[3] Kids Health/Nemours. (2015). *Eczema.* https://kidshealth.org/en/parents/eczema-atopic-dermatitis.html?ref=search

[4] Ibid.

[5] Ibid.

ECZEMA (Atopic Dermatitis) *(continued from previous page)*

[6] Ibid.

[7] National Eczema Association. (n.d.). *Eczema*. https://nationaleczema.org/eczema/

[8] Ibid.

[9] Kids Health/Nemours. (2015). *Eczema.* https://kidshealth.org/en/parents/eczema-atopic-dermatitis.html?ref=search

[10] Ibid.

[11] Ibid.

[12] Ibid.

[13] American Academy of Dermatology/Association. (2018). *Eczema resource center.* https://www.aad.org/public/diseases/eczema/eczema-resource-center

[14] Ibid.

[15] Kids Health/Nemours. (2015). *Eczema.* https://kidshealth.org/en/parents/eczema-atopic-dermatitis.html?ref=search

[16] Mayo Clinic. (2018). *Atopic dermatitis (eczema).* https://www.mayoclinic.org/diseases-conditions/ atopic-dermatitis-eczema/symptoms-causes/syc-2035273

[17] Kids Health/Nemours. (2015). *Eczema.* https://kidshealth.org/en/parents/eczema-atopic-dermatitis.html?ref=search

[18] Ibid.

[19] Ibid.

[20] Mayo Clinic. (2018). *Atopic dermatitis (eczema).* https://www.mayoclinic.org/diseases-conditions/ atopic-dermatitis-eczema/symptoms-causes/syc-2035273

[21] Ibid.

[22] Ibid.

[23] Kids Health/Nemours. (2015). *Eczema.* https://kidshealth.org/en/parents/eczema-atopic-dermatitis.html?ref=search

[24] Ibid.

[25] Mayo Clinic. (2018). *Atopic dermatitis (eczema).* https://www.mayoclinic.org/diseases-conditions/ atopic-dermatitis-eczema/symptoms-causes/syc-2035273 3

[26] Kids Health/Nemours. (2015). *Eczema.* https://kidshealth.org/en/parents/eczema-atopic-dermatitis.html?ref=search

[27] American Academy of Dermatology/Association. (2018). *Eczema resource center.* https://www.aad.org/public/diseases/eczema/eczema-resource-center

[28] Ibid.

[29] Ibid.

ENCOPRESIS

DEFINITION/ETIOLOGY:

Encopresis is defined as stool incontinence by a child of an age that should be able to control bowel movements, usually over 4 years old.[1] Most cases are due to chronic constipation that can result in the stretching of the large intestine. Eventually, the enlarged intestine loses its ability to sense the presence of stool.[2] This leads to involuntary soiling or leakage of liquid stool around the larger stool mass.[3] The incontinence occurs as stool leaks around the impaction and it cannot be controlled by the child.[4]

Encopresis is not a disease but a symptom. It can have several causes.[5] It may be due to physiologic and/or psychological factors. Withholding stool may be related to fear of using toilet, painful bowel movements, not wanting to interrupt play or not enough fiber in diet.[6] It could be related to stress such as premature/difficult toilet training or life changes such as starting school, divorce in family, birth of sibling or schedule changes.[7] Organic causes, or constipation due to a medical origin, are less common, e.g. Hirschsprung or Celiac Disease.[8]

Prevalence: Encopresis occurs in 3-4% of four-year-old children and it decreases with age.[9] It's more common in boys, children with autism, anxiety disorder and those taking medications that cause constipation.[10]

SIGNS AND SYMPTOMS:

- Fecal impaction with leaking of liquefied stool around impaction (most common)[11]
- Large stools that block up the toilet[12]
- Fecal soiling of clothes[13]
- Needing to have a bowel movement with little or no warning or involuntary bowel movement[14]
- Fecal odor[15]
- Loss of appetite[16]
- Abdominal pain[17]
- Urinary symptoms: urinary tract infections, urine incontinence, bedwetting[18]
- Rectal bleeding related to a small tear in skin from passing large, hard stool[19]

<u>EMOTIONAL/BEHAVIORAL FINDINGS:</u>[20]

<u>Some children have significant behavioral and emotional difficulties such as:</u>

- Peer conflicts
- Academic difficulties
- Feelings of shame, embarrassment and low self-esteem
- Family conflicts/issues: family members may get more frustrated and angry over the child's bowel control/lack of control

ENCOPRESIS *(continued from previous page)*

MANAGEMENT/TREATMENT:

- Develop an Individualized Healthcare Plan (IHP) based on medical treatment plan to meet the student's needs during the school day.

- Treatment should always be guided by child's healthcare provider.[21]

- Make change of clothing and wash-up facilities available. Ensure the confidentiality of the child's condition from other children and school personnel as much as possible.

- Disimpaction: Healthcare provider may prescribe a "clean out" that may include stool softeners, enemas, laxatives, suppositories or a combination of things.[22] This clean out period is often planned for weekends or may require child to stay home from school for typically one to two days.

- Disimpaction is followed by mild laxatives, bowel training and increased fiber and fluids in diet. After time, the intestine and rectum will decrease to normal size and the child should be able to have normal bowel movements without the aid of medication.[23] The school nurse should work with the parents/guardians, if possible, so that the mild laxatives do not "work" during school or school bus times.

- Bowel training includes a toileting schedule encouraging the child to sit on the toilet for five to 10 minutes about 15-30 minutes after a meal in a private, non-stressful environment. Consider adding an identified private bathroom for student to use after lunch in the IHP.[24] Have child put feet on a small foot stool when sitting on the toilet to have a bowel movement. This puts pressure on the abdomen, making a bowel movement easier.[25]

- Start school counseling or professional mental health counseling for help with associated emotional/behavioral problems.[26] Include child support and positive reinforcement in the student IHP as directed by the mental health providers.[27]

- Teach and encourage importance of diet and exercise:[28]
  - Increase in fruits, vegetables and whole grains
  - Increase in fluids, especially water
  - Increase in exercise

- Enlist parent or other person in home to assist with diet, prescribed laxatives, and regular bowel training. The home and school plan for times, rewards or behavioral techniques, appropriate foods, etc., should be jointly developed so that the school staff and family are consistent in their management.

ENCOPRESIS *(continued from previous page)*

FOLLOW UP:

- The goal is to prevent constipation and maintain good bowel habits.
- Long term success depends on how well the plan of care is followed.
- Maintain liaison with teacher, parents and healthcare provider.

RESOURCES

Websites for Children:

- Movie: Digestive System - https://kidshealth.org/en/kids/dsmovie.html?ref=search
- Constipation - https://kidshealth.org/en/kids/constipation.html?ref=search
  https://gikids.org/constipation/resources

REFERENCES

---

[1] Kids Health/Nemours. (2018). *Soiling (encopresis).* https://kidshealth.org/en/parents/encopresis.html?ref=search

[2] Boston Children's Hospital. (n.d.). *Encopresis.* http://www.childrenshospital.org/conditions-and-treatments/conditions/e/encopresis

[3] Ibid.

[4] Ibid.

[5] Kids Health/Nemours. (2018). *Soiling (encopresis).* https://kidshealth.org/en/parents/encopresis.html?ref=search

[6] Mayo Clinic. (2019). *Encopresis.* https://www.mayoclinic.org/diseases-conditions/encopresis/symptoms-causes/syc-20354494

[7] Ibid.

[8] Merck Manual. (2018). *Stool incontinence in children.* https://www.merckmanuals.com/professional/pediatrics/incontinence-in-children/stool-incontinence-in-children

[9] Merck Manual. (2018). *Stool incontinence in children.* https://www.merckmanuals.com/professional/pediatrics/incontinence-in-children/stool-incontinence-in-children

[10] Mayo Clinic. (2019). *Encopresis.* https://www.mayoclinic.org/diseases-conditions/encopresis/symptoms-causes/syc-20354494

[11] Kids Health/Nemours. (2018). *Soiling (encopresis).* https://kidshealth.org/en/parents/encopresis.html?ref=search

[12] Ibid.

[13] Ibid.

[14] Boston Children's Hospital. (n.d.). *Encopresis.* http://www.childrenshospital.org/conditions-and-treatments/conditions/e/encopresis

[15] Harvard Health Publishing, Harvard Medical School. (2018). *Encopresis (fecal soiling).* https://www.health.harvard.edu/a_to_z/encopresis-fecal-soiling-a-to-z

ENCOPRESIS *(continued from previous page)*

[16] Kids Health/Nemours. (2018). *Soiling (encopresis).* https://kidshealth.org/en/parents/encopresis.html?ref=search

[17] Ibid.

[18] Mayo Clinic. (2019). *Encopresis.* https://www.mayoclinic.org/diseases-conditions/encopresis/symptoms-causes/syc-20354494

[19] Kids Health/Nemours. (2018). *Soiling (encopresis).* https://kidshealth.org/en/parents/encopresis.html?ref=search

[20] American Academy of Pediatrics. (2015). *Soiling (encopresis).* https://www.healthychildren.org/English/health-issues/conditions/emotional-problems/Pages/Soiling-Encopresis.aspx

[21] Cincinnati Children's. (2016). *Encopresis.* https://www.healthychildren.org/English/health-issues/conditions/emotional-problems/Pages/Soiling-Encopresis.aspx

[22] Kids Health/Nemours. (2018). *Soiling (encopresis).* https://kidshealth.org/en/parents/encopresis.html?ref=search

[23] Boston Children's Hospital. (n.d.). *Encopresis.* http://www.childrenshospital.org/conditions-and-treatments/conditions/e/encopresis

[24] Merck Manual. (2018). *Stool incontinence in children.* https://www.merckmanuals.com/professional/pediatrics/incontinence-in-children/stool-incontinence-in-children

[25] Children's Hospital of Wisconsin. (2017). *Kids and constipation: How to keep things moving.* https://chw.org/newshub/stories/kids-and-constipation-how-to-keep-things-moving

[26] Mayo Clinic. (2019). *Encopresis.* https://www.mayoclinic.org/diseases-conditions/encopresis/symptoms-causes/syc-20354494

[27] Kids Health/Nemours. (2018). *Soiling (encopresis).* https://kidshealth.org/en/parents/encopresis.html?ref=search

[28] Cincinnati Children's. (2016). *Encopresis.* https://www.healthychildren.org/English/health-issues/conditions/emotional-problems/Pages/Soiling-Encopresis.aspx

ENURESIS

DEFINITION/ETIOLOGY:
Enuresis (involuntary urination) is repeated, spontaneous urinary voiding in clothes or in bed after the age when toilet training should be complete (usually age five years or under). Enuresis is typically diagnosed after the age of five. It does not usually indicate a physical or emotional problem. It is twice as common in boys. Enuresis usually takes the form of bed wetting.[1]

CAUSES:[2]

- Idiopathic hereditary type (primary nocturnal enuresis) is the most common
- If both parents had a history of enuresis, the rate of nocturnal enuresis found in children is approximately 80%
- Sleep apnea
- Chronic constipation
- Some children have unusually deep sleep patterns
- Mitral stenosis in boys
- Boys with excessively long foreskin and poor hygiene
- Chronic urinary tract infection
- Small bladder capacity, irritable bladder, poor sphincter control, or other organic conditions
- Various emotional/psychological problems, including sexual abuse
- Stress

SIGNS AND SYMPTOMS:

- Urine-stained and wet clothes
- Odor
- Urgency to void
- Bed wetting
- Emotional/behavioral problems, but not as pervasive or common as in children with encopresis
- Symptoms of chronic infection: poor nutritional status plus anemia, itching, foul odor, low-grade fever, stained underpants from constant dribbling, redness and/or impetigo in genital area
- Small caliber of urinary stream in boys with mitral stenosis
- Infection under an excessively long foreskln

ENURESIS *(continued from previous page)*

MANAGEMENT/TREATMENT:

Bed wetting

- Children may outgrow bed wetting without any intervention.
- Behavior modification with rewards may help.
- Bladder control training.
- Limiting fluids at bedtime alone does not appear to be effective.
- Alarm devices which wake child when the bed is wet – most effective long-term strategy.
- Healthcare provider may prescribe medication – drugs can decrease bed wetting; results are often not sustained after treatment is stopped.
- Oral desmopressin (DDAVP) along with limiting fluids reduces urine production in children with normal bladder capacity.
    - Side effect – DDAVP increases the potential for seizures.
- Anticholinergic agents such as oxybutynin chloride and tolterodine; the combination of desmopressin acetate and oxybutynin chloride may be efficacious in children with overactive bladder or dysfunctional voiding who show daytime response to anticholinergic therapy but continue to wet at night.[3]

At school[4]

- Develop an individualized Healthcare Plan
- Protect privacy of child's condition from other children.
- Eliminate shame, guilt or punishment.
- Make toilet, washing, and change of clothing facilities available.
- Keep extra clothing at school.
- Help child make pre-need trips to bathroom.
- Use clock to help remind child of the need to use the bathroom.
- Liaison with parent/guardian(s) and healthcare provider as necessary.
    - The healthcare provider may request a diary to understand the pattern of daytime urination and bowel movements, diet, etc.
- Educate the child that, during sleep, his/her brain may not "hear" his/her full bladder's signal to help him/her understand the condition and how medication or other interventions (alarm) may help.

ENURESIS *(continued from previous page)*

FOLLOW-UP:

- If prescribed, monitor for side effects of medication.
- Monitor for medical conditions – enuresis may be a symptom of a physical condition (diabetes mellitus, diabetes insipidus, sickle cell anemia, urethral obstruction, renal failure etc.). There may be a correlation between pinworms and nocturnal enuresis.
- If indicated, refer to healthcare provider for further diagnostic workup.
- RED FLAG – enuresis could be a sign of sexual abuse; monitor; if indicated, report to child protective services per school and state guidelines.

POSSIBLE COMPLICATIONS:

- Contributes to poor self-esteem
- Disrupts family interactions
- May disrupt peer/social interactions
- Genital rash

NOTES:

- Children with significant ADHD are more likely to experience nocturnal enuresis.[5]

REFERENCES

[1] American Psychiatric Association (APA). (2013). *Diagnostic and statistical manual of mental disorders (DSM-V)* (5th ed.) https://doi.org/10.1176/appi.books.9780890425596

[2] Dunn, A.M., & McGarry, M. (2017). Elimination patterns. In C. Burns, A.M. Dunn, M.H. Brady, N.B. Starr, C.G. Blosser, & D.L. Garzon (Eds.), Pediatric *primary care* (6th ed., pp.216-233). Elsevier.

[3] American Psychiatric Association. (2013). *Diagnostic and statistical manual of mental disorders (DSM-V)* (5th ed.) https://doi.org/10.1176/appi.books.9780890425596

[4] Jakubowski, T., & Perron, T. (2019). Students with common complaints. In J. Selekman, R.A. Shannon, & C. F. Younkaitis (Eds.), *School Nursing: A comprehensive text* (3rd ed., pp. 335-367). F. A. Davis.

5. American Psychiatric Association (APA). (2013). *Diagnostic and statistical manual of mental disorders (DSM-V)* (5th ed.) https://doi.org/10.1176/appi.books.9780890425596

OTHER REFERENCES CONSULTED

Mayo Clinic. (2019). *Bed-wetting.* https://www.mayoclinic.org/diseases-conditions/bed-wetting/symptoms-causes/syc-20366685

Merck Manual. (2019). *Urinary incontinence in children.* https://www.merckmanuals.com/professional/pediatrics/incontinence-in-children/urinary-incontinence-in-children

EYE TRAUMA

DEFINITION/ETIOLOGY:[1]
Ocular injuries can involve the eyelids, the eyeball and the bones surrounding the eye. Eye injuries in children commonly result from blunt trauma, sharp objects, sport injuries or projectiles. Facial injuries often accompany eye trauma.

Chemical burns to the eye are ophthalmologic emergencies and must be referred for immediate emergency care.

Corneal abrasion may result from a direct contact injury, contact lens, or a foreign body with or without penetration.

Foreign Body injuries to the eye may present as either non-penetrating or penetrating. Penetrating injuries are ophthalmologic emergencies and must be referred for immediate emergency care.

SIGNS AND SYMPTOMS (general):[2]
- Pain
- Difficulty with vision
- Redness in the sclera
- Blood in or around the eye
- Hematoma
- Tearing
- Photosensitivity
- Foreign body in eye or under eyelid
- Sensation of foreign body
- Irregular size or shape of the pupil

Assessment[3]
- Obtain history and nature of physical injury or chemical exposure.
- Assess visual acuity first by using appropriate assessment chart such as the Snellen Chart, "E" test, or LEA symbols chart (pre-school aged children). Each eye should be checked individually. The only exception is an acute chemical exposure/injury that requires immediate irrigation (flush with water).
- If student is unable to open eye, do not force.
- Check for visible contusion/lacerations on lids or eyeball.
- Check for blood in anterior chamber (between iris and cornea), called "hyphema".
- Check extra-ocular movements.
- Check for double vision (diplopia).
- Check for unequal or irregular pupils.
- Check pupil responses.

EYE TRAUMA *(continued from previous page)*

MANAGEMENT/TREATMENT (for all eye injuries)

- Instruct student to not rub eye.
- Do not attempt to remove penetrating objects.

Emergency referral to healthcare provider:

- All cases with chemical burn after irrigation with copious amount of water or saline.
- Impaired vision in any way.
- Painful eye or feels like a foreign object.
- Contusion or laceration on eyelid or eyeball.
- Red eye persists for more than one hour (suggests corneal abrasion or foreign object).

Eye trauma without above symptoms:

- Small abrasion or laceration of skin around the eye- without other symptoms- can be washed and left uncovered.
- Red spot limited to the sclera (white of the eye) is typically related to coughing or vomiting (subconjunctival hemorrhage will resolve spontaneously).[4]
- Cold pack may be useful for minor trauma if healthcare provider referral is not necessary.
- Avoid using any eye drops or ointments.

Chemical Burn[5]

Ophthalmic burns to the cornea and conjunctiva are an ophthalmic emergency and treatment should begin immediately. The eye will be painful, sensitive to light (photophobic) and exhibit excessive tearing (lacrimation).

1. Determine chemical if possible. Alkali burns are generally worse than acid burns. If chemical is known, contact poison control (1-800-222-1222) for further information regarding specific emergency treatment. Send available chemical information (name of chemical and ph) with student to emergency treatment center.
2. *Immediately,* flush/irrigate eye with copious amounts of water or saline solution while both eyelids are held open. If only one eye has been exposed to the chemical, attempt to irrigate the eye with the person lying on his/her side. If possible, pour water from the inner corner flowing toward the outer corner.
3. Notify parent/guardian.
4. Refer for emergency medical treatment. Eye should be examined by an ophthalmologist as soon as possible, no longer than 24 hours after exposure.
5. Cool compress to the surrounding area may provide comfort.

EYE TRAUMA *(continued from previous page)*

Corneal Abrasion [6]

The eye will be painful, sensitive to light (photophobic) and exhibit excessive tearing (lacrimation).

1. Remove contact lens, if present.
2. Examine the eye for the presence of a foreign body. The absence of a *visible* foreign body does not negate the presence of or irritation from a foreign body.
3. Notify parent/guardian.
4. Refer to ophthalmologist for evaluation and necessary treatment.
5. To minimize eye movement, patch both eyes with gauze pads prior to travel to healthcare provider or ophthalmologist.

Foreign Body (non-penetrating)[7]

The eye will be painful, sensitive to light (photophobic), exhibit excessive tearing (lacrimation), and have the sensation of a foreign body presence in the eye.

1. Remove contact lens, if present.
2. Examine the eye for the presence of a foreign body. To visualize foreign object, have student look up and down and from side to side. It may be necessary to invert the upper lid to see the presence of a foreign body.
3. If foreign body (speck of dirt, sand, eyelash, etc.) is obvious, try to remove it by gently flushing with warm water from inner to outer area of eye. If foreign object is visualized in corner of eye or in the lower lid, attempt to remove object by touching object with clean moistened cotton swab.
4. If these attempts and maneuvers fail, notify parents/guardians and refer to the healthcare provider.
5. To minimize eye movement, patch both eyes with gauze pads prior to travel to healthcare provider or ophthalmologist.

Foreign Body (penetrating)[8]

The patient will experience intense pain, sensitivity to light (photophobic), exhibit excessive tearing (lacrimation) and redness. You may be able to visualize the penetrating object.

Penetrating injuries are ophthalmologic emergencies.

- **Do not attempt to remove the object or flush the eye.**
- Cover the injured eye with an eye shield or small paper cup. Anchor in place. Patch the other eye to minimize eye movement.
- Notify parent/guardian.
- Refer to emergency medical center or ophthalmologist for *immediate* care.[9]

EYE TRAUMA *(continued from previous page)*

FOLLOW UP:

- If student returned to class, re-examine eye later that day and on the following day. Continue to monitor for pain and infection.
- For eye trauma without emergency symptoms, re-check visual acuity 3-4 days after treatment and refer to healthcare provider if there is difference from prior screening.
- If seen by the healthcare provider, implement healthcare provider's instructions for care after initial evaluation and treatment.
- Healthcare provider may recommend not wearing contact lens for a few days following eye trauma requiring emergency care. This may have implications for reading and classroom work.

NOTES:

Prevention

Stress the importance of wearing protective eyewear when participating in contact and ball sports, working with metal and glass projects, hammering metal on metal, and handling chemicals.[10]

REFERENCES

---

[1] American Academy of Ophthalmology. (2019). *Recognizing and treating eye injuries.* http://www.geteyesmart.org/eyesmart/living/eye-injuries/index.cfm

[2] Ibid.

[3] Gardiner, M.F. (2019). *Overview of eye injuries in the emergency department.* https://www.uptodate.com/contents/overview-of-eye-injuries-in-the-emergency-department?search=eye%20injury%20children&source=search_result&selectedTitle=1~150&usage_type=default&display_rank=1#H1904749

[4] Merck Manual. (2018). *Subconjunctival hemorrhages.* http://www.merckmanuals.com/professional/eye-disorders/conjunctival-and-scleral-disorders/subconjunctival-hemorrhages

[5] Kuckelkorn, R., Schrage, N., Keller, G., & Redbrake, C. (2002). Emergency treatment of chemical and thermal eye burns. *Acta Ophthalmologica Scandinavica*, *80*(1), 4-10. https://doi.org/10.1034/j.1600-0420.2002.800102.x

[6] Merck Manual. (2017). *Corneal abrasions & foreign bodies.* http://www.merckmanuals.com/professional/injuries_poisoning/eye_trauma/corneal_abrasions_and_foreign_bodies.html?qt=corneal%20abrasions&alt=sh

[7] Jacobs, D. (2019). *Cornea abrasions and corneal foreign bodies: Management.* https://www.uptodate.com/contents/corneal-abrasions-and-corneal-foreign-bodies-management?search=eye%20foreign%20body&source=search_result&selectedTitle=1~112&usage_type=default&display_rank=1#H7154913

[8] Ibid.

[9] Ibid.

[10] American Academy of Ophthalmology. (2013). *Clinical statement: Protective eyewear for young athletes.* http://one.aao.org/CE/PracticeGuidelines/ClinicalStatements_Content.aspx?cid=1fda605b-97b9-47e3-90d1-11b7a9607797

FACTITIOUS DISORDER

DEFINITION/ETIOLOGY:
Factitious Disorder is a condition that was previously referred to as Munchausen and Munchausen by Proxy.

Factitious disorders are mental health conditions in which a person acts as if he or she has an illness by deliberately producing, feigning, or exaggerating symptoms. People with factitious disorders seek painful diagnostic tests and procedures in order to obtain attention. They can deliberately create or exaggerate symptoms. While the cause of factitious disorders is unknown, some theories believe there is both a biological and psychological cause. Frequently there is a history of abuse, neglect, a previous hospitalization and/or professional experience in healthcare.[1] Factitious disorders frequently result in injury, illness, and unnecessary medical tests including possible unnecessary surgical interventions.

There are two types of factitious disorders which include *Factitious Disorder Imposed on Self* and *Factitious Disorder Imposed on Others*.

- **Factitious Disorder imposed on self** includes the falsification of physical or psychological signs and symptoms, injury or disease that is not explained by another disorder, including another mental health disorder. [2]
- **Factitious Disorder Imposed on Another** is the falsification of physical or psychological signs or symptoms, or induction of injury or disease on another.[3] This was previously referred to as Munchausen by Proxy. This is a form of child abuse in which a parent/guardian/caregiver (most often the mother) deliberately produces false physical or psychological symptoms in a child under their care causing the victim to be regarded as ill or impaired by others. The child is presented for medical treatment and the parent or caregiver fails to acknowledge the deception. It often involves physical abuse, neglect, and emotional abuse.[4] The parent often thrives on the attention garnered from health care professionals.[5] **A child who is subjected to this behavior is a victim of child abuse.**

Factitious disorders must be distinguished from **malingering** (faking illness to avoid other responsibilities). In malingering, the individual also produces the symptoms intentionally, but has a *goal that is recognizable* when the circumstances are known. For example, the falsification of symptoms to avoid a math test would be called malingering.[6]

Medical conditions fabricated by children may go undetected or be diagnosed as **somatization**. Somatization refers to the occurrence of a combination of physical complaints and excessive thoughts, feelings and behavior for which medical evaluation reveals no physical pathology, or when pathology is present, the complaints are grossly in excess of what would be expected from the physical findings.[7] Further study of children who falsify symptoms may in some cases help identify earlier experiences of Factitious Disorder Imposed on Another (parent/guardian involvement) or covert parental coaching of illness falsification. Better understanding and identification of these children is likely to help prevent the development of more chronic adult factitious disorders.

FACTITIOUS DISORDER *(continued from previous page)*

SIGNS AND SYMPTOMS:

Factitious Disorder Imposed on Self

- Child may present with an inconsistent medical history
- Child may seek frequent treatment from the school nurse/health office personnel
- May present with reports of symptoms that are not observable
- May demonstrate an extensive knowledge of medical terminology and descriptions of illness
- Presence of bruises or infection
- Causing self-harm
- Evidence of self-bruising or ingestion of substances to cause illness
- Presence of symptoms only when the child is alone or never observed by someone else
- Willingness or eagerness to have medical tests, operations, or other procedures
- Reluctance by the child to have the school nurse speak with their parent/guardian(s) or healthcare providers
- Seeking treatment from multiple doctor's, clinic, hospitals, etc.
- New symptoms after obtaining negative results

Factitious Disorder Imposed by Another

- A parent or caregiver fabricates symptoms of illness in a child
- Most common in children under one and up to age six years old
- The child is presented for medical assessment and care, usually persistently, often resulting in multiple medical procedures and hospitalizations
- Dramatic but inconsistent medical history
- History of frequent hospitalizations, usually for a variety of nonspecific symptoms
- The perpetrator denies the etiology of the child's illness
- Common physical signs include seizures, fever, diarrhea, apnea, nervous system dysfunction, signs of bleeding often seen in urine or stool and rashes which can be reported or actual when caused by perpetrator
- Refusal of psychiatric services
- Forecasting negative medical outcomes
- Symptoms of illness abate upon separation of the child from the perpetrator
- Improvement of symptoms occurs when child is hospitalized but return on discharge
- Parent is often viewed as overprotective and caring[8]

FACTITIOUS DISORDER *(continued from previous page)*

MANAGEMENT/TREATMENT:
Be alert to the possibility of Factitious Disorder.

- If there are concerns regarding illness fabrication or discrepancies between the caregiver's reports of health problems in the child and the school nurse's observations of the child's health, the school nurse should:
  - Review the child's past medical history.
  - Consult with the child's healthcare provider to review the child's diagnosis and health status. Discuss implications for school attendance and participation in school activities. Inform the provider of observations of the child in the school setting.
  - Document child/parent/guardian interactions.
  - Maintain a trusting relationship with the caregiver.
- Information about the child's attendance, school health records, parental reports of medical/health problems, educational testing, and staff observations of health and behavioral issues are relevant and may be requested by the healthcare provider or legal authorities.
- Be prepared to provide information as needed or initiate a referral to Child Protective Services. Follow district policy.
- Factitious disorders are usually treated with psychotherapy and/or family therapy. Behavior modification is the first goal.[9]
- Medication may be used to treat related disorders such as depression or anxiety.[10]

POTENTIAL COMPLICATIONS:
- Absences from school which affect academic success
- Side effects of use of drugs or medical tests used to explore cause of reported physical or psychological symptoms
- Injury from self-inflicted medical conditions or harm
- Fear
- Pain and suffering
- Loss of normal attachment to parent/caregiver
- Loss of normal developmental experiences (i.e., kept out of school or staying home from school in cases of Factitious Disorder)
- Loss of normal social experiences
- Alcohol or substance abuse
- Death

FACTITIOUS DISORDER *(continued from previous page)*

REFERENCES

[1] The Cleveland Clinic Foundation. (2019). *An overview of factitious disorders.* http://my.clevelandclinic.org/health/diseases/9832-an-overview-of-factitious-disorders

[2] American Psychiatric Association. (2013). Diagnostic and statistical manual of mental disorders, (5th ed., pp. 324-326). American Psychiatric Publishing.

[3] Ibid.

[4] The Cleveland Clinic Foundation. (2019). *An overview of factitious disorders.* http://my.clevelandclinic.org/health/diseases/9832-an-overview-of-factitious-disorders

[5] Gordon, S., Selekman, J. (2019). Student victimization. In J. Selekman, R. Adair Shannon, & C. F. Yonkaitis (Eds.), *School nursing: A comprehensive text* (3rd ed., pp. 790-822). F.A. Davis.

[6] Medscape (2017). *Malingering.* https://emedicine.medscape.com/article/293206-overview

[7] American Psychiatric Association. (2013). Diagnostic and statistical manual of mental disorders, (5th ed., pp. 324-326). American Psychiatric Publishing.

[8] Gordon, S., Selekman, J. (2019). Student victimization. In J. Selekman, R. Adair Shannon, & C. F. Yonkaitis (Eds.), *School nursing: A comprehensive text* (3rd ed., pp. 790-822). F.A. Davis.

[9] The Cleveland Clinic Foundation. (2019). *An overview of factitious disorders.* http://my.clevelandclinic.org/health/diseases/9832-an-overview-of-factitious-disorders

[10] Ibid.

OTHER RESOURCES CONSULTED

Mayo Clinic. (2019). *Factious disorder.* https://www.mayoclinic.org/diseases-conditions/factitious-disorder/symptoms-causes/syc-20356028

FEVER

DEFINITION/ETIOLOGY:

Fever is a physiological response to inflammation, viral illness, infection or some other cause, which generally helps the body's defense mechanism. Fever is one of the body's responses to illness or injury; however, it can also be a result from heat exposure. Fever is not always cause for alarm, but sometimes it is a sign of a serious problem. Fever is not an illness but is a sign or symptom of what could be an illness or concern.[1]

Fever can improve the immune response at lower temperatures and impair some microorganisms and viruses. Fever can play a key role in helping the body fight off infection.[2] However, fever can cause dehydration, and may stress the cardio-respiratory system. It can also cause discomfort. An oral temperature of over 100.4 degrees Fahrenheit is considered a fever.[3]

SIGNS AND SYMPTOMS:[4]

- Headache
- Loss of appetite
- Mild irritability
- State they feel cold or shiver
- Signs and symptoms of infectious disease such as:
    - Cough
    - diarrhea
    - vomiting
    - general weakness
    - muscle ache
- Sensitive skin; described as "prickly"
- Eyes may appear glassy
- Face may be flushed
- Skin will be warm or hot to touch
- Dehydration
- Increase of 10 – 15 pulse beats for every degree of fever
- Respirations increase three (3) to five (5) breaths per minute per degree[5]

MANAGEMENT/TREATMENT:

1. **Evaluation and treatment of acute fever could vary depending on the age and accompanying symptoms of the child.[6]**
2. Assess vital signs.
3. Ensure accurate temperature reading; wait several minutes to take temperature if student has been out in cold or if has just consumed hot or cold liquid.
4. Provide comfort measures and cool compress on the forehead.

FEVER *(continued from previous page)*

MANAGEMENT/TREATMENT *(continued)*

5. Remove extra outer clothing (but not to point to create shivering which will increase temperature).
6. Give fluids to drink.
7. Assess for signs of infectious disease and use social distancing.
8. Follow school exclusion policies for elevated temperature.
9. Fever that causes enough discomfort to need medication usually indicates that the student should not be in school.
10. Follow school policy regarding over-the-counter (OTC) medications. Since a low-grade fever may be beneficial, withhold acetaminophen unless healthcare provider/nurse practitioner orders. Recheck the student's temperature 30-60 minutes after giving medication and note if medication was effective.

NOTES:

- Children with fever, headache, neck stiffness, petechiae or purpura may have significant or more serious illness and should be evaluated by a healthcare provider.[7]
- A healthcare provider should evaluate children with fever and who are lethargic, unusually drowsy, altered level of consciousness, or extremely pale or cyanotic.[8]
- Some children, usually between the ages of six (6) months and five (5) years may experience seizures from a high fever.[9] Never give aspirin to a child or teen under 19 during episodes of fever-causing illnesses as aspirin has been linked to the life-threatening disorder Reye's syndrome.[10]
- Children can return to school when the temperature has been normal for 24 hours without medication.[11]

REFERENCES

---

[1] The Nemours Foundation. (2018). *Fevers.* http://Kidshealth.org/en/parents/fever.html#

[2] Merck Manual. (2018). *Fever.* http://www.merckmanuals.com/professional/pediatrics/symptoms-in-infants-and-children/fever-in-infants-and-children

[3] Ibid.

[4] Mayo Clinic. (2018). *Fever.* http://www.mayoclinic.org/diseases-conditions/fever/basics/definition/con-20019229

[5] Jakubowski, T. & Perron, T. (2019). Students with common health complaints. In J. Selekman, R. Adair Shannon, & C. F. Yonkaitis (Eds.), *School nursing: A comprehensive text* (3rd ed., pp. 338-340). F.A. Davis.

[6] Merck Manual. (2018). *Fever.* http://www.merckmanuals.com/professional/pediatrics/symptoms-in-infants-and-children/fever-in-infants-and-children

[7] Ibid.

FEVER *(continued from previous page)*

[8] Mayo Clinic. (2018). *Fever.* http://www.mayoclinic.org/diseases-conditions/fever/basics/definition/con-20019229

[9] Ibid.

[10] Merck Manual. (2018). *Fever.* http://www.merckmanuals.com/professional/pediatrics/symptoms-in-infants-and-children/fever-in-infants-and-children

[11] Centers for Disease Control. (2017). *Parents of childcare and K-12 students.* https://www.cdc.gov/nonpharmaceutical-interventions/school/parents-childcare-k-12-students.html

FIFTH DISEASE (Erythema Infectiosum)

OVERVIEW/DEFINITION:

"Fifth Disease" is named that because it was identified after rubeola, rubella, scarlet fever, and roseola. It is caused by Human Parvovirus (*parvovirus B19)*—related to, but not the same as dog parvovirus. It is a common viral infection and occurs in preschool and school aged children. It is most common in the winter and spring and in children four to 10 years old.[1] Transmission or spread is by droplets from respiratory secretions or secondarily by hands before the rash appears. It can also be transmitted in blood, which although rare, can cause a miscarriage. About 50% of adults have had the disease as children, thus are immune.[2] The incubation period is four to 14 days but can be as long as 21 days.[3] Rash symptoms occur one to three weeks after infection. No vaccine is available. If you have had fifth disease you cannot get it again.

SIGNS AND SYMPTOMS:[4, 5]

- About a week after exposure, the child may develop mild systemic symptoms including but not limited to a low-grade fever, headache, cold symptoms and/or muscle aches which may last seven to 10 days, after which the child recovers with no other symptoms.
- About one to three weeks after the fever goes away, a distinctive rash may appear. The rash has a slapped cheek appearance and a faint, lacy rash on the trunk, arms and legs may develop about 1 day later. At this point the child is no longer contagious.
- Adults, especially women, may have joint pain and swelling at this stage. The rash fades in one to two weeks but may recur for several weeks brought on by exposure to sunlight, heat, exercise, or stress.
- Up to 50% of the time neither fever or rash are seen with this disease (sub-clinical form).[6]

ANTICIPATED CONCERNS/PROBLEMS:

- Children with unusual long-term blood disease such as sickle cell anemia, immunodeficiency, organ transplants, HIV etc. need special consideration.
- Exposed pregnant women need advice from their healthcare provider or an infectious disease specialist.
- Testing for susceptibility may be available.
- Teachers and day care workers are at increased risk of exposure, but a routine policy of exclusion of pregnant women from these workplaces is not recommended.

MANAGEMENT/POTENTIAL INTERVENTIONS:

1. No treatment is usually required.
2. Acetaminophen can be used for joint pain per healthcare provider.
3. The most contagious period is just before onset of fever, gradually declining during the next week and low to absent by the time the rash appears. An outbreak of this disease often occurs in late winter and spring. Therefore, fifth disease may be suspected in the pre-rash, infective stage, if it has occurred in other family members. Transmission of fifth disease is enhanced by household contact. A susceptible parent/guardian has a 50% chance of catching the disease from their child. In contrast, during an extensive school outbreak, about 20% of susceptible teachers may develop the infection.[7]
4. Children with the rash of fifth disease do not need to be isolated because they are *no longer contagious by the time the rash appears* ***unless*** *he/she has a compromised immune system or a blood disorder such as sickle cell anemia.*[8]

FIFTH DISEASE (Erythema Infectiosum) *(continued from previous page)*

FOLLOW-UP:

1. Encourage pregnant family members and staff that expect to have contact with children in school to consult with their health professional about their risk for infection. A blood test to determine if they are already immune may help to alleviate their concern.
2. Teach students and staff cough and sneeze etiquette.[9] *(Refer to COVER YOUR COUGH APPENDIX).*
3. Handwashing and proper tissue disposal should be scrupulously practiced. *(Refer to HANDWASHING APPENDIX).*

NOTES:

1. Available data suggest that a susceptible woman exposed during the first 20 weeks of pregnancy runs an increased risk (about 5%) of having a miscarriage, a stillbirth or the baby develops severe anemia.[10]
2. If the exposure is at school or another job site, the risk is lower because of less intimate contact.

REFERENCES

[1] American Academy of Pediatrics. (2016). Fifth disease. In A. J. Mancini, & D. P. Krowchuk (Eds.), *Pediatric dermatology* (3rd ed., pp. 115-119). American Academy of Pediatrics.

[2] American Academy of Pediatrics, Committee on Infectious Diseases. (2018). Parvovirus 19 (Erythema Infectiosum, Fifth Disease). In D.W. Kimberlin, M.T. Brady, M.T., M.A. Jackson, & S.S. Long (Eds.), *Red Book, (2018-2021): Report of the Committee on Infectious Diseases* (31st ed., pp. 602-606). American Academy of Pediatrics.

[3] American Academy of Pediatrics. (2020). Fifth disease (human parvovirus B19). In S. Aronson, & T. Shope (Eds.), *Managing infectious diseases in child care and schools* (5th ed., pp. 95-96). American Academy of Pediatrics.

[4] Ibid.

[5] Merck Manual Professional Version. *Erythema infectiosm.* https://www.merckmanuals.com/professional/pediatrics/miscellaneous-viral-infections-in-infants-and-children/erythema-infectiosum?query=fifth%20disease

[6] American Academy of Pediatrics. (2016). Fifth disease. In A. J. Mancini, & D. P. Krowchuk (Eds.), *Pediatric dermatology* (3rd ed., pp. 115-119). American Academy of Pediatrics.

[7] American Academy of Pediatrics, Committee on Infectious Diseases. (2018). Parvovirus 19 (Erythema Infectiosum, Fifth Disease). In D.W. Kimberlin, M.T. Brady, M.T., M.A. Jackson, & S.S. Long (Eds.), *Red Book, (2018-2021): Report of the Committee on Infectious Diseases* (31st ed., pp. 602-606). American Academy of Pediatrics.

[8] Ibid.

[9] Centers for Disease Control and Prevention. (2016). *Water, sanitation, & environmentally–related hygiene: Coughing and sneezing.* Retrieved from https://www.cdc.gov/healthywater/hygiene/etiquette/coughing_sneezing.html

[10] American Academy of Family Physicians Disease and Conditions. (2017). *Fifth disease.* https://familydoctor.org/condition/fifth-disease/?adfree=true

FOOD ALLERGY (*Refer to ALLERGIES and ANAPHYLAXIS*)

DEFINITION/ETIOLOGY:

A food allergy is an exaggerated immune system response to a particular protein found in that food (most commonly cow's milk, eggs, peanuts, tree nuts, soy, wheat, fish, shellfish and sesame, or some other specific food).[1] Food intolerance is an adverse reaction to certain foods but which does not involve the immune system.[2] In a true food allergy, the immune system reacts to exposure to a certain food.[3] The body reacts as though that certain food is harmful. As a result, the body's immune system creates antibodies. These antibodies go to work destroying these food allergens by releasing histamines which then trigger the symptoms of an allergic reaction.[4] Food allergies may develop at any time, even after eating the food repeatedly in the past without having problems. Symptoms may occur after that allergic individual consumes or is exposed to even a small amount of the food.[5]

MILD SIGNS AND SYMPTOMS:[6]

- Hives on any part of the body
- Rash or eczema
- Diarrhea and mild abdominal cramping
- Nausea or vomiting
- Nasal congestion, runny nose or sneezing
- Itchy mouth or ear canal
- Odd taste in mouth

SEVERE/ANAPHYLAXIS SIGNS AND SYMPTOMS:[7]

- Sense of impending doom
- Rapid pulse, palpitations, thready, or unobtainable pulse
- Swelling of face, lips, tongue, eyelids, or throat
- Blue or gray color around the lips or nail beds
- Dizziness
- Difficulty breathing, coughing or wheezing
- Trouble swallowing
- Fall in blood pressure
- Fainting, unresponsiveness

Not <u>ALL</u> signs and symptoms need be present in anaphylaxis. Severe symptoms alone or a combination of milder symptoms from two or more body systems may be a sign of life-threatening anaphylaxis and will require epinephrine.[8]

NOTE: Symptoms of anaphylaxis usually appear within minutes of ingesting the allergen and progress rapidly. However, in some cases, the severe reaction may be delayed a few hours.[9]

(Refer to ANAPHYLAXSIS)

FOOD ALLERGY *(continued from previous page)*

MANAGEMENT/TREATMENT:

The school treatment plan should be to avoid the allergen and all foods that contain it.[10] An Individualized Healthcare Plan (IHP) and an emergency care plan (ECP) should be developed for any student with food allergies.[11] Develop an IHP with input from the healthcare provider and family that includes specific actions to prevent exposure, staff training, and the emergency care plan with individualized orders.[12]

- Avoid contact and exposure to foods which trigger allergic reactions. Parents and the food service director should work together as parents need access to food labels for food served at school. [13]
- Work with student's classroom teacher and other school personnel for possible environmental triggers that may cause allergic reactions.[14]
- Suggest to parent/guardian that child wear a Medic Alert bracelet or tag.[15]
- If injectable epinephrine is ordered, educate the student regarding self-management strategies, including self-carrying and self-administering epinephrine when determined that it is developmentally appropriate for the individual student and replace if expired or used.[16]

If you suspect an allergic reaction: Antihistamines might be used to treat mild symptoms such as hives, runny nose, or belly pain from an allergic reaction if directed by healthcare provider on the IHP.[17] However, antihistamines cannot treat a more severe allergic reaction - anaphylaxis.[18] Epinephrine is the only treatment for anaphylaxis and must be administered immediately.

1. ANAPHYLAXIS: Inject Epinephrine medication as quickly as possible, every second counts followed by an **immediate call to Emergency Medical Services (EMS)** and transport to a hospital emergency department. (Despite initial improvement after first injectable epinephrine, a student can experience a bi-phasic response and symptoms often recur).[19] Follow ECP.
2. A copy of the student's record should be sent with the emergency medical services (EMS) and should include:
    - Allergen to which student is reacting, if known
    - Signs and symptoms of distress
    - Emergency measures instituted
    - Student's response to emergency measures
    - Time of all activities, including giving injectable epinephrine
    - Signature of nurse and phone number
    - Give used epinephrine auto injector to EMS
3. **If student's anaphylaxis symptoms have not improved or have relapsed after five (5) minutes after first dose of epinephrine, a repeat dose may be needed.** (Plans need to be made in advance with parents/guardians for two doses of injectable epinephrine to be in place if school does not stock injectable epinephrine).[20] *(Refer to ANAPHYLAXSIS).*

FOOD ALLERGY *(continued from previous page)*

MANAGEMENT/TREATMENT *(continued)*

4. Stay with student and monitor them closely.[21]
5. Lay student down and elevate legs if possible. Roll to side if vomiting or if trouble breathing have them sit or maintain a position of comfort.[22]
6. Notify parents/guardians and healthcare provider.

FOLLOW UP:

- After an allergic reaction at school, the school nurse should communicate with the parents and healthcare provider to make any changes to the IHP or ECP if indicated.
- The school nurse should evaluate the IHP annually or as need needed to determine if any additional preventive measures are indicated.

NOTES:[23]

Controlling Food Allergies

Food allergy reactions and life-threatening anaphylaxis may occur at school or during school-sponsored activities. The risk of accidental exposure to trigger foods can be reduced in the school setting if schools communicate with students, parents, and healthcare providers to minimize risks and provide a safe educational environment for food-allergic students. Schools should see that:

- Staff (i.e., teachers, cafeteria personnel, lunch, playground and bus monitors) and parent/guardian are educated about food allergies and preventive measures, e.g., checking food and container labels.
- IHPs are developed for students known to have a food allergy.
- There is immediate access to emergency medications, including epinephrine, and local emergency medical services.

Children with food allergies are two to four times more likely to have asthma which increases the severity of an anaphylactic reaction.[24]

RESOURCES

- **Food Allergy Research & Education (FARE)** - extensive website with tools and resources for schools including sample action plans http://www.foodallergy.org
- **Food Allergy Anaphylaxis in School: What School Staff Need to Know** – online training module. https://www.allergyhome.org/schools/management-of-food-allergies-in-school-what-school-staff-need-to-know/
- **NASN Allergies and Anaphylaxis** –https://www.nasn.org/nasn/nasn-resources/practice-topics/allergies-anaphylaxis
- **Food Allergy Research and Education (FARE).** (n.d.) *At School*. https://www.foodallergy.org/life-with-food-allergies/managing-lifes-milestones/at-school
- **Allergy and Asthma Network**. https://www.allergyasthmanetwork.org/education/

FOOD ALLERGY *(continued from previous page)*

RESOURCES *(continued)*

- Allergy & Asthma Network: ***Allergy & Anaphylaxis: A Practical Guide for Schools & Families*** https://www.allergyasthmanetwork.org/outreach/publications/special-publications/allergy-anaphylaxis-practical-guide-for-schools-and-families/

- ***Allergy & Anaphylaxis: A Practical Guide for Schools & Families*** https://www.allergyasthmanetwork.org/outreach/publications/special-publications/allergy-anaphylaxis-practical-guide-for-schools-and-families/

REFERENCES

---

[1] American Academy of Allergy, Asthma & Immunology. (2019). *Food allergy overview.* http://www.aaaai.org/conditions-and-treatments/allergies/food-allergies

[2] Ibid.

[3] Ibid.

[4] Kids Health/Nemours. (2018). *Food allergies.* https://kidshealth.org/en/parents/food-allergies.html?WT.ac=p-ra#catqa

[5] Food Allergy Research and Education (FARE). (n.d.) *What is a food allergy?* https://www.foodallergy.org/life-with-food-allergies/food-allergy-101/symptoms-of-an-allergic-reaction-to-food

[6] Ibid.

[7] Ibid.

[8] Kids Health/Nemours. (2018). *Food allergies.* https://kidshealth.org/en/parents/food-allergies.html?WT.ac=p-ra#catqa

[9] American Academy of Allergy, Asthma & Immunology. (2019). *Food allergy overview.* http://www.aaaai.org/conditions-and-treatments/allergies/food-allergies

[10] Kids Health/Nemours. (2018). *Food allergies.* https://kidshealth.org/en/parents/food-allergies.html?WT.ac=p-ra#catqa

[11] Ibid.

[12] American Academy of Pediatrics. (2017). *Allergy and anaphylaxis emergency plan.* https://www.aap.org/en-us/Documents/AAP_Allergy_and_Anaphylaxis_Emergency_Plan.pdf

[13] Centers for Disease Control and Prevention. Healthy Schools. (2019). *Food allergies.* https://www.cdc.gov/healthyschools/foodallergies

[14] Food Allergy Research and Education (FARE). (n.d.) *At school.* https://www.foodallergy.org/life-with-food-allergies/managing-lifes-milestones/at-school

[15] American Academy of Pediatrics. (2017). *Allergy and anaphylaxis emergency plan.* https://www.aap.org/en-us/Documents/AAP_Allergy_and_Anaphylaxis_Emergency_Plan.pdf

[16] Food Allergy Research and Education (FARE). (n.d.) *At school.* https://www.foodallergy.org/life-with-food-allergies/managing-lifes-milestones/at-school

[17] Kids Health/Nemours. (2018). *Food allergies.* https://kidshealth.org/en/parents/food-allergies.html?WT.ac=p-ra#catqa

[18] Mayo Clinic. *Food allergy.* (2017). https://www.mayoclinic.org/diseases-conditions/food-allergy/diagnosis-treatment/drc-20355101

[19] Kids Health/Nemours. (2018). *Food allergies.* https://kidshealth.org/en/parents/food-allergies.html?WT.ac=p-ra#catqa

FOOD ALLERGY *(continued from previous page)*

[20] American Academy of Pediatrics. (2017). *Allergy and anaphylaxis emergency plan*. https://www.aap.org/en-us/Documents/AAP_Allergy_and_Anaphylaxis_Emergency_Plan.pdf

[21] Ibid.

[22] Michigan Association of School Nurses. (n.d.) *Emergency anaphylaxis plan for stock epinephrine.* http://nursingnetwork-groupdata.s3.amazonaws.com/NASN/Michigan_ASN/file/Epinephrine_Training_Toolkit/3.Emergency%20Anaphylaxis%20Action%20Plan%20for%20stock%20Epinephrine%20Auto%20Injection.pdf

[23] Ibid.

[24] Centers for Disease Control and Prevention. Healthy Schools. (2019). *Food allergies.* https://www.cdc.gov/healthyschools/foodallergies

FOREIGN BODIES: Eye, Ear (including earwax), Nose

DEFINITION/ETIOLOGY:

It is not uncommon for children to present with a foreign body in the eye, ear, or nose. A variety of inanimate objects such as toy parts, beads and paper are common as well as foods such as seeds or nuts. Environmental materials such as dust, dirt, sand, and insects can also get in the eyes, ears, and nose.

Students may be embarrassed to admit that they put something in their nose or ear and a careful history will be warranted. It will be important to do a focused history as well as a focused assessment looking for obvious foreign objects and inspecting for related signs and symptoms.

SIGNS AND SYMPTOMS:

- *Eye:* pain, tearing, light sensitivity (with corneal abrasion), irritation, inflammation redness.[1]
- *Ear:* initially usually no discomfort. Later may complain of pain, itching in ear canal or purulent drainage from affected ear.
    - Child may report something in ear.
    - Object may be visible in ear canal.
    - Hearing may be affected
    - An insect may cause pain[2]
- *Nose:* usually no symptoms at first. After few days, a unilateral sero-purulent foul-smelling or bloody discharge may be present.[3]
    - Child may report putting something in nose.
    - May have difficulty breathing through obstructed nostril.
    - Object may be visible in nose.

MANAGEMENT/TREATMENT:

EYE (*Refer to EYE TRAUMA*)

1. Never remove an intraocular foreign body or if history indicates there was a projectile object involved. Shield the eye and have the student close the unaffected eye to avoid eye movement. Refer immediately to an eye specialist or to emergency care.[4]
2. For a nonpenetrating foreign body that is visualized, flush with warm water from the inner to outer part of the eye.[5]
3. If foreign body can be seen in the sac of the lower lid, remove with a moistened cotton swab.[6]
4. If foreign body is in the upper eyelid flush or gently invert upper lid using a cotton tipped applicator over the upper eyelid and pulling eyelid outward and up over the applicator.[7]
5. If not successful in removing object or is student continues to complain of a sensation of an object in the eye, patch the eye and refer to the healthcare provider.[8]

FOREIGN BODIES: Eye, Ear (including earwax), Nose *(continued from previous page)*

MANAGEMENT/TREATMENT *(continued)*

Minor irritation from foreign object, e.g., glitter, sand in eye:

1. Instruct the student not to rub the eye which may cause further damage or a corneal abrasion.
2. Rinse the eye out with water using a paper cup filled with water or flush at an eye station.[9]

EAR

- ***Do not*** *try to remove unless foreign body can be easily seen and grasped with forceps, tweezers or fingers and can be removed safely. Frequently swabs, forceps, tweezers and fingers push the object farther into the ear canal.*
- If the object is an insect, do not attempt to examine with an otoscope as the light may irritate the insect causing it to move and creating discomfort for the student. Take the student into a dark room and shine a flashlight into the ear and the insect may crawl toward the light and out of the ear canal. If school protocol permits you may place the student with the ear upward and place a small amount of mineral oil and the insect may float out. [10]
- If a battery is in the ear it should not be flushed, and the battery should be removed emergently.
- If policy/protocol permits and with parent/guardian's permission, ear wax may be treated by instilling mineral oil into ear and after 10 minutes turn onto affected side and allow draining.
- If these attempts are not successful, refer to healthcare provider.

NOSE

- Try having child blow nose gently while holding the unaffected nostril shut.[11]
- Have the student avoid breathing in sharply.
- ***Do not*** *attempt to remove object unless object can be seen and can be grasped with forceps or fingers and can be removed safely.*
- While removing visible object, press the nose above the object so you cannot push it farther in. If foreign object is visualized in both nares – refer to healthcare provider. Seek immediate medical care if child is having difficulty breathing.
- Refer to healthcare provider if foreign object removal is unsuccessful.

FOLLOW UP:

Eye: Ask teacher to report any further symptoms. Recheck visual acuity three to four days after treatment.

Ear: No, follow up if object has been removed.

Nose: None if object removed. Check for cessation of nasal discharge.

FOREIGN BODIES: Eye, Ear (including earwax), Nose *(continued from previous page)*

REFERENCES

[1] Harvard Health Publishing. (2019). *Foreign bodies in the eye*. https://www.health.harvard.edu/a_to_z/foreign-body-in-eye-a-to-z

[2] Stanford Children's Health. (2019). *Foreign bodies in the ear, nose and airway.* https://www.stanfordchildrens.org/en/topic/default?id=foreign-bodies-in-the-ear-nose-and-airway-90-P02035

[3] Ibid.

[4] Jakubowski, T., Perron,T .(2019).Students with common health complaints. In J. Selekman, R. Adair Shannon, & C. F. Yonkaitis (Eds.), *School nursing: A comprehensive text* (3rd ed.) (pp. 345-347). F. A. Davis.

[5] Ibid.

[6] Ibid.

[7] Ibid.

[8] Ibid.

[9] National Eye Institute. *First aid tips.* https://nei.nih.gov/kids/first_aid_tips

[10] Jakubowski, T., Perron, T. (2019). Students with common health complaints. In J. Selekman, R. Adair Shannon, & C. F. Yonkaitis (Eds.), *School nursing: A comprehensive text* (3rd ed.) (pp. 345-347). F. A. Davis.

[11] Medline Plus, U.S. National Library of Medicine. (2017). *Foreign body in the nose.* http://www.nlm.nih.gov/medlineplus/ency/article/000037.htm

OTHER RESOURCES CONSULTED

Medline Plus, U.S. National Library of Medicine. (2019). *Eye pain.* http://www.nlm.nih.gov/medlineplus/ency/article/003032.htm

Medline Plus, U.S. National Library of Medicine. (2019). *Eye emergencies.* http://www.nlm.nih.gov/medlineplus/ency/article/000054.htm

Medline Plus, U.S. National Library of Medicine. (2019). *Ear emergencies.* http://www.nlm.nih.gov/medlineplus/ency/article/000052.htm

Merck Manual. (2019). *External ear obstructions, foreign bodies.* http://www.merckmanuals.com/professional/ear_nose_and_throat_disorders/external_ear_disorders/external_ear_obstructions.html

Merck Manual. (2019). *External ear obstructions, foreign bodies.* http://www.merckmanuals.com/professional/ear_nose_and_throat_disorders/external_ear_disorders/external_ear_obstructions.html

FRACTURES (including dislocation and subluxation) *(Refer to SPRAIN/STRAIN)*

DEFINITIONS/ETIOLOGY:

A fracture is a broken bone most frequently associated with an injury to its surrounding tissue caused from direct trauma. Fractures nay also be:

- Simple – the bone is lined up and does not need to be set, just immobilized
- Hairline – a fine crack; this may not show immediately on x-ray
- Greenstick – split on one side but not the other
- Displaced – ends of bones are not lined up and may actually overlap
- Impacted – two broken ends are jammed together
- Compound – both ends are apart and one or both protrudes through broken skin

Fractures may also be caused from diseases that weaken the bone such as osteogenesis.[1]
Other types of fractures are depicted in the graphic below:

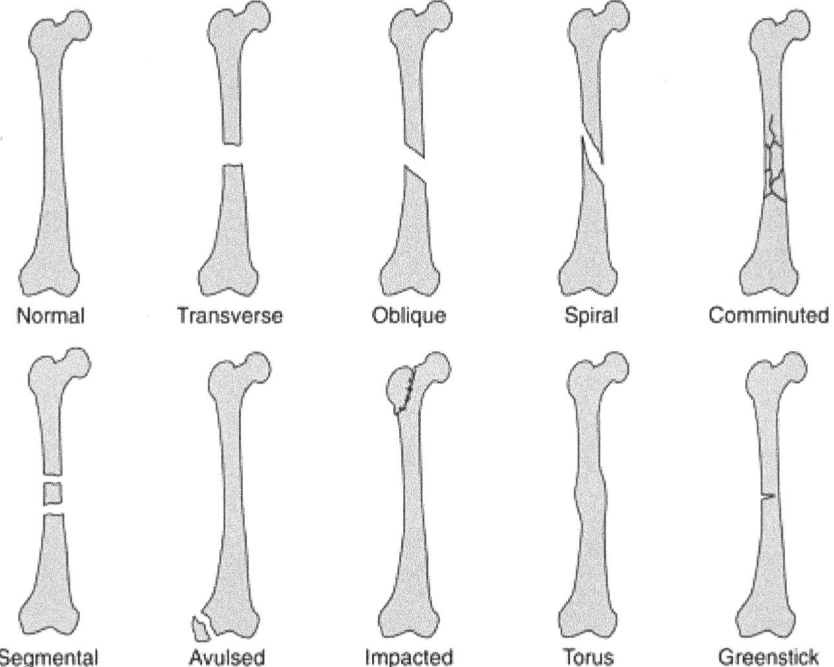

From the Merck Manual Professional Version (Known as the Merck Manual in the US and Canada and the MSD Manual in the rest of the world), edited by Robert Porter. Copyright (2020) by Merck Sharp & Dohme Corp., a subsidiary of Merck & Co., Inc, Kenilworth, NJ. Available at https://www.merckmanuals.com/professional/injuries-poisoning/fractures/overview-of-fractures. Accessed 2-21-20.

FRACTURES (including dislocation and subluxation) *(continued from previous page)*

SIGNS AND SYMPTOMS:

- Asymmetry compared to opposite side, but not always present.
- Deformity is associated with severe pain.
- Swelling and discoloration are not always present, but the likelihood of a fracture is greater if discoloration appears within 30 minutes of injury.
- Suspect "stress" fracture if extremity/bone is painful from excess exercise, jogging, gymnastics, ballet training, etc. Produces pain without swelling at site of fracture, especially on movement.
- Most frequently missed fractures: ribs, fingers/toes (chipped), elbow, knee, and distal radius.
- Other signs of a fracture:
    - Pain and swelling
    - Difficulty moving the affected extremity
    - Tenderness
    - Bruising
    - Numbness
    - Stiffness

MANAGEMENT/TREATMENT:

1. Management and treatment depend on the type and severity of the injury and may include pain relievers and PRICE - protection, rest, ice, compression, and elevation. If using ice, wrap in a towel before applying to the area.
2. Do not move the student until an assessment is complete.
3. Do not move the student if a fracture of the leg bones, pelvis, head, neck or spine is suspected unless the student is in grave danger by being left where he/she is. If a student must be moved under these circumstances, utilize multiple people and devices such as backboards or other large flat items in order to keep the student immobilized.
4. Inspect for deformity, pain, bleeding, protruding bone and edema.
5. Stop bleeding if present.
6. Calm student. Watch for signs of shock and treat symptoms.
7. Check for pulses near injury; if skin color is white/pale or pulse is absent, gently reposition only until circulation improves. If limb resists movement, stop.
8. Immobilize beyond joints above and below ends of suspected fracture, leaving the limb in position.

FRACTURES (including dislocation and subluxation) *(continued from previous page)*

MANAGEMENT/TREATMENT *(continued)*

9. Splint only with a pillow if calling for emergency medical services (EMS). Raise body part above the heart if possible.

10. Cover exposed bone with sterile/clean bandage. DO NOT wash or probe.

11. Summon EMS and notify parent/guardian.
    - Severity and need for special transportation
    - Discolored or numb
    - Limb or joint is deformed
    - Bone is piercing the skin
    - Heavy bleeding

12. Monitor pulse(s) and breathing rate, checking for shock, every five minutes until EMS arrive.

13. If EMS are unnecessary as per the list above, refer to healthcare provider or emergency department.

14. Fingers/Toes:
    - If suspect fracture, tape to adjacent finger/toe ("buddy" splint). Refer to healthcare provider within the day, sooner if deformity is present.
    - Jammed finger: buddy tape to adjacent digit. Check onset of discoloration; usually within 12-15 hours if fractured and more than 15 hours if only "jammed."

FOLLOW-UP:

- Splint/cast care as directed.[2]
- Check fingers/toes for adequate circulation and sensation.
- Assist with modifications for classes, writing, keeping cast dry, etc.
- Participate in Section 504 plan development
- Assess proper crutch use.
- Promote mobility.

POTENTIAL COMPLICATIONS:

- Damage to blood vessels
- Fat embolism
- Nerve damage
- Osteomyelitis
- Compartment Syndrome

FRACTURES (including dislocation and subluxation) *(continued from previous page)*

OTHER MUSCULOSKELETAL CONCERNS:

- Dislocation – injury to a joint in which the ends of bones are forced from their normal positions. Can occur in major joints such as the shoulder, hip, knee, elbow and ankle, and the smaller joints (fingers, thumbs and toes)
- Subluxation – partial dislocation
- Sprain – tearing or stretching of a ligament (caused by injury)
- Strain - tearing or stretching of a muscle or tendon (caused by overuse)

SIGNS AND SYMPTOMS of dislocation or subluxation:

- Joint looks visibly deformed or out of place
- Area swollen
- Immovable
- Area intensely painful

COMPLICATIONS of dislocation or subluxation:

- Nerve damage
- Blood vessel damage

MANAGEMENT/TREATMENT of dislocation or subluxation:

- Refer to healthcare provider.
- Depending on the severity of the injury:
  - Healthcare provider may try to gently maneuver the dislocated bone back into place (this is called reduction).
  - If dislocation is severe – may need local or general anesthesia to move back into place.
- Evaluate the need to immobilize joint with a sling or splint.
- Evaluate need for RICE (rest, ice, compression, elevation).

NOTES:

- Encourage children to wear protective gear such as helmets, elbow pads, kneepads and shin pads while biking, roller blading, and participating in contact sports.
- Repeated fractures can be an indication of other underlying health conditions.
- Child abuse should be considered if there are reoccurring fractures without a medical indication; if the type of fracture is uncommon for a particular age group; or the fracture is inconsistent with reported cause.
- Compartment Syndrome (mostly in lower limbs) is a serious condition that occurs when there's a large amount of pressure inside a muscle compartment. Compartments are groups of muscle tissue, blood vessels, and nerves in your arms and legs surrounded by a very strong membrane called the fascia. Fascia does not expand, so swelling in a compartment can result in an increase in pressure inside the compartment. This results in injury to the muscles, blood vessels, and nerves inside the compartment. Compartment Syndrome can also be caused from a splint or cast.[3]
- The most common fractures in children are the clavicle, distal forearm, ulna, tibia and femur.[4]

FRACTURES (including dislocation and subluxation) *(continued from previous page)*

REFERENCES

[1] Claytor, C.M., & Bazner-Chandler, J. (2017). Musculoskeletal disorders. In C. E. Burns, A.M. Dunn, M.A. Brady, N. B. Starr, Catherine G. Blosser, & D.L. Garzon Maaks, (Eds.) *Pediatric primary care* (6th ed., pp. 1042-1082). Elsevier, Inc.

[2] Medline Plus. (2017). *Creating a sling*. https://medlineplus.gov/ency/presentations/100137_1.htm

[3] Campagne, D. (2019). *Overview of fractures. The Merck Professional Manual.* https://www.merckmanuals.com/professional/injuries-poisoning/fractures/overview-of-fractures

[4] Patterson, M. (2020). Musculoskeletal disorders. In B. Richardson (Ed.), *Pediatric primary care: Practice guideline for nurses* (4th ed., pp. 525-561). Jones & Bartlett Learning, LLC.

OTHER REFERENCES CONSULTED

Cleveland Clinic. (2017). *Bone fractures.* https://my.clevelandclinic.org/health/diseases/15241-bone-fractures

Mayo Clinic. (2019). *Bone fractures.* https://www.mayoclinic.org/search/search-results?q=bone%20fractures

HEADACHE(S)

DEFINITION/ETIOLOGY:
Headaches are common in children and have a wide range of causes with many levels of severity. The pain may be felt anywhere in the head or neck. Headaches can be caused by a variety of triggers or certain infections. In females, occurrence of headaches may be related to hormonal changes. Headaches are thought to be caused by changes in chemicals, nerves, or blood vessels in the area which send pain messages to the brain and bring on a headache.[1]

Headaches can be considered primary or secondary. Primary headaches are most common and are not due to any underlying condition. Secondary or organic headaches are a symptom of another disease or disorder.[2]

The two most common primary headaches in the pediatric population are tension headaches and migraine headaches.

Tension headaches, the most common type of headache seen in children, occur when the head or neck muscles contract and are described as pressing or squeezing of the head. They may be further described as dull, aching, and constant.[3]

Tension-type headaches may also be further classified by frequency:[4]

- Infrequent (less than one headache/month)
- Frequent (headache one to 14 days/month)
- Chronic (headache 15 or more days/month)

Migraine headaches are less common in children. They are characterized by pounding, throbbing pain on one or both sides of the head and often accompanied by dizziness, nausea, and vomiting. Often the child with a migraine will experience an aura (seeing spots or halos) prior to the onset of a migraine.[5]

Cluster headaches occur rarely in children. When present, children will experience unilateral burning pain up to eight times a day.[6]

Secondary headaches are more concerning and may be caused by:

- Tumors
- High blood pressure
- Head injuries
- Sinusitis
- Central nervous system bleeding
- Increased intracranial pressure (ICP)(chronic progressive headache)

HEADACHE(S) *(continued from previous page)*

SIGNS AND SYMPTOMS:[7]

- **Tension-type headache**: the most common type in adolescence, "dull/achy," diffuse, bilateral, radiates to cervical neck, rarely accompanied by nausea, vomiting, abdominal pain or visual disturbances. It is described as a general pain around the head. Precipitating factors include emotional stress and fatigue.

- **Vascular headaches**:
  - **Migraine:** "throbbing/pounding," usually unilateral. It is common to experience nausea, vomiting, and sensitivity to light which makes it difficult to carry out activities of daily living. About 1/3 of migraine sufferers also experience an "aura" prior to the headache which may be described as a visual disturbance such as blinking lights or loss of vision. The **presence of auras is less common in children than adults. Hunger may precede a childhood** migraine. Pain may last for hours or days. Dizziness, light-headedness, pallor, or purple bags around the eyes may also occur. Preschool-age children may have irritability, restlessness, malaise, head banging, head holding, and sensitivity to light and sound. Migraine headaches are often hereditary.
  - **Cluster:** Often described as "burning/stabbing," often felt most around one eye. These headaches generally start suddenly and are of short duration but may reoccur for several months at a time. They are most common in spring and autumn.

- **Rebound or medication overuse:** Pain may be bandlike, over entire head or crushing and occurs several times a week or daily. Rebound headaches increase in frequency over time and recur when medication wears off.

- **Secondary to other conditions**, e.g., sinusitis, dental problem, eye strain. May be associated with other symptoms such as cough, fever or blurred vision. A headache associated with sinusitis may present as a sense of fullness or throbbing in the frontal or temporal areas.

- **Structural headaches**: Caused by space-occupying lesion, hemorrhage, increased ICP. They are chronic and progressive. Severe pain increases in frequency, often in occipital or frontal location. Pain increases with straining (coughing, sneezing, etc.). Vomiting and altered neurologic signs are present. Pain awakens child or is present in morning.

ASSESSMENT:

- History: Ask about occurrences, such as surrounding events (injury, stressor such as lack of food or sleep), frequency, duration, cyclic nature, location, and severity of headache (e.g. interferes with normal activities, such as playing, causes school absenteeism). Determine associated symptoms and use of any medications or other headache treatment.
- Assessment: Check vital signs, noting presence of fever or changes in blood pressure. Utilize a pediatric pain scale to assess severity of pain. Conduct a neurological assessment, noting change in mental status, behavior, vision, speech, balance, and coordination. If exam is abnormal, especially neurological exam and history (e.g., irritability, mental confusion, fatigue or blurred/altered vision), then there is heightened concern for a more serious pathological condition causing the headache, such as the secondary causes noted above.[8]

HEADACHE(S) *(continued from previous page)*

MANAGEMENT/TREATMENT:[9]

- If student has a suspected pathological condition underlying the headache, notify the parent/guardian immediately and refer to the student's healthcare provider or activate the Emergency Medical Service (EMS) if appropriate.
- For benign conditions, headache diaries are useful for evaluation. The school nurse, working with the student's healthcare provider, can suggest a long-term plan.
- Intervention is based on the cause.

Non-medication measures

- Rest in quiet, darkened room
- Assure good hydration
- Cool or warm cloth on forehead
- Stress management/relaxation techniques
- Eliminate precipitating factors or triggers
- Biofeedback, good posture and daily exercise

Medications

- **Tension headache**: Non-prescription analgesics. No food or caffeine restrictions unless the food is a confirmed trigger.
- **Migraine type**: Treat the headache as soon as it starts; do not wait for nausea or other symptoms. Prompt treatment turns off the mediators of inflammation and should be available at school. Over-the-counter analgesics, including acetaminophen, nonsteroidal anti-inflammatory drugs (NSAID) such as ibuprofen and naproxen may be effective if given at the onset of the headache. Triptans and serotonin antagonists are commonly prescribed but should not be used more than four to six times per month. School absences or inability to perform at school due to migraine suggests that prophylactic agents are indicated. Prophylactic agents (such as tricyclic antidepressants (amitriptyline), propranolol, and calcium channel blockers) are used when auras present or in severe cases.
- **Cluster headache**: Children are usually referred to pediatric neurologists.

FOLLOW UP:

- Gauge continuing symptoms with a headache diary.
- Reevaluation is warranted any time initial impressions do not fit, when symptoms persist or worsen with time, or when new symptoms emerge.
- Monitor complications such as side effects of medications and disruption of activities (e.g. school absences, poor academic performance).
- Assist those with migraine or tension headache to follow their medical and non-medical regimens.
- Healthy lifestyle strategies such as adequate sleep, good diet and relaxation techniques can be helpful.

HEADACHE(S) *(continued from previous page)*

POTENTIAL COMPLICATIONS:
Headaches can be painful and debilitating but are generally not due to dangerous conditions. However, occasionally headaches can be a sign of something more serious including very severe high blood pressure greater than 180/110 mm Hg, stroke, brain tumor, or meningitis.

It is critical to seek emergency medical care if a headache[10]
- **gets worse over days or weeks**
- **is accompanied by impaired neurological function**
- **is accompanied by persistent nausea and vomiting**
- **is accompanied by fever or stiff neck**
- **is accompanied by seizure, mental disturbance, or loss of consciousness**
- **is different than usual headaches, strikes suddenly with great intensity, or**
- **wakes the patient from sleep and is worse when laying down**

NOTES: (PREVENTION)
Migraine-specific preventive interventions:
- Meals should not be skipped; a morning snack can help if hunger is a trigger. The role of specific food triggers is controversial, but parents/guardians may want child to avoid one food at a time to see if there is a benefit.
- Stay well hydrated; dehydration is a trigger for some migraines.
- Regular sleep routines and stress management.
- Daily exercise (20-30 minutes).

REFERENCES

[1] Kids Health from Nemours. (2019). *Headaches.* https://kidshealth.org/en/parents/headache.html

[2] Ibid.

[3] Ibid.

[4] Jakubowski, T. & Perron, T. (2019). Students with common health complaints: Neurological problems. In J. Selekman, R. Adair Shannon, & C. F. Yonkaitis (Eds.), *School nursing: A comprehensive text* (3rd ed., pp. 359-360). F.A. Davis.

[5] Kids Health from Nemours. (2019). *Headaches.* https://kidshealth.org/en/parents/headache.html

[6] Jakubowski, T. & Perron, T. (2019). Students with common health complaints: Neurological problems. In J. Selekman, R. Adair Shannon, & C. F. Yonkaitis (Eds.), *School nursing: A comprehensive text* (3rd ed., pp. 359-360). F.A. Davis.

[7] Ball, J., Bindler, R., Cowen, K., & Shaw, M. (Eds.). (2017). *Principles of Pediatric Nursing: Caring for Children* (7th ed., pp. 761-762). Pearson Education, Inc.

[8] Jakubowski, T. & Perron, T. (2019). Students with common health complaints: Neurological problems. In J. Selekman, R. Adair Shannon, & C. F. Yonkaitis (Eds.), *School nursing: A comprehensive text* (3rd ed., pp. 359-360). F.A. Davis.

[9] Ibid.

[10] Kids Health from Nemours. (2019). *Headaches.* https://kidshealth.org/en/parents/headache.html

HEART MURMURS

DEFINITION/ETIOLOGY:
A murmur is defined as an extra or unusual sound heard during a heartbeat. The sounds are made as blood flows through valves and vessels. Murmurs can be functional (innocent) or pathologic (abnormal) indicating possible cardiac disease or a malfunction in the cardiac system.[1]

A heart murmur is a common finding among children, occurring in up to 50% of infants and children. Murmurs may also come and go. Many children will have an innocent murmur at some point in their childhood. Innocent murmurs are often heard in the newborn period, especially in the first few days of life.[2]

Auscultation of heart sounds should be done in a step wise fashion utilizing both the bell and the diaphragm. The diaphragm is better for picking up high pitched sounds heard in S1 and S2 and the bell is better for lower pitched sounds heard with space between S3and S4. Auscultation of the heart to detect the presence of murmurs takes practice and experience. If at any time the school nurse is unsure of the findings a referral should be made.

Auscultation Locations

Cardiac auscultation is performed systematically over five locations on the anterior chest wall. Use the stethoscope's diaphragm, switching to the bell to hear lower pitched sounds.

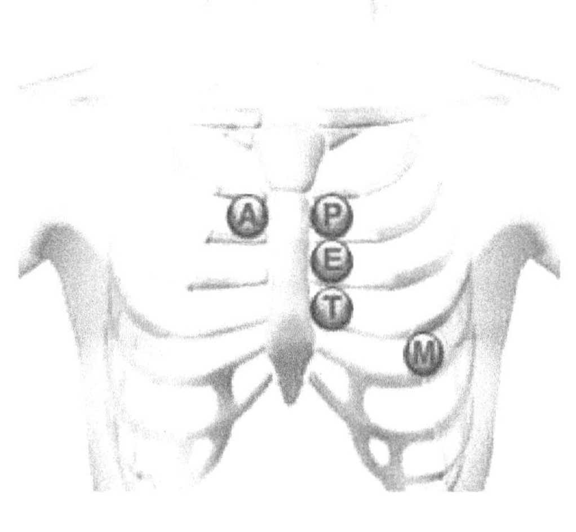

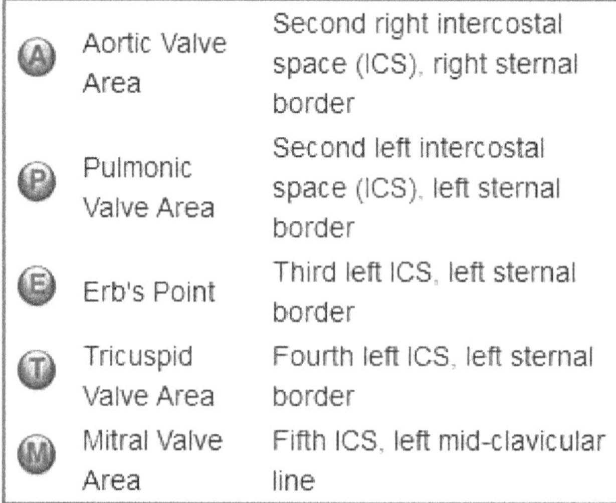

A	Aortic Valve Area	Second right intercostal space (ICS), right sternal border
P	Pulmonic Valve Area	Second left intercostal space (ICS), left sternal border
E	Erb's Point	Third left ICS, left sternal border
T	Tricuspid Valve Area	Fourth left ICS, left sternal border
M	Mitral Valve Area	Fifth ICS, left mid-clavicular line

MedEdu LLC[3]

HEART MURMURS *(continued from previous page)*

Murmurs should be described based on the following characteristics:

- Location and radiation (where the murmur is heard best, usually the origin of the murmur)
- Timing to the cardiac cycle and duration (systolic murmurs are heard between S1 and S2, diastolic murmurs between S2 and S1, continuous murmurs are heard throughout)
- Intensity
    - Grade 1 barely audible
    - Grade 2 soft but easily audible
    - Grade 3 moderately loud with no palpable thrill (a vibratory feeling over the sternum) Moderate load should be defined
    - Grade 4 loud with a thrill
    - Grade 5 audible with the stethoscope barely touching the chest
    - Grade 6 audible with no stethoscope
- Quality (harsh, musical or high, medium or low in pitch)
- Variation with position (audible changes when the student is supine, sitting, standing or squatting
- Pitch (low, medium, high)[4]

SIGNS AND SYMPTOMS:

The following should also be assessed in the presence of a murmur

- Arterial rate and rhythm
    - Tachycardia may be indicative of cardiovascular or respiratory compromise
- Arterial pulse quality and amplitude
    - A bounding pulse can be indicative of a cardiac abnormality
    - A weak or thready pulse can be indicative of poor cardiac output
- Blood pressure in all 4 extremities and in the sitting, lying and standing position
- A decreased blood pressure in the lower extremities can be indicative of a coarctation of the aorta
- Color of skin, nail beds, and lips, respiratory rate and rhythm[5]

Symptoms suggestive of cardiac pathology

- Chest pain associated with shortness of breath or murmur
- Family history of Marfan Syndrome or sudden death of young family members
- Increased precordial activity
- Decreased femoral pulses
- Abnormal second heart sound (a diastolic murmur)
- Increased intensity of a murmur when the student stands
- A murmur of grade 4 or higher especially with harsh quality
- Palpitations
- Lightheadedness or syncope
- Exercise intolerance
- Clubbing of nails indicating arterial desaturation[6]

HEART MURMURS *(continued from previous page)*

SIGNS AND SYMPTOMS *(continued)*

Symptoms suggestive of an innocent murmur:

- Usually grade 1 to 3
- May change with position
- May increase with exercise, anemia, or fever
- Heard between S1 and S2 (systolic)
- Duration is short, musical or vibratory in nature
- Vital signs normal, and student is in good health[7]

MANAGEMENT/TREATMENT:

Any previously undiagnosed murmur heard in the school aged child should be evaluated by the student's healthcare provider. A murmur in the absence of any other abnormal finding is not a medical emergency but evaluation is warranted.

Children with a newly diagnosed murmur will often be referred to a pediatric cardiologist.

Other Diagnostic Tests That May Be Ordered by a Cardiologist

- Chest radiograph
- Electrocardiogram (ECG)
- Echocardiogram
- Complete blood count (CBC)
- Cardiac catherization
- Pulse oximetry[8]

FOLLOW-UP:

When innocent murmurs are found in a child, the parent should be assured that these are normal heart sounds of the developing child. For students with cardiovascular disease, an Individualized Healthcare Plan (IHP) should be developed which includes an Emergency Care Plan (ECP) for heart disease/emergencies.

RESOURCES

Auscultation of Heart Sounds | Assessing Heart Sounds | Listening to the Heart with a Stethoscope
https://www.youtube.com/watch?v=M4PPeBDx9oM

HEART MURMURS *(continued from previous page)*

REFERENCES

[1] American Heart Association. (2019). *Heart murmurs*. https://www.heart.org/en/health-topics/heart murmurs

[2] O'Brien, P. & Evangelista, J. (2018). Heart and vascular assessment In Duderstadt, K. (Ed.), *Pediatric physical examination* (3rd ed., pp.110-130)., Elsevier, Inc.

[3] MedEdu LLC. (n.d.). *Heart murmur sounds*. https://www.easyauscultation.com/heart-murmur

[4]Marrchenke, J., & Rummell, M. (2017). Cardiovascular disorders. In In C. Burns, A.M. Dunn, M.A. Brady, N.B. Starr, C.G. Blosser, & D.L. Garzon (Eds.), *Pediatric primary care* (6th ed., pp.762-765)., Elsevier, Inc.

[5] Ibid.

[6] Ibid.

[7] Ibid.

[8] Tong, E. & O'Brien, P. (2014). Heart and vascular system. In Duderstadt, K. (Ed.) *Pediatric physical examination* (2nd ed., pp.89-93). Elsevier, Inc.

OTHER RESOURCES CONSULTED

Bernstein, D. (2016). In R.M. Kliegman, B.S. Stanton, J. St. Geme, & N.F. Schor (Eds.), *Textbook of pediatrics: Expert consult* (20th ed., pp. 2163-2167). Elsevier, Inc.

Mayo Clinic. (2019). *Heart murmurs.* https://www.mayoclinic.org/diseases-conditions/heart-murmurs/diagnosis-treatment/drc-20373175

National Heart, Lung and Blood Institute, U.S. Department of Health and Human Services. (2012). *Explore heart murmurs*. http://www.nhlbi.nih.gov/health/health-topics/topics/heartmurmur

HEAT-RELATED ILLNESS

DEFINITION/ETIOLOGY:

Heat-related illness occurs when the body's temperature-regulating mechanisms are over-whelmed. Heat-related illnesses occur when the body is unable to properly cool itself.[1] As the body tries to cool itself, blood rushes to the skin surface resulting in decreased blood flow to the brain, muscles and other vital organs. This can lead to heat cramps, heat exhaustion and heatstroke.[2] Initially, electrolyte problems occur with the loss of salt and potassium from heavy perspiring that may lead to **muscle cramps,** referred to as **heat cramps.[3]** **"Heat cramps** are brief, severe cramps of skeletal or abdominal muscles following exertion. Core body temperature is normal or slightly elevated."[4] **Heat exhaustion** may occur after several days of heat exposure and dehydration whereas the most serious form of heat illness is **heatstroke** in which the body temperature may rise above 106° F.[5]

Prolonged exposure to conditions of hot environments such as outdoors on a hot and humid day or indoors in a hot, poorly ventilated area can cause heat-related illness. Contributing factors such as certain medications such as beta-blockers, diuretics, and some medications used to treat depression, psychosis, or ADHD can alter the body's response to heat and sun. Similarly, consumption of alcohol, inappropriate use of drugs, prolonged exertion, dehydration, heart disease, not drinking enough fluids during activity and wearing too much clothing can put a person at great risk.[6]

SIGNS AND SYMPTOMS:

HEAT CRAMPS[7]

- Muscle cramps often in the abdomen or legs that are painful, involuntary, brief, intermittent and are usually self-limited
- Excess perspiration
- Weakness (fatigue), lightheadedness
- Thirst

HEAT EXHAUSTION[8]

- Confusion
- Dark urine
- Dizziness, lightheadedness, or fainting
- Headache
- Muscle or abdominal cramps
- Nausea, vomiting, or diarrhea
- Pale skin
- Profuse sweating
- Rapid heartbeat

HEAT-RELATED ILLNESS *(continued from previous page)*

SIGNS AND SYMPTOMS *(continued)*

HEAT STROKE[9]

- Temperature above 106°F
- Fainting
- Throbbing headache
- Dizziness and lightheadedness
- Red, hot and dry skin,
- Muscle weakness or cramps
- Nausea and vomiting
- Rapid heartbeat that may be strong or weak
- Rapid, shallow breathing
- Confusion, disorientation, or staggering
- Seizures
- Unconsciousness[10]

MANAGEMENT/TREATMENT:
It is crucial to move the person from the extreme environmental temperature and to remove clothing to begin cooling the body. Generally, heat cramps will respond to rest and rehydration, but heat exhaustion requires medical evaluation.[11]

HEAT CRAMPS

1. Move person to cool, shady place and encourage rest.
2. If person is alert, give sips of water, four oz. every 15 minutes.
3. Provide firm, gentle massage to cramp, and passive stretching.[12]
4. Do not give salt tablets.[13]
5. If person does not improve or if status worsens call Emergency Medical Services (EMS).

HEAT EXHAUSTION

1. Move person to cool, shady place.
2. Loosen clothing.
3. If person is alert, give sips of water, 4 oz. every 15 minutes.
4. Apply cool, wet cloths to neck, armpits, and groin.[14]
5. Use fan to cool (evaporation) and/or move to air-conditioned area.
6. If nausea or vomiting occurs, discontinue fluids.
7. If vomiting and prevent aspiration by turning on side.
8. Seek immediate medical attention if symptoms are severe, worsen, or last over 15 minutes.[15]
9. Seek medical attention immediately, if person has high blood pressure or heart problems.

HEAT-RELATED ILLNESS *(continued from previous page)*

MANAGEMENT/TREATMENT *(continued)*

HEAT STROKE

1. Call EMS.
2. Move the person to a cooler environment.
3. Reduce body temperature with cold bath or sponging, wet sheets, or towel.
4. Monitor body temperature and continue cooling efforts until body temperature reaches 101 to 102°F.
5. Remove clothing, use fans, air-conditioners.
6. Apply ice to the person's armpits, groin, neck and back.[16]
7. Do not give fluids to drink.
8. Be alert for vomiting and prevent aspiration by turning on side.[17]
9. Monitor consciousness and prepare to administer CPR, if necessary.

NOTE: Untreated Heat Cramps and Heat Exhaustion may lead to Heat Stroke.

HEAT STROKE IS A SEVERE MEDICAL EMERGENCY. SUMMON EMERGENCY MEDICAL ASSISTANCE OR GET THE VICTIM TO A HOSPITAL IMMEDIATELY. DELAY CAN BE FATAL.[18]

PREVENTION:

1. Provide information about temperature and heat index during extreme heat conditions.
2. Follow local news and weather channels or contact the local health department for health and safety updates.
3. Provide education:[19]
   a. Drink plenty of fluids.
   b. Do not wait until thirsty to drink fluids.
   c. During heavy exercise in a hot environment, drink two to four glasses (16-32 ounces) of cool fluids every hour.
   d. Encourage limiting activities to morning and evening (avoid mid-day sun) and providing opportunities for frequent rest in shady areas.
   e. Wear loose-fitting, lightweight and light-colored clothing.

4. Initiate efforts to promote "Sun Safety" for students, faculty and staff, and parents.
   - Sunburn causes the loss of body fluids and effects the body's ability to cool itself.[20]

HEAT-RELATED ILLNESS *(continued from previous page)*

PREVENTION *(continued)*

- Promote an awareness campaign such as SLIP, SLOP, SLAP, SEEK, SLIDE on days with high temperatures, high heat index, and outdoor activities in bright sunlight.[21]
    - SLIP on a long sleeve shirt.
    - SLOP on sunscreen of SPF 15 or higher (the most effective products marked "broad spectrum" or "UAV/UVB protection" on the labels). Sunscreen must be applied liberally and frequently.
    - SLAP on a hat (a broad brimmed hat gives the most protection).
    - SEEK shade.
    - SLIDE on sunglasses.

5. Recommend programs and efforts to prevent heat-related health emergencies:
    - Hydration and extended "rest/time out" during athletic and sport events/practices.
    - Indoor (air conditioning) classes for physical education on high heat index days.
    - Contribute to playground planning efforts to include areas of shade for respite from heat and sun.

REFERENCES

[1] Centers for Disease Control and Prevention. (2019). *About extreme heat.* https://www.cdc.gov/disasters/extremeheat/index.html

[2] WebMD. (2019). *Understanding heat-related illness the basics.*https://www.webmd.com/first-aid/understanding-heat-related-illness-basics

[3] WebMD. (2019). *Heat cramps.* https://www.webmd.com/fitness-exercise/heat-cramps#1-2

[4] Carney, K. P., & Roswell, K. (2018). Emergencies & injuries. In W.W. Hay, M.J. Levin, R. R. Deterding, & M. J. Abzug (Eds.), *Current diagnosis and treatment: Pediatrics* (24th ed., p.326). McGraw Hill Education.

[5] Medline Plus, U.S. National Library of Medicine. (2019). *Heat illness.* https://medlineplus.gov/heatillness.html

[6] WebMD. (2019). *Understanding heat-related illness the basics.* https://www.webmd.com/first-aid/understanding-heat-related-illness-basics

[7] Voskuil, V., & Selekman, J. (2019). Health issues related to physical activity and athletics. In J. Selekman, R. Adair Shannon, & C. F. Yonkaitis (Eds.), *School nursing: A comprehensive text* (3rd ed., pp. 367-400). F.A. Davis.

[8] WebMD. (2019). *Understanding heat-related illness the basics.* https://www.webmd.com/first-aid/understanding-heat-related-illness-basics

[9] Ibid.

[10] Ibid.

[11] Carney, K. P., & Roswell, K. (2018). Emergencies & injuries. In W.W. Hay, M.J. Levin, R. R. Deterding, & M. J. Abzug (Eds.), *Current diagnosis and treatment: Pediatrics* (24th ed., p.326). McGraw Hill Education.

[12] Voskuil, V., & Selekman, J. (2019). Health issues related to physical activity and athletics. In J. Selekman, R. Adair Shannon, & C. F. Yonkaitis (Eds.), *School nursing: A comprehensive text* (3rd ed., pp. 367-400). F.A. Davis.

HEAT-RELATED ILLNESS *(continued from previous page)*

[13] WebMD. (2019). *Heat cramps*. https://www.webmd.com/fitness-exercise/heat-cramps#1-2

[14] Voskuil, V., & Selekman, J. (2019). Health issues related to physical activity and athletics. In J. Selekman, R. Adair Shannon, & C. F. Yonkaitis (Eds.), *School nursing: A comprehensive text* (3rd ed., pp. 367-400). F.A. Davis.

[15] WebMD. (2019). *Heat exhaustion.*https://www.webmd.com/fitness-exercise/heat-exhaustion#1

[16] WebMD. (2019). *Heat stroke.*https://www.webmd.com/a-to-z-guides/heat-stroke-symptoms-and-treatment#1

[17] Voskuil, V., & Selekman, J. (2019). Health issues related to physical activity and athletics. In J. Selekman, R. Adair Shannon, & C. F. Yonkaitis (Eds.), *School nursing: A comprehensive text* (3rd ed., pp. 367-400). F.A. Davis.

[18] WebMD. (2019). *Heat stroke.*https://www.webmd.com/a-to-z-guides/heat-stroke-symptoms-and-treatment#1

[19] Centers for Disease Control and Prevention. (2019). *Tips for preventing heat-related illness.* https://www.cdc.gov/disasters/extremeheat/heattips.html

[20] Ibid.

[21] Cancer Council Australia. (2019). *Slip slop slap seek slide.*https://www.cancer.org.au/preventing-cancer/sun-protection/campaigns-and-events/slip-slop-slap-seek-slide.html

HEMOPHILIA

DEFINITION/ETIOLOGY:

Hemophilia is usually a genetic, life-long bleeding disorder.[1] In rare cases, hemophilia is also associated with pregnancy, autoimmune conditions, cancer, and multiple sclerosis.[2] These rare cases often resolve themselves with appropriate medical treatment.

Hemophilia is caused by a change or mutation in one of the genes essential for producing the clotting factor proteins used to form blood clots.[3] As a result, people with hemophilia lack sufficient blood-clotting proteins (clotting factor) and may experience spontaneous bleeding and bleeding that is difficult to control following injuries or surgery. The severity of hemophilia, along with the signs and symptoms is determined by the level of clotting factor in a person's blood. A severe deficiency of clotting factor increases the likelihood that excessive and spontaneous bleeding may occur. The greater health concern of bleeding episodes is deep bleeding inside the body, especially in knees, ankles and elbows. This internal bleeding can result in damage to organs, tissues and may be life-threatening.[4]

SIGNS AND SYMPTOMS:

- Unexplained and excessive bleeding from cuts, injuries, after surgery or dental work
- Many large or deep bruises
- Unusual bleeding after vaccinations or injections
- Pain, swelling or tightness in joints (frequently experienced in the elbows, knees, and ankles)
- Blood in urine or stool
- Nosebleeds without a known cause
- Hematoma (build-up of blood in skin, muscle and soft tissue)
- Bleeding of the mouth and gums
- In infants, unexplained irritability [5]
- Bleeding in the head of an infant after a difficult delivery [6]

MANAGEMENT/TREATMENT:

- Replacement of the specific clotting factor that is reduced in the body [7] (injecting treatment products called, clotting factor concentrates, into a person's vein). This procedure is usually done outside of the school environment.
- Secure medications or treatment products for use in the school environment in case of bleeding emergencies, for episodic care or for prophylactic care. Episodic care is used to stop a patient's bleeding episodes; prophylactic care is used to prevent bleeding episodes from occurring.
- Learn how to self-administer (or administer by family members) clotting factor treatment products at home. Bleeding episodes can be treated more efficiently, resulting in less serious bleeding and fewer side effects.[8]
- Seek medical treatment immediately if internal bleeding is suspected; uncontrolled bleeding occurs after an injury; or joints are swollen, painful and hot to the touch.[9]

HEMOPHILIA *(continued from previous page)*

MANAGEMENT/TREATMENT *(continued)*

- First aid for bleeding may include:
  - Applying firm pressure for 10 minutes over skin lacerations or abrasions.
  - Applying ice pack to small bleeds under the skin.
  - Carefully observing student following minor trauma for possible internal bleeding.
  - Notify parent/guardian after all accidents (even if there is no visible sign of injury).
  - Do not administer any medications without a provider's order.
  - Never administer ASPIRIN or IBUPROPHEN (prolongs bleeding time).
  - No injections at school without a healthcare provider's order.
  - Follow healthcare provider's orders for physical education or sports participation.
- Observe for and encourage students to report early bleeding episodes.

FOLLOW UP:

- Refer to healthcare specialist or to a comprehensive hemophilia treatment center regarding education of or the specific care for persons with hemophilia.

POTENTIAL COMPLICATIONS:

- Internal bleeding
- Joint damage
- Infection
- Adverse reaction to clotting factor treatment [10]

NOTES:

- People with hemophilia can live relatively normal lives with proper treatment.
- Provide education regarding hemophilia and safety in school environments and programs (sports, physical education, playground, etc.).
- Specific orders for treatment of bleeding episodes and medication administration must be obtained and followed for all students with a diagnosis of hemophilia.
- Students must have an Individualized Healthcare Plan, Emergency Plans and may be eligible for Section 504 services.
- Provide education to students and families including: signs and symptoms of internal bleeding, injury prevention, and importance of good oral hygiene to prevent dental concerns.

HEMOPHILIA *(continued from previous page)*

REFERENCES

[1] Centers for Disease Control and Prevention. (2018). *Hemophilia.* https://www.cdc.gov/ncbddd/hemophilia/facts.html

[2] Mayo Clinic. (2019). *Hemophilia* https://www.mayoclinic.org/diseases-conditions/hemophilia/symptoms-causes/syc-20373327

[3] Center for Disease Control and Prevention. (2018). *Hemophilia.* https://www.cdc.gov/ncbddd/hemophilia/facts.html

[4] Mayo Clinic. (2019). *Hemophilia.* https://www.mayoclinic.org/diseases-conditions/hemophilia/symptoms-causes/syc-20373327

[5] Ibid.

[6] Ibid.

[7] Ibid.

[8] Centers for Disease Control and Prevention. (2018). *Hemophilia.* https://www.cdc.gov/ncbddd/hemophilia/facts.html

[9] Mayo Clinic. (2019). *Hemophilia.* https://www.mayoclinic.org/diseases-conditions/hemophilia/symptoms-causes/syc-20373327

[10] Ibid.

OTHER REFERENCES CONSULTED

Merck Manual. (2018). *Hemophilia.* http://www.cdc.gov/ncbddd/hemophilia/facts.html

National Heart, Lung, and Blood Institute. (2019). *Bleeding disorders.* https://www.nhlbi.nih.gov/health-topics/bleeding-disorders

John, T. (2019). Children with other chronic conditions. n J. Selekman, R. Adair Shannon, & C. F. Yonkaitis (Eds.), *School nursing: A comprehensive text* (3rd ed., pp. 685-686). F. A. Davis.

HEPATITIS (VIRAL, TYPES A, B, AND C)

DEFINITION/ETIOLOGY:

The term hepatitis describes inflammation of the liver. Although hepatitis may be caused by alcohol, drugs, autoimmune diseases, metabolic diseases and other possible causes, viruses are the most common cause of jaundice (conjugated hyperbilirubinemia) in childhood and adolescence and are responsible for more than to 50% of acute hepatitis in the United States.[1] Three types of hepatitis (A, B, C) are reportable illnesses in most states. These viruses affect the liver and produce similar symptoms.[2] The incubation period, the mode of transmission, and results of serologic tests help to distinguish the different types of viral hepatitis.

The five types of viral hepatitis are Hepatitis A (HAV), Hepatitis B (HBV), Hepatitis C (HCV), Hepatitis D (HDV), and Hepatitis E (HEV). In the United States, HAV is the most common cause of acute hepatitis and HCV is the most common cause of chronic hepatitis. The information provided in this guideline will focus on HAV, HBV, and HCV infections in the pediatric population.

CAUSE:

Hepatitis: Characteristics of Virus Types

	Hepatitis A	**Hepatitis B**	**Hepatitis C**
Transmission	Transmission is almost always person to person via fecal-oral route or from contaminated water/food	Most Common parenteral, blood, blood products Uncommon saliva, vaginal fluids and semen, contact with open sores, direct contact with bites or scratches Sexual contact, drug use or children born to infected mother's during birth	Parenteral, blood , blood product, sexual contact, drug use In children perinatal transmission is the most prevalent mode of transmission
Incubation period	Two to six weeks (average four weeks) Most infectious in the two weeks prior to symptoms	One to six months (average 3 mos.)	two weeks – six months (average six to seven weeks)
Carrier Status	Not long-term	Yes. May carry the virus in the blood for a lifetime.	Yes
Treatment (acute)	Immune globulin within two weeks of exposure	Hepatitis B immunoglobulin after exposure	None
Treatment (chronic)	Supportive	Supportive	Supportive –interferon see below
Vaccine	Available (recommended 2 doses, the second dose 6 to 18 months after the first dose, for all children 12 months and older)[3]	Available (recommended shortly after birth with two additional doses)[4]	Not available[5]

HEPATITIS (VIRAL, TYPES A, B, AND C) *(continued from previous page)*

SIGNS AND SYMPTOMS:

- Fever, malaise, fatigue, headache, joint pain
- Dark urine and lighter-color stools
- Loss of appetite, nausea, vomiting, stomachache
- Jaundice (yellow eyes and skin)
- Enlargement or tenderness of the liver on palpation
- Most cases in young children are mild[6]

HEPATITIS A (HAV)

- **HAV infection occurs throughout the world but is most common in developing countries.**
- HAV has decreased by more than 95% since the vaccine was established in 1995. Most infected children have no jaundice. Among older children and adults, infection usually is symptomatic and typically lasts several weeks.[7]
- The highest titer of HAV in stool occurs during one to two weeks before the onset of illness. HAV is transmitted from person-to-person or by contamination by food and water. The risk of transmission subsequently diminishes by one week after onset of jaundice. However, HAV can be detected in stool for long periods, especially in young children.[8]
- Post-exposure prophylaxis: Immune globulin (IG) is recommended for un-immunized close personal contacts within two weeks after exposure. Giving Hepatitis A vaccine immediately following exposure for those older than 12 months and less than 40 years is considered as effective as giving immunoglobulin.[9] Exposure in a typical daytime school setting is *not* considered a close contact and IG is not recommended except under unusual circumstances.
- Children with hepatitis A should be referred to the healthcare provider and excluded for one week after onset of illness.
- Adults with acute HAV infection who work as food handlers or in child care settings should be excluded until one week after onset of the illness, until the IG prophylaxis program has been completed, or as directed by the health department.
- Active immunization (HAV vaccine) is effective for children age one year and up, and adults.[10]
- Contact the local health department promptly to review the need to treat household contacts.[11]

HEPATITIS B (HBV)

- HBV has two phases, acute and chronic. Acute HBV is new and is short-term, occurring shortly after exposure to the virus. Chronic HBV is ongoing and long-term lasting longer than six months. Chronic HBV may not go away completely.
- Young children usually do not have jaundice or other symptoms. Sometimes, HBV affects other parts of the body resulting in arthritis, rash or thrombocytopenia. More than 90% of infants who are infected perinatally will develop chronic infection, whereas 25%-50% of children infected between one and five years of age and 10% of infected older children and adults develop a chronic case.[12]
- Risk of transmission in schools is very small.[13]

HEPATITIS (VIRAL, TYPES A, B, AND C) *(continued from previous page)*

HEPATITIS B (HBV) *(continued)*

- HBV virus is transmitted through blood and body fluids, including exudates, semen, cervical secretions and uncommonly with saliva. Person-to-person contact can occur in any setting involving interpersonal contact over an extended period. HBV virus can survive in the environment for one week, so transmission from shared objects, such as razor blades or toothbrushes also may occur but is uncommon. Among adolescents and adults, those at highest risk include users of injection drugs and those with multiple sexual partners.[14]
- HBV is almost always preventable. Pre-exposure HBV immunization is the universally recommended preventive measure for infants, un-immunized children and adolescents.
- School nurses, athletic trainers, and teachers of students who are severely developmentally delayed and positive for Hepatitis B surface antigens (HBsAg), and any adult who are expected to come in contact with blood as part of their employment are candidates for immunization.[15]
- Most children with hepatitis B should be admitted to school without restrictions. If the student has weeping sores, or behaviors that would lead to bleeding exclusion may be necessary.[16]
- Post-exposure prophylaxis: Hepatitis B Immune Globulin (HBIG) is indicated for people at risk of developing HBV due to recent exposure of body fluids of someone infected with HBV. This includes babies of mothers infected with HBV, healthcare workers, emergency first responders, and morticians. HBIG is effective because it provides temporary induced immunity by the transfer of immunoglobulin.[17]

HEPATITIS C (HCV)

- Acute disease tends to be mild and insidious in onset and most infections are asymptomatic. Liver disease due to hepatitis C in children is extremely rare.[18]
- Risk factors are bring born to a mother who has hepatitis C, blood transfusions primarily before 1992, long term kidney dialysis, and injected illicit drug use.[19]
- Treatment is with interferon-alfa alone or in combination with ribavirin in chronic hepatitis C in adults.[20]
- Children with chronic infection should be screened periodically for chronic hepatitis because of potential risk of chronic liver disease.
- Risk of transmission in schools is very small.

MANAGEMENT/TREATMENT:

1. Notify the parent/guardian of symptoms of concern and refer to healthcare provider.
2. Follow state regulations and school policy on reporting to health department.
3. Immune globulin is not recommended for phrophylaxis after mild exposure.[21]
4. Use good hand washing techniques at all times and instruct children as necessary.
5. If a child with known hepatitis B or C bites or a child is bitten by a child who is unimmunized they should be referred to their healthcare provider.[22]
6. Drugs such as acetaminophen should be monitored closely.[23]
7. Currently there is no vaccine for hepatitis C.

HEPATITIS (VIRAL, TYPES A, B, AND C) *(continued from previous page)*

FOLLOW UP:

- Educate campus personnel and students on Universal/Standard Precautions. (*Refer to STANDARD PRECAUTION APPENDIX).*
- Educate students with chronic liver disease on the risk of drug and alcohol use.
- Teach about specific routes of transmission, incubation periods, and signs of infection.
- Athletes should cover existing cuts, abrasions, wounds, or other areas of broken skin with a dressing.
- Inquire about other cases in family and after-school care, group or club.
- Inform about requirements and availability of Hepatitis A and Hepatitis B vaccines.

REFERENCES

---

[1] Buggs, A. M. (2017). *Hepatitis: Viral.* http://emedicine.medscape.com/article/185463-overview

[2] American Academy of Pediatrics. (2020). Hepatitis A infection; Hepatitis B infection. In S. Aronson, & T. Shope (Eds.), *Managing infectious diseases in child care and schools* (5th ed., pp.103-106). American Academy of Pediatrics.

[3] Ibid.

[4] Ibid.

[5]Blosser, K, O'Keefe, C., Sanderson, S. (2017). Infectious diseases and immunizations. In C. Burns, A.M. Dunn, M.A. Brady, N.B. Starr, C.G. Blosser, & D.L. Garzon (Eds.), *Pediatric primary care* (6th ed., pp. 500-501). Elsevier, Inc.

[6] American Academy of Pediatrics. (2020). Hepatitis A infection; Hepatitis B infection. In S. Aronson, & T. Shope (Eds.), *Managing infectious diseases in child care and schools* (5th ed., pp.103-106). American Academy of Pediatrics.

[7] Centers for Disease Control and Prevention. (2019). *Viral hepatitis.* http://www.cdc.gov/HEPATITIS/

[8] American Academy of Pediatrics. (2020). Hepatitis A infection; Hepatitis B infection. In S. Aronson, & T. Shope (Eds.), *Managing infectious diseases in child care and schools* (5th ed., pp.103-106). American Academy of Pediatrics.

[9] Ibid.

[10] Immunization Action Coalition. (2019*). Ask the experts.* https://www.immunize.org/askexperts/experts_hepa.asp

[11] Ibid.

[12] Buggs, A. M. (2017). *Hepatitis: Viral.* http://emedicine.medscape.com/article/185463-overview

[13] American Academy of Pediatrics. (2020). Hepatitis A infection; Hepatitis B infection. In S. Aronson, & T. Shope (Eds.), *Managing infectious diseases in child care and schools* (5th ed., pp.103-106). American Academy of Pediatrics.

[14] Ibid.

[15] Ibid.

[16] Ibid.

[17]Blosser, K, O'Keefe, C., Sanderson, S. (2017). Infectious diseases and immunizations. In C. Burns, A.M. Dunn, M.A. Brady, N.B. Starr, C.G. Blosser, & D.L. Garzon (Eds.), *Pediatric primary care* (6th ed., pp. 500-501). Elsevier, Inc.

[18] Children's Hospital of Pitttsburgh (2019). *Hepatitis C in children.* http://www.chp.edu/our-services/transplant/liver/education/liver-disease-states/hepatitis-c

HEPATITIS (VIRAL, TYPES A, B, AND C) *(continued from previous page)*

[19] Ibid.

[20] Blosser, K, O'Keefe, C., Sanderson, S. (2017). Infectious diseases and immunizations. In C. Burns, A.M. Dunn, M.A. Brady, N.B. Starr, C.G. Blosser, & D.L. Garzon (Eds.), *Pediatric primary care* (6th ed., pp. 500-501). Elsevier, Inc.

[21] Ibid.

[22] American Academy of Pediatrics. (2020). Hepatitis A infection; Hepatitis B infection. In S. Aronson, & T. Shope (Eds.), *Managing infectious diseases in child care and schools* (5th ed., pp.103-106). American Academy of Pediatrics.

[23] Blosser, K, O'Keefe, C., Sanderson, S. (2017). Infectious diseases and immunizations. In C. Burns, A.M. Dunn, M.A. Brady, N.B. Starr, C.G. Blosser, & D.L. Garzon (Eds.), *Pediatric primary care* (6th ed., pp. 500-501). Elsevier, Inc.

OTHER REFERENCES CONSULTED

American Academy of Pediatrics, Committee on Infectious Diseases. (2018*).* Hepatitis A, B, C. In D.W. Kimberlin, M.T. Brady, M.T., M.A. Jackson, & S.S. Long (Eds.), *Red Book, (2018-2021): Report of the Committee on Infectious Diseases* (31st ed., pp. 392-434). American Academy of Pediatrics. Hepatitis A, B, C.

Centers for Disease Control and Prevention (CDC). (2018). Hepatitis A. In W. Atkinson, C. Wolfe, & J., Hamborsky (Eds.), *Epidemiology and prevention of vaccine-preventable diseases* (13th ed.). Washington DC: Public Health Foundation. http://www.cdc.gov/vaccines/pubs/pinkbook/hepa.html

Centers for Disease Control and Prevention (CDC) (2018). Hepatitis B. In W. Atkinson, C. Wolfe, & J., Hamborsky (Eds.), *Epidemiology and prevention of vaccine-preventable diseases* (13th ed.). Washington DC: Public Health Foundation. http://www.cdc.gov/vaccines/pubs/pinkbook/hepb.html

Jensen, K. & Balistreri, W. (2016). The digestive system. In R.M. Kliegman, B.F. Stanton, J.W. St. Geme, & N.F. Schor (Eds.), *Nelson textbook of pediatrics (*20th ed.*, p.38*).: Elsevier Saunders

HERPES SIMPLEX - ORAL (cold sore, fever blister)

DEFINITION/ETIOLOGY:

An acute, viral infection with a local primary lesion (cold sore or fever blister occurring on the lips, mouth or gums), which is frequently latent and tends to recur. Most persons are initially infected by school age. During the first infection people may shed the virus for at least a week and possibly several weeks after signs and symptoms appear. The virus remains dormant in the body and recurrent disease may occur because of a variety of triggers such as stress, cold or sunlight.[1] Recurrent episodes are due to reactivation of latent *Herpes simplex virus* (HSV). People with recurrent sores shed the virus for three to four days after symptoms appear.[2] The virus is often spread by people with no signs or symptoms, often adults and is spread by direct contact through kissing or contact with open sores.[3]

Etiology: HSV, type 1 is the usual cause of mouth sores and herpes simplex virus, Type 2 is the usual causative for most genital herpes lesions. At times, type 1 may cause infection in the genital area and type 2 can cause infection in the mouth.[4]

SIGNS AND SYMPTOMS:

- Painful superficial, fluid filled blisters on an erythematous base, usually on the mouth, lips, and face. Vesicles weep clear fluid and may bleed, they often are slow to crust over.
- May have an itchy or tingling sensation before blister appears.
- During an episode the typical duration is seven to 10 days.
- Contagious until the lesion is completely crusted over.

In the initial infection of HSV, the symptoms are more generalized and more severe than in recurrent infections including fever and tender cervical adenopathy. Children may develop 10 or more small ulcers on the buccal mucosa, tonsils, inner lips, tongue, and gingiva. During the first infection the virus can be shed for a week or up to several weeks.[5]

MANAGEMENT/TREATMENT:

- No exclusion from school unless it is a first or primary infection and the child meets other exclusion criteria such as fever or excessive drooling.[6]
- Wrestlers should be excluded from wrestling for active lesions.[7]
- Always use good hand-washing techniques. (*Refer to HANDWASHING APPENDIX).*
- Lesions may be covered if non-mucosal involvement.
- There is no cure for herpes simplex and re-occurrence is common.
- Glyoxide, campho-phenique, and aloe vera relieve burning and itching briefly.
- Blisters should be kept clean to prevent bacterial infection.
- Lesions are contagious (spread by skin to skin contact), so hands should be washed after touching lesions.
- Refrain from kissing when blisters are present.
- Refer to healthcare provider if severe, frequently recurring or long lasting.
- The use of sunscreen on lips may help prevent re-occurrence.

HERPES SIMPLEX - ORAL (Cold sore, fever blister) *(continued from previous page)*

MANAGEMENT/TREATMENT *(continued)*

- Some healthcare providers may prescribe topical or oral anti-viral medications for early use in frequently recurring or severe cases.
- A child with type 2 lesions should be evaluated for possible sexual abuse.

POTENTIAL COMPLICATIONS:

- Avoid cross-contamination. Keep hands away from eyes. Herpes simplex infections of the eye can cause scarring of the cornea which can potentially lead to blindness. Any suspicion of ocular involvement should be immediately referred to an ophthalmologist.[8]
- Can result in secondary bacterial infection.
- Can cause meningitis or encephalitis if the herpes simplex virus spreads to the brain.
- Can result in dehydration due to dysphagia especially in young children.
- Can be spread to other body parts by scratching skin, especially in a child with eczema.

NOTES:

The herpes simplex virus can be life-threatening to a person with a compromised immune system.[9]

For INFORMATION on HERPES SIMPLEX, type 2 refer to *Sexually Transmitted Diseases*.

REFERENCES

[1] American Academy of Pediatrics. (2020). Herpes simplex (cold sores). In S. Aronson, & T. Shope (Eds.), *Managing infectious diseases in child care and schools* (5th[d] ed., pp. 107-108, 137, 237). American Academy of Pediatrics.

[2]Ibid.

[3] Glosser, C., O'Keefe, K., Sanderson, S. (2017). Infectious disease and immunizations. In C. Burns, A.M. Dunn, M.A. Brady, N.B. Starr, C.G. Blosser, & D.L. Garzon (Eds.), *Pediatric primary care* (6th ed., pp. 501-502). Elsevier, Inc.

[4] Ibid.

[5] American Academy of Pediatrics. (2020). Herpes simplex (cold sores). In S. Aronson, & T. Shope (Eds.), *Managing infectious diseases in child care and schools* (5th[d] ed., pp. 107-108, 137, 237). American Academy of Pediatrics.

[6] Ibid.

[7] Glosser, C., O'Keefe, K., Sanderson, S. (2017). Infectious disease and immunizations. In C. Burns, A.M. Dunn, M.A. Brady, N.B. Starr, C.G. Blosser, & D.L. Garzon (Eds.), *Pediatric primary care* (6th ed., pp. 501-502). Elsevier, Inc.

[8] Ibid.

[9] Smith, S. (2017). *Herpes labialis.* http://www.nlm.nih.gov/medlineplus/ency/article/000606.htm

HUMAN IMMUNODEFICIENCY VIRUS (HIV)

DEFINITION/ETIOLOGY:

Human Immunodeficiency Virus (HIV) is a virus that attacks the body's immune system (specifically the CD4 cells or T cells) rendering it ineffective in fighting off infections.[1] No cure currently exists for HIV, however, with use of antiretroviral therapy (ART), HIV can be controlled. If left untreated, HIV reduces the number of CD4 or T cells, making the body vulnerable to getting other infections or infection-related cancers.[2]

HIV is most commonly transmitted through sexual behaviors and needle or syringe use.[3] For HIV transmission to occur, body fluids from a person who has HIV must come in contact with a mucous membrane (found inside rectum, vagina, penis, and mouth), damaged tissue or be directly injected into the bloodstream. These body fluids include blood, semen, pre-seminal fluid, rectal fluids, vaginal fluids, and breast milk.[4] HIV does not survive for a long time outside the human body, and it cannot reproduce outside a human host.[5]

There are three stages of HIV. If taken as prescribed, ART can be used to slow or prevent progression of the disease from one stage to the next.

- The first stage, acute HIV infection, occurs within 2 to 4 weeks after being infected and is the most contagious stage. In this first stage, there are large amounts of virus in the blood.
- During the second stage, clinical latency (as known as HIV inactivity, dormancy or chronic HIV), HIV levels in the blood are very low, but still active in the body.
- Stage 3, acquired immunodeficiency syndrome (AIDS), is the most severe phase of HIV disease. In this stage, the body's immune system has been badly damaged and persons with AIDS are susceptible to getting increased numbers of severe illnesses (i.e., opportunistic illnesses) because of their body's inability to fight off infectious organisms.[6] People with AIDS can, therefore, be very infectious because of their inability to fight off opportunistic illnesses.

SIGNS AND SYMPTOMS:

The symptoms of HIV vary depending on the phase of the infection.

1. **Acute HIV Infection (Primary Infection):[7]**
   - Fever
   - Headache
   - Muscle aches and joint pain
   - Rash
   - Sore throat and painful mouth sores
   - Swollen lymph glands, mainly on the neck
   - Flu-like illness that may last for a few weeks

2. **Clinical latency infection (HIV inactivity, dormancy or chronic HIV):[8]**
   - Fever
   - Fatigue
   - Swollen lymph nodes — often one of the first signs of HIV infection
   - Diarrhea
   - Weight loss
   - Oral yeast infection (thrush)
   - Shingles (herpes zoster)

HUMAN IMMUNODEFICIENCY VIRUS (HIV) *(continued from previous page)*

SIGNS AND SYMPTOMS *(continued)*

3. **AIDS:**[9]
   - Soaking night sweats
   - Recurring fever
   - Chronic diarrhea
   - Persistent white spots or unusual lesions on your tongue or in your mouth
   - Persistent, unexplained fatigue
   - Weight loss
   - Skin rashes or bumps

MANAGEMENT/TREATMENT:

- There's no cure for HIV/AIDS, but ART are available to control the virus, if taken as prescribed. Each class of ART blocks the virus in different ways. The classes of anti-HIV drugs include: Non-nucleoside reverse transcriptase inhibitors; Nucleoside or nucleotide reverse transcriptase inhibitors; Protease inhibitors; and Integrase inhibitors.[10]
- Provide education regarding protection from getting or spreading HIV:
  - Use a new condom every time you have sex. Women can use a female condom. If using lubricant, make sure it is water based. Oil-based lubricants can weaken condoms and cause them to break. During oral sex use a non-lubricated, cut-open condom or a dental dam (a piece of medical-grade latex).
  - Tell sexual partners if you have HIV.
  - Use a clean needle. If a needle is used to inject drugs, make sure it's sterile. Don't share needles. Seek out needle-exchange programs in local your community and consider seeking help for suspected or known drug addiction.
  - If pregnant, get medical care immediately. HIV-positive persons may pass the infection to their babies. If treatment is prescribed and adhered to during pregnancy, a baby's risk of getting HIV significantly decreases.
  - Consider male circumcision. Research has shown that male circumcision may help reduce a man's risk of getting HIV infection.[11,12]

FOLLOW-UP:

- See a healthcare provider as soon as possible if HIV is suspected or if persons are at risk for contracting the virus.
- Students must have an Individualized Healthcare Plan, Emergency Care Plans and may be eligible for Section 504 services.

POTENTIAL RISKS and COMPLICATIONS:

- Infections - tuberculosis, cytomegalovirus, candidiasis, cryptococcal meningitis, toxoplasmosis, cryptosporidiosis [13]
- Cancers - Kaposi's sarcoma, lymphomas [14]
- Other - Wasting Syndrome, neurological complications, kidney disease [15]

HUMAN IMMUNODEFICIENCY VIRUS (HIV) *(continued from previous page)*

NOTES:

- Develop school policy and procedures on confidentiality, including specific privacy and confidentiality on HIV and AIDS, with the advice and expertise of the school nurse and school medical advisor.
- The local school district may include the use of Pre-exposure prophylaxis (PrEP) in the adolescent population to prevent HIV in those at high risk.
- Sexual risk behaviors place youth at risk for HIV infection. Provide health education regarding preventive and safe sexual behaviors.
- Provide annual training for standard/universal precautions, include education about HIV to all school staff at the beginning of the school year.[16] (*Refer to STANDARD PRECAUTIONS APPENDIX*).
- Keep health records, including notes and other documents referencing a student's HIV status, in a secure and locked location. Follow state and federal laws regarding HIV confidentiality.
- Parents/guardians and students are not required to disclose students' HIV status for enrollment in or to attend school.[17]
- If parents/guardians or students choose to disclose their HIV status to named school staff, the confidentiality of this information must be emphasized.

REFERENCES

[1] National Institute of Allergy and Infectious Diseases. (2019). *HIV/AIDS symptoms*. https://www.niaid.nih.gov/diseases-conditions/hivaids

[2] Centers for Disease Control and Prevention. (2019). *About HIV/AIDS*. https://www.cdc.gov/hiv/basics/whatishiv.html

[3] Centers for Disease Control and Prevention. (2019). *HIV transmission*. https://www.cdc.gov/hiv/basics/transmission.html

[4] Ibid.

[5] Ibid.

[6] Centers for Disease Control and Prevention. (2019). *About HIV/AIDS*. https://www.cdc.gov/hiv/basics/whatishiv.html

[7] Mayo Clinic. (2019). *HIV/AIDS*. https://www.mayoclinic.org/diseases-conditions/hiv-aids/symptoms-causes/syc-20373524

[8] Ibid.

[9] Ibid.

[10] Ibid.

[11] Ibid

[12] National Institute of Allergy and Infectious Diseases. (2019). *HIV/AIDS symptoms*. https://www.niaid.nih.gov/diseases-conditions/hivaids

[13] Mayo Clinic. (2018). HIV/AIDS. https://www.mayoclinic.org/diseases-conditions/hiv-aids/symptoms-causes/syc-20373524

HUMAN IMMUNODEFICIENCY VIRUS (HIV) *(continued from previous page)*

[14] Ibid.

[15] Ibid.

[16] United States Department of Labor, Occupational Safety and Health Administration. (2019). *Universal precautions.* https://www.osha.gov/SLTC/etools/hospital/hazards/univprec/univ.html

[17] United States Department of Education. (2018). *Placement of school children with acquired immunodeficiency syndrome.* http://www2.ed.gov/about/offices/list/ocr/docs/hq53e9.html

HUMAN PAPILLOMAVIRUS (HPV)

DEFINITION/ETIOLOGY:

The Human papillomavirus (HPV) is the most common sexually transmitted infection in the United States.[1] HPVs are small, double-stranded DNA viruses that infect the epithelium. While there are more than 40 different strains of HPV that specifically infect the mucosal epithelium affecting the genital area, most of the HPV infections do not lead to cancer.[2] However, some types of genital HPV can cause cancer of the cervix as well as the mouth. HPV vaccines can help protect against certain strains of genital HPV which are most likely to cause genital warts or cervical cancer.

HPV is primarily transferred by skin-to-skin contact. The infection occurs when the virus enters the body through:

- Cut in the skin
- Abrasion
- Small tear in the outer layer of skin
- Anal or vaginal intercourse

SIGNS AND SYMPTOMS:

Most often, the immune system defeats HPV infection before warts are created. However, when warts do appear as a result of HPV infection, the appearance may vary depending on the type of HPV involved.[3] Below are descriptions of the various types of warts resulting from HPV infection:

- **Genital warts** – flat lesions, small cauliflower-like bumps, or tiny stem-like protrusions. In women, genital warts appear on the vulva and may occur on the cervix or in the vagina. In men, genital warts appear on the penis and scrotum or around the anus. Rarely cause discomfort or pain.
- **Common warts** – rough, raise bumps occurring on hands, fingers, and around fingernails. May be painful and susceptible to bleeding/injury.
- **Plantar warts** – hard and grainy growths, commonly appear on heels or balls of feet; may cause discomfort.
- **Flat warts** – flat topped appearance, slightly raised lesions, may appear darker that regular skin color on face, neck, hands, wrists, elbows, or knees. Usually affect children, adolescents, and young adults.
- **Recurrent respiratory papillomatosis (RRP)** – very rare, warts grow on the throat. May occur as in children (juvenile onset) or in adults (adult onset). Growths can block the airway causing hoarse voice and difficulty breathing.

Risk factors for HPV infection include:

- Number of sexual partners.
- Weakened immune system increases the risk of HPV infections. (Note: immune systems may be weakened by HIV/AIDS or by drugs which may suppress the immune system.)
- Damaged skin.
- Personal contact.

HUMAN PAPILLOMAVIRUS (HPV) *(continued from previous page)*

MANAGEMENT/TREATMENT:

HPV can be managed and prevented in several ways:

- HPV vaccines are administered as a series of three shots over six months to protect against HPV infection and the health problems that HPV infection can cause. There are three HPV vaccines (Cervarix®, Gardasil®, and Gardasil 9®).
    - It is recommended that girls and young women receive any of these HPV vaccines.[4]
    - It is recommended that boys receive either Gardasil® or Gardasil® of these HPV vaccines.[5]

Vaccine	Prevents in Girls/Young Women	Prevents in Boys
Cervix®	• Cervical cancer	
Gardasil®	• Cervical vulvar, vaginal and anal cancer • Genital warts	• Anal cancer • Genital warts
Gardasil®	• Cervical, vulvar, vaginal and anal cancer • Genital warts	• Anal cancer • Genital warts

- HPV vaccines offer the best protection to girls and boys who receive all three-vaccine doses and have time to develop an immune response before being sexually active with another person. HPV vaccination is recommended for preteen girls and boys at age 11 or 12 years.
    - Protection for sexually active individuals include the use of condoms, which may lower the risk of HPV infection, and HPV related diseases.
    - Limiting the number of sex partners can lower chances of getting HPV.

FOLLOW-UP:

The school nurse can assist in the management and prevention of HPV infection among children and adolescents in the following ways:

- Conduct health promotion education sessions in the school setting to increase awareness among youth and parents about HPV prevention and available vaccines.
- Promote safe sex education, use of condoms for both males and females.

POTENTIAL COMPLICATIONS:

- Oral and upper respiratory lesions
- Cancer, e.g. cancers of the genitals, anus, mouth, and upper respiratory tract
- Cervical cancer – caused by two specific types of genital HPV; do not cause warts and no signs or symptoms in the early stages of cervical cancer. Annual pap tests are important to detect precancerous changes in the cervix.

HUMAN PAPILLOMAVIRUS (HPV) *(continued from previous page)*

NOTES:

- Genital HPV infections are transmitted through sexual intercourse, anal or vaginal intercourse, and other skin-to-skin contact in the genital area.
- HPV infection is very rarely transmitted from mother to infant during delivery.[6] However, if exposure occurs during delivery, it may cause HPV infection in the baby's genitals and upper respiratory system.

REFERENCES

---

[1] Centers for Disease Control and Prevention (CDC). (2019). *Human papillomavirus.* https://www.cdc.gov/hpv/parents/vaccine.html?CDC_AA_refVal=https%3A%2F%2Fwww.cdc.gov%2Fhpv%2Fvaccine.html

[2] Atkinson, W., Wolfe, S., Hamborsky J., & McIntyre, L. (Eds.). (2018). *Epidemiology and prevention of vaccine-preventable diseases- The pink book: course textbook (13th ed.).* Public Health Foundation. https://www.cdc.gov/vaccines/pubs/pinkbook/supplement.html

[3] Ibid.

[4] Mayo Clinic. (2019). *HPV infection.* https://www.mayoclinic.org/diseases-conditions/hpv-infection/symptoms-causes/syc-20351596

[5] Ibid.

[6] Atkinson, W., Wolfe, S., Hamborsky J., & McIntyre, L. (Eds.). (2018). *Epidemiology and prevention of vaccine-preventable diseases- The pink book: course textbook (13th ed.).* Public Health Foundation. https://www.cdc.gov/vaccines/pubs/pinkbook/supplement.html

HYPOTHERMIA

DEFINITION/ETIOLOGY:

Hypothermia is abnormally low body temperature.[1] When the body is exposed to prolonged cold temperatures, it begins to lose heat faster than it can produce heat. This causes a dangerously low body temperature. Hypothermia most likely occurs at very cold temperatures, however, it can also occur at cool temperatures (above 40°F) if a person becomes chilled from rain, sweat, or submerged in cold water. Normal body temperature is 98.6°F (37°C) and hypothermia occurs as the body temperature decreases below 95°F (35°C).[2] Hypothermia is considered a medical emergency as it affects proper functioning of the brain, heart, nervous system, and other vital organs. If hypothermia is left untreated, complete failure of the heart and respiratory system can occur and lead to death. Children are especially vulnerable to extreme cold weather and can become hypothermic because they are less able to regulate their body temperature than adults.[3]

SIGNS AND SYMPTOMS:

- Shivering (the human body automatically responds to cold weather by shivering in an attempt to create heat and warm up. As hypothermia worsens, shivering stops)
- Exhaustion or feeling very tired
- Very low energy
- Drowsiness
- Confusion
- Inability to think clearly
- Memory loss
- Slurred speech
- Fumbling hands
- Weak pulse
- Loss of consciousness
- Drowsiness[4]
- Bright red, cold skin (in infants)[5]
- Arrhythmias (with severe hypothermia)[6]

MANAGEMENT/TREATMENT:

- Immediately activate emergency medical response if a person exhibits any of the above signs and symptoms and their temperature is below 95° F (Call Emergency Medical Services [EMS]).[7]
- **Rewarming is the top priority**. Focus on treatments to rewarm the body to normal temperature while awaiting emergency assistance.[8]
- Persons with severe hypothermia may become unconscious and appear to not have a pulse or breathing. Perform cardiopulmonary resuscitation (CPR) until the person responds or emergency medical support becomes available, even if the person appears dead.[9]
- If medical assistance is delayed, move the person out of the cold and remove wet clothing, replacing with warm, dry covering such as blankets, clothing, towels, sheets or sleeping bags to trap the heat.
- Initially focus on rewarming the center of a person's body (chest, neck, head and groin).[10]

HYPOTHERMIA *(continued from previous page)*

MANAGEMENT/TREATMENT *(continued)*

- If conscious, give warm drinks to assist in increasing body temperature. **Do not feed unconscious persons.**
- Once body temperature has increased, continue the rewarming process and keep the person's entire body, including head and neck, dry and warm.
- Avoid massaging frostbitten skin as rubbing can cause severe damage to the tissues.
- Medical attention should be accessed as soon as possible for hypothermic conditions.

FOLLOW UP:

Medical attention and assessment are needed in order to determine the severity of hypothermia experienced by individuals. Once diagnosed and if indicated, persons should then be referred to the appropriate medical specialty areas for further treatment.

POTENTIAL RISKS AND COMPLICATIONS:

Risks:

- Age can be a risk factor for hypothermia
  - Older age: The body's ability to regulate temperature may decrease with age. Older adults also have a reduced shivering response.
  - Younger age: Children tend to lose heat faster than adults due to their larger head to body ratio. Under-dressing in cold weather may increase the risk of hypothermia in children.
- People who drink alcohol or use illicit drugs.
- People who remain outdoors for long periods of time, such as hikers, hunters or people who are homeless.[11]
- Certain medical conditions can affect the body's ability to regulate heat, i.e. underactive thyroid gland, poor nutrition, stroke, severe arthritis, chronic conditions affecting sensation, hypoglycemia, trauma, psoriasis and conditions that limit the normal circulation/blood flow.
- Certain medications such as benzodiazepines, tricyclic antidepressants, opioids, barbiturates and phenothiazine's can reduce core temperature and may alter the body's ability to regulate temperature.

Complications:

- Frostbite: freezing of body tissues
- Gangrene: decay and death of tissue due to interrupted blood flow
- Chilblains: damage to the nerves and small blood vessels in the hands or feet due to prolonged exposure to cold temperatures
- Trench foot: damage to nerves and small blood vessels because of prolonged immersion in cold water
- Aspiration pneumonia
- Clotting disorders

HYPOTHERMIA *(continued from previous page)*

PREVENTION:
Educate children and families about outdoor activities during the cold weather to stay warm and prevent hypothermia:

- Cover up with appropriate clothing for cold weather, e.g. hats, mittens, to prevent body heat from escaping.
- Encourage children to wear layers of clothing – loose fitting and lightweight.
- Encourage children to stay as dry as possible and to change wet clothing as soon as possible.
- Limit amount of time spent outside during cold weather.
- Educate youth and adolescents about risky behaviors and the importance to abstain from alcohol and drug use, especially during periods of prolonged cold weather exposure.

REFERENCES

[1] Centers for Disease Control and Prevention. (2019). *Prevent hypothermia & frostbite.* https://www.cdc.gov/disasters/winter/staysafe/hypothermia.html

[2] Mayo Clinic. (2019). *Hypothermia.* https://www.mayoclinic.org/diseases-conditions/hypothermia/symptoms-causes/syc-20352682

[3] American Academy of Pediatrics. (2019*). Children and disasters: Disaster preparedness to meet children's needs.* https://www.aap.org/en-us/advocacy-and-policy/aap-health-initiatives/Children-and-Disasters/Pages/Extreme-Temperatures-Heat-and-Cold.aspx

[4] Ibid.

[5] Mayo Clinic. (2019). *Hypothermia.* https://www.mayoclinic.org/diseases-conditions/hypothermia/symptoms-causes/syc-20352682

[6] American Academy of Pediatrics. (2019). *Extreme temperatures: Heat and cold.* https://www.aap.org/en-us/advocacy-and-policy/aap-health-initiatives/Children-and-Disasters/Pages/Extreme-Temperatures-Heat-and-Cold.aspx

[7] Ibid.

[8] Mayo Clinic. (2019). *Hypothermia.* https://www.mayoclinic.org/diseases-conditions/hypothermia/symptoms-causes/syc-20352682

[9] Ibid.

[10] Ibid.

[11] Ibid.

IMPETIGO

DEFINITION/ETIOLOGY:[1]

Impetigo is a highly contagious bacterial skin infection characterized by eruptions caused by either *Streptococcal* or *Staphylococcal* bacteria. Methicillin-resistant staph aureus (MRSA) is also becoming a common cause. Minor skin injuries, insect bites, and dermatitis may be the portal for the infectious agent. The eruptions may proceed through vesicular, pustular, and encrusted stages. It usually appears as red bumps that form on the face (particularly around the nose and mouth) or extremities. The red bumps fill with pus, break open, and form a honey-colored crust. The lesions are usually itchy and can cause mild discomfort. Infection is spread by direct contact with secretions from lesions. It can also be spread by using an infected person's towel or from sports equipment.[2] It is most common in ages two (2) to six (6). It is more common in the summer months with the heat and humidity.[3]

SIGNS AND SYMPTOMS:

- Begins as a red sore, pimple or fluid-filled blister, most often found on face (most commonly around the nose and mouth) but may be anywhere on body.[4]
- One spot can spread easily due to scratching.[5]
- Itchy blisters, filled with honey-colored fluid that may be oozing and crusting over.[6]
- May have swollen lymph nodes near the infection (lymphadenopathy).[7]

MANAGEMENT/TREATMENT:

- Untreated impetigo often clears in two (2) to four (4) weeks but there is great risk of complications and thus is recommended to treat with antibiotics.
- Infected individuals do not transmit the infection 24 - 48 hours after antibiotic treatment is underway.[8]
- Parents/guardians should keep contagious children home until 24 hours after starting topical or oral antibiotic therapy per district policy for contagious diseases.
- Contacts of cases do not need to be excluded.[9]
- Hygienic measures: Wash the skin several times a day with a mild soap to gently remove crusts and drainage.[10] Keep fingernails trimmed.
- Antibiotic therapy: Mild cases may be treated with prescribed topical antibiotic ointment or antibacterial cream. Before applying the topical medication, gently remove scabs as noted above so the medication can penetrate the lesion. More severe cases may require oral antibiotics.[11]
- Cover a draining lesion with a dressing.

FOLLOW UP:

- Educate parents that if their child is being treated for an impetigo infection to monitor the sores and call their healthcare provider if there is no improvement after three days of treatment or if a fever develops. If the area becomes red, warm or tender to the touch, contact their health care provider immediately.[12]
- Encourage diligence in skin cleansing and nail hygiene (clean and trimmed).
- Monitor completion of antibiotic course even though lesions are healed.
- Have family observe close contacts and family members for lesions.
- Monitor for additional cases.

IMPETIGO *(continued from previous page)*

POTENTIAL COMPLICATIONS:

- Post streptococcal glomerulonephritis (PSGN) (rare)[13]
- Spread of the infection to other parts of the body
- Cellulitis (*Refer to SKIN INFECTION*)[14]
- Methicillin-resistant *Staphylococcus aureus* (*Refer to SKIN INFECTION*)[15]
- Ecthyma (deep skin ulcers)[16]

Prevention:

- Keep skin clean. Washing hands often and take routine baths or showers. [17]
- Pay special attention to any skin injuries (cuts, scrapes, bug bites, etc.) that could potentially become infected.[18]
- Infected person should:[19]
  - Use a clean towel and wash cloth each time.
  - Not share towels, clothing, razors, and other personal care products with others.
  - Wash hands thoroughly after touching skin lesions.
- Caregiver should wear gloves when washing lesions and applying antibiotic medication and wash hands thoroughly after treating.
- May return to school 24 hours after treatment is started with topical or oral antibiotics, per advice of healthcare provider or district protocol.[20]

REFERENCES

[1] Merck Manual. (2017). *Impetigo and ecthyma.* http://www.merckmanuals.com/professional/dermatologic disorders/bacterial skin infections/impetigo and ecthyma.html?qt=impetigo&alt=sh

[2] American Academy of Dermatology, Inc. (2018). *Impetigo.* https://www.aad.org/public/diseases/contagious-skin-diseases/impetigo#symptoms

[3] US Food and Drug Administration. (2016). *How to treat impetigo and control this common skin infection.* https://www.fda.gov/consumers/consumer-updates/how-treat-impetigo-and-control-common-skin-infection

[4] Mayo Clinic. (2019). *Impetigo.* http://www.mayoclinic.org/diseasesconditions/impetigo/basics/definition/con-20024185

[5] Medline Plus, U.S. National Library of Medicine. (2019). *Impetigo.* http://www.nlm.nih.gov/medlineplus/impetigo.html

[6] Ibid.

[7] Ibid.

[8] American Academy of Dermatology, Inc. (2018). *Impetigo.* https://www.aad.org/public/diseases/contagious-skin-diseases/impetigo#symptoms

[9] Ball, J., Binder, R., & Cowen, K. (Eds.). (2017). Alterations in skin integrity. *Principles of pediatric nursing: Caring for children* (7th ed., pp. 900-941). Pearson Education, Inc.

[10] Mayo Clinic. (2019). *Impetigo.* http://www.mayoclinic.org/diseases-conditions/impetigo/basics/definition/con-20024185

[11] Ibid.

IMPETIGO *(continued from previous page)*

[12] Kids Health/Nemours. (2018). *Impetigo*. https://kidshealth.org/en/parents/impetigo.html?ref=search

[13] Medline Plus, U.S. National Library of Medicine. (2019). *Impetigo.* *http://www.nlm.nih.gov/medlineplus/impetigo.html*

[14] Mayo Clinic. (2019). *Impetigo.* *http://www.mayoclinic.org/diseases-conditions/impetigo/basics/definition/con-20024185*

[15] Ball, J., Binder, R., & Cowen, K. (Eds.). (2017). Alterations in skin integrity. *Principles of pediatric nursing: Caring for children* (7th ed., pp. 900-941). Pearson Education, Inc.

[16] American Academy of Dermatology, Inc. (2018). *Impetigo*. *https://www.aad.org/public/diseases/contagious-skin-diseases/impetigo#symptoms*

[17] Kids Health/Nemours. (2018). *Impetigo*. https://kidshealth.org/en/parents/impetigo.html?ref=search

[18] Ibid.

[19] Medline Plus, U.S. National Library of Medicine. (2019). *Impetigo.* *http://www.nlm.nih.gov/medlineplus/impetigo.html*

[20] American Academy of Pediatrics. (2015). *Impetigo*. *https://healthychildren.org/English/health-issues/conditions/skin/Pages/Impetigo.aspx*

INFLUENZA

DEFINITION/ETIOLOGY:

Influenza is a respiratory virus affecting the nose, throat, and lungs. There are two main types of influenza viruses: A and B.[1] The symptoms are typically more severe with Influenza type A and Influenza type B is usually milder.[2] The incubation period is one to four days but typically about two days.[3] It is generally contagious from 1 day before the symptoms start to 5 or more days after the onset of symptoms.[4] Symptoms typically last three to five days.[5] The virus is spread by airborne respiratory droplets, hand-to-hand contact or by contact with contaminated objects. Influenza viruses are constantly changing with new strains every year.[6] Influenza is prevalent in the United States from October to May.[7]

SIGNS AND SYMPTOMS:[8]

- Fever –over 100.4°F; abrupt onset; fever may last three to four days
- Chills/sweats
- Headache
- General muscle or body aches
- Fatigue
- Nasal congestion
- Sore throat
- Cough (nonproductive and persistent)
- Mild conjunctivitis

MANAGEMENT/TREATMENT:

- Diagnosis is typically determined by clinical symptoms. The healthcare provider may do a rapid influenza test to determine type/subtype.[9]
- Encourage fluids and bedrest.[10]
- Healthcare provider may prescribe antiviral medication (Tamiflu® or Relenza®) for five days to shorten the duration of the symptoms and to reduce the risk of complications.[11]
    - Benefit of taking antiviral medication is greatest if started within 48 hours of onset of symptoms.[12]
    - If healthcare provider prescribes antiviral medication, monitor for side effects such as nausea and vomiting. These may be lessened if taken with food.[13]
- May administer acetaminophen or ibuprofen if ordered to help alleviate flu symptoms (body aches, elevated temperature, etc.). Follow medication orders.[14]
- Do not administer aspirin to children under the age of 18. Aspirin can play a role in causing Reye's Syndrome (rare but potentially fatal disease).[15]
- Instruct parent/guardian to keep child home from school until the child is fever free for 24 hours (without the use of antipyretics).[16]
- Educate parent/guardian(s) on potential complications of influenza.

INFLUENZA *(continued from previous page)*

FOLLOW UP:

- Refer to healthcare provider if symptoms worsen or the child experiences trouble breathing, a stiff neck, or a headache that is not relieved with acetaminophen or ibuprofen.[17]
- If need be, reiterate to the parent/guardian that the child should be kept home for 24 hours after the fever subsides (without antipyretic medication).

POTENTIAL COMPLICATIONS:[18]

The following are at higher risk of complications:

- Children under the age of five
- Those with weakened immune systems
- Those with chronic diseases such as asthma, diabetes, heart conditions, kidney or liver disease.

Flu complications[19]

- Pneumonia – most serious complication
- Ear infection
- Febrile seizure
- Bronchitis
- Asthma flare up

NOTES:[20]

Educate on the importance of:

- Yearly influenza vaccine for everyone six months or older. If an allergy to eggs exist talk to the healthcare provider before getting the vaccine.
- Controlling and preventing the spread of influenza
    - Avoid crowds during peak influenza season.
    - Do not share food or drink.
    - Promote good handwashing. (*Refer to HANDWASHING APPENDIX).*
    - Cover mouth and nose with tissue when cough and/or sneeze; dispose of tissue properly; wash hands or use an alcohol-based hand sanitizer to remove germs.
    - If tissue is not available, cough and/or sneeze into shoulder or elbow. (*Refer to COVER YOUR COUGH APPENDIX).*

REFERENCES

[1] Mayo Clinic. (2019). *Influenza (flu)*. https://www.mayoclinic.org/diseases-conditions/flu/symptomes-causes/syc-20351719

[2] Merck Manual. (2018). *Influenza.* https://www.merckmanuals.com/professional/infectious_diseases/respiratory_viruses/influenza

[3] Ibid.

[4] Mayo Clinic. (2019). *Influenza (flu)*. https://www.mayoclinic.org/diseases-conditions/flu/symptomes-causes/syc-20351719

INFLUENZA *(continued from previous page)*

[5] Merck Manual. (2018). *Influenza.* https://www.merckmanuals.com/professional/infectious_diseases/respiratory_viruses/influenza

[6] Mayo Clinic. (2019). *Influenza (flu).* https://www.mayoclinic.org/diseases-conditions/flu/symptomes-causes/syc-20351719

[7] Kids Health/Nemours. (2018). *The flu (Influenza).* https://kidshealth.org/en/parents/flu.html?WT.ac=ctg#catflu-center-about

[8] Mayo Clinic. (2019). *Influenza (flu).* https://www.mayoclinic.org/diseases-conditions/flu/symptomes-causes/syc-20351719

[9] Merck Manual. (2018). *Influenza.* https://www.merckmanuals.com/professional/infectious_diseases/respiratory_viruses/influenza

[10] Mayo Clinic. (2019). *Influenza (flu).* https://www.mayoclinic.org/diseases-conditions/flu/symptomes-causes/syc-20351719

[11] Ibid.

[12] Kids Health/Nemours. (2018). *The Flu (Influenza).* https://kidshealth.org/en/parents/flu.html?WT.ac=ctg#catflu-center-about

[13] Mayo Clinic. (2019). *Influenza (flu).* https://www.mayoclinic.org/diseases-conditions/flu/symptomes-causes/syc-20351719

[14] Ibid.

[15] Ibid.

[16] Ibid.

[17] Kids Health/Nemours. (2018). *The Flu (Influenza).* https://kidshealth.org/en/parents/flu.html?WT.ac=ctg#catflu-center-about

[18] Mayo Clinic. (2019). *Influenza (flu).* https://www.mayoclinic.org/diseases-conditions/flu/symptomes-causes/syc-20351719

[19] Ibid.

[20] Ibid.

OTHER REFERENCES CONSULTED

Centers for Disease Control and Prevention. (2019). *Influenza (flu).* http://www.cdc.gov/flu

KIDNEY DISEASE, CHRONIC (CKD) IN CHILDREN

DEFINITION/ETIOLOGY:

Chronic Kidney Disease (CKD) refers to irreversible anatomic or functional kidney damage.[1] In the United States, the incidence rate of End Stage Renal Disease (ESRD) in children up to nine years was 15.2 per million population.[2] The incidence of CKD increases with age in children. Children under four years have the lowest incidence of ESRD related to CKD.[3] CKD is staged based on glomerular filtration rate. In children it is calculated using the Revised Schwartz formula.

Kidneys that function normally control blood pressure, fluid balance, electrolyte homeostasis, acid/base balance. Normal kidneys also secrete hormones that stimulate bone marrow to produce red blood cells, and hormones that manage parathyroid hormone.

Stages of CKD [4]

Stage 1: Normal renal function with glomerular filtration rate (GFR)>/=90 with known kidney disease
Stage 2: GFR 60-89 (mild)
Stage 3: GFR 30-59 (moderate)
Stage 4: GRF 15-29 (severe)
Stage 5: GFR <15 (ESRD)-time to consider renal transplant or initiation of dialysis

Causes of CKD [5]

- Congenital anomalies (born with kidney abnormalities)
  - Congenital obstructive anomalies: Posterior urethral valves (PUV), ureteropelvic junction obstruction (UPJ), dysplastic kidneys, renal agenesis, cloacal anomaly)
- Hypertension (usually doesn't manifest as CKD until late adolescence or adulthood unless severe and untreated)
- Diabetes (usually doesn't manifest as CKD until late adolescence or adulthood)
- Inherited kidney disease: autosomal recessive polycystic kidney disease (ARPKD), autosomal dominant polycystic kidney disease (ADPKD), Alport syndrome
- Inflammatory diseases (Lupus, Wagener's, IgA nephropathy, Focal Segmental Glomerulosclerosis)
- Renal cancer (Wilms tumor)
- Hydronephrosis
- Recurrent urinary tract infections/pyelonephritis
- Renal toxic medications such as chemotherapy for other cancer treatments
- Sickle Cell Anemia
- Anoxic birth injury

KIDNEY DISEASE, CHRONIC (CKD) IN CHILDREN *(continued from previous page)*

Causes of Progression of CKD

- Natural progression
- Other causes of progression
  - Acute illness
  - Dehydration
  - Renal toxic medications such as some antibiotics, NSAIDS, and antihypertensive medications
  - Urinary tract infections

SIGNS AND SYMPTOMS OF CKD:[6]

Early stages of CKD (Stage 1-early Stage 3) may have few symptoms. As CKD progresses or with an acute kidney injury, symptoms may include:

- fatigue
- shortness of breath
- decreased appetite and weight loss
- nausea and vomiting
- headaches
- hypertension
- constipation
- polyuria
- weight gain associated with edema and fluid retention
- hematuria (bright red or cola colored urine)
- proteinuria with foamy urine

Laboratory Changes are associated with CKD and will be more pronounced as CKD worsens. These may include chemistry panel changes, nutritional lab, and specific renal related labs.

MANAGEMENT/TREATMENT:[7]

Medications and Restrictions: Children with CKD will require a variety of restrictions and medications to replace the deteriorating function of the kidneys. The child's nephrologist or Dialysis Clinic staff should provide an individualized medication list and restrictions as well as what needs the child will have during school hours (*italicized items are more likely to be done at school*). Some children will receive medications, fluids, and formula orally and some may have gastrostomy tubes.

KIDNEY DISEASE, CHRONIC (CKD) IN CHILDREN *(continued from previous page)*

MANAGEMENT/TREATMENT *(continued)*

Possible plans will include a combination of the following:

- *Fluid increase or restrictions*
- *Dietary restrictions of sodium, phosphorus, magnesium and potassium*
- *Formula feedings*
- *Potassium supplement*
- Potassium binder (Kayexalate-sodium polystyrene)
- *Phosphorus supplement (Joulies solution)*
- *Phosphorus binder medications given just before meals (TUMS-calcium carbonate, PhosLo/PhosLyra-calcium acetate, Renvela-sevelamer)*
- Magnesium supplement (magnesium carbonate)
- *Sodium supplement (sodium chloride)*
- Injections of Epogen-erythropoietin alpha or Aranesp-darbepoetin alfa
- *Iron supplements*
- *Bicarbonate supplement-sodium bicarbonate (Bicitra solution)*
- Calcitriol or Zemplar
- Multivitamin and vitamin D supplement -cholecalciferol or ergocalciferol
- *Antiemetic such as Zofran-ondansetron*
- *Acetaminophen*
- *Always avoid NSAID medications i.e. ibuprofen, naproxen unless approved by healthcare provider*
- Antihypertensive (diuretics, lisinopril, losartan, amlodipine, metoprolol, atenolol)
- Laxative medication such as MiraLAX-polyethylene glycol, Senokot, docusate

Treatment for Progression of CKD to ESRD: If CKD progress to ESRD and the child is not eligible for a preemptive renal transplant due to poor adherence or due to specific cause of ESRD, they will need to start dialysis. (*Refer to ORGAN TRANSPLANT*).

Dialysis options: Hemodialysis (HD)[8]

Typically done three times weekly at an outpatient dialysis clinic associated with a specialty children's hospital. Older children who are near 18 years may be able to receive HD locally but often will not be accepted at adult units until their 18th birthday.

Each session lasts three to six hours. This includes a 15-30 minutes pre and post HD prep time that will require placement of a Hemodialysis central line (CIV), fistula (access under the skin created from own vessels), or graft (access under the skin created) for dialysis access.

KIDNEY DISEASE, CHRONIC (CKD) IN CHILDREN *(continued from previous page)*

MANAGEMENT/TREATMENT *(continued)*

Access Type	Advantages	Disadvantages	School Nurse Responsibility
Fistula (Preferred)	• Less risk of infection as a person's own vessels are used to create the access • Can bathe and swim once access is healed from the initial surgery • Less risk of stenosis than a graft • If aware will need to start HD in the future, a fistula can be placed in advance and allow it to mature	• Takes weeks to months to mature and be ready for use • May require a second surgical procedure to "raise" the access so it can be used • Cannot place this type of access in small children • Patient must comprehend being able to hold still during dialysis • Access is via needle sticks • May require surgical revision due to stenosis	• Child may come with complaint of pain or lack of thrill (palpable thrill means blood can be felt moving through the access) • It is an emergency (i.e. contact parents to contact the dialysis clinic) if there is no thrill or if there are signs of infection (i.e. pain, tenderness, redness, fever)
Graft (Next best option)	• Able to use within a few weeks after placement • Infection risk is higher than a fistula as foreign graft material is used to create the access • Can bathe and swim once the access is healed	• Often suffers more stenosis than fistulas • Higher infection risk than fistulas • Cannot place this type access in small children • Patient must comprehend being able to hold still during dialysis • Access is via needle sticks • May require surgical revision for stenosis	• Child may come with complaint of pain or lack of thrill ((palpable thrill means blood can be felt moving through the access) • It is an emergency (i.e. contact parents to contact the dialysis clinic) if there is no thrill or if there are signs of infection (i.e. pain, tenderness, redness, fever)
CIV (Least preferred but most common in children)	• Can be used immediately for dialysis • Best to consider if expect dialysis to be short term	• High risk of infection • Dressing over CIV must always remain intact and clean • Cannot bathe, shower or swim with CIV in place • May require surgical revision or replacement if the line is not working well	• Signs of infection (i.e. fever, redness around the catheter area) are an emergency • Dressing must be intact at all time • If there are signs of infection or the dressing is not intact, notify parents to contact the clinic

KIDNEY DISEASE, CHRONIC (CKD) IN CHILDREN *(continued from previous page)*

MANAGEMENT/TREATMENT *(continued)*

Dialysis option: Peritoneal Dialysis (PD)[9]

Performed daily at home as either Continuous Ambulatory Peritoneal Dialysis (CAPD) or Continuous Cyclic Peritoneal Dialysis (CCPD). CAPD is done as four single exchanges daily typically performed morning, after school, with dinner and at bedtime. Each exchange takes 20-40 minutes to perform. CCPD is done every night while the child sleeps via a Baxter Home Choice Cycler. Each session typically is scheduled for eight to 10 hours. It will require surgical placement of a peritoneal dialysis catheter (Tenckhoff catheter). Following the catheter placement, the site will need to be covered with a sterile dressing for four weeks during which time the child cannot shower or swim.

Description of PD Catheter	PD Advantages	PD Disadvantages	School Nurse Responsibility
• A pliable opaque plastic tube inserted into the abdomen surgically • There will be a connector to the surgically placed tube that connects a "transfer set" • The transfer set will have a cap in place that is filled with a betadine-soaked sponge	• Can typically start PD 1-3 days after catheter placement • Less intrusive for child's usual activities i.e. can attend school other than during clinic visits, initially will be seen weekly in clinic for 2-4 weeks, then every other week, then monthly (clinic visits will always be monthly) • Less intrusion on family life • Less fluid and dietary restrictions • Easier to travel on PD vs. HD • Child can swim (in chlorinated pools and ocean after 1st four weeks) and shower	• Increased responsibility for parents or provider of child's care • Child cannot bathe in tub or swim in lakes, go on water park rides (recommend limited swimming in public pools) • Risk of catheter moving out of optimal position that may require surgical revision or replacement • Requires longer hospitalization for initiation of PD and parent training (although sometimes can be completed as an outpatient) • Risk of infection at the catheter exit site or infection of the peritoneal cavity (peritonitis) • Risk of hernia development especially in infants-this will require surgical repair of the hernia and hospitalization for medical management while child is off PD as the hernia repair heals • Risk of severe peritonitis which may require removal of the peritoneal dialysis catheter and transition to HD either temporarily or permanently	• Parents should provide the nurse with an emergency school kit and will show the nurse what to do if there is an issue with the catheter • These issues are considered an emergency due to infection risk. Contact parents to bring the child to their dialysis clinic. • Child may come with wet clothing and a leak may be evident from the catheter or may not be evident (use the provided clamp to clamp off the catheter between the leak and the child) • The transfer set may come apart from the PD catheter which will most likely cause fluid leaking from the peritoneal cavity (abdomen). Clamp the PD catheter with the provided clamp • The cap may come off the transfer set (clamp the PD catheter with the provided clamp)

KIDNEY DISEASE, CHRONIC (CKD) IN CHILDREN *(continued from previous page)*

FOLLOW-UP:

- Children with CKD who are seen by a nephrologist will require appointments based on the severity of their kidney disease.
- Typical follow up may be as frequent as monthly to once a year.
- Children on HD will receive hemodialysis typically three times a week. In rare cases it may be only twice weekly or up to six times weekly.
- Children PD will initially require weekly follow up for approximately 1 month, then twice monthly then monthly. Of course, an urgent visit will be necessary if there is a complication.
- It is critical that the school nurse has clear orders from the student's healthcare provider as well as guidance from their parent or guardian regarding child's medical plan of care.
- The school nurse should work with the healthcare provider, parents/guardians, and school team to develop an Individualized Healthcare Plan (IHP), an Emergency Care Plan (ECP), and a Section 504 Plan or an Individualized Education Plan (IEP) as necessary.
- The IHP should include any treatments/medications to be administered at school, any restrictions or limitations, possible complications and any education/prevention strategies needed.
- The ECP should include action steps in an emergency including accessibility to medication.
- Monitor for normal growth and development and refer student for IEP if regression or delay is noted.
- Provide psycho-social support and referrals as needed.
- Educate staff on potential complications and medical requirements regarding restrictions and medications.

POTENTIAL COMPLICATIONS:

See HD and PD tables for potential access complications. Additional complications for a child with CKD include:

- infection
- fever
- decreased growth and development
- at risk for bullying as often children with CKD as smaller than their peers
- developmental delays
- poor school performance due to uremia symptoms
- missed school days
- depression associated with a chronic illness

Children who have had a renal transplant are at risk for rejection and post-transplant cancers.

KIDNEY DISEASE, CHRONIC (CKD) IN CHILDREN *(continued from previous page)*

NOTES:

Interventions for the school nurse:

- Plan for school re-entry.
- Refer for social skills training, vocational rehabilitation, cognitive remediation therapy as needed.

SCHOOL RE-ENTRY

A child starting dialysis would be expected to return to school within 30 days. Children on HD will miss school half-days or full days depending on the distance they travel for dialysis treatments on treatment days so may require Homebound assistance to keep pace with their peers. Most Pediatric Dialysis Clinics should have an educator that works with the child while they are receiving treatment and who will coordinate school needs with the classroom teacher. Post-renal transplant the child will be out of school for a significant time period to be determined by the transplant center, so will most likely require Homebound Education. *(Refer to TRANSPLANT RECIPIENTS).* It is recommended that any child with advanced CKD or ESRD have an IEP or a Section 504 Plan to provide the necessary academic accommodations and supports.

IMPLICATIONS FOR LEARNING

Treatment and follow-up appointments will affect attendance.
Emotional, behavioral and learning problems may be more common when children have a chronic medical condition.[10]

NOTE: Most children with CKD or ESRD will survive to adulthood; however, they are considered to be immunocompromised so there is a heightened risk of death due to infection or complications as compared to their healthy peers.

REFERENCES

[1] Mistry, K. (2017). Chronic kidney disease. In K.K. Kher, H.W. Schnaper, & L.A. Greenbaum (Eds.). *Clinical pediatric nephrology* (3rd ed., pp. 601-619). CRC Press, Taylor & Francis Group.

[2] Ibid.

[3] Ibid.

[4] Inkler, L.A. & Levey, A.S. (2014). Staging and management of chronic kidney disease. In S.J. Gilbert, D.W. Weiner, D.S. Gipson, M.A. Perazella & M. Tonelli (Eds.). *National kidney foundation's primer on kidney diseases* (6th ed., pp. 458-466). Elsevier Saunders.

[5] Mistry, K. (2017). Chronic kidney disease. In K.K. Kher, H.W. Schnaper, & L.A. Greenbaum (Eds.). *Clinical pediatric nephrology* (3rd ed., pp. 601-619). CRC Press, Taylor & Francis Group.

[6] Greenbaum, L.A. & Schaefer, F. (2012). The decision to initiate dialysis in a pediatric patient. In B.A. Warady F. Schaefer & S.R. Acexander (Eds.). *Pediatric dialysis* (2nd ed., pp. 85-97). Springer.

KIDNEY DISEASE, CHRONIC (CKD) IN CHILDREN *(continued from previous page)*

[7] Inkler, L.A. & Levey, A.S. (2014). Staging and management of chronic kidney disease. In S.J. Gilbert, D.W. Weiner, D.S. Gipson, M.A. Perazella & M. Tonelli (Eds.). *National kidney foundation's primer on kidney diseases* (6th ed., pp. 458-466). Elsevier Saunders..

[8]Hakim, R.M. (2014). Hemodialysis. In S.J. Gilbert, D.W. Weiner, D.S. Gipson, M.A. Perazella & M. Tonelli (Eds.). *National kidney foundation's primer on kidney diseases* (6th ed., pp. 508-519). Elsevier Saunders.

[9]Vardhan, A. & Hutchison, A.J. (2014). Peritoneal dialysis. In S.J. Gilbert, D.W. Weiner, D.S. Gipson, M.A. Perazella & M. Tonelli (Eds.). *National kidney foundation's primer on kidney diseases* (6th ed., pp. 520-533). Elsevier Saunders.

[10]American Academy of Pediatrics, Healthychildren.org (2015). *Children with chronic illness: Dealing with emotional problems and depression.* https://www.healthychildren.org/English/health-issues/conditions/chronic/Pages/Children-with-Chronic-Illness-Dealing-with-Emotional-Problems-and-Depression.aspx

OTHER REFRENCES CONSULTED

Goldstein-Fuchs, D.J. & LaPierre, A.F. (2014). Nutrition and kidney disease. In S.J. Gilbert, D.W. Weiner, D.S. Gipson, M.A. Perazella & M. Tonelli (Eds.). *National kidney foundation's primer on kidney diseases* (6th ed., pp. 467-475). Elsevier Saunders.

Quarles, L.D. (2014). Bone disorders in chronic kidney disease. In S.J. Gilbert, D.W. Weiner, D.S. Gipson, M.A. Perazella & M. Tonelli (Eds.). *National kidney foundation's primer on kidney diseases* (6th ed., pp. 476-487). Elsevier Saunders.

Weiner, D.E. & Sarnak, M.J. (2014). Cardiac function and cardiovascular disease in chronic kidney disease. In S.J. Gilbert, D.W. Weiner, D.S. Gipson, M.A. Perazella & M. Tonelli (Eds.). *National kidney foundation's primer on kidney diseases* (6th ed., pp. 488-496). Elsevier Saunders.

Wish, J.B. (2014). Anemia and other hematologic complication of chronic kidney disease. In S.J. Gilbert, D.W. Weiner, D.S. Gipson, M.A. Perazella & M. Tonelli (Eds.). *National kidney foundation's primer on kidney diseases* (6th e., pp. 497-506). Elsevier Saunders.

LACERATIONS

DEFINITION/ETIOLOGY:

A laceration is a tearing or jagged wound of the soft tissue.[1] Soft tissue tears/cuts (lacerations) are common in children and are often the result of falls, blows, collisions or contact with sharp objects.[2]

SIGNS AND SYMPTOMS:

- Torn or jagged wound of the soft tissue.[3]
- Wound edges may be separated.[4]

MANAGEMENT/TREATMENT:

1. Don gloves. *(Refer to STANDARD PRECAUTIONS APPENDIX)*
2. Stop bleeding by applying firm pressure with sterile or clean dressing until bleeding stops or at least five minutes. [5]
3. If possible, elevate bleeding area above level of heart.[6]
4. Clean wound and surrounding skin with soap and water.[7]
5. Clean wound away from the injury to prevent dirt from entering the wound.[8]
   Note: *Hydrogen peroxide is not appropriate for fresh wounds.*[9]
6. If debris is in wound, let the water from faucet run over cut for several minutes. May need to refer to healthcare provider for follow-up treatment.[10]
7. If no referral to healthcare provider is needed (as noted below), dry site and apply dressing.
8. Review immunization record. Refer family to take child to healthcare provider if last tetanus immunization has been greater than five years.[11]

REFER TO HEALTHCARE PROVIDER WHEN:

- Laceration is longer than about .75 cm, is on the face, appears deep, or has edges that are not approximated.[12]
- Laceration is located close to eye or a larger cut on the face.[13]
- Laceration continues to bleed even after applying pressure for several minutes.[14]
- The injury was caused by an animal or human bite.[15]
- If there are symptoms of a nerve or tendon injury (e.g., numbness or loss of movement).[16]
- If debris is embedded in the laceration.[17]
- If there are signs and symptoms of infection, such as redness, increasing pain, drainage, warmth or swelling.[18]

FOLLOW UP:

- Change bandage as needed.[19]
- Keep area clean and dry.[20]
- Make sure student avoids activity that could reopen wound.[21]
- Follow healthcare provider orders or school district protocol if treatment is required/needed during the school day.

LACERATIONS *(continued from previous page)*

POTENTIAL COMPLICATIONS:

- Wound infection: signs include redness, swelling and may have purulent drainage. Pain that worsens one or more days after injury may be another sign of impending infection.[22]
- Lymphangitis. Look for red streak from infected area toward armpit or groin.[23]

NOTES:

- Educate student in the proper process to wash, apply pressure and bandage to their wound. Encouraging supervised self-care minimizes bloodborne pathogen exposure and encourages student to become more participatory in their own self-care.
- Wound cleansing and debridement are most important in preventing secondary wound infections.[24]

REFERENCES

[1] Medline Plus. U.S. National Library of Medicine. (2017). *Laceration versus puncture wound.* https://medlineplus.gov/ency/imagepages/19616.htm

[2] Kids Health/Nemours. (2018). *First aid: Cuts.* https://kidshealth.org/en/parents/cuts-sheet.html?WT.ac=p-ra

[3] Medline Plus. U.S. National Library of Medicine. (2017). *Laceration versus puncture wound.* https://medlineplus.gov/ency/imagepages/19616.htm

[4] Kids Health/Nemours. (2018). *First aid: Cuts.* https://kidshealth.org/en/parents/cuts-sheet.html?WT.ac=p-ra

[5] Merck Manual. (2018). *Wounds.* https://www.merckmanuals.com/home/injuries-and-poisoning/first-aid/wounds?query=Lacerations

[6] Ibid.

[7] Children's Hospital of Philadelphia. (2018). *Lacerations with stitches* https://www.chop.edu/conditions-diseases/lacerations-stitches

[8] Jakubowski, T., & Perron, T. (2019). Students with common health complaints. In J. Selekman, R.A. Shannon, & C. F. Younkaitis (Eds.), *School Nursing: A comprehensive text* (3rd ed., pp. 362-363). F.A. Davis.

[9] Mayo Clinic. (2017). *Cuts and scrapes: First aid.* https://www.mayoclinic.org/first-aid/first-aid-cuts/basics/art-20056711

[10] Ibid.

[11] Children's Hospital of Philadelphia. (2018). *Lacerations with stitches.* https://www.chop.edu/conditions-diseases/lacerations-stitches

[12] Merck Manual. (2018). *Wounds.* https://www.merckmanuals.com/home/injuries-and-poisoning/first-aid/wounds?query=Lacerations

[13] Children's Hospital of Philadelphia. (2018). *Lacerations with stitches.* https://www.chop.edu/conditions-diseases/lacerations-stitches

[14] Kids Health/Nemours. (2018). *First aid: Cuts.* https://kidshealth.org/en/parents/cuts-sheet.html?WT.ac=p-ra

[15] Ibid.

[16] Merck Manual. (2018). *Wounds.* https://www.merckmanuals.com/home/injuries-and-poisoning/first-aid/wounds?query=Lacerations

[17] Children's Hospital of Philadelphia. (2018). *Lacerations with stitches.* https://www.chop.edu/conditions-diseases/lacerations-stitches

[18] Mayo Clinic. (2017). *Cuts and scrapes: First aid.* https://www.mayoclinic.org/first-aid/first-aid-cuts/basics/art-20056711

LACERATIONS *(continued from previous page)*

[19] Ibid.

[20] Children's Hospital of Philadelphia. (2018). *Lacerations with stitches*. https://www.chop.edu/conditions-diseases/lacerations-stitches

[21] Ibid.

[22] Merck Manual. (2018). *Wounds*. https://www.merckmanuals.com/home/injuries-and-poisoning/first-aid/wounds?query=Lacerations

[23] Medline Plus. U.S. National Library of Medicine. (2017). *Lymphangitis*. https://medlineplus.gov/ency/article/007296.htm.

[24] Jakubowski, T., & Perron, T. (2019). Students with common health complaints. In J. Selekman, R.A. Shannon, & C. F. Younkaitis (Eds.), *School Nursing: A comprehensive text* (3rd ed., pp. 362-363). F.A. Davis.

LEAD POISONING (Plumbism)

DEFINITION/ETIOLOGY:
Lead is a natural metal occurring in the environment. Lead poisoning occurs when there is a build-up of lead in the body. People are exposed to lead by eating food or drinking water or inhaling air that is contaminated with lead. Old homes may have lead in the water pipes or may be painted with lead based paints. Children may be exposed to lead by playing in soil that has been contaminated with lead or eating lead-based paint chips. Lead poisoning most often occurs in young children under the age of six. Lead poisoning is often considered a chronic disorder; therefore, children should be initially screened a minimum of twice by the age of four; however, most providers will test between 12 months and 24 months. No safe blood lead level in children have been identified, even low levels of lead in blood have been shown to affect IQ, the ability to pay attention, and academic achievement.[1] Therefore, a blood lead reference value of >5ug is used to identify children with elevated lead levels and additional follow-up is required.[2]

PREVENTION:
Childhood lead poisoning, although extremely harmful to children, is 100% preventable. It is recommended that parents and caregivers remove lead hazards from the child's environment before they are exposed. The school nurse can assist families by:

- Educating them on the effects of lead;
- Encouraging them to speak with their child's healthcare provider about a blood lead test;
- Encouraging families to consult with their local health department about testing for paint & dust in homes built prior to 1978; and
- Encouraging families to stay current with recalls on toys and to dispose of them immediately.[3]

SIGNS AND SYMPTOMS:
Children may be asymptomatic or have minimal symptoms at first. Symptoms are not obvious until blood levels become elevated. If not treated, children may have irreversible effects. Lead poisoning can affect every organ in the body.

Lead affects the body in many ways. It is important to know that even exposure to low levels of lead, over any length of time can severely harm children.
In children, exposure to lead can cause:

- Nervous system and kidney damage
- Learning disabilities, attention deficit disorder, and decreased intelligence
- Speech, language, and behavior problems
- Poor muscle coordination
- Decreased muscle and bone growth

LEAD POISONING (Plumbism) *(continued from previous page)*

Signs and symptoms of acute lead poisoning[4]

- Irritable/moody
- Anorexia
- Fatigue
- Difficulty concentrating
- Gastrointestinal symptoms – abdominal pain/vomiting/constipation

If Blood level ≥ 50 µg/dL

- Gastrointestinal symptoms
  - Abdominal cramping (chronic)
  - Constipation
- Hand tremors
- Irritability/changes in mood

If Blood level ≥ 100 µg/dL

- Encephalopathy

Signs and symptoms of chronic lead poisoning[5]

- Developmental delays
- Cognitive deficits (risk increases with whole blood level ≥ 10 µg/dL)
- Seizure disorders
- Aggressive behaviors
- Anemia (lead interferes with hemoglobin formation)
- Hearing loss
- Peripheral neuropathy
- Muscle and joint pain
- Kidney damage
- Hearing damage

MANAGEMENT/TREATMENT:[6, 7]

- Eliminate source of lead exposure.
- Children with a blood lead level of 0-4ug/dl, there is no action needed other than eliminating source.
- Children with a blood lead level of 5-9 ug/dl should have a repeat blood lead level in 3 months and the child's vitamin and nutritional status should be assessed; children with diets low in fat and high in iron and calcium absorb less lead. A referral can be made to the local health department upon parental request.
- Children with a blood lead level of 10-19ug/dl are considered poisoned. The local health department should be notified; in addition, the child's iron level should be reviewed.
- Children with a lead level 20-44ug/dl are considered significantly poisoned, may be chelated between 35-44ug/dl, and will need to have a repeat blood draw in 1 month.
- If the poisoned child has siblings, they should have a blood lead screening also.
- Chelation therapy for children diagnosed with encephalopathy or with blood lead levels greater than 45 ug/dL.

LEAD POISONING (Plumbism) *(continued from previous page)*

FOLLOW-UP:

- For any child with a lead level over 5 ug/dl, a referral to support team is appropriate to evaluate if child is eligible for an Individualized Educational Plan under IDEA or Section 504 accommodations.
- For any chronic health needs, an Individualized Healthcare Plan for the student should be developed.
- **Lead poisoning is 100% preventable**. In addition to the steps above, consider writing a newsletter article educating parent/guardian(s) on lead poisoning prevention and the signs and symptoms of lead poisoning.

POTENTIAL COMPLICATIONS:

- Learning disabilities
- Irreversible organ damage
- Seizures
- Encephalopathy
- Death – high lead levels cause brain damage and kidney failure which ultimately lead to death

NOTES:

Potential sources of lead in foods, cosmetics, and products imported from other countries. The following products *may* contain lead:[8,9]

- Some folk remedies (Greta or Azarcon – Hispanic home remedy)
- Kohl – traditional cosmetic
- Some ethnic health-care products (Litargirio – used as deodorant)
- Imported herbal products/medicinal herbs may contain lead
- Daw tway – digestive home remedy from Thailand
- Some candies and pottery from Mexico
- Toys produced overseas may contain lead

RESOURCE:

CDC Lead Poisoning Prevention found at https://www.cdc.gov/nceh/lead/prevention/default.htm

REFERENCES

---

[1] Centers for Disease Control & Prevention. (2019.) *Lead poisoning prevention.* https://www.cdc.gov/nceh/lead/prevention/default.htm

[2] Centers for Disease Control & Prevention, (2019). *CDC blood lead reference values.* https://www.cdc.gov/nceh/lead/prevention/blood-lead-levels.htm

[3] Centers for Disease Control & Prevention. (2019). *Lead poisoning prevention.* https://www.cdc.gov/nceh/lead/prevention/default.htm

[4] Mayo Clinic. (2019). *Lead poisoning.* https://www.mayoclinic.org/diseases-conditions/lead-poisoning/symptoms-causes/syc-20354717

LEAD POISONING (Plumbism) *(continued from previous page)*

[5] Medline Plus. U.S. National Library of Medicine. (2019) *Lead poisoning.* https://medlineplus.gov/ency/article/002473.htm

[6] Mass.gov. (2019). *Learn about lead testing in Massachusetts and what a result means for your child.* https://www.mass.gov/service-details/learn-about-lead-testing-in-massachusetts-and-what-a-result-means-for-your-child

[7] The Merck Manual. (2019). *Lead poisoning.* https://www.merckmanuals.com/professional/injuries-poisoning/poisoning/lead-poisoning?qt=lead%20poisoning&alt=sh

[8] Environmental Protection Agency. (2017). *Protect your family from lead in your home.* https://www.epa.gov/lead/protect-your-family-exposures-lead

[9] CDC (2019). *Sources of Lead Poisoning*. https://www.cdc.gov/nceh/lead/prevention/sources/foods-cosmetics-medicines.htm

LEUKEMIA

DEFINITION/ETIOLOGY:[1]

Leukemia is the most common childhood cancer, defined as cancer of the white blood cells (WBC). There is an increase in the production of abnormal WBCs in leukemia, which replaces normal bone marrow and spills over into the circulating blood. Leukemic cells may infiltrate any organ: liver, spleen, lymph nodes, kidneys, testes, and the central nervous system (brain and spinal cord). Though initial presentations of leukemia may include elevated WBC counts, healthcare providers must be acutely aware of the symptoms of immunosuppression. Efforts to eradicate abnormal cells (i.e. chemotherapy) may lead to a decreased WBC count making the patient more susceptible to infection.

CAUSES:

The exact cause of leukemia is not fully understood by scientists. Leukemia appears to develop from a combination of genetic and environmental factors. If leukemia is found, further tests will be needed to find out the type and subtype of leukemia and determine a course of treatment.[2]

TYPES:[3, 4]

1. Acute Lymphocytic Leukemia (ALL) accounts for approximately 75% of cases. ALL is most common in ages 2-4 years and has the best prognosis during this time period. The survival rate is 90%. There are several subtypes of ALL which are identified by bone marrow appearance and other blood tests. Treatment and prognosis depend on age of onset, subtypes of ALL, and other blood factors.
2. Acute Myelogenous Leukemia (AML) is also called acute myeloid leukemia, acute myelocytic leukemia or acute non-lymphocytic leukemia. AML accounts for approximately 20% of cases. AML is most common is the teenage years. The survival rate is 65 – 70%.
3. Chronic Myelogenous Leukemia (CML) is rare in children. Survival rates are 60-80%.

SIGNS AND SYMPTOMS:[5, 6]

Symptoms are derived from problems in bone marrow; onset may be insidious or acute.

- Bone and joint pain due to pressure and irritation from infiltration by white blood cells
- Anemia, pallor, fatigue, weakness, lethargy, dizziness, lightheaded (symptoms of low red blood count)
- Increased susceptibility to fevers and recurrent infections due to low white blood cell count and weakened immune system
- Bleeding under the skin; bruising; pinpoint hemorrhages (petechiae) or larger areas; bleeding of nose or gums; blood in stool or urine (symptoms of low platelet count)
- Headache due to infiltration of the brain
- Seizures, balance problems, or abnormal vision
- Vomiting from bleeding in stomach or increased intracranial pressure
- Breathing problems and interference with blood flow to and from the heart
- Enlarged liver, spleen or swollen lymph nodes
- Weight loss

LEUKEMIA *(continued from previous page)*

MANAGEMENT/TREATMENT:[7, 8]

- Drug therapy
- Chemotherapy
- Radiation
- Bone marrow or blood stem transplants (required for aggressive ALL)
- Therapy lasts and average of 30-42 months[9]
- The type of medication and length of therapy is individualized[10]

Side Effects of Treatment[11]

Short-term effects:

- Hair loss from drug therapy
- Weight gain from therapy (prednisone)
- Neutropenia
- High blood pressure
- Breathing problems and interference with blood flow to and from the heart

Long-term effects:

- One third to half of survivors have poor short-term memory, short attention span, or other learning difficulties (consider referral for Section 504 plan or Individualized Education Plan [IEP])
- Blood stem transplants may affect child's growth
- Emotional and psychological problems (which may affect schoolwork)

FOLLOW UP:[12, 13]

An individualized healthcare plan (IHP) should be developed and may include:

- Homebound instruction for limited periods.
- Notify teacher of symptoms to observe for indicating possible illness.
- Emphasize that the condition may make the student vulnerable to contagious viral illnesses of others.
- Notify school district registered dietician if child needs dietary accommodations.
- Obtain immunization exemption from healthcare provider if necessary.
- Coordinate with school staff regarding any limitations or precautions needed for physical activity.
- Accommodation of physical/emotional needs (possible Section 504 plan or IEP).
- Educate classmates before student returns to school (with parental permission).
- Notify parent/guardian(s) and doctors of unusual symptoms and the occurrence of contagious illnesses, e.g., chickenpox, in the school. Special treatment is required for exposure to chicken pox.
- Continuous follow up care is important and essential for the child diagnosed with leukemia as their health will impact their school or extracurricular attendance.

LEUKEMIA *(continued from previous page)*

NOTES:

A diagnosis of leukemia may be devastating for the family of a child who is newly diagnosed, efforts must be made to support to the psychological and psychological health of the family unit.

- Siblings are "at risk" for contracting leukemia.
- Children treated for leukemia have an increased risk for developing cancer in adulthood.
- Some school districts and hospitals have a school re-entry program to assist in transitions.
- Children with Li-Fraumeni syndrome, Down's syndrome, and children who have had an organ transplant and on long-term immune suppressing medication, are at slightly higher risk of developing leukemia.

RESOURCES

- **Returning to School,** Leukemia and Lymphoma Society at http://www.livestrong.org/What-We-Do/Our-Actions/Professional-Tools-Training/For-Educators/Returning-to-School

- **Children Diagnosed with Cancer**, American Cancer Society at http://www.cancer.org/treatment/childrenandcancer/whenyourchildhascancer/children-diagnosed-with-cancer-returning-to-school

REFERENCES

---

[1] American Cancer Society. (2019). *What is childhood leukemia?* http://www.cancer.org/cancer/leukemiainchildren/detailedguide/childhood-leukemia-what-is-childhood-leukemia

[2] American Cancer Society. (2019). *How is childhood leukemia diagnosed? Signs and symptoms of childhood leukemia.* http://www.cancer.org/cancer/leukemiainchildren/detailedguide/childhood-leukemia-diagnosis

[3] American Cancer Society. (2019). *Survival rates for childhood leukemias.* http://www.cancer.org/cancer/leukemiainchildren/detailedguide/childhood-leukemia-survival-rates

[4] American Cancer Society. (2015). *What are key statistics for childhood leukemia?* http://www.cancer.org/cancer/leukemiainchildren/detailedguide/childhood-leukemia-key-statistics

[5] Kids Health. (2019). *Leukemia.* http://kidshealth.org/parent/medical/cancer/cancer_leukemia.html

[6] Mayo Clinic. (2018). *Leukemia.* https://www.mayoclinic.org/diseases-conditions/leukemia/symptoms-causes/syc-20374373

[7] Leukemia and Lymphoma Society. (2019). *Types of AML treatment.* https://www.lls.org/leukemia/acute-myeloid-leukemia/treatment

[8] American Cancer Society. (2019). *Living as a childhood leukemia survivor.* https://www.cancer.org/cancer/leukemia-in-children/after-treatment/follow-up.html

[9] Horton, T.M. (2019*). Overview of acute lymphoblastic leukemia/lymphoma in children and adolescents.* https://www.uptodate.com/contents/overview-of-the-treatment-of-acute-lymphoblastic-leukemia-lymphoma-in-children-and-adolescents

[10] Leukemia and Lymphoma Society. (2019). *Side effects.* https://www.lls.org/leukemia/acute-myeloid-leukemia/treatment/side-effects

[11] Leukemia and Lymphoma Society. (2019). *Side effects.* https://www.lls.org/leukemia/acute-myeloid-leukemia/treatment/side-effects

[12] Ibid.

[13] American Cancer Society. (2019). *Living as a childhood leukemia survivor.* https://www.cancer.org/cancer/leukemia-in-children/after-treatment/follow-up.html

LICE (HEAD) - Pediculosis humanus capitis

DEFINITION/ETIOLOGY:

The head louse, or *Pediculus humanus capitis*, is a parasitic insect that can be found on the head, eyebrows, and eyelashes of people. Head lice feed on human blood several times a day and live close to the human scalp. Head lice are not known to spread disease.[1] Nits are lice eggs which are laid by the adult female and are cemented at the base of the hair shaft nearest the scalp. Nymphs hatch from the eggs in seven to 10 days and grow to adults capable of reproduction (lay eggs) in nine to 12 days, with a life span of 30 days. The female lays about eight to 10 eggs per day (more than 200 in a lifetime), attaching them firmly to the hair shaft near the scalp. Head lice move by crawling; they cannot hop, jump, or fly and pets do not play a role in transmission of human lice.[2] They are spread most commonly by head-to-head contact, for example during slumber parties, sports activities and camp. Although uncommon, lice can be spread by contact with clothing such as hats, scarves, combs, brushes or towels. Only lice, not nits, spread the infestation.[3]

Although head lice can be a nuisance, they should not be considered a medical or public health hazard because they have not been shown to spread disease.[4] Head lice are found worldwide. In the United States, infestation with head lice is most common among pre-school children attending childcare, elementary schoolchildren, and the household members of infested children. Although reliable data on how many people in the United States get head lice each year are not available, an estimated six million to 12 million infestations occur each year in the United States among children three to 11 years of age.[5] In the United States, infestation with head lice is much less common among African Americans than among persons of other races.[6]

SIGNS AND SYMPTOMS:

- Head lice infestations can be asymptomatic, particularly with a first **infestation or when an infestation is light.[7]**
- Itching (pruritus), the most common symptom of head lice infestation, is caused by an allergic reaction to the saliva associated with louse bites. It may take 4-6 weeks for itching to appear the first time a person has head lice.[8]
- The student may report a tickling feeling or a sensation of something moving in the hair.
- Student irritability and sleeplessness may be present.
- Sores on the head may be caused by scratching. These sores and scabs can sometimes become infected with bacteria normally found on a person's skin. These may also be associated with swollen lymph nodes.

The assessment of a child who is suspected of having head lice includes:

- Ensure student privacy and confidentiality.
- In good lighting, use a wood applicator to separate the hair in small sections. Give particular **attention to the scalp behind the ears and at the nape of the neck, areas of optimal temperature for head lice. Dispose of the applicator after each use.**

LICE (HEAD) - Pediculosis humanus capitis *(continued from previous page)*

SIGNS AND SYMPTOMS (*continued)*

- Recognition of head lice and nits to avoid misidentification of dandruff and other debris as nits or lice.
- Viable nits will be found close to the scalp and will not easily be removed from the hair shaft as will dandruff, hairspray droplets and other hair products, dirt particles, other insects (fleas, bedbugs, etc.) and scabs. Magnification may be helpful in making this assessment.

MANAGEMENT/TREATMENT:

Exclusion:

Policies should be based on current scientific evidence and best practice. Administrators, school nurses, local private and public health healthcare providers and concerned parent/guardian(s) can collaborate to develop rationale and epidemiologically sound school policies. Policy can be further supported through faculty and staff in-service and parent/community educational programs. For the school, when evidence-based policies and intervention strategies are not in place, head lice can significantly disrupt the education process.[9] School nurse practice includes the dual roles of child advocate and collaborator in policy development.

- The American Academy of Pediatrics, National Association of School Nurses, and the Centers for Disease Control and Prevention, recommends against a "no-nit" policy.[10,11,12]
- Children with live head lice should be referred to their parent/guardian(s) for treatment. Data and evidence-based practice does not support school exclusion for nits.[13]
- The discovery of nits or live lice should not cause the student to be sent home from school or isolated while at school.
- Notify parent/guardian(s) at the end of the day of the suspected infestation and recommended management.[14]
- Student may be transported home as usual.
- Screenings of entire classes or school have not been found to be cost effective; disrupt the educational process, have not been shown to reduce the incidence and are not recommended.[15]
- Provide parent with information to increase head lice awareness and prevention to ensure that student's education is not disrupted.
- **In cases that involve head lice, as in all school health issues, it is vital that the school nurse prevent stigmatizing and maintain the student's privacy as well as the family's right to confidentiality.**

LICE (HEAD) - Pediculosis humanus capitis *(continued from previous page)*

MANAGEMENT/TREATMENT *(continued)*

TREATMENT:

- Educate and assist families to enable them to be able to effectively and efficiently treat head lice so that the student can return to school the next day.

- Only students with active infestations need treatment with an over the counter (OTC) or prescription medication (pediculicide). Some medications may require 2 treatments (follow manufacturers recommendation). Some resistance to these products has been reported and may require referral to the healthcare provider.[16]

- Parents/caregivers should persistently work to remove nits. All viable nits should be removed to limit newly hatched nymphs (seven to 10 days). Non- viable nits, those more than 1/2 inch away from the head, do not need to be removed except for cosmetic reasons, or to prevent stigmatization.

- "Preventive" use of lice shampoo is NOT advised. Some lice survive sub-lethal doses of residual chemicals and mutate over generations to resist low doses of pediculicide.

- There is no clear evidence to support the use of food-grade oil, salad dressing, tea tree oil, enzymes, hot air blowers, or other "remedies".

- Parent/guardian(s) should check all household members for lice and treat only those with live lice following the product instructions.[17]

- Students with severe or persistent infestation should be referred to their healthcare provider for treatment or to social services to assist with accessing treatment.

- Supplemental Measures:
    - Articles such as clothing, bedding and other items the infested person wore or used during the two days before treatment should be washed at 130 degrees and dried on the hot setting. Items that are not washable can be sealed in a plastic bag for two weeks.
    - Soak combs and brushes in hot water (at least 130°) for five to 10 minutes.[18]
    - Vacuum carpet, pillows, and furniture where the infested person sat or lay. The risk of being infested by a louse that has fallen onto a rug, carpet, or furniture is very small. Head lice survive less than one to two days if they fall off a person and cannot feed; nits cannot hatch and usually die within a week if they do not stay at the warm temperature found close to the human scalp. Spending too much time and money on housecleaning activities is not necessary to avoid re-infestation by lice or nits that may have fallen off the head or crawled onto furniture or clothing.[19]
    - Do not use fumigant sprays or fogs; they are not necessary to control head lice and can be toxic if inhaled or absorbed through the skin.[20]

LICE (HEAD) - Pediculosis humanus capitis *(continued from previous page)*

FOLLOW UP:

- Monitor progress toward effective eradication of live lice and nits.
- "Treatment failure"(finding crawling lice after two treatments or hand lice and viable nit removal episodes) may be due to misdiagnosis or misidentification of nits, non-adherence to directions for treatment, a new exposure after treatment, or inadequate or low residual ovicidal (egg-killing) action of the lice medication used.[21]
- Seek information from reliable, current, evidence-based, science-based sources.

POTENTIAL COMPLICATIONS:

- Secondary bacterial infections (impetigo)
- Enlarged lymph nodes

PREVENTION:

- Educate parent/guardian(s), students and staff about prevention, recognition, and treatment of head lice before cases or outbreaks occur.
- Inform staff about appropriate follow-up and dispel myths (e.g., lice fly or hop).
- Ask teachers to observe and refer children who scratch or have visible lice/nits.
- Educate teachers and students to avoid "head-to-head" contact (e.g., during telling secrets, teamwork, team sports, babysitting, sleepovers, etc.).
- Encourage teachers to minimize student use of dress-up hats. Discourage fabric sofas and pillows in classroom. Watch for head contact with fabric items (e.g., daily vacuuming of carpet if students lie on it). Keep personal use pillows or blankets for naps stored separately.
- Non-fabric items are low risk. Clean headphones, vinyl bus seat backs, and solid helmets for general hygiene. Exhaustive cleaning is not beneficial.
- Do not let children pile their winter coats/hats. Although there is no clear evidence of effectiveness, some schools separate coats and back packs on hooks or chair backs. Hats may be tucked into coat sleeves.
- Offer clear instructions about effective treatment products and safe actions.
- Utilize multiple instructional strategies that are appropriate for intended audience (parent/guardian(s) /students/staff):
  - Verbal instructions/explanations, and videos.
  - Written head lice information, treatment instructions/directions related to treatment, policy, pamphlets, letters, and newsletters. Use appropriate reading level and languages for intended audience(s) when developing or selecting print materials.
  - Hands-on strategies include demonstration-return demonstration for scalp inspection, head lice and nit identification, and nit combing technique.
- Assess family needs for treatment assistance and follow-through with nit combing and re-treatment if necessary.

LICE (HEAD) - Pediculosis humanus capitis *(continued from previous page)*

REFERENCES

[1] Centers for Disease Control and Prevention. (2016). *Parasites: Lice.* https://www.cdc.gove/parasites/lice/head/gen_info/faqs.html

[2] Centers for Disease Control and Prevention. (2016). *Parasites: Lice.* https://www.cdc.gov/parasites/lice/head

[3] Ibid.

[4] Centers for Disease Control and Prevention. (2016). *Parasites: Lice.* https://www.cdc.gov/parasites/lice/head/gen_info/faqs.html#spread

[5] Centers for Disease Control and Prevention. (2016). *Parasites: Lice.* https://www.cdc.gove/parasites/lice/head/gen_info/faqs.html

[6] Centers for Disease Control and Prevention. (2015). *Head Lice: Frequently asked questions.* https://www.cdc.gov/parasites/lice/head/gen_info/faqs.html

[7] Centers for Disease Control and Prevention. (2016). *Parasites: Lice.* https://www.cdc.gov/parasites/lice/head

[8] Ibid.

[9] National Association of School Nurses. (2016). *Head lice management in the school setting* (Position statement). National Association of School Nurses.

[10] Ibid.

[11] Devore, C., Schurtze, G., & The Council on School Health and Committee on Infectious Diseases. (2015). Head lice. *Pediatrics,* E1355-E1365. https://doi.org/10.1542/peds.2015-0746

[12] Centers for Disease Control and Prevention. (2015). *Parasites: Lice.* https://www.cdc.gov/parasites/lice/head/schools.html

[13] National Association of School Nurses. (2016) *Head Lice management in the school setting* (Position Statement). National Association of School Nurses.

[14] American Academy of Pediatrics. (2020). Lice (pediculosis capitis). In S.S. Aronson, & T.R. Shope (Eds.) *Managing infectious diseases in childcare and schools: A quick reference* guide (5th ed., pp.115-117). American Academy of Pediatrics.

[15] Devore, C., Schurtze, G., & The Council on School Health and Committee on Infectious Diseases. (2015). Head lice. *Pediatrics,* E1355-E1365. https://doi.org/10.1542/peds.2015-0746

[16] Ibid.

[17] Centers for Disease Control and Prevention. (2016). *Parasites: Lice.* https://www.cdc.gov/parasites/lice/head/treatment.html

[18] Ibid.

[19] Devore, C., Schurtze, G., & The Council on School Health and Committee on Infectious Diseases. (2015). Head lice. *Pediatrics,* E1355-E1365. https://doi.org/10.1542/peds.2015-0746

[20] Centers for Disease Control and Prevention. (2016). *Parasites: Lice.* https://www.cdc.gov/parasites/lice/head/treatment.html

[21] Devore, C., Schurtze, G., & The Council on School Health and Committee on Infectious Diseases. (2015). Head lice. *Pediatrics,* E1355-E1365. https://doi.org/10.1542/peds.2015-0746

MEASLES (Rubeola) and RUBELLA (German Measles)

DEFINITION/ETIOLOGY:

Measles (Rubeola)

- Measles (Rubeola) is an extremely communicable, Paramyxovirus, with humans as the only natural host.[1]
- The primary site of infection is the nasopharynx.
- Measles are spread by airborne droplets via secretions throughout the prodromal and eruption stages.
- The incubation period for measles averages 10-12 days, from exposure to onset of symptoms.[2, 3]
- Onset averages 14 days from exposure to rash (range: seven to 21 days).
- A person is contagious 4 days before to 4 days after the appearance of the rash.
- Clinical evaluation and serological testing confirm diagnosis. Serological testing is used to identify the geographic origin of the infection.[4]
- The measles virus can live up to 2 hours in the air or on surfaces. It is one of the most contagious vaccine preventable diseases with 90% of susceptible individuals becoming infected after exposure.[5]

Factors Impacting Disease Outbreaks

In 2019, the World Health Organization (WHO) declared vaccine hesitancy as a threat to world health. WHO stated it is "the reluctance or refusal to vaccinate despite the availability of vaccines – threatens to reverse progress made in tackling vaccine-preventable diseases."[6] Reasons for vaccine hesitancy are complex but complacency, inconvenience in accessing vaccines, and lack of confidence are key reasons underlying hesitancy, according to a WHO advisory group.[7] WHO noted that measle cases have increased by 30% globally, in 2019 and vaccinations are the most cost-effective method to prevent vaccine preventable diseases.[8]

In 2000, measles was declared eliminated in the United States (U.S.). A 95% vaccination rate is required to prevent transmission of disease.[9] Since then, outbreaks in the U.S. have occurred when unvaccinated travelers bring the disease from abroad and it is introduced into communities with low vaccination rates.[10] The 2019 outbreak has resulted in more than 1200 cases in 30 states.[11] It has been the largest outbreak since the 1992 and if it continues could threaten the U.S. elimination status.[12]

State laws vary from state to state and those states that limits that reasons to opt out of vaccinations have higher immunity rates than those that permit religious and philosophical exemptions.[13] Federal laws do not provide guidance on immunizations for the states. Trusted healthcare providers in the community are credible sources of vaccine information that can influence vaccination decisions.[14]

MEASLES (Rubeola) and RUBELLA (German Measles) *(continued from previous page)*

DEFINITION/ETIOLOGY *(continued)*

Rubella (German Measles)[15]

- Rubella (German Measles) is a moderately contagious, communicable disease caused by a *Togavirus* and is spread by respiratory droplets of infected persons.
- Transmission can occur seven days before the rash appears until 14 days after eruption of the rash. The incubation period for Rubella is 14-21 days.
- Clinical evaluation and serological testing confirm diagnosis. Symptoms are mild in children.

Congenital Rubella Syndrome (CRS) is the major focus of rubella prevention vaccination programs.[16, 17]

- Infection with rubella in early pregnancy is most severe. It can affect all organs, result in fetal death, pre-term labor or spontaneous abortion or in a multitude of congenital anomalies/manifestations.
- Congenital defects due to maternal infections range from 85% in the first 12 weeks, 50% from 13-16 weeks and 25% during the end of the second trimester.
- Infection in the first trimester with CRS is one of the few know causes of autism. Infection after 20 weeks may have little or no complications although deafness is the most common and often the sole manifestation of congenital rubella infection.
- Prenatal screening for serologic immunity for all pregnant women is recommended and documentation of immunity is recommended for all those who could become pregnant.
- Since many illnesses can mimic rubella, the only reliable method to diagnose an acute rubella infection is through laboratory diagnosis.
- Note: that Infants with CRS shed large quantities of virus from body secretions for up to one year and therefore can transmit rubella to persons caring for them who are susceptible to the disease.[18]
- In 2004, the U.S. achieved elimination status and in 2010, the Americas achieved elimination of rubella and CRS.

MEASLES (Rubeola) and RUBELLA (German Measles) *(continued from previous page)*

SIGNS AND SYMPTOMS:

MEASLES AND RUBELLA---VACCINE PREVENTABLE DISEASES [19, 20]		
Disease	Measles (Rubeola)	Rubella (German Measles)
Cause	Viral (Paramyxovirus, genus Morbillivirus)	Viral (Togavirus, genus Rubivirus)
Transmission	Breathing airborne droplets and touching infected surfaces	Respiratory droplets
Signs and Symptoms	Prodrome: two to four days before rash • Fever range from 103F to 105F • 3 Cs: cough, coryza (runny nose) and conjunctivitis, • Koplik's spots (rash on mucus membranes) Rash: • Develops on average 14 days after exposure • Rash develop persists for 5-6 days • Maculopapular rash begins on the face and neck and spreads from the trunk to the limbs • The rash becomes confluent and fades in the order that is appears **Note: Persons with a compromised immune system may not present with a rash**	Prodrome: one to five days in adults and older children, rare in young children • Low-grade fever (102^0 F or lower). • Malaise, • Headache, • Stuffy or runny nose, • lymphadenopathy may last for weeks • Pharyngeal involvement present Rash: • Begins on the face and neck and spreads to trunk and extremities • Disease is most contagious when the rash appears • Rash lasts for three days and are occasionally pruritic **Note: Up to 50% of cases may be subclinical**
Disease Course/Incubation	The incubation period of measles, from exposure to onset of symptoms, averages 10-12 days. From exposure to rash, onset averages 14 days (range: seven to 21 days).	The incubation period is 14 days with a range of 12-23 days from exposure to onset of symptoms. The rash occurs from 14-17 days after exposure.
Potential Complications	• Diarrhea, otitis media, pneumonia, encephalitis, seizures and death. • Subacute sclerosing panencephalitis (rare, degenerative disease that can result in a gradual, progressive deterioration of behavior and intellect, followed by ataxia, seizures and death. Average onset is seven years after the measles infection).	• Usually mild, in rare cases can cause ear infections, thrombocytopenic purpura and encephalitis. • 70% of females develop arthralgia • **CRS:** Infection during pregnancy can cause spontaneous abortion, stillbirth, congenital defects (hearing impairment, eye defects, cardiac defects, microcephaly, intellectual disabilities, bone alteration and liver and spleen damage).

MEASLES (Rubeola) and RUBELLA (German Measles) *(continued from previous page)*

Rubeola (Measles)

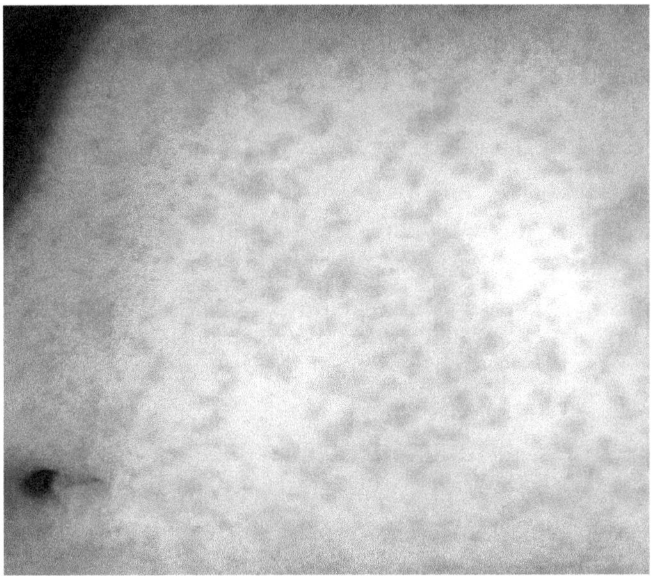

CDC
https://www.cdc.gov/measles/symptoms/photos.html?CDC_AA_refVal=https%3A%2F%2Fwww.cdc.gov%2Fmeasles%2Fabout%2Fphotos.html

Rubella (German Measles)

distinction is less red

CDC *https://www.cdc.gov/rubella/about/photos.html*

MEASLES (Rubeola) and RUBELLA (German Measles) *(continued from previous page)*

MANAGEMENT/TREATMENT:

- Supportive/symptomatic
- Vitamin A is recommended for all children with severe measles (requiring hospitalization).[21]

FOLLOW-UP:

- Both measles and rubella are reportable to the local health department.
- Follow state and local health department recommendations for school exclusion/ attendance.
- If an outbreak occurs at school – exclude unvaccinated students and staff from school/work as directed by the health department.
- In the event of an outbreak at school – exclude unvaccinated students and staff from school/work from the onset of the first diagnosed case through the last confirmed case as directed by local or state health departments.

NOTES:

- It is important to educate staff (especially, those of child-bearing age) about the need to assess their immunity to childhood diseases prior to travel, pregnancy or exposure to disease with their healthcare provider.
- Make susceptible (unvaccinated) pregnant women aware of the presence of measles or rubella and urge to contact their healthcare provider or obstetrician.
- Provide accurate, reliable vaccine information for staff and families.
- Support school located vaccination programs to increase vaccination rates.
- Tuberculin skin test (TST) or Interferon Gamma Release Assay (IGRA) may be administered at the same time as MMR vaccine. If they are not administered with the MMR vaccine, the TST or IGRA must be delayed for 28 days.[22]
- It is critical for all international travelers to be protected against measles. Those who are travelling internationally can consult *https://www.cdc.gov/measles/plan-for-travel.html*.

RESOURCES

The Centers for Disease Control and Prevention (CDC) has information for:

- Healthcare providers at:
  - *https://www.cdc.gov/measles/hcp/index.html*
  - *https://www.cdc.gov/measles/toolkit/healthcare-providers.html*
- Toolkits for Outbreaks:
  - at camps: *https://www.cdc.gov/measles/resources/camp-guidance.html*
  - and local and state health departments: *https://www.cdc.gov/measles/toolkit/state-health-departments.html*

The Immunization Action Coalition provides information on:

- Individual state requirements as of February 2019 *http://www.immunize.org/states/*
- Exemptions Permitted for State Immunization Requirements as of June 2019 *http://www.immunize.org/laws/exemptions.asp*

MEASLES (Rubeola) and RUBELLA (German Measles) *(continued from previous page)*

RESOURCES *(continued)*

- U.S. Map Exemptions Permitted to School and Child Care Immunization Requirements as of June 2019 *http://www.immunize.org/laws/exemptions.pdf*
- American Academy of Pediatrics. (2016). Rubella. In A. J. Mancini, & D. P. Krowchuk (Eds.), *Pediatric dermatology* (pp. 147-150. Author.
- American Academy of Pediatrics. (2016). Measles. In A. J. Mancini, & D. P. Krowchuk (Eds.), *Pediatric dermatology* (pp. 13-138). Author.

The National Association of School Nurses provides information at:

- Immunization Transition Toolkit (n.d.) *https://www.nasn.org/nasn/nasn-resources/practice-topics/immunizations/immunization-transition-toolkit*
- Immunizations Position statement at: *https://www.nasn.org/nasn/advocacy/professional-practice-documents/position-statements/ps-immunizations*

REFERENCES

[1] American Academy of Pediatrics. (2017). Measles. In S. Aronson, and T. Shope (Eds.) In *Managing infectious diseases in childcare and schools: A quick reference guide,* (4th ed., pp. 117-118). American Academy of Pediatrics.

[2] Center for Disease Control (CDC) and American College of Obstetrics and Gynecology (ACOG). (2019). *The 2019 measles outbreak: The latest CDC recommendations and ACOG practice advisory.* https://www.obgproject.com/2019/05/01/the-2019-measles-outbreak-the-latest-cdc-recommendations-and-acog-practice-advisory

[3] Center for Disease Control and Prevention (CDC), National Center for Respiratory Diseases and Immunizations. (2019 August 14). *Epidemiology and prevention of vaccine-preventable diseases Pink Book Webinar Series: measles, mumps, rubella- 2019.* https://www2.cdc.gov/vaccines/ed/pinkbook/2019/downloads/pb9/2019_MMR_PB_Webinar.

[4] American Academy of Pediatrics. (2018). Measles. In D. W. Kimberlin, M. T. Brady, M.A. Jackson, & S.S. Long (Eds.) *Red Book: 2018 Report of the committee on infectious diseases* (31st ed., pp. 537-550). American Academy of Pediatrics.

[5] Ibid.

[6] World Health Organization (WHO). (2019) *Ten threats to world health in 2019.* Vaccine Hesitancy (p. 14, para 1). https://www.who.int/emergencies/ten-threats-to-global-health-in-2019

[7] Ibid.

[8] Ibid.

[9] Crowcroft, N. S., and Bolotin, S. (2019). *Measles outbreaks demand systems-level action locally, nationally and globally. CMAJ: Canadian Medical Association Journal*, 15 July 2019, p. E777-E778. https://doi.org/10.1503/cmaj.190559

[10] Centers for Disease Control and Prevention (CDC). (2019). *Measles Cases and Outbreaks.* https://www.cdc.gov/measles/cases-outbreaks.html

[11] Ibid.

MEASLES (Rubeola) and RUBELLA (German Measles) *(continued from previous page)*

[12] Centers for Disease Control and Prevention (CDC), National Center for Respiratory Diseases and Immunizations. (2019 August 14). *Epidemiology and prevention of vaccine-preventable diseases Pink Book Webinar Series: measles, mumps, rubella- 2019.* https://www2.cdc.gov/vaccines/ed/pinkbook/2019/downloads/pb9/2019_MMR_PB_Webinar

[13] American Federation of Teachers (AFT). (n.d.) *Ten things to know about immunizations.* https://www.aft.org/sites/default/files/fs_10-things-immunizations.pdf.

[14] World Health Organization (WHO). (2019) *Ten Threats to World Health in 2019.* p. 14, Vaccine Hesitancy, para 1. https://www.who.int/emergencies/ten-threats-to-global-health-in-2019

[15] Centers for Disease Control and Prevention (CDC). (2015). The Pink Book: Chapter 20: Rubella. In J. Hamborsky, A. Kroger,& S. Wolfe (Eds.). *Epidemiology and Prevention of Vaccine-Preventable Diseases (*13th ed., 325-340). Public Health Foundation. https://www.cdc.gov/vaccines/pubs/pinkbook/downloads/rubella.pdf

[16] Ibid.

[17] American Academy of Pediatrics. (2018). Rubella. In D. W. Kimberlin, M. T. Brady, M.A. Jackson, & S.S. Long (Eds.) *Red Book: 2018 Report of the committee on infectious diseases* (31st ed., pp. 705-711). American Academy of Pediatrics.

[18] American Academy of Pediatrics. (2017). Rubella (German Measles). In S. Aronson, S and T. Shope (eds.) In *Managing infectious diseases in childcare and schools: A quick reference guide* (4th ed., p. 147). American Academy of Pediatrics.

[19] Centers for Disease Control and Prevention (CDC). (2015). The Pink Book: Chapter 13: Measles. In J. Hamborsky, A. Kroger, & S. Wolfe (Eds.) *Epidemiology and Prevention of Vaccine-Preventable Diseases* (13th ed., 209-230). Public Health Foundation. https://www.cdc.gov/vaccines/pubs/pinkbook/downloads/meas.pdf

[20] Centers for Disease Control and Prevention (CDC). (2015). The pink book: Rubella. In J. Hamborsky, A. Kroger, & S. Wolfe (Eds). *Epidemiology and Prevention of Vaccine-Preventable Diseases* (13th ed., pp. 325-340). Public Health Foundation. https://www.cdc.gov/vaccines/pubs/pinkbook/downloads/rubella.pdf

[20] American Academy of Pediatrics. (2018). Rubella. In D. W. Kimberlin, M. T. Brady, M.A. Jackson, & S.S. Long (Eds.) *Red Book: 2018 Report of the committee on infectious diseases* (31st ed., pp. 705-711). American Academy of Pediatrics.

[21] American Academy of Pediatrics. (2018). Measles. In D. W. Kimberlin, M. T. Brady, M.A. Jackson, & S.S. Long (Eds.) *Red Book: 2018 Report of the committee on infectious diseases* (31st ed., pp. 537-550). American Academy of Pediatrics.

[22] Centers for Disease Control and Prevention (CDC), National Center for Respiratory Diseases and Immunizations. (2019 August 14). *Epidemiology and prevention of vaccine-preventable diseases Pink Book Webinar Series: measles, mumps, rubella- 2019.* https://www2.cdc.gov/vaccines/ed/pinkbook/2019/downloads/pb9/2019_MMR_PB_Webinar

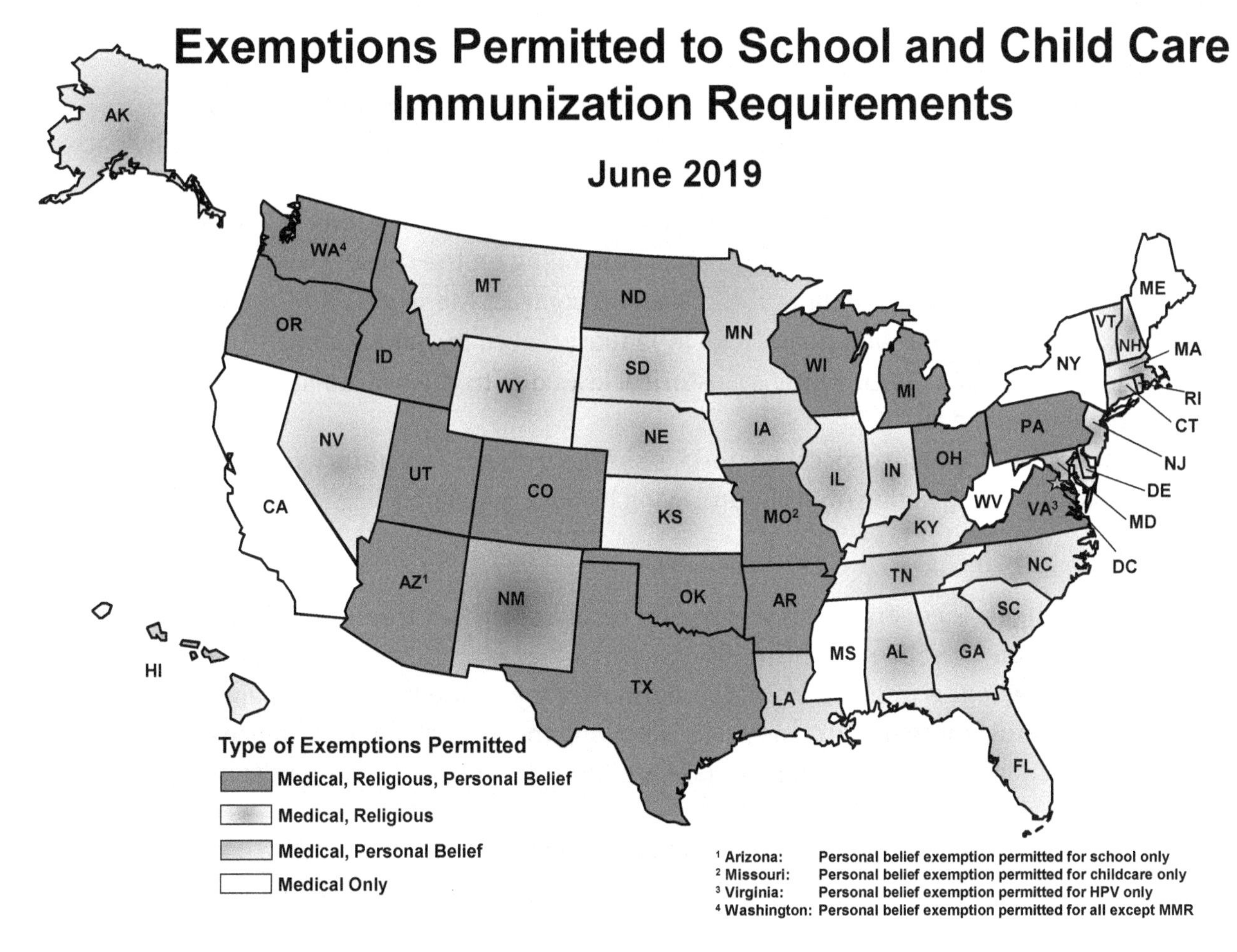
Exemptions Permitted to School and Child Care Immunization Requirements
June 2019
AK
WA4
OR
ID
MT
ND
MN
SD
WY
NV
CA
UT
CO
NE
IA
WI
MI
IL
IN
OH
PA
NY
VT
NH
ME
MA
RI
CT
NJ
DE
MD
DC
KS
MO2
KY
WV
VA3
NC
TN
SC
AZ1
NM
OK
AR
MS
AL
GA
TX
LA
FL
HI
Type of Exemptions Permitted
Medical, Religious, Personal Belief
Medical, Religious
Medical, Personal Belief
Medical Only
1 Arizona: Personal belief exemption permitted for school only
2 Missouri: Personal belief exemption permitted for childcare only
3 Virginia: Personal belief exemption permitted for HPV only
4 Washington: Personal belief exemption permitted for all except MMR

MENINGITIS

DEFINITION/ETIOLOGY:[1]
Meningitis is an inflammation of leptomeninges, a covering of the brain and spinal cord. Meningococcemia is a meningococcal blood stream infection. Meningitis may be caused by bacteria, viruses or, rarely, fungi.

- It is important to know whether meningitis is caused by viral or bacterial infection because the severity of illness and treatment differ depending on the cause.
- College students are three times more likely to contract Meningitis B.[2]
- Meningitis is seasonal with peaks seen in January, February, and March.
- Rates of meningitis are currently at historical lows due to the availability the Meningitis B vaccine beginning in 2014.[3]
- Transmission of meningococcal bacteria is spread through respiratory recreations (coughing or kissing), sharing eating utensils, and living in close quarters.[4]

<u>CAUSES</u>

- **Viral** meningitis is generally less severe and resolves without treatment. Enteroviruses are the most common causative organism (85-95%).[5]
- **Bacterial** meningitis (meningococcal) progresses rapidly and its severity depends on host immune status, route of entry, and age. Knowing the type of bacteria causing the meningitis is important in providing the appropriate antibiotic treatment to prevent some types from spreading and infecting other people.[6]
    - In children 2 months to 12 years of age, meningitis is traditionally the result of infection with *Streptococcus pneumoniae*, *Haemophilus influenzae* or *Neisseria meningitides*.
    - In children 9 years old or older, *Streptococcus pneumoniae* or *Neisseria meningitides* are the common causative organisms.
    - Increased immunizations rates have directly led to decrease of disease associated with *Streptococcus pneumoniae* and *Haemophilus influenza.*
    - In children who have ventriculoperitoneal (VP) shunt, meningitis is commonly the result of *Staphylococcus epidermidis* and, less commonly, *Staphylococcus aureus.*
- **Fungal and Mycobacterium** tuberculosis are uncommon but should be considered in the immuno-compromised host.

SIGNS AND SYMPTOMS:[7, 8]

- Classic triad for suspicion: sudden high fever, severe headache, and stiff neck which can typically be rotated but not flexed are most common in children > 2 years of age
- Signs of brain dysfunction include altered mental status or consciousness, seizures
- Signs of increased of intracranial pressure (ICP) include headache, vomiting or papilledema
- Photosensitivity
- Rash
- Sepsis (meningococcemia)
- Paradoxical irritability, in which cuddling and consoling by a parent irritates rather than comforts

MENINGITIS *(continued from previous page)*

ANTICIPATED CONCERNS/PROBLEMS:[9]

Poor prognosis is associated with young age, long duration of illness before effective antibiotic therapy, immuno-compromised status and the development of late onset seizures, coma, or shock. Those with bacterial meningitis may sustain complications including:

- Hearing loss
- Kidney damage
- Seizures
- Brain damage
- Learning disabilities
- Blindness
- Ataxia
- Hydrocephalus
- Limb loss
- Brain, nerve, or death increase in young children and adults over 60 when treatment is delayed.[10]
- Approximately 10-15% of people with bacterial meningitis will die.[11]
- Approximately 11-15% of people with bacterial meningitis will have long term disabilities.[12]

MANAGEMENT/POTENTIAL INTERVENTIONS:[13]

1. **Meningitis is an emergency condition** and requires diagnosis and appropriate treatment as soon as possible to prevent serious complications.

2. Suspected cases should be referred to a healthcare provider with concomitant notification of parents/guardians.

3. Closely monitor vital signs and physical findings, especially neurological findings such as level of consciousness.

4. Specific treatment of meningitis depends on confirmed diagnosis:
   - For suspected viral meningitis: supportive care may be done as an outpatient, *except* herpes meningitis (for which antiviral therapy occurs with close supervision in hospital setting). Most children with non-herpetic viral meningitis recover completely.

   - For suspected bacterial meningitis, treatment is initially directed to the most common pathogens based on child's age and setting. All children need to be admitted for close monitoring. Delay in treatment may result in brain damage or death.

5. Chemoprophylaxis of close contacts (usually roommates, members of same household, or person in direct contact of oral secretions of an infected person) are considered, and based on the type of pathogen that was cultured (*Haemophilus influenzae* or *Neisseria meningitides*), age, and other aspects of the situation surrounding exposure.[14] Contact local and state health departments with details and for guidance on management of close contacts.[15]

MENINGITIS *(continued from previous page)*

MANAGEMENT/POTENTIAL INTERVENTIONS *(continued)*

6. Work closely with health department and school officials to reduce public anxiety.
7. Follow local and state public health officials' decisions regarding reporting, outbreak control and management.

FOLLOW-UP:

- All children with meningitis should have a hearing evaluation before hospital release and follow-up visit.
- After hospitalization, children need to be transitioned to rehabilitation at home until there is complete recovery.
- When children return to school: monitor for mental, social, and functional and cognitive alterations that may be present and provide planning with a multi-disciplinary team, e.g., Section 504 plan.
- Monitor side effects of medical therapy (i.e., anticonvulsant drugs).

NOTES:[16, 17]

- Vaccines to prevent some types of meningitis include: Haemophilus Influenza Type B (Hib) and Meningococcal Conjugate vaccine.
- Meningococcal conjugate vaccine recommendations include all children 11-12 years and a booster at 16 years.
- Serogroup B meningococcal vaccine is recommended for ages 16-23 but can be used for anyone 10 or older who is at risk for the disease.
- If there is a threat of an epidemic, vaccines are used for groups living in close quarters, (dorms, military, etc.) who are not immunized.
- Risk of contracting meningitis increases if vaccinations are not up to date.
- Following good hand, respiratory, and contaminated surface cleaning and hygiene practices is effective in reducing the spread of infection. *(Refer to HANDWASHING and COUGH & COVER APPENDIX).*
- Proper hand hygiene and respiratory etiquette can reduce the spread of viral infections such as viral meningitis.
- Clean contaminated surfaces and avoid sharing items with sick people.

REFERENCES

[1] Merck Manual, Consumers Version. (2019). *Introduction to meningitis.* https://www.merckmanuals.com/home/brain,-spinal-cord,-and-nerve-disorders/meningitis/introduction-to-meningitis?query=meningitis

[2] Centers for Disease Control and Prevention (CDC). (2017). *Surveillance.* https://www.cdc.gov/meningococcal/surveillance/index.html

[3] Ibid.

MENINGITIS *(continued from previous page)*

[4] Centers for Disease and Prevention. (2019). *Meningococcal disease -Causes and spread to others.* https://www.cdc.gov/meningococcal/about/causes-transmission.html

[5]American Academy of Pediatrics. (2020). *Meningitis.* In S. Aronson, (Ed.), *Managing infectious diseases in child care and schools* (5[th]ed., pp. 125-126). American Academy of Pediatrics.

[6] Mayo Clinic. (2019). *Meningitis.*http://www.mayoclinic.org/diseases-conditions/meningitis/basics/definition/con-20019713

[7] Ibid.

[8] American Academy of Pediatrics. (2020). *Meningitis.* In S. Aronson, (Ed.), *Managing infectious diseases in child care and schools* (5[th]ed., pp. 125-126). American Academy of Pediatrics.

[9] Mayo Clinic. (2019). *Meningitis.*http://www.mayoclinic.org/diseases-conditions/meningitis/basics/definition/con-20019713

[10] Merck Manual. (2018). *Acute bacterial meningitis.* https://www.merckmanuals.com/home/brain,-spinal-cord,-and-nerve-disorders/meningitis/acute-bacterial-meningitis?query=Acute%20Bacterial%20Meningitis

[11] Centers for Disease Control and Prevention (CDC). (2018). *Meningococcal disease.*https://www.cdc.gov/vaccines/pubs/pinkbook/mening.html#supplement-mening01

[12] Ibid.

[13] Mayo Clinic. (2019). *Meningitis.*http://www.mayoclinic.org/diseases-conditions/meningitis/basics/definition/con-20019713

[14] Centers for Disease and Prevention. (2019). *Meningococcal disease*: *Causes and spread to others.* https://www.cdc.gov/meningococcal/about/causes-transmission.html

[15] Centers for Disease Control and Prevention (CDC). (2018). *Meningococcal disease.*https://www.cdc.gov/vaccines/pubs/pinkbook/mening.html#supplement-mening01

[16] Centers for Disease Control and Prevention (CDC). (2017). *Vaccines and immunizations.* https://www.cdc.gov/vaccines/vpd/mening/index.html

[17] American Academy of Pediatrics. (2020). *Meningitis.* In S. Aronson, (Ed.), *Managing infectious diseases in child care and schools* (5[th]ed., pp. 125-126). American Academy of Pediatrics.

OTHER REFERENCES CONSULTED

Ball, J., Binder, R., & Cowen, K. (Eds.). (2017). Immunizations and Communicable Disease. In *Principles of pediatric nursing: Caring for children (7th ed.)* (pp. 353). Upper Saddle River, NJ: Pearson Education, Inc.

Boyer-Chu, L., & Yonkaitis, C.F. (2019). Disease prevention in schools. In J. Selekman, R. Adair Shannon, & C. F. Yonkaitis (Eds.), *School nursing: A comprehensive text* (3rd ed., pp. 330-331). F.A. Davis.

Roa, S. (2018). Infections: bacterial and spirochetal. In W.W. Hay, M.J. Levin, R. R. Deterding, & M. J. Abzug (Eds.), *Current diagnosis and treatment: Pediatrics* (24th ed., pp. 1261-1264). McGraw Hill Education.

MENSTRUAL DISORDERS

DEFINITION/ETIOLOGY:

Menstrual disturbances can include a variety of conditions such as irregularity, heavy flow, pain and delayed onset. It is estimated that up to 75% of females experience a disturbance such as these in adolescence.[1] Frequently these are minor variations from normal menarche. The term abnormal uterine bleeding (AUB) is used to describe any pattern that beyond what is considered normal and can be described as mild, moderate or severe.[2] Below are some additional terms used to more specifically describe the condition.

Term	Definition
Amenorrhea	Absence of menstruation. Primary amenorrhea is defined as absence of menarche by 16 years old with normal pubertal growth and development or absence of menarche by 14 years old in the absence of secondary characteristics. Secondary amenorrhea is defined as the absence of menstruation of at least 3 cycles in females who have an established menstrual pattern.[3]
Dysmenorrhea	Defined as painful menstruation with cramping in the lower abdomen. Usually during the onset and first few days of the menstrual period. Primary dysmenorrhea is in the absence of pelvic pathology. Secondary dysmenorrhea is painful uterine contractions related to an identified cause, e.g. endometriosis, pelvic inflammatory disease. Typically occurs in the first three years after initial menstruation.[4]
Menorrhagia	Excessive bleeding in amount and duration, at regular intervals.[5]
Menarche	Onset of menses. Average age is between 12 and 13 years, but may occur from 8-15 years. Menstrual periods are often irregular during first six months to two years.[6]
Menometrorrhagia	Excessive and prolonged bleeding, frequent and irregular intervals.[7]
Metrorrhagia	Irregular frequency of cycles with bleeding between cycles.[8]
Mittelschmerz	Intermenstrual pain and/or bleeding, lasting a few hours to 3 days. Pain is usually associated with ovulation and is considered a normal gynecologic variation.[9]
Oligomenorrhea	Infrequent, irregular episodes of bleeding, usually occurring at intervals greater than 40 days.[10]
Polymenorrhea	Frequent but regular episodes of bleeding, occurring at intervals of 21 days or less.[11]

MENSTRUAL DISORDERS *(continued from previous page)*

SIGNS AND SYMPTOMS:

Dysmenorrhea[12]

- Primary dysmenorrheal - pain, usually shortly before menstrual flow lasting one to three days
- "Crampy" pelvic/Suprapubic pain radiating to the thigh and lower back
- Associated nausea, vomiting, and diarrhea
- Breast tenderness
- Headache, fatigue, sleep disturbances
- Dizziness, syncope

Amenorrhea [13]

Requires evaluation when:

- Menarche delayed beyond age 15
- No secondary sexual characteristics develop by age 13 (breasts, pubic and axillary hair)
- Three years after developing secondary sexual characteristics if menstruation has not begun

Persons at risk:[14]

- Runners, gymnasts, ballet dancers associated with excessive exercise
- Girls with too little body fat, eating disorders, undernutrition, weight loss
- Possible development of osteoporosis due to lack of estrogen (female hormone)
- Girls with systemic disease such as inflammatory bowel disease
- Girls with thyroid disorders
- Girls with polycystic ovary disease

Note: Amenorrhea is part of the female athlete triad which is a concern among competitive athletes: amenorrhea, anorexia, and osteoporosis

Abnormal Uterine Bleeding[15]

- It is helpful to divide cases in to mild, moderate or severe to determine treatment.
- Hemoglobin < 10 gm/dL with would indicate a severe case.
- Hemoglobin between 10-12 gm/dL would indicate moderate anemia.
- In mild cases, there is no anemia.

MENSTRUAL DISORDERS *(continued from previous page)*

MANAGEMENT/TREATMENT:

It may be 18-24 months after menarche before females develop a regular ovulatory cycle. Anovulatory cycles where there is a lack of a progesterone peak, are present in the majority of girls within 24 months of menarche and are responsible for irregular menses. Irregular cycles after 24 months post menarche should be evaluated.[16]

Primary dysmenorrhea

- Analgesic medication specifically NSAIDS (non-steroid anti-inflammatories) which reduce prostaglandin level.
- Educate on proper use of NSAIDS to avoid stomach irritation or overdose.
- Warm pad to lower abdomen and position of comfort.
- Encourage physical exercise and balanced diet.
- Refer severe disorders for healthcare evaluation.
- Hormonal contraception can be used to treat dysmenorrhea when NSAIDS are ineffective.

Amenorrhea

- Complete a focused history including age of onset of pubertal changes and sexual history to rule out pregnancy or sexually transmitted infections and refer as indicated.
- Refer for healthcare evaluation as indicated.

Abnormal Uterine Bleeding[17]

- For severe cases, where there is hemodynamic instability, or a hemoglobin less than 8 gm/dL hospitalization and transfusion may be necessary.
- Oral hormonal therapy may be used to regulate cycles and decrease bleeding.
- Reassurance, a high iron diet, and the use of a multivitamin with iron should be encouraged.

NOTES:

- Educate the student on normal menstruation. Heavy menstrual bleeding can be described as needing more than eight (8) pads or 12 tampons/day.[18]
- Educate students that tampons should be changed at least every eight (8) hours.
- Educate students to keep diary of menstrual cycles to share with parent/guardian and healthcare provider.
- Encourage students to keep sanitary napkins/tampons at school. An emergency supply of sanitary napkins and tampons should be kept in health room.
- Students may keep medication for discomfort at school following school policy and guidelines for medication at school.
- Be alert to history and signs that suggest pregnancy or secondary dysmenorrhea, e.g., PID (pelvic inflammatory disease).
- Irregular menstrual cycles in a girl within two years of menarche can usually be observed before an extensive work up. Provide reassurance.
- Students should be encouraged to continue to participate in usual sports and activities.
- Although rare, refer to the healthcare provider for sudden fever and illness which may be toxic shock syndrome related to tampon use.

MENSTRUAL DISORDERS *(continued from previous page)*

REFERENCES

[1] Sucato, G., & Burstein, G. (2016). Menstrual problems. In R.M. Kliegman, B.S. Stanton, J. St. Geme, & N.F. Schor (Eds.), *Textbook of pediatrics: Expert consult* (20th ed., pp.963-965). Elsevier, Inc.

[2] Ibid.

[3] Gerlt, T., & Starr, N. (2017). Gynecologic disorders. In C. Burns, A.M. Dunn, M.A. Brady, N.B. Starr, C.G. Blosser, & D.L. Garzon (Eds.), *Pediatric primary care* (6th ed., pp.971-975). Elsevier, Inc.

[4] Jakubowski, T., & Perron, T. (2019). Students with common health complaints. In J. Selekman, R. Adair Shannon, & C. F. Yonkaitis (Eds.), *School nursing: A comprehensive text* (3rd ed., pp. 357-359). F.A. Davis.

[5] Gerlt, T., & Starr, N. (2017). Gynecologic disorders. In C. Burns, A.M. Dunn, M.A. Brady, N.B. Starr, C.G. Blosser, & D.L. Garzon (Eds.), *Pediatric primary care* (6th ed., pp.971-975). Elsevier, Inc.

[6] Jakubowski, T., & Perron, T. (2019). Students with common health complaints. In J. Selekman, R. Adair Shannon, & C. F. Yonkaitis (Eds.), *School nursing: A comprehensive text* (3rd ed., pp. 357-359). F.A. Davis.

[7] Gerlt, T., & Starr, N. (2017). Gynecologic disorders. In C. Burns, A.M. Dunn, M.A. Brady, N.B. Starr, C.G. Blosser, & D.L. Garzon (Eds.), *Pediatric primary care* (6th ed., pp.971-975). Elsevier, Inc.

[8] Ibid.

[9] Ibid.

[10] Mayo Clinic. (2019). *Women's wellness.* https://newsnetwork.mayoclinic.org/discussion/womens-wellness-abnormal-menstruation-happens-in-a-variety-of-ways/

[11] Gerlt, T., & Starr, N. (2017). Gynecologic disorders. In C. Burns, A.M. Dunn, M.A. Brady, N.B. Starr, C.G. Blosser, & D.L. Garzon (Eds.), *Pediatric primary care* (6th ed., pp.971-975). Elsevier, Inc.

[12] Sucato, G., & Burstein, G. (2016). Menstrual problems. In R.M. Kliegman, B.S. Stanton, J. St. Geme, & N.F. Schor (Eds.), *Textbook of pediatrics: Expert consult* (20th ed., pp.963-965). Elsevier, Inc.

[13] Ibid.

[14] Ibid.

[15] Gerlt, T., & Starr, N. (2017). Gynecologic disorders. In C. Burns, A.M. Dunn, M.A. Brady, N.B. Starr, C.G. Blosser, & D.L. Garzon (Eds.), *Pediatric primary care* (6th ed., pp.971-975). Elsevier, Inc.

[16] Ibid.

[17] Sucato, G., & Burstein, G. (2016). Menstrual problems. In R.M. Kliegman, B.S. Stanton, J. St. Geme, & N.F. Schor (Eds.), *Textbook of pediatrics: Expert consult* (20th ed., pp.963-965). Elsevier, Inc.

[18] Jakubowski, T., & Perron, T. (2019). Students with common health complaints. In J. Selekman, R. Adair Shannon, & C. F. Yonkaitis (Eds.), *School nursing: A comprehensive text* (3rd ed., pp. 357-359). F.A. Davis.

MOLLUSCUM CONTAGIOSUM

DEFINITION/ETIOLOGY:
Molluscum contagiosum virus (MCV) is a cutaneous (skin) infection caused by a poxvirus that is somewhat similar to warts. It is more common in toddlers and younger children. In adults and adolescents, it may be seen in the genital area and may be considered a sexually transmitted infection.[1] It is spread person to person through close contact and can also be spread by the sharing of inanimate objects although only mildly contagious. More commonly it is spread from one part of the infected person's body to another. The incubation period is usually between 2-7 weeks but may be as long as 6 months.[2]

SIGNS AND SYMPTOMS:[3]
- Usually asymptomatic although can be itchy
- Lesions are one to six mm, discrete, dome shaped, skin colored, erythematous or translucent
- Lesions commonly have an indented (umbilicated) center
- Lesions can be solitary or multiple
- Can occur anywhere but commonly on the face, eyelids, neck, chest, axillae, folds of extremities and genital region

UNIQUE FINDINGS OF MOLLUSCUM CONTAGIOSUM:[4]

In immunosuppressed individuals lesions may be widespread or "giant" eight to 15mm.

MANAGEMENT/TREATMENT:[5]
- Encourage good hand hygiene especially after touching the bumps.
- Discourage children from picking at the bumps as this may cause spreading or a secondary infection.
- Discourage sharing of clothes or other skin contact articles.
- A cold compress can be effective in resolving the itch.
- Cover the lesions when possible or during water activities.
- Treatments can include cryotherapy, topical creams, curettage but these treatments may cause pain or scarring, and lesions will typically resolve over time.[6]

FOLLOW-UP:

The lesions generally resolve on their own in six to 12 months but may last for years.[7]

POTENTIAL COMPLICATIONS:
- Children with atopic dermatitis may develop extensive lesions.[8]
- Immunocompromised children may develop hundreds to thousands of lesions.[9]
- Molluscum dermatitis may occur which is a surrounding red itchy patch around the lesion.[10]

NOTES:
Children with molluscum contagiosum should not be excluded from school.

MOLLUSCUM CONTAGIOSUM *(continued from previous page)*

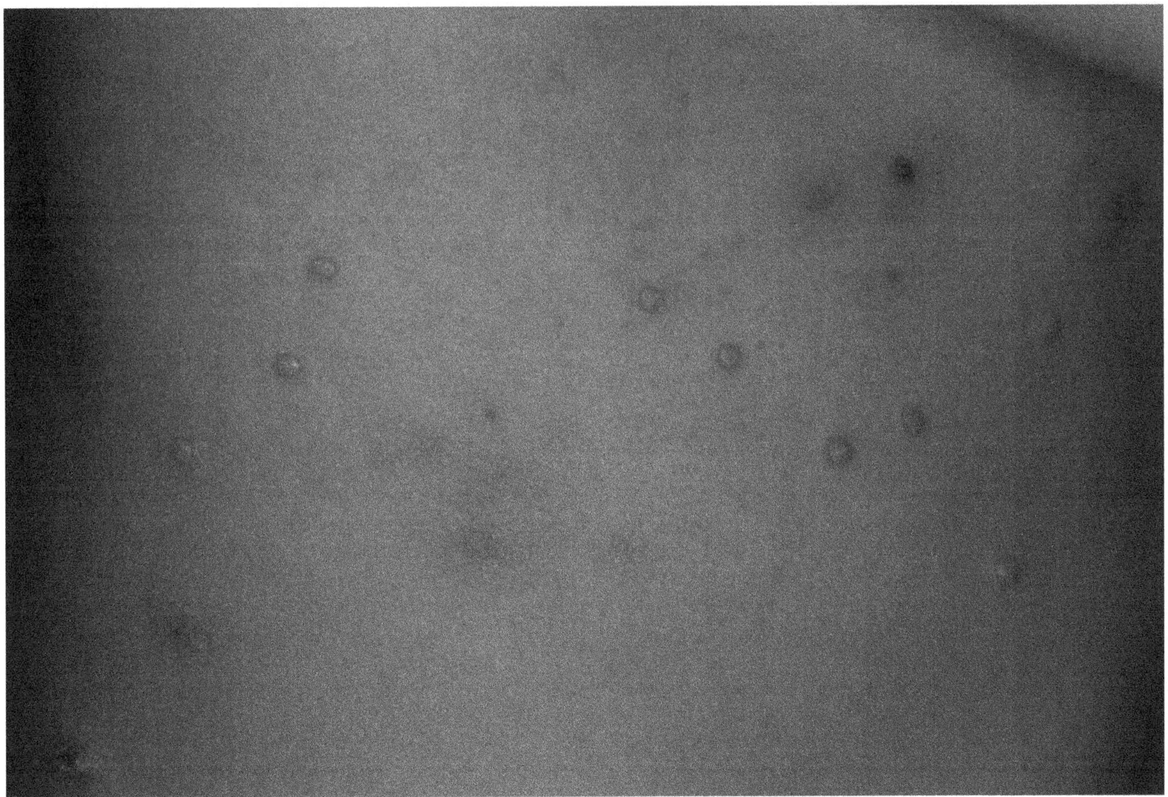

Image courtesy of James G.H. Dinulos, MD. From the Merck Manual Professional Version (Known as the Merck Manual in the US and Canada and the MSD Manual in the rest of the world), edited by Robert Porter. Copyright 2020 by Merck Sharp & Dohme Corp., a subsidiary of Merck & Co., Inc, Kenilworth, NJ. Available at http://www.merckmanuals.com/professional. Accessed 3-3-2020.

REFERENCES

[1] Newell, B. (2017). Warts and molluscum contagiosum. In Feld, L., Mahan, J. (Eds.), *Succinct pediatrics* (pp. 636-638). American Academy of Pediatrics.

[2] American Academy of Pediatrics. (2020). Molluscum contagiosum. In S. Aronson, & T. Shope (Eds.), *Managing infectious diseases in child care and schools* (5th[d] ed., p. 127). American Academy of Pediatrics.

[3] American Academy of Pediatrics. (2016). Molluscum contagiosum. In A. J. Mancini, & D. P. Krowchuk (Eds.), *Pediatric dermatology (*3rd ed., pp. 103-106). American Academy of Pediatrics.

[4] Ibid.

[5] American Academy of Pediatrics. (2020). Molluscum contagiosum. In S. Aronson, & T. Shope (Eds.), *Managing infectious diseases in child care and schools* (5th[d] ed., p. 127). American Academy of Pediatrics.

[6] American Academy of Pediatrics. (2016). Molluscum contagiosum. In A. J. Mancini, & D. P. Krowchuk (Eds.), *Pediatric dermatology* (3rd ed., pp. 103-106). American Academy of Pediatrics.

[7] American Academy of Pediatrics. (2020). Molluscum contagiosum. In S. Aronson, & T. Shope (Eds.), *Managing infectious diseases in child care and schools* (5th[d] ed., p. 127). American Academy of Pediatrics.

[8] American Academy of Pediatrics. (2016). Molluscum contagiosum. In A. J. Mancini, & D. P. Krowchuk (Eds.), *Pediatric dermatology* (3rd ed., pp. 103-106). American Academy of Pediatrics.

[9] Newell, B. (2017). Warts and molluscum contagiosum. In L. Feld, & J. Mahan (Eds.), *Succinct pediatrics* (pp. 636-638). American Academy of Pediatrics.

[10] Ibid.

MONONUCLEOSIS (Infectious Mono)

DEFINITION/ETIOLOGY:

An acute viral infection caused by the Epstein-Barr virus (EBV). Incubation period is four to six weeks. The virus is present in pharyngeal secretions and is most commonly spread by saliva.[1] The virus can be excreted for some months after infection and remains with the host for life.[2] It can occur at any age but is most common in adolescents.[3]

SIGNS AND SYMPTOMS (COMMON):[4]

- Milder and often undiagnosed in young children, more severe in high school and college age youth
- Fever, malaise, headache, and fatigue
- Sore throat and enlarged, red, exudative tonsils. Occasionally strep infection is associated with the sore throat.
- Lymph nodes swollen in axilla, groin, and especially in neck (post cervical)
- Enlarged spleen
- Maculopapular confluent rash if treated with penicillin
- Fever and sore throat lessen within a couple weeks; fatigue and malaise may last four to six weeks
- Periorbital edema and jaundice are less likely[5]

MANAGEMENT/TREATMENT:

Treatment is aligned with supporting the symptoms; most patients recover in 4-6 weeks without medication.

1. Refer to healthcare provider; laboratory tests may be needed to confirm diagnosis; strep throat may accompany. Healthcare provider may prescribe oral steroids if symptoms are severe.[6]
2. Symptomatic support for sore throat (gargle), fever (fluids) and fatigue (rest).[7]
3. Return to school on advice of healthcare provider.[8]
4. May be in school during illness if temperature is below 100° and able to tolerate activity.[9]
5. Rest and contact sports restrictions may be needed for a month or longer.[10]

FOLLOW UP:[11]

Monitor one to two weeks after return to school for full recovery.

- May need to avoid physical education class until splenomegaly resolved.
- May need to modify school schedule due to fatigue.

POTENTIAL COMPLICATIONS:[12]

- Complications are rare and can include encephalitis, meningitis, Guillain-Barré syndrome, anemia, myocarditis.
- Danger of ruptured spleen. Must be asymptomatic before return to activity. Protect from contact sports for 1 month or until splenomegaly has resolved.
- Liver conditions such as hepatitis (liver inflammation) or jaundice

MONONUCLEOSIS (Infectious Mono) *(continued from previous page)*

NOTES:

Health education:[13, 14]

- Teach youth mode of transmission and duration: person-to-person via saliva. Virus may remain in saliva for months during and after convalescence.
- Avoid kissing on the mouth and sharing food from the same container or by sharing things like eating utensils, glasses, toothbrushes, and lipstick or lip gloss.
- Always use good handwashing techniques. (*Refer to HANDWASHING APPENDIX).*

REFERENCES

[1] Centers for Disease Control and Prevention (CDC), National Center for Infectious Diseases. (2018). *Epstein-Barr virus and infectious mononucleosis.* http://www.cdc.gov/epstein-barr/index.html

[2] Merck Manual. (2018). *Infectious mononucleosis.*https://www.merckmanuals.com/professional/infectious-diseases/herpesviruses/infectious-monnucleosis

[3] Centers for Disease Control and Prevention (CDC), National Center for Infectious Diseases. (2018). *Epstein-Barr virus and infectious mononucleosis.* http://www.cdc.gov/epstein-barr/index.html

[4] Mayo Clinic. (2018). *Mononucleosis.*https://www.mayoclinic.com/diseases-conditions/mononucleosis/symptoms-causes/syc-20350328

[5] Merck Manual. (2018). *Infectious mononucleosis.*https://www.merckmanuals.com/professional/infectious-diseases/herpesviruses/infectious-monnucleosis

[6] Mayo Clinic. (2018). *Mononucleosis.*https://www.mayoclinic.com/diseases-conditions/mononucleosis/symptoms-causes/syc-20350328

[7] Ibid.

[8] Ibid.

[9] Kids Health/Nemours. (2016). *Mononucleosis.* https://kidshealth.org/en/teens/mononucleosis.html

[10] Ibid.

[11] Kids Health/Nemours. (2014). *Mononucleosis special needs fact sheet.* https://kidshealth.org/en/parents/mono-fact-sheet.html?ref=search

[12] Mayo Clinic. (2018). *Mononucleosis.*https://www.mayoclinic.com/diseases-conditions/mononucleosis/symptoms-causes/syc-20350328

[13] Mayo Clinic. (2018). *Mononucleosis.*https://www.mayoclinic.com/diseases-conditions/mononucleosis/symptoms-causes/syc-20350328

[14] Kids Health/Nemours. (2016). *Mononucleosis.* https://kidshealth.org/en/teens/mononucleosis.html

MOSQUITO-BORNE DISEASES

DEFINITION/ETIOLOGY:

A mosquito-borne disease is transmitted by mosquitos infected with a virus or parasite. Mosquitoes become infected by feeding from birds, mammals or people who are infected with the virus or parasite. The severity of mosquito-borne disease in human's ranges from mild, flu like symptoms to severe illness and even death.[1]

Some examples include:

Eastern equine encephalitis (EEE)[2]	A rare illness in humans and an average of 7 cases are reported annually. **EEE is considered the most serious mosquito-borne disease in the United States.** Most cases occur in Atlantic and Gulf coast states.
Western equine encephalitis[3]	Illness caused by Western equine encephalitis virus is very rare in the United States. Cases are most commonly reported from states and Canadian provinces west of the Mississippi River.
La Crosse encephalitis [4]	Most cases of La Crosse encephalitis occur in the southeastern, upper mid-Western, and mid-Atlantic states. Children under the age of 16 usually have the most severe cases.
West Nile virus (WNV)[5]	Most cases of WNV occur in the summer to fall months in North America. Risk is highest July through September. WNV has also been known to spread through organ transplants, blood transfusions, breast-feeding and during pregnancy from mother to baby.
Dengue[6]	Dengue viruses are uncommon in United States, but local transmission has been reported in Texas, Florida, and Hawaii. Suspect Dengue fever if individual suddenly develops symptoms and has recently travelled to Puerto Rico, Southeast Asia and/or the Caribbean. Dengue is vaccine-preventable.
Malaria[7]	Infection with malaria parasites may result in a wide variety of symptoms, ranging from absent or very mild illness to severe disease and even death. Cases in the United States are travel-related.
Zika[8]	Zika is spread mostly by the bite of an infected Aedes species mosquito. These mosquitoes bite during the day and night. Zika can be passed from a pregnant woman to her fetus. Infection during pregnancy can cause certain birth defects. Zika can be passed through sex from a person who has Zika to his or her sex partners. Condoms can reduce the chance of getting Zika from sex. There is no vaccine or medicine for Zika. The mosquitoes that can spread Zika are found throughout the United States.

MOSQUITO-BORNE DISEASES *(continued from previous page)*

SIGNS AND SYMPTOMS:

- Range from none to severe
- Depends on the virus or parasite transmitted
- Mild, flu-like (fever, body aches, headache, vomiting, nausea)
- Stiff neck
- Rash
- High fever
- Altered mental status
- Swollen lymph glands
- Convulsions
- Encephalitis
- Meningitis
- Coma, paralysis, death

MANAGEMENT/TREATMENT:

- No specific treatment unless malaria – supportive care
- Based on symptoms
- Pain control
- Over the counter medications to alleviate flu like symptoms
- Avoid ibuprofen, naproxen sodium, which may increase bleeding disorders
- Close medical monitoring is required for severe symptoms

PREVENTION/CONTROL:

Educate students, families, staff, and the community on prevention:

- Wear protective clothing (i.e., long pants, long sleeves and socks).
- Use U.S. Environmental Protection Agency (EPA)-registered insect repellents– follow manufacturer instructions.
- Install screens on windows and doors.
- Remove standing water around your home (i.e., flowerpots, buckets, pool covers, bird baths, pet dishes, etc.).
- Avoid shaded and wooded areas.
- Limit outdoor activity dusk to dawn.
- Be aware of community-wide mosquito prevention programs.
- Establish a protocol for school sponsored outdoor field-trip planning that includes advanced notice to the school nurse and the provision of relevant mosquito [or insect] disease prevention strategies for attendees.

MOSQUITO-BORNE DISEASES *(continued from previous page)*

REFERENCES

[1] American Academy of Pediatrics. (2018). Prevention of mosquito borne and tick-borne diseases. *Red Book Report on Infectious Disease 2018-2021* (31st ed., pp. 195-200). American Academy of Pediatrics.

[2] Centers for Disease Control and Prevention. (2019). *Division of vector-borne diseases.* https://www.cdc.gov/ncezid/dvbd/a-z-index.html

[3] American Academy of Pediatrics. (2018). Prevention of mosquito borne and tick-borne diseases. *Red Book Report on Infectious Disease 2018-2021* (31st ed., pp. 195-200). American Academy of Pediatrics.

[4] Centers for Disease Control and Prevention. (2019). *Division of vector-borne diseases.* https://www.cdc.gov/ncezid/dvbd/a-z-index.html

[5] Mayo Clinic. (2019). *West nile virus.* https://www.mayoclinic.org/diseases-conditions/west-nile-virus/symptoms-causes/syc-20350320

[6] Merck Manual. (2019). *Dengue.* https://www.merckmanuals.com/professional/infectious-diseases/arboviridae-arenaviridae-and-filoviridae/dengue

[7] Centers for Disease Control and Prevention. (2019). *Malarias.* https://www.cdc.gov/parasites/malaria/index.html

[8] Centers for Disease Control and Prevention. (2019). *Zika.* https://www.cdc.gov/zika/prevention/index.html

OTHER REFRENCES CONSULTED

Centers for Disease Control and Prevention. (2019). *West nile virus.* https://www.cdc.gov/westnile/

Centers for Disease Control and Prevention. (2019). *Zika.* https://www.cdc.gov/zika/prevention/index.html

Mayo Clinic. (2019). *West nile virus.* https://www.mayoclinic.org/diseases-conditions/west-nile-virus/symptoms-causes/syc-20350320

MUMPS

DEFINITION/ETIOLOGY:
Mumps an acute viral illness characterized by swelling of one or more of salivary glands, usually the parotid glands.

Mumps is caused by *Rubulavirus* that infects the respiratory tract. The virus is spread by direct contact with respiratory droplets and saliva. The incubation period is generally 16-18 days (range 12-25 days) from time of exposure to onset of symptoms. Mumps virus has been isolated from saliva from between 2 and 7 days before symptom onset until 9 days after onset of symptoms.[1] When person is ill with mumps, they should avoid any contact with others until five days after the parotitis begins by staying home from school and other activities.[2] Mumps has a 12-24-day incubation period.[3]

Mumps is a vaccine preventable disease (VPD).

SIGNS AND SYMPTOMS:

- Non-specific prodrome, which may include myalgia and/or joint pain, nausea, decreased appetite, malaise, headache, and fever for three to five days.[4]
- Unilateral or bilateral tender swelling of parotid or other salivary glands that can last two days but can continue for 10 or more days.[5]
- These glands can be especially painful when chewing or eating foods that stimulate the release of salivary juices, such as eating citrus foods.[6]

MANAGEMENT/TREATMENT:

- Rapidly identify infected and susceptible persons and report to local and state health departments.
- If a case of mumps is identified, educate school staff on signs and symptoms and how to prevent the spread of the virus.
- There is no specific treatment for mumps. The healthcare provider may recommend that parent/guardian(s) apply ice or heat packs to the neck and the administration of non-aspirin analgesics.[7] Use soft diet if pain with chewing, drink extra fluids and get plenty of rest.[8]
- Infected student should be excluded for five days from onset of parotid glands swelling.[9] Adults without evidence of immunity, should have at least one dose of MMR vaccine. A second dose should be given, at least 28 days later, to school children and adults at high risk of mumps exposure (e.g. health care personnel, students at post high school educational institutions and international travelers).[10]

MUMPS *(continued from previous page)*

MANAGEMENT/TREATMENT *(continued)*

- Mumps vaccine has not been effective in preventing of infection after exposure; however, immunization will provide protection to subsequent exposures.[11]
- Recommend that unimmunized, pregnant females exposed to mumps consult with their healthcare provider. Pregnant women who are infected with mumps may be at risk for complications.[12]
- Follow local and/or state public health officials' decisions regarding outbreak control and management.[13]

Potential Complications:[14]

- Aseptic meningitis
- Orchitis (in post-pubertal males)
- Hearing loss
- Encephalitis
- Pancreatitis
- Mumps during pregnancy could lead to miscarriage especially early in pregnancy
- Oophoritis (inflammation of the ovaries)[15]

NOTES:

PREVENTION

- Mumps is a vaccine preventable disease.[16]
- Mumps immunization status should be assessed. Mumps vaccine is given as an MMR for students and staff who have not already had mumps or mumps vaccine.
- In children the first MMR is given on or after first birthday (recommended between 12 and 15 months of age). Second dose is given between ages four and six.[17]
- The effectiveness of MMR against mumps is approximately 78% after one dose and approximately 88% after two doses.[18]
- Because the vaccine is not 100% effective, some cases can occur in vaccinated persons.
- Students should be kept home until five days after the onset of parotid swelling.[19]

MUMPS *(continued from previous page)*

REFERENCES

---

[1] Centers for Disease Control and Prevention. (2019). *Mumps.* http://cdc.gov/mumps

[2] Ibid.

[3] Merck Manual. (2018). *Mumps (epidemic parotitis). https://www.merckmanuals.com/professional/pediatrics/miscellaneous-vial-infections-in-infants-and-children/mumps*

[4] American Academy of Pediatrics. (2015). *Mumps. https://www.healthychildren.org/English/health-issues/vaccine-preventable-diseases/Pages/Mumps.aspx*

[5] Centers for Disease Control and Prevention. (2019). *Mumps.* http://cdc.gov/mumps

[6] Ibid.

[7] Mayo Clinic. (2018.) *Mumps. https://www.mayoclinic.org/diseases-conditions/mumps/diagnosis-treatment/drc-20375366*

[8] Ibid.

[9] Centers for Disease Control and Prevention. (2019). *Mumps.* http://cdc.gov/mumps

[10] Centers for Disease Control and Prevention. (2018). *Measles, mumps, and rubella (MMR) vaccination: What Everyone Should Know. https://cdc.gov/vaccines/vpd/mmr/public/index.html*

[11] Centers for Disease Control and Prevention. (2019). *Mumps.* http://cdc.gov/mumps

[12] Ibid.

[13] Ibid.

[14] Mayo Clinic. (2018.) *Mumps. https://www.mayoclinic.org/diseases-conditions/mumps/diagnosis-treatment/drc-20375366*

[15] Merck Manual. (2018). *Mumps (epidemic parotitis). https://www.merckmanuals.com/professional/pediatrics/miscellaneous-vial-infections-in-infants-and-children/mumps*

[16] American Academy of Pediatrics. (2015). *Mumps. https://www.healthychildren.org/English/health-issues/vaccine-preventable-diseases/Pages/Mumps.aspx*

[17] Centers for Disease Control and Prevention. (2019). *Mumps. http://cdc.gov/mumps*

[18] Ibid.

[19] Mayo Clinic. (n.d.) *Mumps. https://www.mayoclinic.org/diseases-conditions/mumps/diagnosis-treatment/drc-20375366*

OTHER REFERENCES CONSULTED

Boyer-Chu, L., & Yonkaitis, C.F. (2019). Disease prevention in schools. In J. Selekman, R. Adair Shannon, & C. F. Yonkaitis (Eds.), School nursing: A comprehensive text (3rd ed., pp. 313-334). F.A. Davis.

Kids Health/Nemours. (2016). *Mumps. https://kidshealth.org/en/parents/mumps.html?ref=search*

MUSCULAR DYSTROPHY

DEFINITION/ETIOLOGY:

Muscular dystrophy is a group of genetic, degenerative diseases primarily affecting voluntary muscles. Muscles become progressively weaker. In the late stages of muscular dystrophy, fat and connective tissue often replace muscle fibers. Some types of muscular dystrophy affect heart muscles, other involuntary muscles, and organs. The most common types of muscular dystrophy appear to be due to a genetic deficiency of the muscle protein dystrophin. There is no cure for muscular dystrophy. Supportive care, therapy, and medications can prolong functionality and slow the course of the disease.

SIGNS AND SYMPTOMS: [1, 2]

Duchenne Muscular Dystrophy

- Most common and most severe form of muscular dystrophy.
- Occurs mostly in males. Typically affects the legs first. A child may experience delay in walking, disease is usually evident by age 3 and obvious by 5-6. [3]
- May exhibit language delays.
- *Gower sign,* the process used by the child to move from the floor to a standing position.[4]
- Early symptoms are clumsiness, toe walking, swayback, frequent falling, difficulty with stairs and getting up from floor, weakness in lower leg muscles resulting in difficulty running and jumping, waddling gait, and constipation.
- Always progressive, leading to need for leg braces, wheelchair dependency, contractures, obesity, respiratory complications (may progress to need for oral suctioning, tracheostomy and ventilator), and cardiac symptoms. Some may exhibit curvature of the spine (scoliosis).
- Calf and some other muscles enlarge due to fatty infiltration.
- Intellectual impairment is often present.
- Life expectancy age is 20-30s, death often the result of pneumonia, respiratory muscle weakness, or cardiac complications.

Other forms of muscular dystrophy

Becker's muscular dystrophy

- Signs and symptoms similar to Duchenne Muscular Dystrophy
- Milder form of muscular dystrophy
- Symptoms may be seen in older boys and young men but may not occur until mid-20s or later.[5]
- Most are able to walk through their teens and into adulthood.

Myotonicdystrophy (Steinert's Disease), Facioscapulohumeral muscular dystrophy (Landouzy-Dejerine dystrophy), Emery-Dreifuss muscular dystrophy, Limb-Girdle muscular dystrophy, congenital muscular dystrophy, oculopharyngeal muscular dystrophy are other forms of muscular dystrophy. All vary in age onset, severity, rapidity of progression, associated intellectual impairment, and years of life.

MUSCULAR DYSTROPHY *(continued from previous page)*

ANTICIPATED CONCERNS: [6]

- Breathing difficulties
- Obesity
- Contractures and spinal curvature
- Diminished fine motor skills
- Compromised skin integrity
- Urinary tract infections
- Constipation
- Respiratory infections
- Decline in independence with Activities of Daily Living (ADL's)
- Swallowing difficulties
- Cardiac inefficiency
- Emotional/mental health issues secondary to condition itself, medications, or living with a chronic illness
- Sense of helplessness and hopelessness (depression)

MANAGEMENT/TREATMENT: [7, 8, 9] (Treatment emphasizes the need for nursing assessment)

- Fever and respiratory difficulty must be reported to the family, parent, or immediately and seen by a healthcare provider.
- Vomiting must be reported to the family if the student is taking steroids.
- **Medication -** Corticosteroids, immunosuppressive drugs, anticonvulsants, skeletal muscle relaxants and antiarrhythmic drugs may be used improve muscle strength and delay progression of muscle weakness; delay the damage to dying muscle cells; and to manage the muscle spasms, rigidity and affected cardiac muscles in certain types of muscular dystrophy. A medport may be in place for medications administered via intravenous therapy. If so, precautions must be taken when moving or repositioning a student.
- **Physical therapy** to keep joints flexible and delay the progression of contractures.[10]
- **Dietary Considerations** include high fiber and fluid to prevent constipation. Diet may change as disease progresses requiring soft foods or possibly a gastrostomy feeding tube to prevent aspiration.
- **Assistive devices** such as braces, walkers, canes, and wheelchairs improve mobility and independence. Ventilators assist with oxygenation if muscles used to facilitate respiration become weakened.
- **Surgery** may be necessary to relieve painful contractures. Curvatures of the spine, significant enough to compromise respiratory function may warrant surgical interventions. Consider homebound school services while recovering after surgery.
- Cardiac muscle may become compromised; treated with medication or pacemaker.
- When swallowing is affected, the family may opt for gastrostomy tube placement for nutrition. Collaborate with Speech and Language Pathologist to develop specialized feeding protocol for oral intake (if indicated).
- As respiratory muscles weaken, respiratory support in the form of Nocturnal Nasal Intermittent Positive Pressure Ventilation (NNIPPV) or a ventilator may be used.

MUSCULAR DYSTROPHY *(continued from previous page)*

MANAGEMENT/TREATMENT *(continued)*

- Altered cough secondary to neuromuscular weakness may require manual or mechanical cough assist.
- May require oral suctioning to clear the airway.

FOLLOW-UP:

- Continually monitor for progress toward goals and watch for signs and symptoms of complications.
- Update the Individualized Healthcare Plan (IHP) as necessary. Update appropriate faculty and staff of changes in the IHP and Emergency Care Plan (ECP).[11]
- Individualized Education Plan (IEP) or Section 504 plan for special services and accommodations, if needed.
- Recommend up to date immunizations, including the flu vaccine for staff and other students to prevent respiratory illness which can cause setbacks and hospitalizations.[12]

NOTES:

- As the disease progresses the student may be followed by a palliative care team or hospice and may have a DNAR in place. Often these students wish to continue to attend school. Accommodations can be made to make the child comfortable and have optimal quality of life while at school.

Refer to ***Do Not Attempt Resuscitation (DNAR)*** *for further information, if needed.*

- A sample IHP and ECP is available in *School Nursing: A Comprehensive Text*, for a student with muscular dystrophy.[13]

Role of the School Nurse:

- Staff development/in-service.
- Child and family advocate.
- Partner with the healthcare provider, parents/guardians, and other members of the school team to develop the IHP, ECP, and other school plans, such as IEP or Section 504 plan.
- The team may include a school healthcare provider, school nurse, physical therapist, occupational therapist, speech/language therapist, school counselor, social worker, director of transportation, and educational specialist.

MUSCULAR DYSTROPHY *(continued from previous page)*

RESOURCES

- **Education Matters: A Teacher's Guide to Duchenne Muscular Dystrophy**. Downloadable from: https://www.parentprojectmd.org/wp-content/uploads/2018/04/EdMatters_Teachers.pdf
- **Nursing Management, Health Promotion**: (A sample of Nursing Management Plan on health promotion is available in *Principles of Pediatric Nursing: Caring for Children.)* [14]
- **Learning and Behavior in Duchenne Muscular Dystrophy for Parents and Educators**. Downloadable from: http://www.columbia.edu/cu/md/Learning_and_Behavior_Guide.pdf
- **Muscular Dystrophy Association**: Research, information, support at http://mda.org
- **Parent Project Muscular Dystrophy**: 1-800-714-5437

REFERENCES

[1] American Academy of Pediatrics. (2019). Muscular dystrophy. In E.A. Donoghue, & C.A. Kraft (Eds.), *Managing chronic health needs in child care and schools* (2nd ed., pp. 165-16). American Academy of Pediatrics.

[2] National Institute of Neurological Disorders and Stroke. (2019). *NINDS muscular dystrophy information page*. http://www.ninds.nih.gov/disorders/md/md.htm

[3] Ibid.

[4] John, J. (2019). Students with other chronic conditions In J. Selekman, R. Adair Shannon, & C. F. Yonkaitis (Eds.), *School nursing: A comprehensive text* (3rd ed., pp.673-720). F.A. Davis.

[5] Mayo Clinic. (2018). *Muscular dystrophy.* http://www.mayoclinic.com/health/muscular-dystrophy/DS00200

[6] Ibid.

[7] Muscular Dystrophy Association (MDA). (2017). *Duchenne muscular dystrophy: Medical management.* https://www.mda.org/disease/duchenne-muscular-dystrophy

[8] National Institute of Neurological Disorders and Stroke. (2019). *NINDS muscular dystrophy information page*. http://www.ninds.nih.gov/disorders/md/md.htm

[9] American Academy of Pediatrics. (2019). Muscular dystrophy. In E.A. Donoghue, & C.A. Kraft (Eds.), *Managing chronic health needs in child care and schools* (2nd ed., pp. 165-16). American Academy of Pediatrics.

[10] Muscular Dystrophy Association (MDA). (n.d.). Diagnosis: *Duchenne muscular dystrophy (DMD).* Muscular Dystrophy Association (MDA).

[11] John, J. (2019). Students with other chronic conditions In J. Selekman, R. Adair Shannon, & C. F. Yonkaitis (Eds.), *School nursing: A comprehensive text* (3rd ed., pp.673-720). F.A. Davis.

[12] American Academy of Pediatrics. (2019). Muscular dystrophy. In E.A. Donoghue, & C.A. Kraft (Eds.), *Managing chronic health needs in child care and schools* (2nd ed., pp. 165-16). American Academy of Pediatrics.

[13] John, J. (2019). Students with other chronic conditions In J. Selekman, R. Adair Shannon, & C. F. Yonkaitis (Eds.), *School nursing: A comprehensive text* (3rd ed., pp.673-720). F.A. Davis

[14] Ball, J., Binder, R., & Cowen, K. (Eds.). (2017). Alteration in musculoskeletal function. In *Principles of pediatric nursing: Caring for children* (7th ed., pp. 849-851). Pearson Education, Inc.

MUSCULAR DYSTROPHY *(continued from previous page)*

OTHER REFERENCES CONSULTED

Centers for Disease Control. (2015). *Muscular dystrophy*. http://www.cdc.gov/ncbddd/musculardystrophy/

Merck Manual, Consumers Version. (2019). *Duchenne muscular dystrophy and Becker muscular dystrophy.* https://www.merckmanuals.com/home/children-s-health-issues/muscular-dystrophies-and-related-disorders/duchenne-muscular-dystrophy-and-becker-muscular-dystrophy?query=Duchenne%20Muscular%20Dystrophy%20and%20Becker%20Muscular%20Dystrophy

Muscular Dystrophy News. (2019). *Approved medications muscular dystrophy.* https://musculardystrophynews.com/muscular-dystrophy-medications/

National Center of Advancing Translational Science. (2019). *Becker muscular dystrophy.* https://rarediseases.info.nih.gov/diseases/5900/becker-muscular-dystrophy

NOROVIRUS

DEFINITION/ETIOLOGY:

Norovirus is an acute highly contagious virus that causes acute inflammation of the stomach and intestines (gastroenteritis). It is the most common cause of acute gastroenteritis in the United States. It spreads easily through contact with an infected person, contaminated food or water or by touching contaminated surfaces.[1]

SIGNS AND SYMPTOMS: [2]

Symptoms typically begin 12 – 48 hours after exposure and may include:

- Diarrhea
- Vomiting
- Nausea
- Stomach pain/cramps
- Fatigue/malaise
- Low grade fever
- Headache
- Muscle aches

MANAGEMENT/TREATMENT:[3]

There is no treatment for norovirus. Management is to provide support for symptoms. Norovirus symptoms, in most people, resolve without treatment in one to three days.

- Rehydrate with oral rehydration fluids, sport drinks and broths. Avoid liquids with a lot of sugar as this can make diarrhea worse.
- Infected persons should wash hands and surfaces touched frequently to prevent spreading virus to others.
- Wash fruits and vegetables before eating them.
- Wash hands before preparing food.
- Clean contaminated surfaces with bleach-based cleansers.
- Exclude from school until symptoms are completely resolved (children should not go to daycare or school while they have diarrhea or vomiting). Recommend that student or staff stay home two days after symptoms stop and in accordance with district policies for "returning to school" following an illness.
- Norovirus can be found in the stool for at least two weeks after symptoms resolve.

FOLLOW-UP:[4]

- Any outbreak of norovirus in the school should be reported to the local health department for surveillance purposes and for guidance in school procedures and student exclusion.
- Practice standard/universal precautions when changing diapers or any contact with stool. (*Refer to STANDARD PRECAUTIONS APPENDIX*).

POTENTIAL COMPLICATIONS:[5]

Young children, older adults and those immunocompromised are at greater risk for dehydration, malnutrition and even death.

NOROVIRUS *(continued from previous page)*

NOTES:[6]

The way to prevent getting norovirus is to practice good hand washing in every situation. Norovirus spreads quickly and easily when people are in close proximity such as hotels, resorts, cruise ships, nursing homes, schools (especially with dormitories) and childcare centers.

REFERENCES

---

[1] Centers for Disease Control and Prevention (CDC). (2019). *Norovirus.* http://www.cdc.gov/norovirus/index.html

[2] American Academy of Pediatrics. (2020). Norovirus. In S. Aronson, & T. Shope (Eds.), *Managing infectious diseases in child care and schools* (5th[d] ed., pp. 139-140). American Academy of Pediatrics.

[3] Centers for Disease Control and Prevention (CDC). (2019). *Norovirus.* http://www.cdc.gov/norovirus/index.html

[4] American Academy of Pediatrics. (2020). Norovirus. In S. Aronson, & T. Shope (Eds.), *Managing infectious diseases in child care and schools* (5th[d] ed., pp. 139-140). American Academy of Pediatrics.

[5] Mayo Clinic. (2017). *Norovirus Infection.* http://www.mayoclinic.org/diseases-conditions/norovirus/symptoms-causes/syn-20355296

[6] Ibid.

OTHER REFERENCES CONSULTED

American Academy of Pediatrics, Committee on Infectious Diseases. (2018). Norovirus. In D.W. Kimberlin, M.T. Brady, M.T., M.A. Jackson, & S.S. Long (Eds.), *Red Book, (2018-2021): Report of the Committee on Infectious Diseases* (31st ed., pp. 577-580). American Academy of Pediatrics.

NOSEBLEED (Epistaxis)

OVERVIEW/DEFINITION:
A nosebleed can be a common problem in children ages two to ten especially boys and the outcomes can range from a minor irritation to life-threatening.[1,2,3] Most nosebleeds come from the anterior blood vessels in the front of the nose where the tissue separates the sides of the nose and can be stopped with direct pressure. Posterior nosebleeds are less common, harder to control, usually appear in older people and are considered more serious.

A nosebleed can be caused by trauma, scratching the nose, picking the nose, repeated nose blowing that irritates the mucous membranes, or colds. It may start with sudden temperature change, dry air, mucosal infection, inflammation associated with allergic rhinitis, or upper respiratory infections. Students with nosebleeds may have a foreign body in the nose.

SIGNS AND SYMPTOMS:
- Blood coming from the nose
- Complaint of tasting blood or swallowing blood

ANTICIPATED CONCERNS/PROBLEMS:
- Choking on blood
- Vomiting from swallowed blood
- Anemia with frequent nosebleeds
- Suspect posterior bleeding if there was been blunt trauma to the head[4]

MANAGEMENT/POTENTIAL INTERVENTIONS:[5]

1. Instruct person to breathe through their mouth. Reassure the young or anxious child that he can still breathe through the mouth.
2. Have the person sit down and lean forward. This minimizes the amount of blood swallowed that may cause nausea or hematemesis.
3. Assist the student to firmly pinch anterior nose (nostrils closed) below the bone continuously for five minutes (timed by clock).
4. If bleeding continues, hold nose closed an additional 10 minutes. If bleeding continues for more than 15 to 20 minutes, contact the parent/guardian to refer to healthcare provider, e.g., vasoconstricting nose drops.
5. Additionally, a cold compress or ice applied to the bridge of the nose may help.
6. Seek medical help if the person is dizzy, light-headed, pale, has a rapid heart rate, or is taking anticoagulant or aspirin therapy (blood thinner).
7. A child with a recent nosebleed is more susceptible to recurring bleeding. For three to four days avoid bending, stooping, hot drinks, hot bath or shower. Elevate the head while sleeping and humidify the room.[6]
8. Posterior nosebleeds usually do not respond to outside direct pressure and blood will run down the throat even if standing or sitting forward.
9. Posterior nosebleeds usually require packing or cautery.

NOSEBLEED (Epistaxis) *(continued from previous page)*

FOLLOW-UP:[7]

- For the rest of the day, avoid blowing, sniffing, probing/picking the nose and dislodging the clot.
- Inquire about any clotting abnormalities and use of aspirin or anticoagulants.
- Repeated nosebleeds: refer to healthcare provider.
- Assess if family history of bleeding disorders.
- Assess if there is possible substance abuse by nasal snorting.
- Assess if history of other types of frequent or excess bleeding, for example with menstruation.
- Assess if history of blood in stool (black or tarry appearance).
- Assess aspirin or ibuprofen use.
- Educate parents about increasing humidity to prevent or decrease nosebleeds.

NOTES:

- Room or individual humidifiers, petroleum jelly or bacitracin (consult healthcare provider) can be applied three times per day or saline nasal spray may also be used to keep the lining of the nose moist.[8]
- Young children have more nosebleeds because the blood vessels are more fragile.
- Most nosebleeds that occur in children are not serious and usually stop within a few minutes.
- Frequent nosebleeds are considered more than once a week.
- High blood pressure does not cause nosebleeds, but it may increase the severity.[9]
- Frequent heavy, hard to stop nose bleeds may be due to an absence of clotting factors, possible Von Willebrand's disease.[10]

REFERENCES

[1]American Academy of Otolaryngology – Head and Neck Surgery. (2018). *ENT health. Nosebleeds.* https://www.enthealth.org/conditions/nosebleeds/

[2] American Academy of Otolaryngology – Head and Neck Surgery. (2018). *ENT health. Nosebleeds.* https://www.enthealth.org/conditions/nosebleeds/

[3] Merck Manual. *Epistaxis.* (2018). https://www.merckmanuals.com/professional/ear-nose-and-throat-disorders/approach-to-the-patient-with-nasal-and-pharyngeal-symptoms/epistaxis?qt=nosebleeds&alt=sh

[4] Ball, J., Binder, R., & Cowen, K. (Eds.). (2017). Alterations of the eye, ear, nose, and throat functions. In *Principles of pediatric nursing: Caring for children* (7th ed., pp. 465-66). Pearson Education, Inc.

[9] Mayo Clinic. (2017). *Nosebleeds: First aid.* https://www.mayoclinic.org/first-aid/first-aid-nosebleeds/basics/art-20056683

[5] Ibid.

[6] Cleveland Clinic. (2018). *Nosebleeds (Epistaxis).* https://my.clevelandclinic.org/health/diseases/13464-nosebleed-epistaxis

[7] American Academy of Otolaryngology – Head and Neck Surgery. (2018). *ENT health. Nosebleeds.* https://www.enthealth.org/conditions/nosebleeds/

NOSEBLEED (Epistaxis) *(continued from previous page)*

[8] Mayo Clinic. (2017). *Nosebleeds: Home remedies:4 tips to stop a nosebleed.* https://newsnetwork.mayoclinic.org/discussion/home-remedies-4-steps-to-stop-a-nosebleed/

[9] Mayo Clinic. (2017). *Nosebleeds: First aid.* https://www.mayoclinic.org/first-aid/first-aid-nosebleeds/basics/art-20056683

[10] Kids Health from Nemours. (2019). *Von Willebrand disease.* https://kidshealth.org/en/parents/vwd.html

OTHER REFERENCES CONSULTED

American Academy of Pediatrics. (n.d.) *Nosebleeds: What to do?* https://www.healthychildren.org/English/health-issues/conditions/ear-nose-throat/Pages/Chronic-Nosebleeds-What-To-Do.aspx

Kids Health from Nemours. (2015). *Nosebleeds.* https://kidshealth.org/en/kids/nosebleeds.html

Medline Plus. (2019). *Nosebleed.* https://medlineplus.gov/ency/article/003106.htm

ORAL HEALTH

Poor oral health can have a detrimental effect on children's quality of life, their performance at school, and their success later in life.[1] Because tooth decay is preventable, students having preventive oral health services in school is important to help them stay healthy and ready to learn.

TOOTH DECAY/DENTAL CARIES

DEFINITION/ETIOLOGY:
Tooth decay (cavities) is one of the most common chronic conditions of childhood in the United States. About one in five (20%) children aged five –11 years have at least one untreated decayed tooth, and about one in seven (13%) adolescents aged 12–19 years have at least one untreated decayed tooth.[2] The percentage of children and adolescents aged five –19 years with untreated tooth decay is twice as high for those from low-income families (25%) compared with children from higher-income households (11%).[3] Dental sealants prevent tooth decay and stop cavities from growing—they result in a large reduction in tooth decay among school-aged children five –16 years of age.[4]

SIGNS AND SYMPTOMS:[5]

- Toothache
- Tooth sensitivity
- Pain when biting or when eating or drinking something sweet, hot or cold
- Visible holes or pits in teeth
- Brown, black or white staining on any surface of a tooth

MANAGEMENT/TREATMENT of tooth decay and accompanying pain:

- Rinse mouth with warm water.
- Floss teeth to remove food particles trapped between teeth.
- All toothaches/tooth pain should be referred to a dentist; severity will dictate the time frame for the dental visit (e.g., immediate or within a few days).

FOLLOW UP:

- Educate regarding good dental care.
- Refer to dentist if family does not have one.

ORAL HEALTH *(continued from previous page)*

PERIODONTAL DISEASE

DEFINITION/ETIOLOGY:

Periodontal disease is a serious bacterial infection that destroys the gums and supporting structures of the teeth. It is also called gum disease. The main cause is plaque buildup on the teeth.
Certain things may raise a child's risk for periodontal disease. These include:

- Genetically predisposed
- Food lodged in the gums
- Mouth breathing, which may lead to severe drying of the gums and teeth in the front of the mouth
- Poor diet
- Smoking and using smokeless tobacco
- Autoimmune or systemic diseases
- Diabetes
- Hormonal changes in the body, such as during puberty
- Repeated clenching or grinding of the teeth unable to be controlled (bruxism)
- Certain medicines causing an overgrowth of the gums
- Poor oral hygiene e.g., lack of tooth brushing and proper flossing

SIGNS AND SYMPTOMS:

Periodontal disease can range from mild to severe. Most children with gum disease have the mildest form, called gingivitis. It causes the gums to become red, swollen, and sore. More advanced cases of gum disease are not common in children. Most common symptoms of gum disease include:

- Red, swollen, sore gums
- Bleeding while brushing or flossing
- Gums that pull away from the teeth (receding gums)
- Loose or separating teeth creating abnormal spacing
- Bad breath that won't go away
- Pus between the teeth and gums
- A change in bite and jaw alignment

MANAGEMENT/TREATMENT of Periodontal Disease:

- Have student rinse mouth thoroughly with a warm salt-water solution (1/4 teaspoon of table salt to four oz. glass of water).
- Instruct student to repeat rinses every two hours, and after eating or tooth brushing, and before bedtime.
- Check for abscesses below the tooth line.

If no improvement in one to two days, refer to healthcare provider or dentist. Treatment is dependent on the symptoms, age, general health and the severity of the condition. Early treatment is important, left untreated, underlying bone around the teeth may dissolve.

ORAL HEALTH *(continued from previous page)*

ORAL PIERCING[6]

DEFINITION/ETIOLOGY:

Oral piercing of the tongue, lip, cheek, or other soft tissues is a form of body art and self-expression. Oral piercings are more typically seen in adolescents and young adults, and the tongue is considered the most common site for oral-piercing placement.

- Complications associated with oral piercing include:
  - swelling
  - bleeding
  - infection
  - chipped or damaged teeth
  - gingival recession
  - lacerations/scarring
  - embedded oral jewelry (requiring surgical removal)
  - airway obstruction
  - hypersalivation
  - palatal erythema
  - keloid formation
  - purulent or unusual discharge from the pierced region

Tongue splitting is a less common form of body modification within the oral cavity. By definition, the tongue-splitting process is one in which an individual's tongue is severed into two pieces using various techniques. The procedure is inherently invasive and dangerous, with significant risks of severe bleeding, infection, inflammation, lingual nerve damage or other complications.

The American Dental Association (ADA) advises against the practices of cosmetic intraoral/perioral piercing and tongue splitting, and views these as invasive procedures with negative health sequelae that outweigh any potential benefit.

ORAL HEALTH *(continued from previous page)*

ORTHODONTIA RELATED ISSUES

The following orthodontic issues/emergencies and their treatments are listed in the order of the least severe to the most severe. Only the most severe emergencies may require immediate attention by an orthodontist. The majority of these are easily treated with a follow-up by the patient's orthodontist. [7]

FOOD CAUGHT BETWEEN TEETH - remove using dental floss, toothpick or interproximal brush.

LIGATURES COME OFF

- Tiny rubber bands or small, fine wires, known as ligatures, hold the wire to the bracket.
- Put it back in place using sterile tweezers.
- If a wire ligature comes loose, simply remove it with sterile tweezers.
- If the wire ligature is sticking out into the lip but is not loose, it may be bent back down with a Q-tip or pencil eraser to eliminate the irritation.
- Notify parent/guardian, who should then inform the orthodontist.
- If a rubber or wire ligature is lost, notify the parent/ guardian so that the orthodontist may advise whether the patient should be seen.

DISCOMFORT

- It's normal for a patient to have discomfort for a day or two after braces or retainers are adjusted.
- Encourage soft foods.
- Rinse the mouth with warm saltwater.

MOUTH SORES

- While braces do not cause mouth sores, they may be precipitated or exacerbated by an irritation from braces.
- Prompt relief may be achieved by applying a small amount of topical anesthetic directly to the ulcerated surface using a cotton swab (as directed by the student's healthcare provider or if permitted by standing orders).

IRRITATION OF LIPS OR CHEEKS

- Apply a small amount of non-medicinal relief wax.
- Pinch off a small piece and roll it into a ball the size of a small pea. Flatten the ball and place it completely over the area of the braces causing irritation.

ORAL HEALTH *(continued from previous page)*

ORTHODONTIA RELATED ISSUES *(continued)*

PROTRUDING WIRE

- Protruding wire from a brace can be gently bent out of the way to relieve discomfort by using a tongue depressor or pencil eraser. If the wire cannot be bent easily, apply dental wax or place a small piece of gauze or cotton over the end to prevent irritation to cheek or gum. Do not try to remove any wire embedded in the cheeks, gum, or tongue. (Local orthodontists often donate care kits).
- Obtain orthodontic care same day.

LOOSE BRACKETS, WIRES OR BANDS

- If the braces have come loose in any way, the parent/guardian needs to be notified.
- Obtain orthodontic care.
- If the bracket is off center, the adhesive may have failed. Call the parent/guardian and recommend that they immediately notify the orthodontist.
- If the loose bracket has rotated on the wire and is sticking out and the patient cannot immediately be taken to the orthodontist, you can do a temporary fix to alleviate discomfort and prevent further damage, taking care to prevent swallowing or other injury.
- To put the bracket back in place, use sterile tweezers to slide the bracket along the wire until it is between two teeth. Rotate the bracket back to the proper position, then slide it back to the center of the tooth.

PIECE OF APPLIANCE IS SWALLOWED

- If the patient is coughing excessively or having difficulty breathing, the piece could have been aspirated. If you can see the piece, you may carefully attempt to remove it. Do not make the attempt if you could cause harm.
- If appropriate under the circumstances, examine the patient's braces for problems that may result from the missing piece, such as looseness or irritation, and treat as specified above.
- If you are unable to see the piece and believe it may have been aspirated, notify the parent/guardian and the orthodontist immediately.

PREVENTION:
Protecting Student's Teeth

Even though tooth decay—or cavities—has been on the decline for the past 30 years, it is still one of the most common chronic diseases for youth from age six to 19.[8]

ORAL HEALTH *(continued from previous page)*

ORTHODONTIA RELATED ISSUES *(continued)*

Prevention Education

Good dental habits can prevent dental caries and gum disease. Children at increased risk of getting cavities can be higher if:

- Family members (older brothers, sisters, or parents) have cavities.
- They eat and drink a lot of sugary foods and drinks, like soda, especially between meals.
- They have special health care needs.
- They wear braces or orthodontics or oral appliances.

Teach children to:

- Brush his or her teeth twice a day.
- Use a toothbrush that is the right size based on the child's age and size.
- Floss daily.
- See the dentist regularly.
- Eat healthy foods, limiting those high in sugar and starch.

Dental Sealants

School-based sealant programs provide sealants to children in a school setting, and school-linked programs screen the children in school and refer them to private dental practices or public dental clinics that place the sealants. These programs have been shown to increase the number of children who receive sealants at school and are especially important for reaching children from low-income families who are less likely to receive private dental care.[9]

COMMONLY ASKED DENTAL QUESTIONS:

1. **What should school nurses know about tooth development?**
   Most importantly, the permanent teeth form very close to the apices (roots) of the primary teeth. Any injury to a primary tooth has the potential to damage the permanent tooth below. Primary tooth injuries range in damage from as minor as a small spot on the crown of the tooth to as severe as aborting further development of the permanent tooth bud. Consequently, all primary tooth injuries need evaluation by a dentist. School nurses should also be aware of other things that can affect tooth development such as excessive fluoride, tetracyclines, congenital defects, metabolic diseases and high fever. These can have deleterious effects on the quality of dental hard tissues, especially the enamel.

2. **What about students with disabilities?**
   Students with disabilities seem to have special problems because of systemic problems (cognitive impairment, poor muscle control, diminished reflexes, etc.) or because of the secondary effects of diet, medications or the because of difficulty in maintaining good oral hygiene.[10] Referral to a pediatric dentist or another dentist who has had advanced training in working with patients with special needs is extremely important. After dental work, monitor the child closely to prevent chewing on anesthetized surfaces.

ORAL HEALTH *(continued from previous page)*

REFERENCES

[1] Centers for Disease Control and Prevention. (2017). *Oral health in schools.* https://www.cdc.gov/healthyschools/npao/oralhealth.htm

[2] Ibid.

[3] Ibid.

[4] Ibid.

[5] Mayo Clinic. (2017). *Cavities/tooth decay.* https://www.mayoclinic.org/diseases-conditions/cavities/symptoms-causes/syc-20352892

[6] American Dental Association. (n.d.). *Oral health topics: Oral piercing.* https://www.ada.org/en/member-center/oral-health-topics/oral-piercing

[7] American Association of Orthodontists. (n.d.). *Handling orthodontic emergencies.* https://www.aaoinfo.org/system/files/media/documents/OrthoEmergency-FLYER-13-hl.pdf

[8] Centers for Disease Control and Prevention, Division of Oral Health, National Center for Chronic Disease Prevention and Promotion. (2019). *Protecting your child's teeth.* https://www.cdc.gov/oralhealth/basics/childrens-oral-health/fl_caries.htm

[9] Griffin, S.O., Wei, L., Gooch, B.F., Weno, K., & Espinoza, L. (2016). Vital signs: Dental sealant use and untreated tooth decay among U.S. school-aged children. *Morbidity and Mortality Weekly Report, 65*(41), 1141-1145. https://www.cdc.gov/mmwr/volumes/65/wr/mm6541e1.htm

[10] U.S. Department of Health and Human Services, National Institute of Dental and Craniofacial Research. (2016). *Oral conditions in children with special needs: A guide for health care providers.* https://www.nidcr.nih.gov/sites/default/files/2017-09/oral-conditions-children-special-needs.pdf

PANDAS/PANS

DEFINITION/ETIOLOGY:
PANDAS is an acronym for Pediatric Autoimmune Neuropsychiatric Disorders Associated with Streptococcal infections. The term PANDAS is used to describe a subset of children and adolescents who following a strep infection have worsening symptoms of Obsessive-Compulsive Disorder (OCD) or tic disorders. PANS is an acronym for Pediatric Acute Onset Neuropsychiatric Syndrome and is a newer term used to describe a larger class of acute onset OCD which has been proposed to have multiple etiologies including infectious, autoimmune, or metabolic.[1] Children who develop PANS or PANDAS have a genetic predisposition for these syndromes.[2]

SIGNS AND SYMPTOMS: (Sudden, Dramatic and Often Episodic)[3]

- Motor or vocal tics
- Obsessions or compulsions (OCD like behaviors)
- Heightened anxiety
- Increased urinary frequency
- Impulsivity, inattention, poor concentration
- Handwriting changes and deterioration in school performance
- Sensory issues
- Selective eating and food refusal
- Sleep disruptions
- Emotional lability, depression, or aggression

Diagnosis for PANDAS and PANS is based on clinical presentation.

PANDAS diagnosis criteria include:[4]

- Presence of OCD or tics
- Onset between three years of age and puberty
- Abrupt onset and episodic course of symptom severity, neurological abnormalities, and an association with Group A Streptococcal infection.

NOTE: Anti-streptococcal antibody titers may be drawn to determine evidence of a previous strep infection.

PANS diagnosis criteria include:[5]

- Abrupt onset of OCD or restricted food intake
- No age requirement
- Symptoms that are explained by a known neurological or medical disorder such as Tourette's Disorder or Lupus
- An abrupt onset of at least two of the following comorbid symptoms:
    - Anxiety
    - Depression
    - Aggression
    - Behavioral regression
    - Motor or sensory abnormalities
    - Deterioration in school performance
    - Sleep problems and or urinary symptoms

PANDAS/PANS *(continued from previous page)*

MANAGEMENT/TREATMENT:

The best treatment for PANDAS/PANS is individualized treatment. If a strep infection is present, a single course of antibiotics may help reduce or eliminate the PANDAS symptoms.[6] Long term use of antimicrobial prophylaxis and plasmapheresis has been effective for some children affected by PANDAS or PANS.[7] Cognitive behavioral therapy and the use of medications to treat OCD and tic disorders may be used. In addition, anti-inflammatory medication as well as steroids or intravenous immunoglobulin (IVIG) may be helpful.[8]

FOLLOW-UP:

- School nurse should collaborate with parents and healthcare provider to develop a plan for frequent but sporadic missed days as well as extended absences. Some students may require temporary educational services in the home or hospital.
- School nurses can be essential in assisting families of children with sudden behavioral changes in the identification of a possible PANDAS/PANS case. The nurse may also be the first one to link the behavior to a recent strep case and can contact parents or guardians of other cases of strep in the classroom.
- Educating school staff on PANDAS/PANS is an important role of the school nurse.
- Develop an Individualized Healthcare Plan and Emergency Care Plan for the student.
- Be a part of the Section 504/Individualized Educational Plan (IEP) team to develop a plan for the student.
- A Section 504 plan or an IEP should be considered.[9]
    - Academic accommodations may need to be re-evaluated after PANDAS/PANS symptoms have lessened and student's functions improve.[10]
    - During flares numerous accommodations can be instituted such as rest periods, modified schedules, extended time for work, copies of notes, use of computer for classwork, seating preference, breaking assignments in smaller tasks, and using visual and non-visual cueing to stay on task.[11]
- Positive behavioral classroom supports should be put in place.

POTENTIAL COMPLICATIONS:

Exacerbations and times of remissions may occur, the longer the student remains untreated the greater the effects of the symptoms.

PANDAS/PANS *(continued from previous page)*

REFERENCES

[1] Calaprice, D., Tona, J., Parker-Athill, E. C., & Murphy, T.K. (2017) A survey of pediatric acute-onset neuropsychiatric syndrome characteristics and course. *Journal of Child and Adolescent Psychopharmacology*, *27*(7), 607-618. https://doi.org/ 10.1089/cap.2016.0105

[2] Stanford Chidren's Health. (2018). *Q&A: Sudden symptoms are first sign of PANS and PANDAS*. https://healthier.standordchilrens.org/en/q-sudden-symptoms-first-sign-pans-pandas/

[3] Thienemann, M., Murphy, T., Leckman, J., Shaw, R., Williams, K., Kapphahn, C., & Swedo, S. (2017). Clinical management of pediatric acute-onset neuropsychiatric syndrome: Part I—Psychiatric and behavioral interventions. *Journal of Child and Adolescent Psychopharmacology*, *27*(7), 566–573. https://doi.org/10.1089/cap.2016.0145

[4] PANDAS Physicians Network. (2019). *PANDAS Diagnostic Guidelines.* https://www.pandasppn.org/pandas/

[5] PANDAS Physicians Network. (2019). *PANS Diagnostic Guidelines.* https://www.pandasppn.org/pans/

[6] Cooperstock, M. S., Swedo, S. E., Pasternack, M. S., Murphy, T. K., & Consortium, F. T. P. (2017). Clinical management of pediatric acute-onset neuropsychiatric syndrome: Part III—treatment and prevention of infections. *Journal of Child and Adolescent Psychopharmacology*, *27*(7), 1-13. https://doi.org/10.1089/cap.2016.0151

[7] Ibid.

[8] Sigra, S., Hesselmark, E., & Bejerot, S. (2018). Treatment of PANDAS and PANS: A systematic review. *Neuroscience and Biobehavioral Reviews*, *86*(2018), 51-65. https://doi.org/ 10.1016/j.neurbiorev.2018.01.001

[9] Thienemann, M., Murphy, T., Leckman, J., Shaw, R., Williams, K., Kapphahn, C., & Swedo, S. (2017). Clinical management of pediatric acute-onset neuropsychiatric syndrome: Part I—Psychiatric and behavioral interventions. *Journal of Child and Adolescent Psychopharmacology*, *27*(7), 566–573. https://doi.org/10.1089/cap.2016.0145

[10] Ibid.

[11] Ibid.

PERTUSSIS (WHOOPING COUGH)

DEFINITION/ETIOLOGY:

Pertussis is a highly contagious bacterial infection caused by *Bordetella pertussis*.[1] Pertussis is a vaccine preventable disease (VPD) that is increasing in incidence.[2] Incubation period for *Bordetella pertussis* is usually seven-10 days, but can be as long as 21 days and is spread from person to person through airborne droplets in close contact (coughing and sneezing).[3]

SIGNS AND SYMPTOMS:

- Pertussis is divided in three stages:
    1. The catarrhal stage lasts one to two weeks and may not be recognized or may include non-specific symptoms such as rhinorrhea (runny nose), sneezing, watery eyes, mild cough, hoarseness, and rarely fever. Without appropriate treatment, pertussis is most contagious from catarrhal stage until two weeks after onset of cough.[4]
    2. The paroxysmal stage lasts two to four weeks or longer and is characterized by paroxysmal cough or whooping cough (cough with whoop at the end). The cough may increase in severity, vomiting may occur during or after coughing episodes.[5] The affected individual may become exhausted.[6]
    3. The convalescent stage begins about week four of illness onset and lasts one to two weeks as cough becomes milder and less often. Cough may persist for several months. [7]
- The duration of classic pertussis is seven weeks but can range from three weeks to three months.[8]

MANAGEMENT/TREATMENT:

1. Refer to healthcare provider for diagnosis and appropriate treatment. Diagnosis is made on history and possible nasopharyngeal culture.[9]
    a. Treatment includes antibiotics. They are most effective in shortening the length of infection when given in the catarrhal stage. After the catarrhal stage, antibiotics cannot shorten the duration of the illness, but may reduce the amount of time an infected person can transmit the bacteria to others.[10]
2. Implement state health regulations/school policy for control measures.
    a. Students and staff with pertussis should be excluded from school and may return five days after they begin appropriate therapy.[11]
    b. Those who do not receive antimicrobial therapy should be excluded from school for 21 days after onset of symptoms (coughing).[12]
    c. School-wide or classroom chemoprophylaxis generally has *not* been recommended because of the delay in recognition of outbreak and related overuse of antibiotics.[13]
    d. People who have been in contact with an infected person should be monitored closely for respiratory tract symptoms for 21 days after last contact.[14]
    e. Implement surveillance for community health reporting. [15]

PERTUSSIS (WHOOPING COUGH) *(continued from previous page)*

MANAGEMENT/TREATMENT *(continued)*

f. For household contacts: Immunization recommended according to schedule for adolescents 11 – 18, adults 19 and older and children 7-10 who are not fully vaccinated against pertussis (fewer than 4 doses). Children 4-6 years old who have not received the 5th DTaP should be vaccinated.[16]

3. A course of antibiotics may be recommended to be administered to close contacts.[17]
4. Cough medicine will not likely help and should not be given unless instructed by the healthcare provider.[18]
5. Rest and a cool mist vaporizer may help to loosen secretions.[19]
6. Encourage good handwashing.[20]
7. Encourage fluids and watch for signs of dehydration.[21]
8. Keep environment free of irritants that can trigger coughing, such as tobacco smoke, and/or wood burning fireplace/stove.[22]

FOLLOW-UP:[23]

- Monitor nutritional status. To avoid vomiting after coughing, advise eating smaller, more frequent meals, instead of large meals.
- Adults and teens generally have milder symptoms.

POTENTIAL COMPLICATIONS:[24]

- Pertussis causes disease in every age group but has the most significant impact on un-immunized young children, particularly infants.
- Major complications are most common among infants and young children. Complications include bacterial pneumonia, seizure, encephalopathy, and death. Most deaths occur among unvaccinated children or children too young to be vaccinated.
- Other complications may include difficulty sleeping, weight loss, urinary incontinence, syncope, pneumonia and rib fracture during violent coughing.
- Previously immunized adolescents can become susceptible when immunity wanes, but they can receive a booster (Tdap) if they previously received only the tetanus-diphtheria toxoids (Td) booster at age 11-13 years. Secondary schools, in most states, require a Tdap, for this age group.

PERTUSSIS (WHOOPING COUGH) *(continued from previous page)*

REFERENCES

[1] Center for Disease Control and Prevention. (2017). *Pertussis.* https://www.cdc.gov/pertussis/about/index.html

[2] Merck Manual. (2018). *Pertussis.* https://www.merckmanuals.com/professional/infectious-diseases/gram-negative-bacilli/pertussis

[3] Kids Health/Nemours. (2016). *Whooping cough (Pertussis).* https://kidshealth.org/en/parents/whooping-cough.html?ref=search

[4] Merck Manual. (2018). *Pertussis.* https://www.merckmanuals.com/professional/infectious-diseases/gram-negative-bacilli/pertussis

[5] Ibid.

[6] Center for Disease Control and Prevention. (2017). *Pertussis.* https://www.cdc.gov/pertussis/about/index.html

[7] Merck Manual. (2018). *Pertussis.* https://www.merckmanuals.com/professional/infectious-diseases/gram-negative-bacilli/pertussis

[8] Ibid.

[9] Kids Health/Nemours. (2016). *Whooping cough (Pertussis).* https://kidshealth.org/en/parents/whooping-cough.html?ref=search

[10] Ibid.

[11] New York State Department of Health. (2016). *Pertussis or whooping cough fact sheet* https://www.health.ny.gov/publications/2171/

[12] Ibid.

[13] Centers for Disease Control and Prevention. (2017). *Postexposure antimicrobial prophylaxis.* https://www.cdc.gov/pertussis/outbreaks/pep.html

[14] Centers for Disease Control and Prevention. (2017). *Pertussis.* https://www.cdc.gov/pertussis/about/index.html

[15] Ibid.

[16] Centers for Disease Control and Preventions. (2018). *Pertussis.* https://www.cdc.gov/vaccines/pubs/pinkbook/pert.html

[17] Kids Health/Nemours. (2016). *Whooping cough (Pertussis).* https://kidshealth.org/en/parents/whooping-cough.html?ref=search

[18] Ibid.

[19] Ibid.

[20] Centers for Disease Control and Prevention. (2017). *Pertussis.* https://www.cdc.gov/pertussis/about/index.html

[21] Kids Health/Nemours. (2016). *Whooping Cough (Pertussis).* https://kidshealth.org/en/parents/whooping-cough.html?ref=search

[22] Ibid.

[23] Ibid.

[24] Centers for Disease Control and Prevention. (2017). *Pertussis.* https://www.cdc.gov/pertussis/about/index.html

PINWORM INFECTION (Enterobiasis)

DEFINITION/ETIOLOGY:

Pinworms are the most common of all roundworm infections. They are small thread-like roundworms measuring about 1/4 to 1/2 inch in length.[1] The ova of the parasite transfers from the perineal area to fomites (i.e., objects), are picked up by a new host, transferred to the mouth, and swallowed. The lifecycle of the pinworm - egg, larva (immature stage), and mature worm takes place inside the colon and requires 3-6 weeks to complete. Eggs can be carried to the mouth by contaminated food, drink, or fingers and are capable of clinging to bedding, clothes, toys, doorknobs, furniture, or faucets for up to two weeks.[2] Pinworms are found more commonly among people living in crowded conditions, day-care facilities, and schools.[3]

SIGNS AND SYMPTOMS:[4]

- More common in children; especially five to 10 years old
- Many people have no symptoms at all
- Itching around the anus and vagina
- Intense itching that may interfere with sleep
- Irritability from lack of sleep
- Intermittent abdominal pain and nausea

MANAGEMENT/TREATMENT:

- Eggs may be collected with a strip of sticky, clear tape placed on the anal opening and identified by a healthcare provider.[5] The tape method is usually performed at home by a parent or guardian and should be conducted on three consecutive mornings before washing.[6]
- Infestations are typically harmless. Treatment is reserved for symptomatic patients.[7]
- If medication (Mebendazole, Pyrantel Pamaoate, or Albendazole (Albenza) is indicated, the entire household should be treated.
- Medication works by keeping the worm from absorbing sugar (glucose) causing the death of the worm or by causing sudden contraction, followed by paralysis, of the parasite, causing the worm to "lose its grip" on the intestinal wall.[8, 9]
- Antipruritic creams and ointments may be recommended to relieve anal itching.

FOLLOW UP:

- Monitor for sleepiness and weight loss.
- Clean classroom as indicated - pinworm eggs can survive for two to three weeks on surfaces.

PINWORM INFECTION (Enterobiasis) *(continued from previous page)*

POTENTIAL COMPLICATIONS:[10]

- Infection of the female genitalia and reproductive system
- Cutaneous infection secondary to excoriation
- Abdominal pain
- Weight loss

NOTES: Prevention[11]

- Bathe after waking.
- Wash nightclothes and bedding often using hot water.
- Frequent hand washing, and always after using the bathroom or changing diapers, and before eating. *(Refer to HANDWASHING APPENDIX).*
- Change underclothes each day.
- Avoid nail biting.
- Avoid scratching anal area.

REFERENCES

[1] Mayo Clinic. *Pinworm infection.* (2018). https://www.mayoclinic.org/diseases-conditions/pinworm/symptoms-causes/syc-20376382

[2] Ibid.

[3] Ibid.

[4] Centers for Disease Control and Prevention. (2013). *Parasites- enterobaisis disease.* https://www.cdc.gov/parasites/pinworm/disease.html

[5] Merck Manual. *Pinworm infestation.* (2019). http://www.merckmanuals.com/professional/infectious_diseases/nematodes_roundworms/pinworm_infestation.html?qt=pinworms&alt=sh

[6] Centers for Disease Control and Prevention. (2013). *Parasites- enterobaisis diagnosis.* https://www.cdc.gov/parasites/pinworm/diagnosis.html

[7] Merck Manual. *Pinworm infestation.* (2019). http://www.merckmanuals.com/professional/infectious_diseases/nematodes_roundworms/pinworm_infestation.html?qt=pinworms&alt=sh

[8] Centers for Disease Control and Prevention. (2013). *Parasites- enterobaisis (also known as pinworm infection).* http://www.cdc.gov/parasites/pinworm/treatment.html

[9] Drug.com. (2015). *Pyrantel pamoate.* http://www.drugs.com/cdi/pyrantel-pamoate.html

[10] Centers for Disease Control and Prevention. (2013). *Parasites- enterobaisis diagnosis.* https://www.cdc.gov/parasites/pinworm/diagnosis.html

[11] Merck Manual. *Pinworm infestation. (2019).* http://www.merckmanuals.com/professional/infectious_diseases/nematodes_roundworms/pinworm_infestation.html?qt=pinworms&alt=sh

PNEUMONIA

DEFINITION/ETIOLOGY:
Pneumonia is an inflammation or infection of the bronchioles and alveolar spaces which may occur in one or both lungs.[1] When pneumonia occurs, the air sac of one or both lungs become inflamed. During the pneumonia infection, the air sacs may fill with fluid or pus, causing cough with phlegm or pus, fever, chills and difficulty breathing.[2] Pneumonia may be caused by bacteria, viruses, and fungi.

Pneumonia can range from mild to life-threatening and is most serious for infants and young children, as well as adults older than 65 years of age.[3] Additionally, people with underlying health problems or weakened immune systems are at increased risk of pneumonia complications. Antibiotics and antiviral medications are used to treat many common forms of pneumonia.

CAUSES OF PNEUMONIA
The main causes of pneumonia:
- Bacteria
- Viruses
- Mycoplasmas[4]

Other less common causes:
- Fungi and other infectious agents
- Various chemicals [5]

TYPES OF PNEUMONIA
Pneumonia is classified according to the location where the infection is acquired. Below are four types of pneumonia based on the specific acquired location and the specific organisms associated with the cause.

- Community-acquired pneumonia – most common type. [6] Usually preceded by an upper respiratory infection including rhinitis and cough.[7] There is significant risk of pneumonia as a complication of the flu.[8] May be caused by the following:
    - Bacteria: Streptococcus pneumoniae [9]
    - Bacteria-like organisms: Mycoplasma pneumoniae produces milder signs and symptoms and more common in children 5 years and older.[10] The term "Walking Pneumonia" may result from Mycoplasma pneumoniae.[11]
    - Viruses: Most common cause of pneumonia in children younger than five years of age.[12] Usually mild and can become severe.
        - Fungi: Common in people with chronic health problems or weakened immune systems, as well as those who have inhaled large doses of organisms. The fungi that cause it can be found in soil or bird droppings.[13]
- Hospital-acquired pneumonia –bacterial infection
    - Bacteria causing this type of pneumonia may be resistant to antibiotics
    - People who are assisted by a ventilator for breathing are at higher risk for hospital-acquired pneumonia[14]

PNEUMONIA *(continued from previous page)*

TYPES OF PNEUMONIA *(continued)*

- Healthcare-acquired pneumonia – bacterial infection; generally, occurs among people when living in a long-term care facility, after discharge from hospital, or after exposure at an outpatient center/clinic
    - Bacteria may be resistant to antibiotic treatment[15]

- Aspiration pneumonia - occurs when food, drink, vomit, or saliva are inhaled into the lungs
    - May occur if the normal gag reflex is disturbed by brain injury, swallowing problems, or excessive use of drugs and alcohol[16]

SIGNS AND SYMPTOMS OF PNEUMONIA:

- Fever and shaking chills
- Sweating and clammy skin
- Lower than normal temperature in people with weakened immune system or poor health[17]
- Cough - which may produce phlegm.
- Chest pain with deep breathing and coughing
- Shortness of breath[18]
- Wheezing (may be more common in viral pneumonia)
- Muscle aches and muscle fatigue
- Nausea, vomiting, and diarrhea especially in small children[19]
- Headache[20]
- Confusion in the elderly[21]

POTENTIAL RISKS AND COMPLICATIONS:

- Chronic health conditions (asthma, COPD, heart disease, etc.)
- Weak, compromised or suppressed immune system
- Smoking because it damages the body's natural defenses against bacteria and viruses causing pneumonia
- Using ventilator assistance for breathing while hospitalized[22]

Complications:

- Bacteremia – bacteria in the bloodstream can cause organ failure
- Abscess in the lung due to formation of pus in the lung cavity
- Pleural effusion – fluid accumulation around the lungs; chest tube may be necessary to drain infected fluid
- Difficulty breathing [23]

PNEUMONIA *(continued from previous page)*

MANAGEMENT/TREATMENT:

General Information

- Hospitalization is recommended for severe cases of pneumonia
- Immunizations provide protection against pneumonia, e.g. pertussis, influenza and pneumococcal vaccines[24]
- Adequate nutrition helps to improve the natural immunity of children
- Promote good hygiene practices, e.g. handwashing[25]
- Teach students and staff cough and sneeze etiquette *(Refer to COVER YOUR COUGH APPENDIX)*
- Pain, fever control rest and fluids[26]

Bacterial Pneumonia

- Treated with oral antibiotics
- Proper diet
- Oxygen as needed
- Acetaminophen/ibuprofen for fever and discomfort[27]

Viral Pneumonia

- May be treated with antiviral medication
- Usually improves in one to three weeks
- Symptom management and rest[28]

Mycoplasma Pneumonia

- May be weak for extended period of time
- Adequate rest is important for progression toward full recovery

PREVENTION:[29,30]

1. Annual flu shots
2. Vaccination against vaccine preventable diseases
3. Handwashing
4. No smoking

REFERENCES

[1]Ball, J., Binder, R., & Cowen, K. (Eds.). (2017). Alterations in respiratory function. In *Principles of pediatric nursing: Caring for children* (7th ed., pp. 491-492). Pearson Education, Inc.

[2] American Lung Association. (2019). *Pneumonia symptoms and diagnosis.* https://www.lung.org/lung-health-and-diseases/lung-disease-lookup/pneumonia/symptoms-and-diagnosis.html

[3] Mayo Clinic. (2018). *Pneumonia.* https://www.mayoclinic.org/diseases-conditions/pneumonia/symptoms-causes/syc-20354204

[4] Children's Hospital of Philadelphia. (2018). *Pneumonia in children.* https://www.chop.edu/conditions-diseases/pneumonia-children

[5] Ibid.

PNEUMONIA *(continued from previous page)*

[6] Mayo Clinic. (2018). *Pneumonia.* https://www.mayoclinic.org/diseases-conditions/pneumonia/symptoms-causes/syc-20354204

[7] Ball, J., Binder, R., & Cowen, K. (Eds.). (2017). Alterations in respiratory function. In *Principles of pediatric nursing: Caring for children* (7th ed., pp. 491-492). Pearson Education, Inc.

[8] American Lung Association. (2019). *Pneumonia symptoms and diagnosis.* https://www.lung.org/lung-health-and-diseases/lung-disease-lookup/pneumonia/symptoms-and-diagnosis.html

[9] Mayo Clinic. (2018). *Pneumonia.* https://www.mayoclinic.org/diseases-conditions/pneumonia/symptoms-causes/syc-20354204

[10] Children's Hospital of Philadelphia. (2018). *Pneumonia in children.* https://www.chop.edu/conditions-diseases/pneumonia-children

[11] Ball, J., Binder, R., & Cowen, K. (Eds.). (2017). Alterations in respiratory function. In *Principles of pediatric nursing: Caring for children* (7th ed., pp. 491-492). Pearson Education, Inc.

[12] Mayo Clinic. (2018). *Pneumonia.* https://www.mayoclinic.org/diseases-conditions/pneumonia/symptoms-causes/syc-20354204

[13] Ibid.

[14] Ibid.

[15] Ibid.

[16] Ibid.

[17] Ibid.

[18] Centers of Disease Control and Prevention (CDC). (2018). *Pneumonia: An infection of the lungs.* https://www.cdc.gov/pneumonia/index.html

[19] American Lung Association. (2019). *Pneumonia symptoms and diagnosis.* https://www.lung.org/lung-health-and-diseases/lung-disease-lookup/pneumonia/symptoms-and-diagnosis.html

[20] Children's Hospital of Philadelphia. (2018). *Pneumonia in children.* https://www.chop.edu/conditions-diseases/pneumonia-children

[21] American Lung Association. (2019). *Pneumonia symptoms and diagnosis.* https://www.lung.org/lung-health-and-diseases/lung-disease-lookup/pneumonia/symptoms-and-diagnosis.html

[22] Mayo Clinic. (2018). *Pneumonia.* https://www.mayoclinic.org/diseases-conditions/pneumonia/symptoms-causes/syc-20354204

[23] Ibid.

[24]American Academy of Pediatrics. (2020). Pneumonia. In S. Aronson, & T. R. Shope, (Eds.), *Managing chronic health needs in child care and schools: A quick reference guide* (5th ed., pp.145). American Academy of Pediatrics.

[25] Centers of Disease Control and Prevention (CDC). (2018). *Pneumonia: An infection of the lungs.* https://www.cdc.gov/pneumonia/index.html

[26] American Lung Association. (2019). *Pneumonia symptoms and diagnosis.* https://www.lung.org/lung-health-and-diseases/lung-disease-lookup/pneumonia/symptoms-and-diagnosis.html

[27] Mayo Clinic. (2018). *Pneumonia.* https://www.mayoclinic.org/diseases-conditions/pneumonia/symptoms-causes/syc-20354204

[28] American Lung Association. (2019). *Pneumonia symptoms and diagnosis.* https://www.lung.org/lung-health-and-diseases/lung-disease-lookup/pneumonia/symptoms-and-diagnosis.html

[29] Ibid.

[30] Mayo Clinic. (2018). *Pneumonia.* https://www.mayoclinic.org/diseases-conditions/pneumonia/symptoms-causes/syc-20354204

POISON IVY/OAK (Contact Dermatitis)

OVERVIEW/DEFINITION:

Poison ivy/oak is a skin reaction (contact dermatitis) due to the allergen, urushiol, which is found in all parts (stem, flowers, berries, and roots) of the poison ivy, oak and sumac (rhus) plant, which usually occurs in the spring, summer, and fall. Poison ivy/oak grows as a low-lying shrub and a short or high trailing vine. Leaves appear in groups of three with white berries and greenish flowers. A rash only occurs in people sensitive to these plants when the skin directly touches the urushiol from the plant, contaminated objects or smoke from burning plants.[1] About 60-80% of people will have an allergic reaction.[2] A reaction is most commonly seen on the hands, forearms, and face.

SIGNS AND SYMPTOMS:[3,4]

Reaction typically begins 12- 48 hours after exposure but can also take as long as a week.

- Red, itchy rash
  - Small papules and vesicles
  - Rash may have a linear appearance were the plant brushes against the skin.
- May have large blisters and generalized weeping of skin.
- Localized swelling.
- Dryness, crusting and gradual shedding of crusts and scabs is a sign of healing which may take one to two weeks.
- Difficulty breathing if smoke from burning poison ivy is inhaled.

ANTICIPATED CONCERNS/PROBLEMS:

- Scratching the rash with dirty fingernails can cause a secondary infection.

MANAGEMENT/POTENTIAL INTERVENTIONS:[5, 6, 7]

1. Wash skin and fingernails thoroughly with a degreasing detergent (dishwashing soap) and cool water within 10 minutes of exposure or with a commercial product (e.g., Tecnu® or Zanfel® cleansers) as soon as possible to prevent or decrease a reaction.
2. Continue to rinse the area frequently to prevent wash solutions from drying on the skin and the spread of urushiol.
3. To relieve itching, apply cool packs (every 15-20 minutes, 3-4 times daily), and/or a warm baking soda or colloidal oatmeal bath. Avoid hot water that will exacerbate the symptoms.
4. Plain calamine lotion may be applied to dry lesions, do not apply to face or genitals.
5. Topical corticosteroid cream may be used to reduce inflammation.
6. Healthcare provider may prescribe oral steroids for extensive cases.
7. Avoid oral antihistamines as they are usually not helpful for itch, but hydroxyzine (Atarax®) may be prescribed.
8. Applying a loose dressing may help discourage scratching.
9. Refer to healthcare provider if itching is distracting child from attention to tasks, rash is extensive, or involving eye, face, genitals or mucous membranes.

POISON IVY/OAK (Contact Dermatitis) *(continued from previous page)*

FOLLOW-UP: Observe for infection and treat as needed.

- Wear disposable rubber gloves to:
  - Promptly wash contaminated clothing such shoes, shoelaces, socks, pants, and shirts in detergent and hot water.
  - Clean additional contaminated objects used outdoors such as garden tools and jewelry with hot water and detergent.
  - If objects are not cleaned thoroughly, urushiol may remain active for up to five years and be the source of a future reaction.[8]
- Educate regarding how to identify poison ivy/oak and to avoid re-exposure.
- If on school or public play property, report location for safe removal (without burning).

NOTES:

- Do not exclude from school; educate staff on transmission of urushiol.
- Contents of blisters and weepy skin CANNOT cause rash in another individual or even in another location on patient.
- Inhaling smoke from burning poison ivy/oak plants may cause a severe respiratory reaction. A reaction may also occur if burning particles land on your skin. See a healthcare provider.
- To prevent a potential exposure, an over the counter barrier cream containing bantoquatam may be used. However, avoidance is the best protection.
- Urushiol can remain active for five years. If contaminated objects are not cleaned, contact with them at a later date may cause a reaction.[9]
- Consider pet fur as possible source of exposure.

REFERENCES

[1] Mayo Clinic. (2018). *Poison ivy rash.* http://www.mayoclinic.com/health/poison-ivy/DS00774

[2] Kids Health from Nemours. (2018). *First aid: Poison ivy, oak. Sumac.* https://kidshealth.org/en/parents/poison-ivy-sheet.html?WT.ac=ctg

[3] Mayo Clinic. (2018). *Poison ivy rash.* http://www.mayoclinic.com/health/poison-ivy/DS00774

[4] Kids Health from Nemours. (2018). *First aid: Poison ivy, oak. Sumac.* https://kidshealth.org/en/parents/poison-ivy-sheet.html?WT.ac=ctg

[5] Centers for Disease Control and Prevention/ The National Institute for Occupational Safety and Health (NIOSH). (2014). *NIOSH Fast facts: Protecting yourself from poisonous plants.* https://www.cdc.gov/niosh/docs/2010-118/default.html

[6] American Academy of Dermatology. (2018). *Poison ivy, oak, and sumac.* https://www.aad.org/public/diseases/itchy-skin/poison-ivy-oak-and-sumac

[7] Kids Health from Nemours. (2018). *First aid: Poison ivy, oak. Sumac.* https://kidshealth.org/en/parents/poison-ivy-sheet.html?WT.ac=ctg

[8] Centers for Disease Control and Prevention/ The National Institute for Occupational Safety and Health (NIOSH). (2014). *Fast facts: Protecting yourself from poisonous plants.* https://www.cdc.gov/niosh/docs/2010-118/default.html

[9] Ibid.

PUBERTAL GROWTH AND DEVELOPMENT

DEFINITION/ETIOLOGY:

Puberty is a sequence of stages affecting the skeletal, muscular, reproductive, and almost every other body system, that ultimately leads to fertility. During this time there is rapid growth in height and weight. The normal age of onset of puberty is considered to be between eight and 13 years in the general population of girls and between the ages of nine and 14 years in the general population of boys.[1] The sequences of body changes are visible and predictable. The onset of these changes is influenced by nutritional status, genetics and environmental factors and can vary greatly from person to person. Tanner staging, also recognized as the Sexual Maturity Rating (SMR) system, provides a means to document a child's progression through puberty. Separate scales are used for breast size and shape (female), genitalia size and shape (male) and pubic hair development and distribution (both sexes). There are five stages of puberty for both males and females.[2] A pubertal assessment includes a physical assessment in addition to any information provided by the child or parent. Generally with pubertal development there are also changes in cognition and social development.

STAGES OF NORMAL DEVELOPMENT:

A. Females - Pubic hair development

Tanner Stage 1- pre-pubertal, pubic hair is absent

Tanner Stage 2- fine sparse, straight hair along the vulva

Tanner Stage 3-darker, coarser, and slightly curly that extends over the mid pubis

Tanner Stage 4-adult type hair that covers the eternal genitalia but does not extend to the thighs

Tanner Stage 5-adult type hair that extends to the medial thighs

B. Females - Breast Development

Tanner Stage 1- flat appearance with only the papilla (nipple) raised

Tanner Stage 2- a breast "bud" under the enlarging areola

Tanner Stage 3- further enlargement of the breast tissue beyond the margins of the areola

Tanner Stage 4- formation of a secondary mound of the widening and darkening areola above the breast tissue (considered sexual maturity)

Tanner Stage 5- recession of the areola to the same level of skin overlying breast tissue and projection of the papilla beyond the areola and breast (some normal adult women only reach stage 5 in pregnancy)

PUBERTAL GROWTH AND DEVELOPMENT *(continued from previous page)*

STAGES OF NORMAL DEVELOPMENT *(continued)*

C. Males - Pubic Hair Development

Tanner Stage 1- pre-pubertal pubic hair is absent

Tanner Stage 2-fine sparse straight hair at the base of the penis

Tanner Stage 3-darker, coarser, slightly curly hair over the mid pubis

Tanner Stage 4- thicker, more curled adult like hair but covers eternal genitalia but not thighs

Tanner Stage 5-adult like hair that extends to the medial thigh

D. Males – Genitalia

Tanner Stage 1 – pre-pubertal, testes, scrotum and penis are the same as early childhood

Tanner Stage 2 – enlargement of testes and scrotum but no enlargement of the penis

Tanner Stage 3 – continued enlargement of the testes and scrotum along with penile growth

Tanner Stage 4 – continued growth of testes, scrotum and penis, with enlargement of the glans

Tanner Stage 5 – mature genitalia[3]

NOTES:

FEMALES

- Pubertal growth spurt for girls is just before menarche and then growth slows. They can gain approximately 4 pounds per year during this time.[4]
- Pubertal development is considered precocious in those who show signs of early pubertal development in African American girls younger than six and Caucasian girls younger than seven.[5]
- The pubertal growth spurt in girls begins shortly after breast budding. Approximately 99% of girl's growth is complete at a bone age of 15 years.[6]
- Menstruation usually starts about two 1/2 years after the onset of puberty at an average age of 12.5.[7]
- Obesity advances the onset of puberty in girls.
- Asymmetric breast development is a normal variation in pubertal progression.
- It may be 18 to 24 months after menarche before there are regular ovulatory cycles.[8]
- Bone health is very important for girls entering puberty and greatly impacts bone health later in life.

PUBERTAL GROWTH AND DEVELOPMENT *(continued from previous page)*

NOTES *(continued)*

MALES

- The pubertal growth spurt for boys begins an average of two years later than girls. In males, linear growth accelerates during the period of late *mid-puberty* to early late-*puberty*, generally between 12 and 16 years old, but males can continue to grow beyond their teenage years.[9]
- Testicular enlargement is the first clinically significant pubertal event in boys.[10] (see scale below)
- Approximately one half to one third of boys develop gynecomastia (visible or palpable development of breast tissue in males) during mid- puberty that may last 12 to 18 months and resolves in almost all by late puberty.[11]
- Boys can add 13-14 inches and forty pounds in three to four years.
- Voice changes, wet dreams, involuntary erections, breast enlargement and having one testicle lower than the other are all part of the normal growth process.

POTENTIAL COMPLICATIONS:

- The absence of menses after a female has achieved breast development to Stage 4 and has completed a growth spurt may be a cause for concern and indicates a referral to a healthcare provider.
- The onset of vaginal bleeding without a growth spurt or breast development may be a cause for concern and indicates a referral to a healthcare provider.
- Breast development in a boy before puberty is abnormal.
- Delayed puberty is defined as a lack of breast development by age 13 years in girls,[12] and a lack of pubertal testicular development (genital stage 2) by age 14 in boys.[13]
- Girls are vulnerable to the reproductive effects of undernutrition and stress. Decreased body fat is a major cause of pubertal delay in girls. It can be seen in girls who are very athletic or in girls with anorexia nervosa.[14]
- Missing a menstrual cycle for 90 or more days or having an average cycle length less than 21 days is abnormal for a girl of any age. An average cycle length of more than 45 days by two years after menarche is a risk factor. (*Refer to MENSTRAUL DISORDERS*).
- Abrupt testicular pain should be an immediate referral for evaluation of potential testicular torsion.
- Boys with gynecomastia that is unresolved or resembles the breasts of a female in Stage 3-5 of development should be evaluated for a potential pathological condition.
- Boys are more likely than girls to have an underlying pathology for a cause for early puberty.[15]
- Boys with chronic illnesses such as inflammatory bowel disease, sickle cell disease or cystic fibrosis may mature later.
- The physical and psychological changes of puberty add to the challenges of diabetes management. Throughout puberty, the response to insulin decreases and may cause insulin requirements to rise.[16] (*Refer to DIABETES TYPE 1).*

PUBERTAL GROWTH AND DEVELOPMENT *(continued from previous page)*

RESOURCE

Maturity Sexual Chart (Tanner). Vermont Department of Health (n.d.). *The Tanner Stages.* https://www.medschool.lsuhsc.edu/medical_education/undergraduate/spm/SPM_100/documents/tannerstagescard.pdf

REFERENCES

[1] American Academy of Pediatrics. (2015). *Physical changes during puberty.* https://www.healthychildren.org/English/ages-stages/gradeschool/puberty/Pages/Physical-Development-of-School-Age-Children.aspx

[2] Garzon, D. & Dunn, A. (2017). Developmental management of adults. In C. Burns, A.M. Dunn, M.A. Brady, N.B. Starr, C.G. Blosser, & D.L. Garzon (Eds.), Pediatric *primary care* (6th ed., pp. 121-125). Elsevier, Inc.

[3] Ibid.

[4] Mattey, E. (2019). Growth and development: Preschool through adolescence. In J. Selekman, R. Adair Shannon, & C. F. Yonkaitis (Eds.), *School nursing: A comprehensive text* (3rd ed., pp. 202- 239). F.A. Davis.

[5] Ibid.

[6] Garzon, D. & Dunn, A. (2017). Developmental management of adults. In C. Burns, A.M. Dunn, M.A. Brady, N.B. Starr, C.G. Blosser, & D.L. Garzon (Eds.), *Pediatric primary care* (6th ed., pp. 121-125). Elsevier, Inc.

[7] Ibid.

[8] Ibid.

[9] Ibid.

[10] Ibid.

[11] Ibid.

[12] American Academy of Pediatrics. (2015) *Delayed puberty in girls: Information for parents.* https://www.healthychildren.org/English/ages-stages/gradeschool/puberty/Pages/Delayed-Puberty-in-Girls-Information-for-Parents.aspx

[13] American Academy of Pediatrics. (2015). *Delayed puberty in boys: Information for parents.* https://www.healthychildren.org/English/ages-stages/gradeschool/puberty/Pages/Delayed-Puberty.aspx

[14] American Academy of Pediatrics. (2015) *Delayed puberty in girls: Information for parents.* https://www.healthychildren.org/English/ages-stages/gradeschool/puberty/Pages/Delayed-Puberty-in-Girls-Information-for-Parents.aspx

[15] Mattey, E. (2019). Growth and development: Preschool through adolescence. In J. Selekman, R. Adair Shannon, & C. F. Yonkaitis (Eds.), *School nursing: A comprehensive text* (3rd ed., pp. 202- 239). F.A. Davis.

[16] Trast, J. (2014). Diabetes and puberty: A glycemic challenge. *American Journal of Nursing, 111*(7), 26-35. https://doi.org/10.1097/01.NAJ.0000451674.51200.6e

PUBERTAL GROWTH AND DEVELOPMENT *(continued from previous page)*

OTHER REFERENCES CONSULTED

American Academy of Pediatrics. (2015). *Concerns boys have about puberty.* https://www.healthychildren.org/English/ages-stages/gradeschool/puberty/Pages/Concerns-Boys-Have-About-Puberty.aspx

American Academy of Pediatrics. (2015). *Concerns girls have about puberty.* https://www.healthychildren.org/English/ages-stages/gradeschool/puberty/Pages/Concerns-Girls-Have-About-Puberty.aspx

American Academy of Pediatrics. (2015). *Physical development: What's normal? What's not?* Healthychildren.org. https://www.healthychildren.org/English/ages-stages/gradeschool/puberty/Pages/Physical-Development-Whats-Normal-Whats-Not.aspx

American Academy of Pediatrics. (2015). *Physical development: What's normal? What's not?* Healthychildren.org. https://www.healthychildren.org/English/ages-stages/gradeschool/puberty/Pages/Physical-Development-Whats-Normal-Whats-Not.aspx

Rasmussen, A.R., Wohlfahrt-Veje, C., Tefre de Renzy-Martin, K., Hagen, C.P., Tinggaard, J., Mouritsen, A., Mieritz, M.G., & Main, K.M. (2015). Validity of self-assessment of pubertal maturation. *Pediatrics 135*(1), 86-93. https://doi.org/10.1542/peds.*2014-0793*

PUNCTURE WOUNDS

DEFINITION/ETIOLOGY:

Small but deep hole produced by penetrating object.[1] Sharp pointed objects such as nails, tacks, pencils, knife and teeth can cause puncture wounds. Most often occurs in hands and feet but can be any body surface area.[2] Object may penetrate the skin and leave a hole or remain partially or completely in wound. Puncture wounds are typically deeper than lacerations or abrasions.[3]

SIGNS AND SYMPTOMS:

If small object:

- Small hole at puncture site
- Little to no bleeding
- Potential for retained foreign body
- History of injury

If larger object:

- May be medical emergency
- May cause heavy bleeding and injury to areas beneath puncture site

Puncture wounds to the head, genital areas, eye, neck, chest or abdomen are serious. Seek immediate medical treatment. If necessary, call Emergency Medical Services (EMS).

MANAGEMENT/TREATMENT:[4]

1. Use standard/universal precautions. (*Refer to STANDARD PRECAUTIONS APPENDIX*).
2. Contact parent/guardian per school or district policies. Puncture wounds to the head, genital areas, eye, neck, chest or abdomen are serious. Seek immediate medical treatment. If necessary, call Emergency Medical Services (EMS) first, then immediately contact parent/guardian.
3. Apply pressure with a clean cloth or bandage for several minutes to stop bleeding.
4. Once bleeding has stopped, wash around the wound with antibacterial soap and water.
5. Irrigate the wound with running water to remove debris.
6. If debris remains in wound after irrigation with water, do not probe or pull debris from a wound as it may splinter and leave pieces; refer to healthcare provider for follow-up care.
7. If embedded object in wound, minimize movement and leave object in place.
8. Do not try to clean a major wound as it may cause heavy bleeding.
9. Do **NOT** clean the wound with h*ydrogen peroxide. Hydrogen peroxide is not appropriate for fresh wounds; it damages tissues and interferes with healing.*
10. Apply antibiotic ointment and bandage per school district policy. Do not seal the hole with non-porous bandage.
11. Determine cause of puncture, e.g., nail, glass, wood, human, or animal bite, etc.
12. Seek medical treatment if puncture wound is caused by an animal bite. Follow state, school or district protocol regarding reporting animal bites.
13. Determine date of last tetanus booster and refer to healthcare provider if booster is needed. If needed, should have tetanus booster within 48 hours of injury.
14. Seek emergency medical services if wound is deep, bleeding heavily or a large object is embedded in the wound.

PUNCTURE WOUNDS *(continued from previous page)*

FOLLOW-UP:

- Monitor for signs of infection. Signs and symptoms of infection that require a referral to healthcare provider include:
  - Early signs and symptoms: increased pain, redness around the edge of wound, swelling, fever and tenderness
  - Late signs and symptoms: fever, purulent drainage and infected lymph nodes (lymphangitis) caused by a bacterial infection which will cause a red streak from infected area to armpit or groin.
  - Educate student and family on how to care for the wound such as:[5]
    - Clean the wound with antibacterial soap and water.
    - Watch for possible signs and symptoms of infection (i.e. hot, warm to touch, red, pus or colored discharge).
    - Apply antibiotic ointment, over the counter (such as Polysporin®). No prescription is needed. Then, cover with a bandage (such as Band-Aid®). This helps to reduce the risk of infection.
    - Re-wash the wound and put on antibiotic ointment every 12 hours. Do this for 2 days.
    - **If it looks infected call healthcare provider immediately for further instructions**.

POTENTIAL COMPLICATIONS:

- Puncture wounds may be hard to clean resulting in increased risk of infection.
- Wounds can often be deep with little bleeding so there is an increased risk of infection due to germs being embedded and not washed out by the flow of blood.
- Tetanus is a danger with puncture wound because tetanus bacteria (*Clostridium tetani)* grow well in a deep wound with little oxygen.[6]
- Puncture wounds obtained by stepping on a nail has increased risk of contracting a pseudomonas infection.[7]
- Wounds resulting from an animal or human bite are at increased risk of becoming infected.[8]

NOTES:

- Pencils are not made of lead but nontoxic graphite. Pencil lead is rarely embedded after puncture but more likely the "tattoo" from the graphite leaving a mark.[9]

PUNCTURE WOUNDS *(continued from previous page)*

REFERENCES

[1] Mayo Clinic. (2019*). Puncture wounds: First aid.* https://www.mayoclinic.org/search/search-results?q=puncture%20wounds

[2] Boston Children's Hospital. (2019) *Treatments for puncture wounds in childre*n. http://www.childrenshospital.org/conditions-and-treatments/conditions/p/puncture-wounds/treatments

[3] Mayo Clinic. (2019*). Puncture wounds: First aid.* https://www.mayoclinic.org/search/search-results?q=puncture%20wounds

[4] Jakubowski, T., & Perron, T. (2019). Students with common complaints. In J. Selekman, R. Adair Shannon, & C. F. Yonkaitis (Eds.), *School nursing: A comprehensive text* (3rd ed., pp.335-367). F. A. Davis.

[5] Kids Clinic (2019). *Is your child sick? Puncture wound*. Schmitt Pediatric Guidelines. http://kidsclinic.pediatricweb.com/Is-Your-Child-Sick/Is-Your-Child-Sick/Puncture-Wound

[6] Boston Children's Hospital. (2019) *Treatments for puncture wounds in childre*n. http://www.childrenshospital.org/conditions-and-treatments/conditions/p/puncture-wounds/treatments

[7] Mayo Clinic. (2019*). Puncture wounds: First aid.* https://www.mayoclinic.org/search/search-results?q=puncture%20wounds

[8] Kids Clinic. (2019). *Is your child sick? Puncture wound*. Schmitt Pediatric Guidelines. http://kidsclinic.pediatricweb.com/Is-Your-Child-Sick/Is-Your-Child-Sick/Puncture-Wound

[9] Ibid.

OTHER REFERENCES CONSULTED

MedlinePlus. U.S. National Library of Medicine. (2019). *Cuts and puncture wounds.* http://www.nlm.nih.gov/medlineplus/ency/article/000043.htm

WebMD. (2019*). First aid & emergencies.* http://firstaid.webmd.com/tc/cuts-topic-overview

RASHES

Differential Diagnosis of Common Childhood Disease Associated with Rash

	Hand, Foot, & Mouth Disease[1]	Pityriasis rosea[2]	Roseola[3]	Scarlet Fever (scarlatina)[4]	Fifth Disease[5]	Shingles[6]
Etiology	Enterovirus most often caused by coxsackievirus A16	Unknown	Viral, Human Herpes virus & herpes	Streptococcus Bacteria	Human Parvovirus B19	Reactivation of latent varicella-zoster virus
Characteristics of Rash	Vesicles on a erythematous base that erode to form ulcers Deep seated vesico-pustules thtat are white gray on the palms and soles	A generalized eruption of individual lesions, erythematous papules and small oval plaques with scales	Small flat pink spots or patches not usually itchy Last 2-3 days	Bright red rash, feels like sandpaper prominent on the armpits and groin lasts 2-5 days Tongue may appear strawberry-like When rash fades, skin peels from tips of fingers and toes	Red, patchy facial rash ("slapped cheek") Exanthem may spread to include trunk and extremities 1-4 days after the facial rash appears ("lacy looking") Cold-like symptoms may precede rash May be asymptomatic	Grouped erythematous papules or circumscribed erythematous patches that evolve to discreat grouped vesilcels
Part of body rash first appears on	Most common on buccal mucosa and tongue	First occurs with a round or oval erythematous patch with a scaling border and central clearing know as a "herald patch"	Chest, abdomen and back	Neck, face, palms of hands and tips of fingers and toes	Face, cheeks and trunk	Usually unilateral, following dermatones and may be preceeded by pain and itching
Spreads to	Typically lesions are limited to the palms and soles but may involve lateral surfaces of hands and feet, buttocks, elbow, knees and perimeum	Within 2 weeks of the herald patch, the lesions usually are concentrated on the trunk, back with an alignment that resembles a Christmas tree distribution	Neck and arms	Chest, back, and rest of body	May spread to rest of body in lace-like pattern	Vesicles may become cloudy before rupturing and cause crusts
Progression and time intervals for diagnosis	Blisters generally last a little more than one week	New lesions may appear for 2-3 weeks and the resolves typically over several weeks to months	Usually 10 days; range 5-15 days	1-3 days, can be up to 5 days	Variable, 4-20 days	Process lasts 1-3 weeks

School Nurse Guidelines For

Severity of illness	Generally mild	Generally mild	Usually mild to moderate	Mild to moderate	Mild, resolves on its own	Symptoms can be mild but can also be extensive especially in immune-suppressed patients
Associated symptoms other than rash	May be preceded by fever and malaise and less frequently cough and diarrhea	May be a mild itch	Sudden fever up to 103°, cough, runny nose, sore throat fever which may last 3-5 days and prior to the rash	Sudden onset of fever and sore throat/tonsillitis with tender, enlarged lymph nodes, abdominal pain, vomiting, headache and foul odor from the mouth	Fever, headache, runny nose Joint swelling and pain is more common is adults	May be preceded by fever, headache, malaise, pain and itching
Complications	Usually none	Usually none	Usually none Can cause febrile seizures in children and is a risk for those with weak immune system	Rare with appropriate treatment but may include, rheumatic fever, carditis, painful joints, otitis media, sinus infection, kidney infection, meningitis, sepsis and pneumonia	Usually none Can cause Pneumonia Can be serious with weak immune system, anemia, cancer or pregnancy	Scarring, viral dissemination may occur in extensive disease predominately with immunocompro-mised persons
Period of Infectivity	Virus may be shed for weeks to months in the stool although respiratory shedding is limited to 1-3 weeks	none	Unknown Contagious even if no rash is present.	Infectious for 10-21 days if untreated or until 12 hours after start of antibiotic treatment	Most infectious before the onset of rash; not contagious after rash appears	Spread through direct contact with blisters and infectious until the vesicles are scabbed
Additional information	The child can attend school as exclusion will not reduce disease transmission as some children may shed the virus withought being ill and others may shed the virus in the stool for week[7]	Benign and self limiting common in children and young adults	No specific control or preventive measures indicated Most children have had Roseola by the time they enter kindergarten	Curable with penicillin control measures: Emphasize respiratory etiquette ("cover your cough") and frequent hand washing Common in 5-15-year olds About 25% of school children carry the bacteria in their nose and mouth and are not ill. The risk of transmission from a carrier is low	Proper hand hygiene encouraged Although very rare, pregnant women who are immune may develop fetal complications such as severe anemia for the fetus. As this is very common in the school aged populations pregnant staff should be referred to their healthcare provider	Vaccination with 2 doses of the vaccine is key preventive measure Although rare, some children who have had the vaccine may still develop a mild case of chicken-pox Do not use aspirin to treat symptoms The child can attend school as long as the rash can be covered[8]

RASHES *(continued)*

NOTES:

Infection control measures should be considered in regards to the anticipated contact to prevent the spread of communicable diseases. In general, children may be excluded from school for medical reasons related to communicable diseases or due to program or staffing requirements.

Follow local health department directives and school policy in regard to exclusion from school. In general, exclusion should be considered based on the following criteria:

- If children are not able to fully participate in the program
- If elevated temperature
- When the level of care during and illness is not able to be met without jeopardizing the safety of other children
- When the risk or spread of disease to other children cannot be avoided with the appropriate environmental or individual management

> NOTE: Vaccine preventable rashes (Rubeola, rubella, varicella) - If an outbreak occurs at school unvaccinated students and staff may need to be excluded from school/work per health department guidelines.

(Refer to MEASLES/RUBELLA, VARICLLEA, FIFTH DISEASE and SHINGLES for additional information).

REFERENCES

[1] American Academy of Pediatrics. (2016). Hand, foot, & mouth disease (HFMD) and other enteroviral exanthems. In A. J. Mancini, & D. P. Krowchuk (Eds.), *Pediatric dermatology* (3rd ed., pp. 125-132). American Academy of Pediatrics.

[2] American Academy of Pediatrics. (2016). Pityriasis rosea. In A. J. Mancini, & D. P. Krowchuk (Eds.), *Pediatric dermatology* (3rd ed., pp. 331-334). American Academy of Pediatrics.

[3] Mayo Clinic. (2019). *Roseola*. https://www.mayoclinic.org/diseases-conditions/roseola/symptoms-causes/syc-20377283

[4] American Academy of Pediatrics. (2020). Strep throat (streptococcal pharyngitis) and scalet fever. In S. Aronson, & T. Shope (Eds.), *Managing infectious diseases in child care and schools* (5th ed., pp. 163). American Academy of Pediatrics.

[5] Centers for Disease Control and Prevention. (2015). *Parvovirus 19 and fifth disease*. https://www.cdc.gov/parvovirusb19/fifth-disease.html

[6] American Academy of Pediatrics. (2016). Herpes zoster. In A. J. Mancini, & D. P. Krowchuk (Eds.), *Pediatric dermatology* (3rd ed., p. 99-102). American Academy of Pediatrics.

[7] American Academy of Pediatrics. (2020). Hand-foot- and- mouth disease. In S. Aronson, & T. Shope (Eds.), *Managing infectious diseases in child care and schools* (5th ed., pp. 101-102). American Academy of Pediatrics.

[8] American Academy of Pediatrics. (2020). Shingles. In S. Aronson, & T. Shope (Eds.), *Managing infectious diseases in child care and schools* (5th ed., pp. 163). American Academy of Pediatrics.

RINGWORM – TINEA

DEFINITION/ETIOLOGY:
Ringworm is caused by a fungus which can affect the skin, nails and hair. The fungi are microscopic organisms that live on the skin and usually cause no concern or harm. When they cause a skin infection they are known as tinea infections.[1]

Tinea corporis:	Ringworm of the body (face, trunk and extremities)[2]
Tinea capitis:	Ringworm of the scalp
Tinea cruris:	Ringworm of the groin area (also called jock itch)
Tinea pedis:	Ringworm of the feet (also called athlete's foot)
Onychomycosis:	Ringworm of the nails

Symptoms often depend on area of the body that is infected but general symptoms are itchy skin; ring shaped rash; red, scaly, cracked skin; and hair loss.[3] Ringworm spreads easily from people and animals.[4] It also spreads from one part of the body to another.[5] The fungi that cause ringworm thrive in warm, moist environments.[6] Ringworm can be spread through shared towels, clothing and bedding. It can be spread via hard moist surfaces such as shower stall, locker room floors and pool areas.[7]

Incubation period is typically four to 14 days after exposure to fungi that causes ringworm.[8]
Most mild cases of ringworm typically clear up in 2 to 4 weeks with treatment.[9] Treatment may be needed for up to three months if the infection affects the nails or the scalp.[10]

SIGNS AND SYMPTOMS:
Tinea pedis: Red, swollen, itchy, peeling, scaly lesions, between toes and on plantar surface of foot.[11] Vesiculo-papular (blisters or tiny pimples) seen in more severe cases.[12] Lesions may become infected due to scratching.[13] It is most commonly seen in males, those who frequently wear damp socks and tight-fitting shoes and those who walk barefoot in public areas such as locker rooms.[14]

Tinea cruris: Redness, flaking, peeling or cracking of the skin between upper thighs extending onto groin, buttocks and may involve scrotum in males. The rash can look circular, and sometimes with raised edges. Also referred to as "jock itch". Typically seen in males and rarely in females. Jock itch often spreads from athletes' foot.[15]

Tinea corporis: Small, scaly, red lesion on the body or face that as it enlarges it becomes ring-like with a raised erythematous border and clear center. The lesions may be single or multiple, frequently itchy and can become infected. Tinea corporis is not uncommon in student wrestlers because of prolonged skin to skin contact.[16]

Tinea capitis: Red, scaly, itchy, rash on scalp with patches of hair loss. Can be very contagious among children. Mostly seen in children ages two to 10. Rare in adults. Can develop into a kerion, a large tender lesion over the area of ringworm, which is from a hypersensitivity reaction to the fungus.[17]

Onychomycosis: Thick and yellowed nails. It frequently affects toenails rather than fingernails. It occurs more often in adolescents and adults and is rare in young children.[18]

RINGWORM – TINEA *(continued from previous page)*

MANAGEMENT/TREATMENT:

1. Keep skin and feet clean and dry. Change socks regularly.[19]
2. When used as directed, over the counter (OTC) anti-fungal medications (creams) can effectively treat mild cases of ringworm. More severe cases or cases that do not respond in 2-4 weeks with OTC medications should be referred to the healthcare provider for additional medication.[20]
3. Topical antifungal medications are **NOT** effective for the treatment of tinea capitis. Systemic antifungal medication is required for up to 4-8 weeks and should be continued for 2 weeks after resolution.[21]
4. Students with tinea capitis should be instructed not to share combs, hats, hair ribbons, or brushes.[22] <u>They should not be excluded from school once treatment is started</u>.[23]
5. Students should avoid contact sports, such as wrestling, for 72 hours after treatment was started.[24]
6. Students with tinea cruris, tinea corporis, or tinea pedis should be excluded at the end of the school day and be readmitted once treatment is initiated or per district policy.[25]
7. Students with tinea pedis should be prohibited from walking barefoot on locker room and shower floors until treatment has been initiated. They should be encouraged to always wear waterproof shoes or flip-flops when walking around in locker rooms, public showers, and public pool areas.[26]
8. Siblings and household contacts should be evaluated.

FOLLOW-UP:

- Symptoms of ringworm may resemble other skin conditions. Healthcare provider should be contacted if ringworm is suspected.[27]
- Refer severe cases (those which do not improve after 1 week of starting OTC treatment) to healthcare provider or if the rash lasts more than 4 weeks.[28]
- Inform parent/guardian to check contacts, family members, and pets.
- Work with maintenance personnel, teachers, and coaches to assure proper cleaning of headphones, swimming pool and locker areas, gym mats, wrestling headgear, and other equipment with which skin contact is common.

POTENTIAL COMPLICATIONS:

Infection. Especially in those with weaken immune systems.[29]

NOTES:[30, 31, 32, 33]

Prevention should include:

- Wash hands thoroughly with soap and water after petting or playing with pets.
- Keep skin dry and clean.
- Shampoo hair regularly, especially after haircuts
- Do not share clothing, shoes, towels, hairbrushes, combs, headgear, or other personal care items.
- Avoid walking barefoot in public places.
- Wear waterproof shoes or "flip-flops" in public showers and swimming pool areas.
- Change socks and underwear daily and more often if damp with sweat.

RINGWORM – TINEA *(continued from previous page)*

NOTES *(continued)*

- Use powder on feet to absorb moisture.
- Keep shared areas (especially gym) clean. Shower after sports and keep uniform and gear clean.
- Stay cool and dry and change clothing that becomes sweaty or wet.
- Make sure safety mats and other surfaces that might be home to infectious bacteria, such as Methicillin-resistant Staphylococcus aureus (MRSA), ringworm and impetigo, are disinfected often (preferably daily).[34]

REFERENCES

[1] Kids Health/Nemours. (2018). *Ringworm.* https://kidshealth.org/en/parents/fungal-ringworm.html?ref=search

[2] Merck Manual Professional Version. (2018). *Tinea corporis.* https://www.merckmanuals.com/professional/dermatologic-disorders/fungal-skin-infections/tinea-corporis?query=tinea

[3] Centers for Disease Control and Prevention. (2018). *Symptoms of ringworm infections.* https://www.cdc.gov/fungal/diseases/ringworm/symptoms.html

[4] Centers for Disease Control and Prevention. (2018). *Ringworm Information for healthcare professionals.* https://www.cdc.gov/fungal/diseases/ringworm/health-professionals.html

[5] Ibid.

[6] Kids Health/Nemours. (2018). *Ringworm.* https://kidshealth.org/en/kids/ringworm-infection.html?ref=search

[7] Centers for Disease Control and Prevention. (2018). *Ringworm information for healthcare professionals.* https://www.cdc.gov/fungal/diseases/ringworm/health-professionals.html

[8] Centers for Disease Control and Prevention. (2018). *Symptoms of ringworm infections.* https://www.cdc.gov/fungal/diseases/ringworm/symptoms.html

[9] Kids Health/Nemours. (2018). *Ringworm.* https://kidshealth.org/en/parents/fungal-ringworm.html?ref=searchpr

[10] Ibid.

[11] Centers for Disease Control and Prevention. (2018). *Symptoms of ringworm infections.* https://www.cdc.gov/fungal/diseases/ringworm/symptoms.html

[12] Ibid.

[13] Kids Health/Nemours. (2018). *First aid: Ringworm.* https://kidshealth.org/en/parents/ringworm-sheet.html?ref=search

[14] Kids Health/Nemours. (2018). Athletes Foot. https://kidshealth.org/en/parents/athletes-foot.html

[15] Kids Health/Nemours. (2018). *Jock itch.* https://kidshealth.org/en/parents/jock-itch.html?ref=search

[16] American Academy of Pediatrics. (2016). Tinea corporis. In A. J. Mancini, & D. P. Krowchuk (Eds.), *Pediatric dermatology* (3rd ed., p. 263). American Academy of Pediatrics.

[17] Boston Children's Hospital. (n.d.). *Ringworm.* http://www.childrenshospital.org/conditions-and-treatments/conditions/r/ringworm/symptoms-and-causes

[18] Ibid.

[19] Mayo Clinic. (2019). *Ringworm (body).* https://www.mayoclinic.org/diseases-conditions/ringworm-body/symptoms-causes/syc-20353780

[20] Ibid.

RINGWORM – TINEA *(continued from previous page)*

[21] Mayo Clinic. (2018). Ringworm (scalp). https://www.mayoclinic.org/diseases-conditions/ringworm-scalp/symptoms-causes/syc-20354918

[22] Mayo Clinic. (2019). *Ringworm (body).* https://www.mayoclinic.org/diseases-conditions/ringworm-body/symptoms-causes/syc-20353780

[23] American Academy of Pediatrics. (2016). Tinea capitis. In A. J. Mancini, & D. P. Krowchuk (Eds.), *Pediatric dermatology* (3rd ed., pp. 261). American Academy of Pediatrics.

[24] Seattle Children's Hospital. (2019). *Ringworm.* https://www.seattlechildrens.org/conditions/a-z/ringworm/

[25] Ibid.

[26] Teens Health/Nemours. (2018). *Athlete's foot.* https://kidshealth.org/en/teens/athletes-foot.html?ref=search

[27] Boston Children's Hospital. (n.d.). *Ringworm.* http://www.childrenshospital.org/conditions-and-treatments/conditions/r/ringworm/symptoms-and-causes

[28] Seattle Children's Hospital. (2019). *Ringworm.* https://www.seattlechildrens.org/conditions/a-z/ringworm/

[29] Mayo Clinic. (2019). *Ringworm (body).* https://www.mayoclinic.org/diseases-conditions/ringworm-body/symptoms-causes/syc-20353780

[30] Centers for Disease Control and Prevention. (2018). *Ringworm risk & prevention.* https://www.cdc.gov/fungal/diseases/ringworm/risk-prevention.html

[31] Mayo Clinic. (2018). *Ringworm (scalp).* https://www.mayoclinic.org/diseases-conditions/ringworm-scalp/symptoms-causes/syc-20354918

[32] Teens Health/Nemours. (2018). *Athlete's foot.* https://kidshealth.org/en/teens/athletes-foot.html?ref=search

[33] Mayo Clinic. (2019). *Ringworm (body).* https://www.mayoclinic.org/diseases-conditions/ringworm-body/symptoms-causes/syc-20353780

[34] Mayo Clinic. (2019). *MRSA: Protecting student athletes.* https://www.mayoclinic.org/diseases-conditions/mrsa/in-depth/mrsa/art-20047876

ROTAVIRUS

DEFINITION/ETIOLOGY:

Rotavirus is a contagious virus that may result in gastroenteritis or inflammation of the intestines and stomach.[1] Severe diarrhea, abdominal pain, fever and vomiting are among the classic symptoms of rotavirus. While adults can be infected, the highest rates of this disease occur among young children and infants. A child's first infection with rotavirus is usually by five years old and tends to cause the most severe symptoms.[2]

A laboratory testing of stool specimen is required to diagnose rotavirus disease, which has an incubation period of approximately two days. Although the virus is stable in the environment, annual epidemics of Rotavirus in the United States occurs mostly from December through June. During the winter and spring seasonal pattern, it is not uncommon for children to experience multiple episodes of rotavirus disease since neither vaccine nor natural infection provide full immunity from future infections.[3]

The primary mode of transmission is fecal-oral. Additionally, transmission is usually through direct contact between people; may occur through contact with contaminated surfaces or objects; and ingestion of contaminated food or water.[4]

SIGNS AND SYMPTOMS:

- Watery diarrhea and vomiting (usually lasting three to eight days)
- Abdominal pain
- Fever
- Loss of appetite
- Dehydration:[5]
    - Decreased urination
    - Dry mouth and throat
    - Feeling dizzy when standing up
    - Crying with few or no tears and
    - Unusual sleepiness or fussiness

MANAGEMENT/TREATMENT:

- There is no specific treatment for rotavirus infection. Treatment is based on symptoms.
- Oral rehydration to prevent dehydration during rotavirus infection is the primary focus.
- Severe dehydration may require hospitalization for intravenous fluids.[6]

FOLLOW UP:

Two vaccines are available for preventing rotavirus disease among infants and children:[7]

1. RotaTeq® (RV5) is given in three doses at ages 2 months, 4 months, and 6 months.
2. Rotarix® (RV1) is given in two doses at ages 2 months and 4 months.[8]

The first dose of either vaccines above should be given before 15 weeks of age, with all doses of rotavirus vaccine administered to children before they turn 8 months of age.[9]

ROTAVIRUS *(continued from previous page)*

POTENTIAL COMPLICATIONS:

- Severe dehydration from rotavirus disease.
- Although very rare, some studies suggest that one side effect of the rotavirus vaccinations include a small increase in the risk of intussusception (a type of bowel blockage).[10]

NOTES:

- Proper hand hygiene can reduce the spread of rotavirus infection. Hands should be washed thoroughly after each use of toilet, in assisting children to use the toilet, and after diapering. *(Refer to HANDWASHING APPENDIX).*
- Contaminated surfaces should be disinfected.[11]
- Babies should not get the rotavirus vaccine if they have a life-threatening allergy to a dose of the vaccine, have severe combined immunodeficiency, and have had intussusception. Additionally, babies who are experiencing moderate or severe diarrhea or vomiting should first recover, before the vaccine is given.[12]
- The healthcare provider should be called if a child has:
    - Diarrhea for more than 24 hours
    - Severe or bloody diarrhea
    - Frequent episodes of vomiting
    - Temperature of 104°F or higher
    - Seems lethargic, irritable, or in pain
    - Has signs or symptoms of dehydration, e.g. dry mouth, crying without tears, little or no urination, unusual sleepiness or unresponsiveness[13]

REFERENCES

[1] Centers for Disease Control and Prevention. (2018). *Rotavirus*. https://www.cdc.gov/rotavirus/index.html

[2] Centers for Disease Control and Prevention. (2018). *Rotavirus: Clinical information*. https://www.cdc.gov/rotavirus/clinical.html

[3] Ibid.

[4] Ibid.

[5] Ibid.

[6] Ibid.

[7] Centers for Disease Control and Prevention. (2018). *Rotavirus: Vaccination*. https://www.cdc.gov/rotavirus/vaccination.html

[8] Ibid.

[9] Ibid.

[10] Centers for Disease Control and Prevention. (2015). *Rotavirus vaccine safety*. https://www.cdc.gov/vaccinesafety/vaccines/rotavirus-vaccine.html?CDC_AA_refVal=https%3A%2F%2Fwww.cdc.gov%2Fvaccinesafety%2Fvaccines%2FRotaVSB.html

[11] Mayo Clinic. (2019). *Rotavirus*. https://www.mayoclinic.org/diseases-conditions/rotavirus/symptoms-causes/syc-20351300

[12] Centers for Disease Control and Prevention. (2018). *Vaccine information statements*. https://www.cdc.gov/vaccines/hcp/vis/vis-statements/rotavirus.html

[13] Mayo Clinic. (2019). *Rotavirus*. https://www.mayoclinic.org/diseases-conditions/rotavirus/symptoms-causes/syc-20351300

SCABIES

DEFINITION/ETIOLOGY:[1]

Scabies is caused by a tiny, eight-legged burrowing mite called *Sarcoptes scabiei var hominis*. It is a highly contagious infection spread through direct, prolonged, skin-to-skin contact and shared clothing or linen of someone who has scabies. A person infected for the first time may not exhibit symptoms for two to six weeks and can transmit scabies to another person during that time. A person previously infected with scabies may exhibit symptoms as early as one to four days after exposure. In addition, the mite can survive 48-72 hours without human contact. Animals do not spread human scabies.[2]

Crusted scabies is also called Norwegian scabies and is by identified by the increased number of mites. Although crusted scabies is unusual, it is seen in children with long term steroid therapy, and in people with immune deficiencies and developmental disabilities.[3] Scabies is not related to personal hygiene, it affects people regardless of age, sex, or socioeconomic status.[4]

SIGNS AND SYMPTOMS:[5]

- The most common symptom is intense itching, especially at night and the appearance of rash.
- Typical lesion is a "burrow": a tiny, pale, irregular line that marks the path of the scabies mite.
- Rash: tiny (1-2 mm) erythematous papules, vesicles, pustule and scabs, sometimes with tiny, linear dark scabs (0.5-1) mm long.
- Location: webbing between the fingers, flexor surface of wrist and elbow, axillary –skin folds, waist, and thighs and can also spread to breasts and penis.
- **The face, neck, palms and soles** may be involved in infants and very young children **(a good assessment clue).**
- Frequently found in other family members.
- Itching is related to an allergic reaction to mites and may persist a month after successful treatment until top layers of skin are shed.[6]

Diagnostic hints:

1) Appearance and distribution of rash and the presence of burrows.
2) Microscopic examination of skin scrapings for mites, eggs or fecal matter.

ANTICIPATED CONCERNS/PROBLEMS:

- Vigorous scratching can cause breaks in the skin, potentially leading to secondary bacterial infections.

MANAGEMENT/POTENTIAL INTERVENTIONS:[7]

- Exclude from school for prompt treatment. May return next day after proper treatment has been initiated.
- Steroid ointments or lotions are contraindicated.
- Instruct parent/guardian to wash clothes, towels, and bed linen used by the infected person within the previous two days in hot water and dry in hot dryer.
- "Starve the mites". Place items you can't wash in a sealed plastic bag for two weeks.[8]

SCABIES *(continued from previous page)*

MANAGEMENT/POTENTIAL INTERVENTIONS *(continued)*

- MEDICATIONS:[9]
  - Over the counter (OTC) products have not been approved to treat human scabies.
  - Scabacides are available by prescription from the healthcare provider. The medication is usually applied at home by a parent or guardian.
  - The usual prescription product is permethrin 5% cream (Elimite®). Crotamiton 10% cream (Eurax®) for scabies nodules is approved only for adults. Lindane 1% lotion is available but is rarely used due to side effects.
  - Apply scabacide lotions to the entire body (chin-line to toes.) NEVER ON THE FACE. The lotions should be left on the skin as recommended on the package insert and then washed off thoroughly with soap and water.
  - Use anti-scabetic lotions/creams no more than twice in a month.

FOLLOW-UP:

- Assess each day or two after first treatment.
- Watch for new lesions. A second treatment may be necessary.
- Watch for secondary infection and refer accordingly.
- Check siblings in school.
- Educate staff about scabies and transmission.

NOTES:[10]

- May be asymptomatic the first two to six weeks of an **initial** infection of scabies. However, even though the person is asymptomatic, they remain contagious during this time period.
- Itching may continue after medication treatment.
  - If so, apply cool compresses or soak in an oatmeal bath or cool water.
  - Check with your healthcare provider about using over the counter lotions and/or antihistamines.

REFERENCES

[1] Center for Disease Control and Prevention, Parasites. (2017). *Fact sheet scabies.* https://www.cdc.gov/parasites/scabies/fact_sheet.html

[2] Center for Disease Control and Prevention. (2018). *Scabies frequently asked questions.* https://www.cdc.gov/parasites/scabies/gen_info/faqs.html

[3] American Academy of Pediatrics. (2018). *Scabies.* In D. Kimberlin, (Ed.), *Red Book 2018: Report of the Committee on Infectious Diseases* (31st ed., pp. 718-721). American Academy of Pediatrics.

[4] American Academy of Pediatrics. (2020). Scabies. In S. Aronson, & T. Shope (Eds.), *Managing infectious diseases in child care and schools* (5th ed., p. 159-60). American Academy of Pediatrics.

[5] Mayo Clinic. (2018). *Scabies.* https://www.mayoclinic.org/diseases-conditions/scabies/symptoms-causes/syc-20377378

[6] American Academy of Pediatrics. (2020). Scabies. In S. Aronson, & T. Shope (Eds.), *Managing infectious diseases in child care and schools (5th ed.)* (p. 159-60). Elk Grove Village, IL: American Academy of Pediatrics.

SCABIES *(continued from previous page)*

[7] Ibid.

[8]Mayo Clinic. (2018). *Scabies.* https://www.mayoclinic.org/diseases-conditions/scabies/symptoms-causes/syc-20377378

[9] Centers for Disease and Prevention Parasites, Resources for Health Professionals. (2018). *Medications.* https://www.cdc.gov/parasites/scabies/health_professionals/meds.html

[10] Mayo Clinic. (2018). *Scabies.* https://www.mayoclinic.org/diseases-conditions/scabies/symptoms-causes/syc-20377378

OTHER REFERENCES CONSULTED

American Academy of Dermatology. (n.d.). *Scabies.* www.aad.org/public/diseases/contagious-skin-diseases/scabies#overview

Merck Manual. (2018). *Scabies infestation.* https://www.merckmanuals.com/home/skin-disorders/parasitic-skin-infections/scabies-infestation

SEIZURES - EPILEPSY

DEFINITION/ETIOLOGY:

A seizure results from a sudden abnormal change in the electrical activity in the brain that leads to a change of consciousness, motor activity, behavior, or sensation.[1] Most seizures last 30 seconds to two minutes.[2] Some seizures may go unnoticed because they are brief and only cause a person to stare.[3] Seizures can happen after a stroke, a head injury or an infection, such as meningitis. Other causes may include high fever, lack of sleep, low serum sodium levels, certain medications, brain tumor, use of illegal or recreational drugs, or alcohol abuse. Sometimes the cause is unknown. [4] About 0.6% of children under the age of 17 have active epilepsy.[5]

Four types of seizure include:
1) generalized seizures (absence, atonic, and tonic-clonic)
2) partial seizures (simple and complex)
3) non-epileptic seizures (febrile)
4) status epilepticus (a prolonged seizure without recovery of consciousness requiring immediate medical attention).[6] The area in the brain where the seizure originates will determine the type of seizure.[7] A seizure is not a diagnosis but a symptom of a diagnosis.[8] Epilepsy is diagnosed when you have two or more seizures or a tendency to have recurrent seizures.[9]

SIGNS AND SYMPTOMS:

- Signs and symptoms are dependent on where the problem in the brain is located[10]
- Below are signs and symptoms specific to each type of seizure. Some children may exhibit only a few of these signs while others may have multiple signs.
- When creating an Individualized Healthcare Plan (IHP)/Emergency Care Plan (ECP) it is helpful to note what symptoms are typical for the student.

<u>GENERALIZED: ABSENCE (Non-Motor)</u>[11]

- Abrupt onset and very brief (10-20 seconds) period of cessation of motion
- Unresponsive but no loss of consciousness
- May appear to be staring into space
- Occasional brief muscular twitches
- Chewing motion or blinking of eyes
- Once seizure ends, the child resumes activity and has little or no memory of the event

<u>GENERALIZED: CLONIC-TONIC and ATONIC (Motor)</u>[12]

- Clonic-Tonic = generalized, violent muscle contractions
- Atonic = drop seizures
- Affects most of the body
- Loss of consciousness
- Incontinence of urine/stool
- Sometimes the seizure is preceded by an aura of light, noise or odor
- Dusky facial skin color
- Upward eye deviation
- Post-convulsive state: drowsy to deep sleep, awakened to confusion, headache or speech difficulty

SEIZURES - EPILEPSY *(continued from previous page)*

SIGNS AND SYMPTOMS *(continued)*

PARTIAL SEIZURES

A. Focal Onset Aware (Simple Partial)[13]

- Seizure to one part of the brain
- Awake, alert, and able to recall events that happened during the seizure
- Brief, lasting less than two minutes

B. Focal Onset Impaired Awareness (Complex Partial)[14]

- Purposeful but inappropriate motor acts, often repetitive; running, chewing, swallowing
- Seizure that starts in one area or side of the brain
- Not aware of their surroundings during the seizure
- Can involve involuntary movements like rubbing of the hands, lip-smacking, and chewing
- Impaired consciousness
- Disorientated or confused
- Often sleepy after the seizure
- Last 30 seconds to three minutes

PSYCHOGENIC NON-EPILEPTIC SEIZURES (PNES)[15]

- Not caused by abnormal electrical activity in brain
- May be associated with psychological conditions or other physical problems
- May be triggered by Post Traumatic Stress Disorder (PTSD) or other abnormally high stress situations
- May look like any other seizure activity (generalized or focal seizures)
- Psychological in nature but not purposely produced

STATUS EPILEPTICUS [16]

- The active part of a tonic-clonic seizure lasts five minutes or longer.
- A person goes into a second seizure without recovering consciousness from the first one.
- A person has repeated seizures for 30 minutes or longer.
- Emergency help should be called after a seizure lasting more than five minutes.
- Increased chance of brain and other organ damage.

MANAGEMENT/TREATMENT:

PHARMCOLOGICAL TREATMENT[17]

- Antiepileptic medications are the most common treatment for epilepsy.
- The choice of antiepileptic medications depends on the type of seizure, the age of the person, and the effectiveness of the medication.
- Medication must be taken consistently to maintain therapeutic levels, thus decreasing the chance of a seizure.
- The names of benzodiazepines that are most commonly used as rescue medications include: diazepam (Valium®), lorazepam (Ativan®), and midazolam (Versed®).

SEIZURES - EPILEPSY *(continued from previous page)*

MANAGEMENT/TREATMENT *(continued)*

- Some benzodiazepines can be swallowed in pill form, some can be placed under the tongue or placed between the cheek and the gum, and some can be given rectally or by a nasal spray.
- Rescue medications are administered according to the healthcare provider instructions, the state nursing practice act or directives, and the school district policy usually administered after three to five minutes of continuous seizure. May be considered if student is experiencing multiple seizures that do not have a recovery period between and it has been three to five minutes since initial seizure episode.

NON-PHARMACEUTICAL TREATMENTS

KETOGENIC DIET or Modified Atkins diet[18,19]

- A treatment option for children and adults with seizures that do not respond to antiepileptic drugs (AEDs).
- A high fat, **very low carbohydrate** diet that works by burning stored fat (producing a state of ketosis) versus burning glucose for energy.
- Ketosis prevents or reduces seizures. Side effects include increased serum cholesterol levels, constipation, kidney stones, gallstones, gastrointestinal upset (vomiting, diarrhea), low blood sugar, and weight loss.
- Requires checking urine ketones several times a week.
- Requires supervision by a healthcare provider and a dietitian.
- The complexities of the ketogenic diet require collaboration with the school nurse, healthcare provider, school dietitian, parent or caregiver, and teacher to develop a plan for school.
- Schools must not allow carbohydrate ingestion outside of dietary restrictions. Could result in seizure and negate gains from diet.

VAGAL NERVE STIMULATOR (VNS)[20,21]

- Approved for children four years and older to treat focal or partial seizures that do not respond to seizure medications (also called drug-resistant epilepsy or refractory epilepsy).
- Implanted battery-operated device (similar in concept to a pacemaker), about the size of a silver dollar, that is implanted typically in the chest wall. Battery life is approximately six years.
- Small wires are threaded under the skin and wound around the vagus nerve in the neck.
- The device works by sending regular small pulses of electrical energy to the brain.
- When a person feels a seizure coming on (aura), they can activate an extra dose of stimulation by passing a small magnet over the device to hopefully prevent or shorten the seizure
- The device may also be turned off by holding the magnet over the implanted device.
- Side effects include hoarseness, voice alteration, coughing, and increased salivation.

SURGICAL INTERVENTION[22]

- Removes affected area of the brain
- Performed when other options are not successful
- Reduces or stops seizures

SEIZURES - EPILEPSY *(continued from previous page)*

MANAGEMENT/TREATMENT *(continued)*

IMMEDIATE *FIRST AID* FOR SEIZURE (tonic clonic or atonic seizure)

1. Never leave the student alone during a seizure.[23]
2. Keep calm and reassure other people who may be nearby. Keep onlookers away. [24]
3. DO NOT hold the student down or try to stop movements.[25]
4. Time the seizure.[26]
5. Gently lower the student to the floor.[27]
6. Position the student on his/her the side with the mouth toward the floor to prevent the aspiration of saliva or vomitus.[28]
7. Clear the area around the student of sharp objects or items that may lead to secondary injury.[29]
8. Loosen anything around the student's neck that may interfere with breathing.[30]
9. Place something soft under the student's head.[31]
10. DO NOT try to force the student's mouth open.
11. DO NOT insert any objects into the student's mouth.[32]
12. Reassure the student as consciousness returns.[33]
13. Allow to the student to rest following the seizure.[34]
14. Remain with student until the student is entirely awake.[35]
15. Include in the ECP communication plan and plan for evacuating other students.
16. It's important to observe and document, on a seizure log, what is happening before, during and after a seizure.
17. Note onset time and duration. Include noted alteration in motor, autonomic and sensory functions.[36]

WHEN TO SEEK IMMEDIATE MEDICAL ATTENTION:[37]

- First-time seizure
- Generalized tonic-clonic seizures lasting more than five minutes unless otherwise instructed by the healthcare provider
- Repeated seizures without regaining consciousness between seizures
- A change in seizure pattern or an increase in seizure activity
- Seizure that occurs in the water
- Injury that occurs as a result of the seizure
- Some students will have a healthcare provider order for rectal valium (Diastat® AcuDial™) or Intranasal Midazolam (Versed®) for a seizure lasting a specific amount of time (individual orders vary but often given for seizures lasting over three to five minutes)
- Seek immediate medical attention for students who have the following medical conditions:[38]
  - Diabetes (follow emergency health plan)
  - Brain infection
  - Pregnancy
  - Head injury

SEIZURES - EPILEPSY *(continued from previous page)*

FOLLOW UP:[39]

- Obtain an accurate detailed history including triggers, such as lack of sleep, stress, and not taking prescribed seizure medications etc.
- Develop an IHP/ECP and Section 504 plan or Individualized Education Plan (IEP) if needed.
- Provide an emergency plan for school and Emergency medical services (EMS) personnel.
- Assess school environment for triggers (bright lights, loud noises, etc.).
- Monitor the student for medication effectiveness and untoward side effects.
- Educate all staff including bus drivers on all aspects of seizure care after consulting with parents.
- Educate parent or caregivers about quality of life issues including emotional concerns, driving, cognitive abilities, employment, and securing medical insurance.[40]

NOTES:[41]

- Seizure management/emergencies vary from student to student and should be outlined in IHP and ECP.
- The most frequent cause of a breakthrough seizure is the failure to take prescribed seizure medication(s).
- Febrile seizures are common in young children.
- Some students can stop taking antiepileptic medications after remaining seizure free for a specified length of time. Healthcare provider may consider if after two years seizure free.
- Epilepsy, in rare situations, can cause death.
- Death commonly results from Sudden Unexpected Death in Epilepsy (SUDEP)[42] SUDEP usually occurs immediately after a seizure. Although exact cause of SUDEP is unknown, some factors may be prolonged apnea during seizure, abnormal heart rhythms, or a combination of both.[43]
- The school nurse is responsible for seizure training of school personnel. The school nurse and school personnel must recognize seizures and respond appropriately with seizure first aid.
- Families may choose to use non-conventional, non-FDA approved therapies. The school nurse should be in collaborative communication with family and healthcare provider about student's plan of care. The school nurse must always use sound judgement to deliver care to the student at school within the nurse's scope of practice.
- School nurse should be aware of any federal laws/regulations related to non-conventional therapies.

SEIZURES - EPILEPSY *(continued from previous page)*

REFERENCES

[1] Medline Plus/U.S. National Library of Medicine. (2018). *Seizures.* https://medlineplus.gov/ency/article/003200.htm

[2] Ibid.

[3] Ibid.

[4] Mayo Clinic. (2019). *Seizures.* https://www.mayoclinic.org/diseases-conditions/seizure/symptoms-causes/syc-20365711

[5] Centers for Disease Control and Prevention. (2018). *Epilepsy fast facts.* https://www.cdc.gov/epilepsy/about/fast-facts.htm

[6] Quinn, B.L., & Lepkowski, A. (2019). Students with seizures and epilepsy. In J. Selekman, R.A. Shannon, & C. F. Younkaitis (Eds.), *School Nursing: A comprehensive text* (3rded., pp. 652-672). F.A. Davis Company.

[7] Cosby, M.A., Lyons, E., & Prestidge, L. (2019). Students with acute illness and injury. In J. Selekman, R.A. Shannon, & C. F. Younkaitis (Eds.), *School Nursing: A comprehensive text* (3rded., pp. 439-440). F.A. Davis Company.

[8] Quinn, B.L., & Lepkowski, A. (2019). Students with seizures and epilepsy. In J. Selekman, R.A. Shannon, & C. F. Younkaitis (Eds.), *School Nursing: A comprehensive text* (3rded., pp. 652-672). F.A. Davis Company.

[9] Mayo Clinic. (2019). *Seizures.* https://www.mayoclinic.org/diseases-conditions/seizure/symptoms-causes/syc-20365711

[10] Cosby, M.A., Lyons, E., & Prestidge, L. (2019). Students with acute illness and injury. In J. Selekman, R.A. Shannon, & C. F. Younkaitis (Eds.), *School Nursing: A comprehensive text* (3rded., pp. 439-440). F.A. Davis Company.

[11] Ibid.

[12] Ibid.

[13] Epilepsy Foundation. (2017). *Focal onset aware seizures (simple partial seizures).* https://www.epilepsy.com/learn/types-seizures/focal-onset-aware-seizures-aka-simple-partial-seizures

[14] Ibid.

[15] Cleveland Clinic. (n.d.) *What are non-epileptic seizures?* https://my.clevelandclinic.org/-/scassets/files/org/neurological/epilepsy/patient-guides/1-guide-non-epileptic-seizures.ashx?la=en

[16] Merck Manual. (2018). *Seizures in children.* https://www.merckmanuals.com/home/children-s-health-issues/neurologic-disorders-in-children/seizures-in-children?query=status%20epilepticus

[17] Epilepsy Foundation. (2014). *Using Rescue Treatments.* https://www.epilepsy.com/learn/managing-your-epilepsy/using-rescue-treatments

18 Quinn, B.L., & Lepkowski, A. (2019). Students with seizures and epilepsy. In J. Selekman, R.A. Shannon, & C. F. Younkaitis (Eds.), *School Nursing: A comprehensive text* (3rded., pp. 652-672). F.A. Davis Company.

[19] Merck Manual. (2018). *Seizures in children.* https://www.merckmanuals.com/home/children-s-health-issues/neurologic-disorders-in-children/seizures-in-children?query=status%20epilepticus

[20] Quinn, B.L., & Lepkowski, A. (2019). Students with seizures and epilepsy. In J. Selekman, R.A. Shannon, & C. F. Younkaitis (Eds.), *School Nursing: A comprehensive text* (3rded., pp. 652-672). F.A. Davis Company.

[21] Epilepsy Foundation. (2018). *Vagus Nerve Stimulation (VNS).* https://www.epilepsy.com/learn/treating-seizures-and-epilepsy/devices/vagus-nerve-stimulation-vns

[22] Mayo Clinic. (2019). *Seizures.* https://www.mayoclinic.org/diseases-conditions/seizure/symptoms-causes/syc-20365711

SEIZURES - EPILEPSY *(continued from previous page)*

[23] Quinn, B.L., & Lepkowski, A. (2019). Students with seizures and epilepsy. In J. Selekman, R.A. Shannon, & C. F. Younkaitis (Eds.), *School Nursing: A comprehensive text* (3[rd]ed., pp. 652-672). F.A. Davis Company.

[24] Ibid.

[25] Cosby, M.A., Lyons, E., & Prestidge, L. (2019). Students with acute illness and injury. In J. Selekman, R.A. Shannon, & C. F. Younkaitis (Eds.), *School Nursing: A comprehensive text* (3[rd]ed., pp. 439-440). F.A. Davis Company.

[26] Ibid.

[27] Ibid.

[28] Ibid.

[29] Ibid.

[30] Centers for Disease Control. (2019). *Seizure first aid.* https://www.cdc.gov/epilepsy/about/first-aid.htm

[31] Ibid.

[32] Ibid.

[33] Ibid.

[34] Ibid.

[35] Ibid.

[36] Quinn, B.L., & Lepkowski, A. (2019). Students with seizures and epilepsy. In J. Selekman, R.A. Shannon, & C. F. Younkaitis (Eds.), *School Nursing: A comprehensive text* (3[rd]ed., pp. 652-672). F.A. Davis Company.

[37] Cosby, M.A., Lyons, E., & Prestidge, L. (2019). Students with acute illness and injury. In J. Selekman, R.A. Shannon, & C. F. Younkaitis (Eds.), *School Nursing: A comprehensive text* (3[rd]ed., pp. 439-440). F.A. Davis Company.

[38] Centers for Disease Control. (2019). *Seizure first aid.* https://www.cdc.gov/epilepsy/about/first-aid.htm

[39] Quinn, B.L., & Lepkowski, A. (2019). Students with seizures and epilepsy. In J. Selekman, R.A. Shannon, & C. F. Younkaitis (Eds.), *School Nursing: A comprehensive text* (3[rd]ed., pp. 652-672). F.A. Davis Company.

[40] Merck Manual. (2018). *Seizure disorders.* https://www.merckmanuals.com/home/brain,-spinal-cord,-and-nerve-disorders/seizure-disorders/seizure-disorders

[41] Quinn, B.L., & Lepkowski, A. (2019). Students with seizures and epilepsy. In J. Selekman, R.A. Shannon, & C. F. Younkaitis (Eds.), *School Nursing: A comprehensive text* (3[rd]ed., pp. 652-672). F.A. Davis Company.

[42] Merck Manual. (2018). *Seizure disorders.* https://www.merckmanuals.com/professional/neurologic-disorders/seizure-disorders/seizure-disorders?query=sudep

[43] Centers for Disease Control and Prevention (2018). *Sudden unexpected death in epilepsy (SUDEP).* https://www.cdc.gov/epilepsy/about/sudep/index.htm

SELF-INJURY, NON-SUICIDAL (NSSI)

DEFINITION/ETIOLOGY:

School nurses have become increasingly aware of NSSI, especially at the middle and high school level. In fact, schools are often a common site for identification, referral and intervention for students with mental health concerns. NSSI can be defined as the deliberate, self-harm of one's body without suicidal intent.[1] It has been referred to as self-injury, self- harm and commonly "cutting," although the self- injurious behaviors often encompass more than cutting behaviors. It is important that school nurses understand intentional self- harm and know how to respond.

Although cutting is the most common form of NSSI, burns, placing objects under the skin, rubbing the skin raw with erasers or using any other methods such as razor blades or paper clips can be included. Individuals who engage in NSSI may persistently pick at wounds to interfere with the healing process.

A student who engages in self-injury has a different intent than a student engaging in suicide-related behaviors. NSSI is considered a coping mechanism that provides relief to the student and is often considered a form of self- soothing. Students describe it as a quick fix to address loneliness, emotional pain, intense anger and frustration. Intentional self- injury is not a suicide attempt but with self-injury comes the potential of more serious and even fatal self-aggressive actions.[2] Students who engage in NSSI have an increased risk of suicide. Students may also be seeking to gain the attention of parents or other significant others or to identify with a peer group.[3]

Students are often referred to the school nurse by other students, or by faculty who have witnessed the event. It may also be noted during a physical assessment or a student may self-disclose to the school nurse or other staff.

SIGNS AND SYMPTOMS:[4, 5]

- Unexplained markings or injuries on the skin
- Fresh cuts or scratches, often in patterns
- Long sleeved clothing worn during warm weather
- Constant use of wrist coverings or wrist bands
- Behavioral and emotional instability, impulsivity and unpredictability
- Signs of depression, hopelessness and dissociation
- Refusal to participate in things such as swimming due to unwillingness to expose skin

MANAGEMENT/TREATMENT:

- Identify students who may be engaging in NSSI behaviors.
- Assess injuries, noting old scars or injuries, and provide first aid as needed.
- Identify any injuries that may require immediate attention or more advanced medical care.
- Assess the student in a calm, kind, non-judgmental manner, asking questions in a direct and honest way about a student's self-harm behaviors and history.
- Involve the school crisis team and/or counselors or psychologists to illicit counseling supports in the school itself as appropriate.

SELF-INJURY, NON-SUICIDAL (NSSI) *(continued from previous page)*

MANAGEMENT/TREATMENT *(continued)*

- Refer to a mental health professional who has experience in treating individuals with self-injury behaviors.
- Provide parents with the release of information forms to communicate with any outside providers.

FOLLOW-UP:

- Schools should develop protocols to help all school staff respond appropriately to NSSI in the school setting. School nurses can be integral in, not only developing protocols, but also in educating staff and being a resource for parents and the community.[6] *Refer to Mental Health Management.*
- Although NSSI is not generally associated with suicide, a suicide assessment should be completed by trained staff if there is any indication the student may be suicidal.
- A list of referral resources or contact information should be maintained.
- Students should be encouraged to call their parents/caregivers to make them aware of what has occurred. A point person in the school may be utilized to help the student in disclosing this to the parent and assisting the parent in obtaining outside assistance.
- State and local laws may differ in regards to parental/guardian notification. Each school nurse should be aware of these laws as well as specific district policy.

POTENTIAL COMPLICATIONS:[7]

- Life threatening wounds
- Wound infection
- Scarring/disfigurement
- Increased feelings of shame, guilt, and low self-esteem
- Worsening of potential underlying mental health condition
- Severe, possible fatal injury

REFERENCES

[1] Mayo Clinic. (2018). *Self-injury/cutting*. http://www.mayoclinic.org/diseases-conditions/self-injury/basics/definition/con-20025897

[2] Ibid.

[3] Merck Manual Professional. (2019). *Nonsuicidal Self-Injury (NSSI) in Children and Adolescents.* https://www.merckmanuals.com/professional/pediatrics/mental-disorders-in-children-and-adolescents/nonsuicidal-self-injury-nssi-in-children-and-adolescents?query=self%20injury

[4] American Psychological Association. (2015). *Who self-injures?* https://www.apa.org/monitor/2015/07-08/who-self-injures

[5] Merck Manual Professional. (2019). *Nonsuicidal self-injury (NSSI) in children and adolescents.* https://www.merckmanuals.com/professional/pediatrics/mental-disorders-in-children-and-adolescents/nonsuicidal-self-injury-nssi-in-children-and-adolescents?query=self%20injury

[6] Burrick, K., Goodwin, J., & Whitlock J. (n.d.). *Non –suicidal self-injury in schools: Developing and implementing school protocol.* http://www.selfinjury.bctr.cornell.edu/documents/schools.pdf

[7] Ibid.

SEXUALLY TRANSMITTED DISEASES/INFECTIONS

DEFINITION/ETIOLOGY:

Sexually transmitted infections (STIs), sometimes referred to as sexually transmitted diseases (STDs), are infections acquired by sexual contact. Considered an epidemic, STIs have the highest rates in adolescents accounting for about one-half of all new STIs in the United States.[1] Men who have sex with men have higher rates of STIs.[2] STIs can be passed to a person anytime they have unprotected sex with a partner who is already infected. It can be spread during vaginal, anal, or oral sex. The organisms that cause STIs may pass from person to person through blood, semen, or vaginal fluids. Human Papillomavirus (HPV) and Herpes Simplex Virus (HSV) can be spread by contact in the area of the skin not covered by a condom (skin to skin). Adolescents are at increased risk for many STIs due to physiologic characteristics of this age group.[3]

Multiple organisms are responsible for STIs in adolescents and children, the most common being gonorrhea, chlamydia, syphilis, HSV and HPV.[4] These common STIs will be reviewed in this document.

Chlamydial Infections

Chlamydia is the most frequently reported infectious disease in the United States and prevalence is highest among those under 25 years of age. It is caused by the organism *C. trachomatis*. Adolescent women are at a particular risk for C. trachomatis. Annual screening of all sexually active adolescents is recommended.[5]

Gonococcal Infections

Gonorrhea (GC) is the second most commonly reported bacterial STI and is caused by *N. gonorrhoeae*. Symptoms usually develop 2-21 days after having sex. Genital GC generally causes local infection of the urethra, vagina, rectum and cervix, but may ascend into the upper genital tract in women or infect the testicles or prostate in men.[6]

SIGNS AND SYMPTOMS (for chlamydia and gonorrhea):[7]

- Asymptomatic infection is common
- Vaginal, penile, rectal and cervical discharge (Usually white or yellow with chlamydia and green and purulent with gonorrhea)
- Pain/burning with urination
- Unusual vaginal bleeding, between periods or after sex
- Abdominal pain, sometimes with fever or nausea
- Enlarged inguinal or femoral lymph node.
- Swollen testicles
- Rectal pain or discharge

SEXUALLY TRANSMITTED DISEASES/INFECTIONS *(continued from previous page)*

Treatment/ Management (for chlamydia and gonorrhea):[8]

- Students with possible chlamydial and gonococcal infections should be referred to a healthcare provider for testing and treatment.
- Chlamydial and gonococcal infections or suspected infections should be treated with antibiotics.
- C. trachomatis is generally treated with a single dose of oral azithromycin.
- Often presumptive treatment of chlamydial infection for students with gonococcal infections is indicated.
- Uncomplicated gonorrhea is treated with a one-time intramuscular dose of ceftriaxone.
- Students should be re-tested in three to four months.
- Students should be instructed to refer their sex partners to a healthcare provider if they have had sexual contact within 60 days of onset of the symptoms. In some instances, expedited partner treatment (EPT) may be initiated by the practitioner by which a second prescription is given to the client for their partner.
- Students should be educated to refrain from sex until all partners have completed treatment.

Genital Herpes Simplex Virus (HSV)

Genital herpes is a chronic, life- long viral infection. Two types have been identified, HSV-*1* and *HSV-2.* Most cases of genital herpes are caused by *HSV-2.* It is spread by direct contact.[9] Many persons have mild or asymptomatic infection but shed the virus intermittently in the genital tract. Asymptomatic HSV infections are responsible for most transmissions.[10] Herpes episodes may be characterized as primary, first episode of infection, or re-current in a student with a past history of symptomatic HSV infection.

Signs and Symptoms (for genital herpes simplex):[11]

- A flu-like feeling, including fever, may be present with a primary infection.
- Small painful vesicles on an erythematous base on the genitals, rectum or mouth, generally where the virus has entered the body.
- Vesicles become ulcers in one to three days.
- Itching or burning before the symptoms occur.
- Inguinal lymphadenopathy.
- Ulcerations may last one to three weeks.
- Symptoms may return throughout the lifespan but generally occurrences decrease over time.

Treatment/Management (for genital herpes simplex):[12]

- Anti-viral medication may be ordered by the healthcare provider for initial and episodic infections and for suppression. This will shorten the outbreak.
- Warm baths may be helpful.
- Students should understand that although it can be treated, herpes cannot be cured.
- Daily suppression therapy may also decrease the risks of transmission.

SEXUALLY TRANSMITTED DISEASES/INFECTIONS *(continued from previous page)*

Genital Human Papillomavirus (HPV)

HPV is the most common sexually transmitted infection in the U.S today. Almost all sexually active women and men are infected at some point in their lives.[13] There are more than 100 different strains of HPV with 40 that are sexually transmitted and affect the mucosal surfaces of the genital area.[14] The virus is transmitted through skin-to-skin contact. It is associated with genital warts and cervical cancers although most infections do not result in cancer.

Signs and symptoms (for HPV):[15]

- Many people have no symptoms.
- Genital warts in the genital area.
- Warts may be alone or in groups, flat or rounded, pink or skin colored.
- Abnormal cervical cytology.

Treatment/Management (for HPV):[16]

- Students with genital warts should be referred to their healthcare provider.
- In 90% of infections the body's immune system will clear the infection in two years.
- Although there is no cure for genital warts, they can be treated.
- Genital warts may spontaneously resolve without treatment.
- Warts can be treated with ointments, surgical or laser removal.
- Warts may recur after treatment.
- Screening for cervical cancer is only recommended for those 30 years and older.
- Vaccines for the prevention of HPV are available and approved for both males and females and are recommended at 11-12 years.

POTENTIAL COMPLICATIONS of untreated STIs:[17]

- Infertility
- Pelvic Inflammatory Disease (PID)
- Ectopic pregnancy
- Many STIs may be transmitted to newborns during birth or have an adverse effect on pregnancy
- Epididymitis, prostatitis, urethral scarring
- Neisseria gonorrhea bacterium can spread via the bloodstream to heart valves, joints or the brain[18]
- Infection with certain STIs can increase the risk of getting and transmitting Human Immunodeficiency Virus (HIV)[19]

If a student had sexual contact with someone who had or has any of the above symptoms related to an STI, it is important to **see a healthcare provider.**

SEXUALLY TRANSMITTED DISEASES/INFECTIONS *(continued from previous page)*

FOLLOW-UP:

- Encourage student to continue full course of prescribed treatment and obtain necessary tests.
- Abstinence from sexual activity for 7 days is encouraged following treatment.
- Encourage student to cooperate in locating sexual contacts.
- Educate students in regard to prevention, re-infection, and complications.
  - HIV is easier to acquire if one already has another sexually transmitted disease.
  - Many infections are asymptomatic in boys but may cause serious infection in girls (e.g. chlamydia).
- Latex condom use has been shown to prevent transmission of most bacterial infections and is helpful in limiting some transmission of HSV and HPV.[20]
- Students should be aware that abstinence is the only way to prevent a STI with 100% accuracy.
- All 50 states permit treatment of a minor with STIs without parental consent or notification.[21]
- In student's younger than 13 with a sexually transmitted disease there should be involvement with child protective authorities.
- Nurses should be aware of their own state laws and regulations regarding confidentiality.
- Students should be encouraged to involve a parent or responsible adult in the process.

NOTES:

- According to the Centers for Disease Control and Prevention (CDC), the reporting of STIs in an accurate and timely manner is important for assessing morbidity trends, targeting limited resources, and assisting local health authorities in partner notification and treatment. Cases related to STI, HIV, and acquired immune deficiency syndrome (AIDS) should be reported in accordance with state and local statutory requirements. Additionally, Syphilis, Gonorrhea, Chlamydia, Chancroid, HIV infection, and AIDS are reportable diseases in every state. The reporting requirements for other STIs differ by state, thus clinicians should be familiar with state and local reporting requirements.[22]

> Any suspicion of a child younger than 13 with an STI requires a prompt referral to local child protective services. Specific diseases, e.g. Gonorrhea, Syphilis, and Chlamydia, if acquired after the neonatal period, are indicative of sexual contact.

- Minor consent laws may vary from state to state. With a few exceptions, all adolescents in the United States can legally consent to confidential diagnosis and treatment of STIs. In all 50 states and the District of Columbia, adolescents can receive medical care for STIs without parental consent or knowledge. Additionally, adolescents can consent to HIV counseling and testing in the majority of states.[23]

- It is important for the school nurse to promote an environment that the adolescent feels comfortable discussing any reproductive health concerns. Most teens will not seek information or help with seeking treatment if they feel that their parents or guardians will be notified. Offering a private space and non-judgmental attitude and clearly respecting the confidentiality rights of teens will help foster prompt and appropriate access to health care.

SEXUALLY TRANSMITTED DISEASES/INFECTIONS *(continued from previous page)*

REFERENCES

---

[1] Gerlt, T., & Starr, N. (2017). Gynecologic disorders. In C. Burns, A.M. Dunn, M.A. Brady, N.B. Starr, C.G. Blosser, & D.L. Garzon (Eds.), *Pediatric primary care* (6th ed., pp. 976-982). Elsevier Inc.

[2] Center for Disease Control and Prevention. (2019). *Sexually transmitted diseases.* https://www.cdc.gov/STD/

[3] Ibid.

[4] Ibid.

[5] Ibid.

[6] Johnson, K., & Selekman, J. (2019). Students engaging in high risk behavior. In J. Selekman, R. Adair Shannon, & **C. F.** Yonkaitis (Eds.), *School nursing: A comprehensive text* (3rd ed., pp. 847-851). F.A. Davis.

[7] Gerlt, T., & Starr, N. (2017). Gynecologic disorders. In C. Burns, A.M. Dunn, M.A. Brady, N.B. Starr, C.G. Blosser, & D.L. Garzon (Eds.), *Pediatric primary care* (6th ed., pp. 976-982). Elsevier Inc.

[8] Johnson, K., & Selekman, J. (2019). Students engaging in high risk behavior. In J. Selekman, R. Adair Shannon, &**C. F.** Yonkaitis (Eds.), *School nursing: A comprehensive text* (3rd ed., pp. 847-851). F.A. Davis.

[9] U.S National Library of Medicine. (2018*). Herpes simplex.* https://medlineplus.gov/herpessimplex.html

[10] Gerlt, T., & Starr, N. (2017). Gynecologic disorders. In C. Burns, A.M. Dunn, M.A. Brady, N.B. Starr, C.G. Blosser, & D.L. Garzon (Eds.), *Pediatric primary care* (6th ed., pp. 976-982). Elsevier Inc.

[11] Johnson, K., & Selekman, J. (2019). Students engaging in high risk behavior. In J. Selekman, R. Adair Shannon, &**C. F.** Yonkaitis (Eds.), *School nursing: A comprehensive text* (3rd ed., pp. 847-851). F.A. Davis.

[12] Gerlt, T., & Starr, N. (2017). Gynecologic disorders. In C. Burns, A.M. Dunn, M.A. Brady, N.B. Starr, C.G. Blosser, & D.L. Garzon (Eds.*), Pediatric primary care* (6th ed., pp. 976-982). Elsevier Inc.

[13] Ibid.

[14] Ibid.

[15] Ibid.

[16] Ibid.

[17] Johnson, K., & Selekman, J. (2019). Students engaging in high risk behavior. In J. Selekman, R. Adair Shannon, &**C. F.** Yonkaitis (Eds.), *School nursing: A comprehensive text* (3rd ed., pp. 847-851). F.A. Davis..

[18] Gerlt, T., & Starr, N. (2017). Gynecologic disorders. In C. Burns, A.M. Dunn, M.A. Brady, N.B. Starr, C.G. Blosser, & D.L. Garzon (Eds.), *Pediatric primary care* (6th ed., pp. 976-982). Elsevier Inc.

[19] National Institute of Allergy and Infectious Diseases. (2015). *Sexually transmitted diseases.* : https://www.niaid.nih.gov/diseases-conditions/sexually-transmitted-diseases

[20] Center for Disease Control (2019). *How you can prevent sexually transmitted diseases.* : https://www.cdc.gov/std/prevention/default.htm

[21] Gerlt, T., & Starr, N. (2017). Gynecologic disorders. In C. Burns, A.M. Dunn, M.A. Brady, N.B. Starr, C.G. Blosser, & D.L. Garzon (Eds.), *Pediatric primary care* (6th ed., pp. 976-982). Elsevier Inc.

[22] Center for Disease Control and Prevention. (2018). *STD data management and information technology.* : https://www.cdc.gov/std/program/data-mgmt.htm

[23] Centers for Disease Control and Prevention. (2018). *Minors consent laws for STDs and HIV services.* : https://www.cdc.gov/hiv/policies/law/states/minors.html

OTHER REFERENCES CONSULTED

U.S. Department of Health and Human Services, Office of Adolescent Health. (2019). *Sexually transmitted diseases.* http://www.hhs.gov/ash/oah/adolescent-health-topics/reproductive-health/stds.html

SHINGLES (VZV) - also called Herpes Zoster (HZV), Postherpetic neuralgia (PHN)

OVERVIEW/DEFINITION:[1, 2]

Shingles is a disease caused by varicella-zoster virus, the same virus that causes chickenpox. The virus of clinical chickenpox remains dormant in the body in the nervous system and can reactivate years later causing shingles.

1. Shingles can develop in any age group. Most often shingles occur in people over 60 years old, but anyone who has had chickenpox is at risk. Even children can get shingles.
2. Many who have chicken pox the case is so mild that they may not be aware that they have the varicella zoster virus.
3. Those with weakened immune systems are more susceptible.
4. The virus spreads through direct contact with the rash (transmission of the shingle virus is not airborne).
5. An adult or child, who has direct contact with the shingles rash and did not have chickenpox as a child or did not receive the chickenpox vaccine, can develop chickenpox, not shingles.[3]

SIGNS AND SYMPTOMS: [4, 5]

- Characteristically, the first symptoms of shingles are burning or shooting pain and tingling or itching, usually on one side of the body or face.
- Sensitive to touch.
- A rash or blisters appear one to 14 days later and usually involves a narrow area from the spine around to the front of the abdomen of chest.
- The blisters break, forming small lesions that begin to dry and form crusts. The crusts fall off in two to three weeks.
- Scarring is rare.
- The pain of shingles may last for weeks, months, or even years.
- Some may experience sensitivity to light, fatigue, fever and/or headache.

Other symptoms may include:

- General feeling of "not well", headache, fever and chills, enlarged lymph nodes, and/or joint pain.
- With pain, there may be accompanying muscle weakness, and a rash involving different parts of the body and face. Usually the rash is limited to one side of the body's midline.
- If the shingles virus affects a nerve in the face, some of the following symptoms may occur: difficulty moving some of the muscles in the face, drooping eyelid (ptosis), loss of eye motion and other vision problems, hearing loss, taste problems.

ANTICIPATED CONCERNS/PROBLEMS:[6, 7]

- Postherpetic pain is the most common complication experience by 10-13%.
- Recurrences of shingles.
- Bacterial skin infections.
- Permanent vision loss (if shingles occur in the eye).
- Permanent hearing loss and/or balance problems (if shingles occur in the ear).
- Infections that include encephalitis or sepsis in those with compromised immune systems.
- Ramsay Hunt Syndrome (facial paralysis or weakness) may occur if shingles virus affects the face or ear.[8]

SHINGLES *(continued from previous page)*

MANAGEMENT/POTENTIAL INTERVENTIONS:[9]

- The healthcare provider may prescribe an oral antiviral drug to reduce the pain, prevent complications, and shorten the course of the disease.
- The medication should be started as soon as possible of first appearance of pain and itching and it is best to begin the antiviral treatment before the blisters appear.
- Do not give children aspirin which although rare can lead to Reye Syndrome.[10]
- Follow healthcare provider's instructions for home care.
- The application of cool, wet compresses to reduce pain and soothing baths and resting in bed until the fever subsides
- Cover the rash and avoid touching the area.
- A person with shingles infection should stay away from others while the lesions are oozing to avoid infecting:
    - those who have never had chickenpox or chickenpox vaccine,
    - pregnant women and those with compromised immune systems.[11]
- Children should be excluded from school until the blisters are scabbed over or if the rash can't be completely covered.

FOLLOW-UP:

Refer to healthcare provider if:

- Signs and symptoms suggest shingles.
- Symptoms worsen.
- Alert those with a compromised immune system (i.e. chemotherapy, Human Immunodeficiency Virus (HIV) positive, other immune- suppressed, taking medication to prevent rejections of organ transplant) and recommend they seek advice from their healthcare provider.[12]
- Identify those who have not had chickenpox or the chickenpox vaccine.
- Women who are pregnant or might become pregnant should contact their healthcare provider for a blood test.[13]

NOTES:

- Children appear to have a lower risk or less serious case of shingles if they received the varicella vaccine compared to those who were infected by the varicella virus.[14]

PREVENTION:

- Always use and encourage good handwashing. (*Refer to HANDWASHNG APPENDIX*)
- Do not touch the rash or blisters on a person with shingles if you have never had chickenpox or the chickenpox vaccine.
- Herpes zoster vaccine is available. The Centers for Disease Control and Prevention (CDC) recommends that people over 50 years old get the shingles vaccine to prevent shingles or PHN. This is a different vaccine than chickenpox vaccine.

SHINGLES *(continued from previous page)*

REFERENCES

[1] Academy of Pediatrics. (2020). *Meningitis.* In S. Aronson, (Ed.), *Managing infectious diseases in child care and schools* (5th ed., pp. 161). American Academy of Pediatrics.

[2] Centers for Disease Control and Prevention. (2017). *Shingles (herpes zoster).* https://www.cdc.gov/shingles/index.html

[3] National Institute of Neurological Disorders and Stroke. (2019). *NINDS shingles information page.* https://www.ninds.nih.gov/Disorders/All-Disorders/Shingles-Information-Page

[4] Medline Plus. (2017). *Shingles.* https://medlineplus.gov/shingles.html#cat_93

[5] Mayo Clinic. (2018). *Shingles.* https://www.mayoclinic.org/diseases-conditions/shingles/symptoms-causes/syc-20353054

[6] Centers for Disease Control and Prevention. (2017). *Shingles (herpes zoster).* https://www.cdc.gov/shingles/index.html

[7] Mayo Clinic. (2018). *Ramsey Hunt Syndrome.* https://www.mayoclinic.org/diseases-conditions/ramsay-hunt-syndrome/symptoms-causes/syc-20351783

[8] Medline Plus. (2017). *Shingles.* https://medlineplus.gov/shingles.html#cat_93

[9] Mayo Clinic. (2018). *Shingles.* https://www.mayoclinic.org/diseases-conditions/shingles/symptoms-causes/syc-20353054

[10] Kids Health from Nemours. (2015). *Diseases & conditions: Shingles for parents.* https://kidshealth.org/en/parents/shingles.html?ref=search

[11] National Institute of Neurological Disorders and Stroke. (2019). *NINDS shingles information page.* https://www.ninds.nih.gov/Disorders/All-Disorders/Shingles-Information-Page

[12] Mayo Clinic. (2018). Shingles. https://www.mayoclinic.org/diseases-conditions/shingles/symptoms-causes/syc-20353054

[13] Beigi, R. (2018). *Patient education: Avoiding infections in pregnancy (beyond the basics).* https://www.uptodate.com/contents/avoiding-infections-in-pregnancy-beyond-the-basics#!

[14] Kids Health from Nemours. (2015). *Diseases & conditions: Shingles for parents.* https://kidshealth.org/en/parents/shingles.html?ref=search

OTHER REFERENCES CONSULTED:

American Academy of Pediatrics. (2016). Herpes zoster. In A. J. Mancini, & D. P. Krowchuk (Eds.), *Pediatric dermatology* (3rd ed., pp. 99-102). American Academy of Pediatrics.

Centers for Disease Control and Prevention. (2018). *Shingles vaccination: What everyone should know.* https://www.cdc.gov/vaccines/vpd/shingles/public/shingrix/index.html

SICKLE CELL DISEASE

DEFINITION/ETIOLOGY:
Sickle cell disease (SCD) is a hereditary disorder present at birth in which red blood cells change shape. The term *sickle cell disease* refers to a group of genetic disorders where Hemoglobin S is more prevalent than the normal Hemoglobin A in the blood. The red blood cells take on a sickle shape, become sticky and hard, and fail to function well. The sickle cells die early causing chronic anemia. As they travel through small blood vessels, they often get stuck due to their sticky composition. The blocked flow of blood is called vaso-occlusive crisis (VOC). If the student develops a fever, dehydration or a decreased oxygen level, the sickling will become enhanced. A trauma or infection (viral or bacterial) may precipitate a sickle cell crisis.[1, 2]

There are several types of sickle cell disease. The most common and severe form is sickle cell anemia (HbSS). Other types of SCD include HbSC and HbS beta thalassemia. HbSD, HbSE, and HbSO are considered rare.[3]

Sickle cell disease is most common among those of African descent but also affects children from Central America, the Mediterranean, South America, and the Caribbean. It rarely affects white children.[4]

SIGNS AND SYMPTOMS:[5, 6, 7]
Symptoms usually appear around 5-6 months of age. Children are born with this condition and have it for life.

- Hand and foot syndrome, swelling of the hands and feet (may be the first sign) along with fatigue, fussiness, anemia and jaundice
- Pain episode or "crisis" caused by the sickle cells obstructing the circulation (the hallmark sign). Pain may be severe and include joint pain, chest pain, headache, abdominal pain, nausea or vomiting
- Frequently occurring infections
- Fever
- Anemia
  - Fatigue
  - Pallor
  - Tachycardia
  - Delayed growth
  - Irritability
- Leg ulcers
- Vision loss
- Hematuria

SICKLE CELL DISEASE *(continued from previous page)*

MANAGEMENT/TREATMENT:[8, 9]

Preventive measures for the pain crisis should include prevention of an episode with plenty of fluids, avoiding hot and cold temperatures, and avoiding high altitudes or extreme exercising.

Treatment includes:

- Monitor immunization status. Refer to healthcare provider as necessary to ensure that student is up to date on vaccine preventable diseases.[10]
- An Individualized Healthcare Plan (IHP) should be developed with the child with sickle cell disease. Consult the child and parent/guardian on specific symptoms experienced before, during, and after pain episodes.
- Refer to the Section 504/Individualized Educational Plan (IEP) team as necessary.
- team as necessary.
- During the school day, the child should receive extra fluids and rest periods during times of physical activity.[11]
- Fluid therapy is initiated during a crisis to restore circulating blood volume.
- Clearance for using a cold pack for 1st aid should be obtained from the healthcare provider. A cold pack should never be applied to a pain site during a SCD pain episode.[12]
- At the first sign of an infection, it is important for children to see a healthcare provider.[13]
- Prophylactic antibiotics are often given to prevent infection such as penicillin.[14]
- Blood transfusions are sometimes needed for severe anemia.[15]

POTENTIAL COMPLICATIONS:

- Impaired growth and development.
- Acute Splenic Sequestration: Because the sickled cells are trapped, a large amount of blood accumulates in the spleen. The spleen can become very big and break open and this is a life-threatening emergency. This usually occurs in the young child as the spleen commonly stops functioning in early childhood.[16]
- Aplastic Crisis: Episodes of bone marrow suppression that cause the red blood cell production to be decreased. [17] Often occurs after a viral or bacterial infection including parvovirus B19 (e.g., Fifth's Disease). The child can appear very pale and tired.
- High risk for sepsis, meningitis, pneumonia, and other severe infections.[18]
- Possible damage to internal organs.
- Acute chest syndrome: Similar to pneumonia with sudden onset of chest pain, difficulty breathing and fever. It should be treated in the hospital. Occurs most often in children.[19]
- Cerebral stroke: Can occur in 10% of children with SCD due to the clogged blood flow to the brain.[20]

SICKLE CELL DISEASE *(continued from previous page)*

POTENTIAL COMPLICATIONS *(continued)*

- Pulmonary emboli/Deep vein thrombosis: Sickling of the red blood cells increases the risk of forming blood clots.[21]
- Priapism – painful erection of the penis - occurs most often in young men. This is related to poor blood flow and requires emergency treatment.[22]

FOLLOW UP:

The child with SCD should be managed by an interdisciplinary healthcare team with ongoing maintenance and regular visits to the healthcare provider.

NOTES:

- Newborn screening for sickle cell is mandated in the United States. All infants should undergo testing between 24 and 72 hours of age. If sickle cell is suspected in an older child, hemoglobin electrophoresis is used to confirm the diagnosis.[23]
- Children with SCD should have their eyes examined yearly to check for retinal damages.
- The school nurse can assist the child and family by providing information to the staff about the child and the condition. The staff should be aware of the need for prompt medical care in the event of a "crisis" or infection.[24]

REFERENCES

[1] Centers for Disease Control and Prevention, National Center on Birth Defects and Developmental Disabilities/Division of Blood Disorders. (n.d.). *Tips for supporting students with sickle cell disease*. https://www.cdc.gov/ncbddd/sicklecell/documents/tipsheet_Supporting_Students_with_SCD.pdf

[2] Donoghue, E. A., & Kraft, C. A. (Eds.). (2019). Sickle cell disease. *Managing chronic health needs in child care and schools: A quick reference guide* (2nd ed., *pp. 183-185).* American Academy of Pediatrics.

[3] Ibid.

[4] Centers for Disease Control and Prevention, National Center on Birth Defects and Developmental Disabilities/Division of Blood Disorders. (n.d.). *Tips for supporting students with sickle cell disease*. https://www.cdc.gov/ncbddd/sicklecell/documents/tipsheet_Supporting_Students_with_SCD.pdf

[5] Donoghue, E. A., & Kraft, C. A. (Eds.). (2019). Sickle cell disease. *Managing chronic health needs in child care and schools: A quick reference guide* (2nd ed., *pp. .183-185).* American Academy of Pediatrics.

[6] Merck Manual. (2019). *Sickle cell disease.* http://www.merckmanuals.com/professional/hematology-and-oncology/anemias-caused-by-hemolysis/sickle-cell-disease

[7] National Heart, Lung and Blood Institute. (2019). *Sickle cell disease* https://www.nhlbi.nih.gov/health-topics/sickle-cell-disease

[8] Centers for Disease Control and Prevention, National Center on Birth Defects and Developmental Disabilities/Division of Blood Disorders. (n.d.). *Tips for supporting students with sickle cell disease*. https://www.cdc.gov/ncbddd/sicklecell/documents/tipsheet_Supporting_Students_with_SCD.pdf

[9] Donoghue, E. A., & Kraft, C. A. (Eds.). (2019). Sickle cell disease. *Managing chronic health needs in child care and schools: A quick reference guide* (2nd ed., *pp. 183-185).* American Academy of Pediatrics.

SICKLE CELL DISEASE *(continued from previous page)*

[10] Centers for Disease Control and Prevention, National Center for Infectious Diseases. (2019). Sickle *cell disease (SCD).* http://www.cdc.gov/ncbddd/sicklecell/treatments.html

[11] Centers for Disease Control and Prevention, National Center on Birth Defects and Developmental Disabilities/Division of Blood Disorders. (n.d.). *Tips for supporting students with sickle cell disease*. https://www.cdc.gov/ncbddd/sicklecell/documents/tipsheet_Supporting_Students_with_SCD.pdf

[12] Ibid.

[13] Donoghue, E. A., & Kraft, C. A. (Eds.). (2019). Sickle cell disease. *Managing chronic health needs in child care and schools: A quick reference guide* (2nd ed., *pp. 183-185).* American Academy of Pediatrics.

[14] Centers for Disease Control and Prevention, National Center on Birth Defects and Developmental Disabilities/Division of Blood Disorders. (n.d.). *Tips for supporting students with sickle cell disease*. https://www.cdc.gov/ncbddd/sicklecell/documents/tipsheet_Supporting_Students_with_SCD.pdf

[15] Centers for Disease Control and Prevention, National Center for Infectious Diseases. (2019). Sickle *cell disease (SCD).* http://www.cdc.gov/ncbddd/sicklecell/treatments.html

[16] Ibid.

[17] Donoghue, E. A., & Kraft, C. A. (Eds.). (2019). Sickle cell disease. *Managing chronic health needs in child care and schools: A quick reference guide* (2nd ed., *pp. 183-185).* American Academy of Pediatrics.

[18] Centers for Disease Control and Prevention, National Center on Birth Defects and Developmental Disabilities/Division of Blood Disorders. (n.d.). *Tips for supporting students with sickle cell disease* https://www.cdc.gov/ncbddd/sicklecell/documents/tipsheet_Supporting_Students_with_SCD.pdf

[19] Donoghue, E. A., & Kraft, C. A. (Eds.). (2019). Sickle cell disease. *Managing chronic health needs in child care and schools: A quick reference guide* (2nd ed., *pp. 183-185).* American Academy of Pediatrics.

[20] Centers for Disease Control and Prevention, National Center on Birth Defects and Developmental Disabilities/Division of Blood Disorders. (n.d.). *Tips for supporting students with sickle cell disease*. https://www.cdc.gov/ncbddd/sicklecell/documents/tipsheet_Supporting_Students_with_SCD.pdf

[21] Ibid.

[22] Centers for Disease Control and Prevention, National Center for Infectious Diseases. (2019). Sickle *cell disease (SCD).* http://www.cdc.gov/ncbddd/sicklecell/treatments.html

[23] Ibid.

[24] National Heart, Lung and Blood Institute. (2019). *Sickle cell disease.* https://www.nhlbi.nih.gov/health-topics/sickle-cell-disease

SINUSITIS

DEFINITION/ETIOLOGY:

Sinusitis is inflammation of the mucous membranes that line the paranasal sinuses and is commonly referred to as rhinosinusitis. A bad cold is often mistaken for sinusitis. Although many symptoms are the same, including headache or facial pain, runny nose and nasal congestion, sinusitis is usually caused by a bacterial infection, or less commonly a fungal infection.[1]

Sinusitis can be described as acute or chronic:

- Acute sinusitis: abrupt onset of infection of one or more of the paranasal sinuses that resolves following therapy, usually within 30 days.[2]
- Chronic sinusitis: episodes of prolonged inflammation or may be repeated acute infection. Clinical symptoms last more than 90 days.[3]

CAUSES:

Sinusitis is almost always preceded by an upper respiratory infection, although allergies may also be a predisposing condition. Normal sinuses have a protective layer of mucous that traps dust, germs and other particles from the air. Tiny hair-like projections in the sinuses sweep the mucus toward the back of the throat and into the stomach. When infections or allergies interrupt this process, the hair-like projections become blocked and nasal tissues swell, trapping mucous in the sinuses.[4] Mucous stasis creates a good environment for pathogens to grow.

- Other factors that increase risk of sinusitis include:[5]
    - smoke exposure
    - swimming
    - school aged siblings
    - gastroesophageal reflux
    - cystic fibrosis
    - immunodeficiency
    - ciliary dyskinesia
    - anatomical abnormalities
- Sinusitis is more commonly seen in adults or older children.

SIGNS AND SYMPTOMS:[6]

- Nasal and throat inflammation
- Cough (worsening at night) or throat clearing
- Fever (not usually seen in chronic sinusitis)
- Purulent rhinorrhea (runny nose) usually yellow or green
- Halitosis (bad breath) or loss of smell
- Headache/face pain/toothache
- Head pain with bending over or sudden movements
- Snoring
- Earache
- Nasal speech
- Facial swelling

SINUSITIS *(continued from previous page)*

SIGNS AND SYMPTOMS *(continued)*

A clinical diagnosis is generally made after upper respiratory signs and symptoms are present for greater than 10-14 days and with symptoms such as facial swelling, facial pain, and fever. The maxillary and ethmoid sinuses are most commonly involved.[7]

MANAGEMENT/TREATMENT:

- If student has fever, reports feeling ill, and complains of symptoms related to sinusitis, such as facial pain, headache, and nasal discharge, notify parent/guardian(s) and refer to healthcare provider.
- A cool compress on the forehead may make the student more comfortable.
- Encourage fluids.
- Monitor students to be sure they complete the antibiotics regimen and for any side effects.
- If recommended by healthcare provider, normal saline nose drops to assist with drainage and ventilation that can be done both at home and at school.
- Monitor for complications such as orbital cellulitis, exacerbation of asthma, cavernous sinus thrombosis and optic neuritis.[8]
- Prevention: avoid allergens and treat allergies when appropriate.

FOLLOW UP:

Because of the proximity of the paranasal sinuses to the brain, intracranial complications can result and progress rapidly. Symptoms of intracranial complications include acute headache, fever, lethargy, change in mental status, seizure, and coma.

Sinus infections are usually curable with medical treatment and self-care measures. Recurrent sinus attacks require follow up with a healthcare provider to assess for underlying causes such as nasal polyps or allergies.

School nurses can help with prevention by encouraging hand washing, use and disposal of tissues and cough etiquette. *(Refer to HANDWASHING and COVER YOUR COUGH APPENDIX).*

REFERENCES

---

[1] American College of Asthma, Allergy, and Immunology. (n.d.). *Sinus Infection.* https://acaai.org/allergies/types/sinus-infection

[2] Medline Plus/ U.S. National Library of Medicine. (2018). *Sinusitis.* http://www.nlm.nih.gov/medlineplus/ency/article/000647.htm

[3] Medline Plus/ U.S. National Library of Medicine. (2018). *Sinusitis.* http://www.nlm.nih.gov/medlineplus/ency/article/000647.htm

[4] American College of Asthma, Allergy, and Immunology. (n.d.). *Sinus Infection.* https://acaai.org/allergies/types/sinus-infection

SINUSITIS *(continued from previous page)*

[5] Mayo Clinic. (2019). *Acute sinusitis.* https://www.mayoclinic.org/diseases-conditions/acute-sinusitis/symptoms-causes/syc-20351671

[6] Ball, J.W., Binder, R. C., Cowen, K. J., & Shaw, M.R. (Eds.). (2017). Alterations in eye, ear, nose and throat function. *Principles of pediatric nursing: Caring for children, (7th ed.) (pp. 440-473).* Hoboken, NJ: Pearson Education.

[7] Yoon, P.J., Scholes, M.A., & Friedman, N.R. (2018). Ear, nose and throat. In W.W. Hay, M.J. Levin, R. R. Deterding, & M. J. Abzug (Eds.), *Current diagnosis and treatment: Pediatrics* (24th ed., pp. 478-508). McGraw Hill Education.

[8] Ibid.

SKIN AND SOFT TISSUE INFECTION (Boils, Cellulitis, Lymphangitis and Methicillin-Resistant Staphylococcus Aureus [MRSA])

DEFINITIONS/ETIOLOGY:
Acute infection of the skin and soft tissues (subcutaneous tissue, fascia, and muscles) may occur secondary to a wound, abrasion, insect bite, impetigo, pustule, furuncle or carbuncle. Skin and soft tissue infections are classified as uncomplicated or complicated. Uncomplicated skin and soft tissue infections respond well to oral antibiotics and local wound care. Uncomplicated skin infections can become a complicated skin infection. Complicated skin and wound infections do not respond to conventional antibiotic therapy. A complicated skin and wound infection typically involve deeper tissue (subcutaneous tissue, fascia or muscle). Complicated skin infections may require multiple antibiotics and surgical intervention.[1]

Types of skin and soft tissue infections include:

A furuncle (boil) is a skin infection, consisting of a walled off, pus-filled mass that is most commonly staph (*S. aureus*), involving the entire hair follicle and the adjacent subcutaneous tissue. They occur most commonly on sites of friction and swelling such as under the belt, groin, armpit, buttocks and thighs. Some people are afflicted with many, with little success at prevention. Boils can range from a small bump to a large abscess filled with pus.[2]

Cellulitis – acute infection of skin and soft (subcutaneous) tissue. Cellulitis indicates an acute spreading infection of the dermis and subcutaneous tissues. *Staphylococcal aureus* and *Group A Streptococus* are the most common causes of cellulitis.[3]

Lymphangitis is a bacterial infection in the lymphatic vessels. Most often results from *Group A Streptococus* infection of the skin, less frequently from *Staphylococcal aureus*. Lymphangitis may be an indication that a skin infection is worsening. This should raise concern that bacteria may have spread into the bloodstream, which can cause life-threatening problems.[4]

Methicillin-resistant *Staphylococcus aureus* (MRSA) is a type of *staphylococcus aureus* (staph) infection that is resistant to beta-lactams antibiotics (such as methicillin, penicillin and amoxicillin). MRSA is usually transmitted by direct skin-to-skin contact or contact with shared items or surfaces that have come into contact with someone else's infection (e.g., towels, used bandages, wrestling mats). MRSA skin infections can occur anywhere on the body as well as in the environment.[5]

SIGNS AND SYMPTOMS:

<u>Boils</u>

- Pain, swelling and redness
- May be about the size of a marble (1-2 cm) or larger
- May be firm or fluctuant
- Redness progresses to yellowish center of pus

SKIN AND SOFT TISSUE INFECTION *(continued from previous page)*

SIGNS AND SYMPTOMS *(continued)*

Cellulitis

- First appears as a tiny edge of redness encircling a primary lesion.
- Redness spreads in circular fashion, indicating that local body defenses are not limiting the infection. There is pain or tenderness, redness, warmth and/or swelling at the site.
- The sore or rash (macule) appears suddenly, grows quickly in the first 24 hr., and usually has sharp borders.
- If the infection is around a skin wound, there may be swelling and drainage.
- There may be enlarged lymph nodes near the cellulitis.
- May be seen in children on the face, genital area or involving a joint or an extremity.

Lymphangitis

- Painful, red streak below the skin surface leading away from primary lesion to the axilla or to the groin
- Lymph nodes or red streaks above the area (elbow, axilla, or groin) may be enlarged or painful
- May have chills, fever (100°-104°), and malaise

MRSA

- Abscess, pimple, boil, or area on skin
- Redness/swelling around lesion
- Painful around lesion
- Warm to touch
- Lesion may be full of pus or other drainage
- Fever

MANAGEMENT/TREATMENT:[6]

- Gentle skin cleansing of new wounds.
- May apply warm, moist compresses to reduce inflammation and discomfort.
- Refer to healthcare provider immediately if circle or redness is 1/2 cm (dime size) or larger, over a joint or on the face.[7]
- Antibiotic ointment is not generally considered effective but may help eradicate a carrier
  - state. A healthcare provider may recommend an antibiotic for eradicating nasal carriage of staphylococcus.
- Lesion may require incision and drainage for healing.
- Healthcare provider may prescribe oral antibiotics for the infection and an analgesic for pain.
  - If antibiotic is prescribed, contact healthcare provider if condition worsens or there is no improvement after three days on antibiotic.[8]
  - **Cellulitis – if no improvement or condition worsens, the child may need hospitalization and intravenous antibiotic therapy; refer to healthcare provider for immediate follow-up.**

- **Refer suspected lymphangitis to healthcare provider for emergency care immediately**.
  - Prompt treatment with antibiotics typically result in complete recovery.

SKIN AND SOFT TISSUE INFECTION *(continued from previous page)*

MANAGEMENT/TREATMENT *(continued)*

- **Contact healthcare provider immediately if suspect MRSA.**
    - Most MRSA infections are treated with oral antibiotics.
    - May be treated by draining the abscess or boil; drainage is done by a healthcare professional.
    - If indicated, provide wound care per healthcare provider's orders (may include topical antibiotic).
    - Cover the wound with an appropriate bandage.
    - MRSA infections may reoccur.
        - Prevention steps are necessary to avoid reoccurrence of infection (avoid sharing towels or athletic gear, regular disinfectant cleaning of wrestling mats, etc.).

FOLLOW UP:

- MONITOR CAREFULLY!
- To prevent recurrence, the role of good hygiene should be stressed to student and family.
- Washing with an antibacterial soap may be helpful in the event of frequent episodes.
- If antibiotic is prescribed, all doses must be completed unless otherwise directed by the healthcare provider to discontinue medication.
- MRSA – the decision to close a school for any communicable disease should be made by school officials in consultation with local and/or state public health officials.[9]
    - In most cases, it is not necessary to close schools because of a MRSA infection in a student.
    - Generally, students with MRSA should not be excluded from school unless the wound is draining and cannot be covered.

POTENTIAL COMPLICATIONS:

- Methicillin-resistant *Staphylococcus aureus* (MRSA)
- Lymphangitis (abscess, cellulitis, sepsis)
- Meningitis (if cellulitis is on the face)
- Gangrene
- Sepsis

NOTES:

<u>Prevention</u>

Educate student, family and school staff:

- Keep skin clean and hydrated (use lotions) to prevent cracking.
- Give meticulous attention to cuts and wounds (cleaning, bandaging, and observing for signs of infection).
- Give special attention to foot care (trimming nails and wear properly fitted shoes).
- Wear protective clothing for work and sports.
- MRSA transmission can be prevented by simple habitual measures such as good handwashing hygiene, avoid sharing of personal items, and cleaning of athletic gear after each use.
- Discuss and implement preventive measures if student participates in any contact sport, or sports that use mats (gymnastics, wrestling, martial arts).

SKIN AND SOFT TISSUE INFECTION *(continued from previous page)*

REFERENCES

[1] Marcelin, J.R., Schooneveld, T.V., & Bergman, S. (2018). *Skin and soft tissue infections: Treatment guidance.* Nebraska Medicine. https://www.nebraskamed.com/sites/default/files/documents/for- providers/asp/ssti-guidelines-2018.pdf

[2] Medline Plus. U.S. National Library of Medicine. (2019). *Boils.* http://www.nlm.nih.gov/medlineplus/ency/article/001474.htm

[3] Mayo Clinic. (2019). *Cellulitis.* http://www.mayoclinic.com/print/cellulitis/DS00450/DSECTION=all&METHOD=print

[4] Merck Manual. (2019). *Bacterial infections.* https://www.merckmanuals.com/professional/dermatologic-disorders/bacterial-skin-infections

[5] Centers for Disease Control. (2019). *Methicillin-resistant staphylococcus aureus (MRSA) infections.* http://www.cdc.gov/mrsa/

[6] American Academy of Pediatrics, Committee on Infectious Diseases. (2018). Staphylococcal infections. In D.W.Kimberlin, M. T. Brady, M.A. Jackson, & S.S. Long (Eds.), *Red Book: 2018 report of the committee on infectious diseases* (31st ed., pp. 733-746). American Academy of Pediatrics.

[7] Ibid.

[8] Marcelin, J.R., Schooneveld, T.V., & Bergman, S. (2018). *Skin and soft tissue infections: Treatment guidance*. Nebraska Medicine. https://www.nebraskamed.com/sites/default/files/documents/for- providers/asp/ssti-guidelines-2018.pdf

[9] Ross, L. & Selekman, J. (2019). Skin disorders. In J. Selekman, R. Adair Shannon, & C. F. Yonkaitis (Eds.), *School nursing: A comprehensive text* (3rd ed., pp. 401-417). F. A. Davis.

OTHER REFERENCES CONSULTED

American Academy of Pediatrics, Committee on Infectious Diseases. (2018). Staphylococcal infections. In D.W. Kimberlin, M. T. Brady, M.A. Jackson, & S.S. Long (Eds.), *Red Book: 2018 report of the committee on infectious diseases* (31th ed., pp. 733-746). American Academy of Pediatrics.

Merck Manual. (2019). *Cellulitis.* https://www.merckmanuals.com/professional/dermatologic-disorders/bacterial-skin-infections/cellulitis

SORE THROAT (PHARYNGITIS including Streptococcal Infection)

DEFINITION/ETIOLOGY:

Pharyngitis is defined as inflammation of the pharynx and the surrounding lymph tissue causing pain, scratchiness or irritation.[1] It is often caused by a viral (influenza or common cold), bacterial (streptococcus) infection, and/or non- infectious causes such as an irritation (air pollution, allergens, sinus drainage, persistent cough). The most common causes are viruses. Only 15% to 30% of infections are caused by group A streptococcus.[2] The viruses are spread by oral and respiratory secretions and occur more commonly in fall, winter or spring.

SIGNS AND SYMPTOMS OF VIRAL PHARYNGITIS:

- Dry, scratchy throat
- Complaints of pain with swallowing
- Frequent swallowing and sniffing (from sinus drainage)
- Presence/absence of fever and signs of systemic illness
- Irritability in the younger child
- Conjunctivitis
- Increased drooling in the young child
- Symptoms associated with the common cold such as runny nose , cough, and congestion[3]

SIGNS AND SYPMTOMS OF BACTERIAL PHARYNGITIS (COMMONLY STREP THROAT)

"Strep" throat is due to *Group A Streptococcus bacterium.*

- Sudden onset of sore throat
- Fever (often > 101° F)
- Headache, nausea, abdominal pain, occasionally vomiting
- Marked inflammation of throat and tonsils; bright red tonsils may have thin white exudate
- Petechiae on the soft palate and posterior pharynx
- Initially a white swollen tongue which may progress to a "strawberry tongue"
- Enlarged anterior cervical lymph nodes
- A foul odor from the mouth
- Absence of diarrhea or coryza, cough, runny nose and conjunctivitis [4]

Scarlet Fever is a vascular response usually associated with streptococcal pharyngitis.

UNIQUE FINDINGS OF SCARLET FEVER:

- A fine diffuse red rash usually prominent in the armpits, groin and upper chest which makes the skin feel like "goose flesh" or "fine sandpaper".
- The rash spreads and, in five to 10 days, skin peels. Most cases are mild, lasting a few days, but severe cases occur.[5]

Primary oral herpes simplex virus may cause a sore throat due to the presence of ulcerating vesicles throughout the anterior pharynx and the lips. High fever and difficulty taking fluids are common and may last up to 14 days. *(Refer to HERPES SIMPLEX-ORAL).*

SORE THROAT (PHARYNGITIS) *(continued from previous page)*

MANAGEMENT/TREATMENT OF MINOR, VIRAL, AFEBRILE SORE THROAT:

- Warm, salty (1/4 teaspoon of salt to 8 oz. water) gargles
- Warm fluids (broth; hot water with melted lemon drop or warm lemonade)
- Over-the-counter lozenges (if school guidelines/policy allow)
- Analgesics such as acetaminophen or ibuprofen if medication orders are in place
- May attend school if feeling well enough unless other exclusion criteria are present such as fever, excessive drooling or difficulty swallowing[6]

MANAGEMENT/TREATMENT (Streptococcal Infection):

- Refer to healthcare provider for diagnosis by rapid strep test and culture in students with a sudden development of sore throat, fever, headache, nausea, vomiting, and enlarged tender lymph nodes. Some school clinics are equipped to provide the rapid strep test. If positive, it confirms group A strep infection. If the test result is negative, a regular culture (read in 12-24 hours) is still required to rule out strep, so many prefer to refer all suspected cases directly to healthcare provider.
- Encourage adequate fluid to keep mucus thin.
- Treatment of choice is penicillin. Treatment is aimed at preventing complications such as rheumatic heart disease.
- Return to school after 12 hours on antibiotic treatment and fever-free. For many children, three to five days absence may occur.[7]
- Treatment of scarlet fever is no different from the treatment of streptococcal infection[8]

FOLLOW-UP (Strep and Scarlet Fever):

- Monitor for a completed course of antibiotic therapy to prevent complications and carrier state.
- Encourage student to replace toothbrush.
- Two major complications: acute rheumatic fever (joints, heart) occurs in 1% of group A strep cases, and acute self-limiting glomerulonephritis (kidney disease) can be serious. Children younger than three years are very unlikely to develop rheumatic heart disease. Monitor for complications (high fever, joint pain, blood in the urine) and <u>refer immediately to healthcare provider.</u>

POTENTIAL COMPLICATIONS:

- Ear infection
- Glomerulonephritis
- Rheumatic Heart Disease
- Sinusitis
- Tonsillitis
- Peritonsillar abscess (A tonsil displaced anteriorly is a sign of peritonsillar abscess and should be referred immediately).[9]

NOTES:

Avoid giving aspirin under the age of eighteen. Aspirin can play a role in causing Reye's Syndrome. 25% of schoolchildren may carry the bacteria that cause strep throat and be asymptomatic. The risk of transmission from these children is low.[10]

SORE THROAT (PHARYNGITIS) *(continued from previous page)*

REFERENCES

[1] Mayo Clinic. (2019). *Sore throat.* http://www.mayoclinic.com/health/sore-throat/DS00526

[2] Jakubowski, T. & Perron, T. (2019). Students with common health complaints. In J. Selekman, R. Adair Shannon, & C. F. Yonkaitis (Eds.), *School nursing: A comprehensive text* (3rd ed., pp. 347-348). F.A. Davis.

[3] Ibid.

[4] Ibid.

[5] American Academy of Pediatrics. (2020). Strep throat (streptococcal pharyngitis). In S. Aronson, & T. Shope (Eds.), *Managing infectious diseases in child care and schools* (5th ed., pp. 59, 167-168). American Academy of Pediatrics.

[6] Ibid.

[7] Ibid

[8] Ibid.

[9] Jakubowski, T. & Perron, T. (2019). Students with common health complaints. In J. Selekman, R. Adair Shannon, & C. F. Yonkaitis (Eds.), *School nursing: A comprehensive text* (3rd ed., pp. 347-348). F.A. Davis.

[10] American Academy of Pediatrics. (2020). Strep throat (streptococcal pharyngitis). In S. Aronson, & T. Shope (Eds.), *Managing infectious diseases in child care and schools* (5th ed., pp. 59, 167-168). American Academy of Pediatrics.

OTHER REFERENCES CONSULTED

Medline Plus, U.S. National Library of Medicine. (2019). *Sore throat.* http://www.nlm.nih.gov/medlineplus/sorethroat.html

SPIDER BITE (Brown Recluse and Black Widow)

DEFINITION/ETIOLOGY: Most spider bites are harmless. Occasionally, spider bites can cause allergic reactions. However, bites by the venomous black widow and brown recluse spiders can be very dangerous to people.[1]

Brown Recluse spider bites produce poisonous venom that contains both a toxin and an enzyme that spreads the toxin through tissue. Ten species, six of which are poisonous, live in the United States. They are most common in the southern and midwestern U.S.[2] The spiders are non-hairy, yellowish-tan to dark brown, and have a violin pattern on their back. They prefer dark, dry spaces (under porches, attic, closet, woodpiles). They are not aggressive but bite defensively.[3]

Black Widow spiders produce potent, protein venom that attacks the central nervous system. The Southern species are about ½-inch long, shiny, black, globular shape with distinctive red hourglass shape on the underside. The Northern species have a row of red spots down the middle of the upper surface of the abdomen and two cross bars on the underside. They are seen mostly in the southern and western United States.[4] The Black Widow spider is nocturnal, prefers dark corners and crevices, and bites defensively, usually when the victim comes in contact with the web.[5]

SIGNS AND SYMPTOMS:

General signs and symptoms:[6]

- A mark indicating a bite
- Pain, redness, and swelling in bite area
- Nausea and vomiting
- Chills or fever
- Itching or rash
- Muscle pain or cramping
- Joint pain or stiffness
- Reddish to purplish color or blister
- Increased sweating
- Difficulty breathing
- Headache
- Anxiety or restlessness

These symptoms are also indicative of other health concerns. Diagnosis is based on thorough history of location, activities, and physical signs. Spider bites and the identification of the type of spider are difficult to confirm because they usually not witnessed.

SPIDER BITE (Brown Recluse and Black Widow) *(continued from previous page)*

SIGNS AND SYMPTOMS *(continued)*

Brown Recluse

- Painless initially; then pain, which can be severe and involve the entire extremity, develops within one to four hours. Pain begins as local stinging or burning.[7]
- Initially, the lesion is red and swollen or blanched, and may develop a blue-gray halo around the puncture (due to hemolysis and vasospasm). The lesion may change to bluish pustules or large blistering surrounded by purpura discoloration.
- Within 12 hours, fever, chills, nausea/vomiting, scarlatiniform rash, arthralgia, diarrhea and weakness may develop.[8]
- Centrally, necrosis or a "sinking center" develops. The ulcer may take weeks to months to heal.[9]

Black Widow

- Immediate, sharp, stinging sensation, progressing to persistent local pain, diaphoresis, erythema at the site.
- Localized to generalized severe muscle cramps, abdominal pain, weakness, and tremor may occur.[10]
- Nausea and vomiting, dizziness, headache, chest pain, and respiratory difficulty may follow.[11]

MANAGEMENT/TREATMENT:

General spider bites [12]

- Clean the wound with mild soap and water.
- Apply ice and elevate.
- OTC analgesics for pain management.
- Limit movement of affected area and avoid vigorous activity.
- **Seek emergency medical attention if black widow or brown recluse bite is suspected.**[13]

FOLLOW UP:

- Re-assess in 48 hours; may need referral for debridement.
- Continue to monitor. Wound may need skin grafting.
- Healthcare provider may recommend a tetanus booster if needed.

PREVENTION:

Educate staff and students regarding poisonous spider recognition:

- Brown Recluse: About one inch long, non-hairy, yellowish-tan to dark brown, and have a violin pattern on their back. They prefer dark, dry spaces (under porches, attic, closet, woodpiles. They are not aggressive but bite defensively.

- Black Widow*:* The Southern species are about ½-inch long, shiny, black, globular shape with distinctive red hourglass shape on the underside. The Northern species have a row of red spots down the middle of the upper surface of the abdomen and 2 cross bars on the underside. The Black Widow spider is nocturnal, prefers dark corners and crevices, and bites defensively.[14]

SPIDER BITE (Brown Recluse and Black Widow) *(continued from previous page)*

PREVENTION *(continued)*

Educate school staff about prevention of spider bites:

- Avoid areas such as wood piles, fences, and areas where debris has collected.

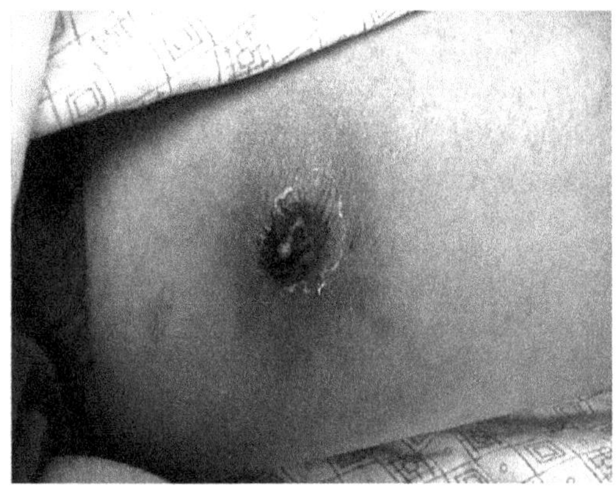

Brown Recluse Spider Bite

From the Merck Manual Professional Version (Known as the Merck Manual in the US and Canada and the MSD Manual in the rest of the world), edited by Robert Porter. Copyright (2020) by Merck Sharp & Dohme Corp., a subsidiary of Merck & Co., Inc, Kenilworth, NJ. Available at https://www.merckmanuals.com/professional/injuries-poisoning/bites-and-stings/spider-bites?qt=spider%20bites&alt=sh Accessed 2-21-20.

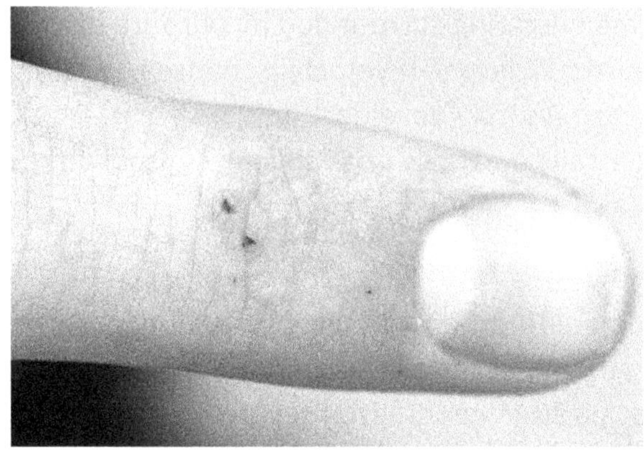

Double fang bite of Black Widow Spider Bite [15]

EMedicineHealth.com (2016). Permission to reprint granted by WebMD as educational resource only.

SPIDER BITE (Brown Recluse and Black Widow) *(continued from previous page)*

REFERENCES

[1] MedlinePlus, U.S. National Library of Medicine. (2018). *Spider bites*. https://medlineplus.gov/spiderbites.html#summary

[2] Centers for Disease Control. (2018*). NIOSH safety and health topic: Venomous spiders.* http://www.cdc.gov/niosh/topics/spiders/

[3] EMedicine Health. (2016). *Spider bites: Black widow vs. brown recluse first aid.* https://www.emedicinehealth.com/slideshow_black_widow_brown_recluse_spiders/article_em.htm

[4] Ibid.

[5] Centers for Disease Control. (2018*). NIOSH safety and health topic: Venomous spiders.* http://www.cdc.gov/niosh/topics/spiders/

[6] Merck Manual, Professional Edition. *Spider bites.* (2018). http://www.merckmanuals.com/professional/injuries_poisoning/bites_and_stings/spider_bites.html?qt=spider%20bites&alt=sh

[7] Ibid.

[8] MedlinePlus, U.S. National Library of Medicine. (2018). *Spider bites*. https://medlineplus.gov/spiderbites.html#summary

[9] Merck Manual, Professional Edition. *Spider bites.* (2018). http://www.merckmanuals.com/professional/injuries_poisoning/bites_and_stings/spider_bites.html?qt=spider%20bites&alt=sh

[10] Crosby, M., Lyons, E., & Prestidge, L. (2019). Students with acute illness and injury. In J. Selekman, R. Shannon, & C.Yonkaitis (Eds.), *School nursing: A comprehensive text* (3rd ed., p. 448). F.A. Davis Company.

[11]Merck Manual, Professional Edition. *Spider bites.* (2018). http://www.merckmanuals.com/professional/injuries_poisoning/bites_and_stings/spider_bites.html?qt=spider%20bites&alt=sh

[12] Centers for Disease Control. (2018*). NIOSH safety and health topic: Venomous spiders.* http://www.cdc.gov/niosh/topics/spiders/

[13] Crosby, M., Lyons, E., & Prestidge, L. (2019). Students with acute illness and injury. In J. Selekman, R. Shannon, & C. Yonkaitis (Eds.), *School nursing: A comprehensive text* (3rd ed., p. 448). F.A. Davis Company.

[14] Centers for Disease Control. (2018*). NIOSH safety and health topic: Venomous spiders.* http://www.cdc.gov/niosh/topics/spiders/

[15] EMedicine Health. (2016). *Spider bites: Black widow vs. brown recluse first aid.* https://www.emedicinehealth.com/slideshow_black_widow_brown_recluse_spiders/article_em.htm

SPINA BIFIDA

DEFINITION/ETIOLOGY:

Spina bifida means "cleft spine", it is the most common neural tube defect and is characterized by the incomplete development of the brain, spinal cord, and/or meninges.[1, 2]
There are four types of spina bifida: occulta, closed neural tube defects, meningocele, and myelomeningocele.

- Occulta is the most common form and mildest that causes one or more vertebrae to be malformed, and a layer of skin covers it.
- Closed neural tube defects is a group of defects in the spinal cord that are malformations of fat, bone or meninges.
- Meningocele is when spinal fluid and meninges protrude through an abnormal vertebra opening, contains no neural elements and may or may not be covered with skin.
- Myelomeningocele is the most severe type and occurs when the spinal cord/neural elements are exposed through an opening in the spine.[3,4]

There are multiple factors that can cause spina bifida including genetics, nutritional, and environmental factors. Research studies indicate that an insufficient intake of folic acid in the mother's diet is a key factor, as well as other vitamins.[5] Spina bifida can be diagnosed during pregnancy or after the baby is born. Spina bifida occulta might not be diagnosed until childhood, or later in life.[6]

SIGNS AND SYMPTOMS:

- Closed neural defect can sometimes be recognized with abnormal clump of hair or a small dimple on the skin at the site of spinal malformation.[7]
- Visible signs of an meningocele and myelomeningocele involve fluid filled sac protruding from the spinal canal. This can be repaired sometimes in utero at various medical centers, but usually surgery is performed after the birth of the child.[8]
- If a student has a diagnosis of spina bifida, that student (depending on the type, and level of malformation) might have hydrocephalus, that will require placement of a shunt.
- Students with the diagnosis of spina bifida might exhibit abnormal gait, neurogenic bowel and bladder, or might be confined to a wheelchair.[9]
- Some students might also have signs and symptoms of intellectual disabilities, that can range from mild to severe.[10]

MANAGEMENT/TREATMENT:

- The management and treatment of a student with spina bifida can include physical therapy, occupational therapy, braces, orthotics, and treatment for bowel and bladder problems that might include catheterization and bowel management regimes. Some students might require further surgeries for problems with their feet, hip and spine, as well as repair or replacement of their shunt if the shunt fails.[11] *(Refer to URINARY CATHETERIZATION).*

SPINA BIFIDA *(continued from previous page)*

MANAGEMENT/TREATMENT *(continued)*

- Shunt care: The school nurse should be aware of where the shunt is placed and are there any limitations to activities. If the student is post -operative of shunt placement or repair, it is important for the school nurse to be aware of any signs and symptoms of post-operative infections, at the surgical site(s) as well as any fevers.

POTENTIAL COMPLICATIONS:

- Signs and symptoms of tethered cord, decrease loss of muscle function in the legs, changes in bowel and bladder function[12, 13]
- Signs and symptoms of shunt failure, such as severe headache, vomiting, lethargy, change in personality[14]
- Urinary infections due to bladder not being emptied completely or student is not self-cathing or not correctly self-cathing
- Constipation due to lack of bowel regime
- Skin integrity if student is wheelchair bound and not performing pressure relief, or if student is incontinent of feces and urine
- Signs and symptoms of student being bullied or questioning why they are different than peers
- Chiari II malformation, which can impact respiratory status[15]

FOLLOW-UP:

- The school nurse should also be aware of signs and symptoms of tethered cord syndrome since there is a chance a student with spina bifida myelomeningocele type might develop this syndrome.[16]
- Monitor for potential health needs (e.g. shunt malfunction, UTIs, constipation, and skin integrity).
- The student should be followed by a neurologist, orthopedist, or spina bifida clinic at least yearly to monitor for concerns.[17]
- Consider a referral to the Section 504/Individualized Education Plan (IEP) team.
- Develop an Individualized Healthcare Plan (IHP).
- Provide relevant education to other students (with parent approval) and for staff.
- Plan for student's access to water at all times.
- **Prevention:** The school nurse should have resources for female students that might be sexually active on the importance of good nutrition, and folic acid needs, as well as prenatal care.[18]

NOTES:

- Women of childbearing age should consume 400 micrograms of folic acid daily.[19]
- Women who already have a child with spina bifida are at greater risk for having another child with spina bifida or neural tube defect.[20]
- Hispanic women have a higher rate of giving birth to a child with spina bifida.[21]

SPINA BIFIDA *(continued from previous page)*

REFERENCES

[1] National Institute of Neurological Disorders and Stroke. (2019). Spina bifida fact sheet. https://www.ninds.nih.gov/Disorders/Patient-Caregiver-Education/Fact-Sheets/Spina-Bifida-Fact-Sheet

[2] Centers for Disease Control and Prevention. (2019). *Data & statistics on spina bifida.* https://www.cdc.gov/ncbddd/spinabifida/data.html

[3] Ibid.

[4] National Institute of Neurological Disorders and Stroke. (2019). Spina bifida fact sheet. https://www.ninds.nih.gov/Disorders/Patient-Caregiver-Education/Fact-Sheets/Spina-Bifida-Fact-Sheet

[5] Ibid.

[6] Centers for Disease Control and Prevention. (2019). *Data & statistics on spina bifida.* https://www.cdc.gov/ncbddd/spinabifida/data.html

[7] National Institute of Neurological Disorders and Stroke. (2019). Spina bifida fact sheet. https://www.ninds.nih.gov/Disorders/Patient-Caregiver-Education/Fact-Sheets/Spina-Bifida-Fact-Sheet

[8] Ibid.

[9] Centers for Disease Control and Prevention. (2019). *Data & statistics on spina bifida.* https://www.cdc.gov/ncbddd/spinabifida/data.html

[10] National Institute of Neurological Disorders and Stroke. (2019). Spina bifida fact sheet. https://www.ninds.nih.gov/Disorders/Patient-Caregiver-Education/Fact-Sheets/Spina-Bifida-Fact-Sheet

[11] Merck Manual. (2018). *Spina bifida.* https://www.merckmanuals.com/professional/pediatrics/congenital-neurologic-anomalies/spina-bifida

[12] National Institute of Neurological Disorders and Stroke. (2019). Spina bifida fact sheet. https://www.ninds.nih.gov/Disorders/Patient-Caregiver-Education/Fact-Sheets/Spina-Bifida-Fact-Sheet

[13] National Organization of Rare Diseases (NORD). (2007). Spina bifida. https://rarediseases.org/rare-diseases/spina-bifida/

[14] Merck Manual. (2018). *Spina bifida.* https://www.merckmanuals.com/professional/pediatrics/congenital-neurologic-anomalies/spina-bifida

[15]Spina Bifida Association. (2019). *We're improving the lives of those living with spina bifida.* https://www.spinabifidaassociation.org/

[16] National Institute of Neurological Disorders and Stroke. (2019). Spina bifida fact sheet. https://www.ninds.nih.gov/Disorders/Patient-Caregiver-Education/Fact-Sheets/Spina-Bifida-Fact-Sheet

[17] Spina Bifida Association. (2019). *We're improving the lives of those living with spina bifida.* https://www.spinabifidaassociation.org/

[18] Centers for Disease Control and Prevention. (2019). *Data & statistics on spina bifida.* https://www.cdc.gov/ncbddd/spinabifida/data.html

[19] Ibid.

[20] Ibid.

[21] National Organization of Rare Diseases (NORD). (2007). Spina bifida. https://rarediseases.org/rare-diseases/spina-bifida/

SPONTANEOUS PNEUMOTHORAX

DEFINITION/ETIOLOGY:

Pneumothorax is air in the pleural space (the space around the lungs) causing partial or complete lung collapse.[1] Spontaneous pneumothorax is the sudden onset of a collapsed lung without any apparent cause, such as a traumatic injury to the chest or a known lung disease.[2] The collapsed lung is caused by the collection of air in the space around the lungs.

Primary spontaneous pneumothorax is a pneumothorax that occurs without any apparent cause in people without a known lung disorder.[3] Primary spontaneous pneumothorax usually occurs when a small weakened area of lung (bulla) ruptures. The condition is most common in tall men younger than age 40 who smoke.[4] It generally occurs at rest, although some cases occur during activities involving reaching or stretching. Primary spontaneous pneumothorax also occurs during diving and high-altitude flying.[5]

Secondary spontaneous pneumothorax occurs in people with an underlying lung disorder. This type of pneumothorax most often occurs when a bulla ruptures in an older person who has chronic obstructive pulmonary disease (COPD), but it also occurs in people with other lung conditions, such as cystic fibrosis, asthma, pulmonary Langerhans cell histiocytosis, sarcoidosis, lung abscess, tuberculosis, and Pneumocystis pneumonia. Because of the underlying lung disorder, the symptoms and outcome are generally worse in secondary spontaneous pneumothorax. The recurrence rate is like that of primary spontaneous pneumothorax.[6]

Many researchers believe that genetic factors may play a role in the development of primary spontaneous pneumothorax. In addition, several genetic disorders have been linked to primary spontaneous pneumothorax, including Marfan syndrome, homocystinuria, and Birt-Hogg-Dube syndrome.[7]

SIGNS AND SYMPTOMS:

Spontaneous pneumothorax most commonly presents without severe symptoms and a student with a small pneumothorax may be asymptomatic.[8] Patients with a collapsed lung may experience a sudden onset of the following symptoms:[9]

- Sharp chest pain, made worse by a deep breath or a cough
- Shortness of breath
- Decreased or absent breath sounds on the affected side
- Absent tactile fremitus (vibration of the chest wall felt while a patient is speaking). Assess by asking the patient to say “99”. Palpate the chest comparing one side to the other while the patient is speaking.[10]
- Hyperresonance to percussion

A larger pneumothorax will cause more severe symptoms, including:[11]

- Chest tightness
- Easy fatigue
- Rapid heart rate
- Bluish color (cyanosis) of the skin caused by lack of oxygen
- Nasal flaring
- Chest wall retractions
- Affected side may be enlarged with the trachea visibly shifted to the opposite side

SPONTANEOUS PNEUMOTHORAX *(continued from previous page)*

SIGNS AND SYMPTOMS *(continued)*

Note: Dyspnea may be sudden or gradual in onset depending on the rate of development and size of the pneumothorax. Pain can simulate pericarditis, pneumonia, pleuritis, pulmonary embolism, musculoskeletal injury (when referred to the shoulder), or an intra-abdominal process (when referred to the abdomen). Pain can also simulate cardiac ischemia, although typically the pain of cardiac ischemia is not pleuritic.[12]

MANAGEMENT/TREATMENT:

- Prompt recognition of symptoms of sudden onset of shortness of breath or sharp chest pain that is worsened by breathing.
- Emergency transport and care including air removal from the pleural space.
- Diagnosis is suspected in stable patients with dyspnea or pleuritic chest pain and is confirmed with upright inspiratory chest x-ray.
- Treatment of spontaneous pneumothorax depends on the duration, severity of symptoms and size of pneumothorax.[13]
- A small, primary spontaneous pneumothorax usually requires no treatment.[14] It usually does not cause serious breathing problems, and the air is absorbed in several days.
- Students may be given oxygen through the nose or a face mask to help speed the absorption of air. The full absorption of air in a larger pneumothorax may take 2 to 4 weeks.
- Primary spontaneous pneumothorax that is < 20% and that does not cause respiratory or cardiac symptoms can be safely observed without treatment if follow-up chest x-rays done at about 6 and 48 hours show no progression.[15]
- Larger or symptomatic primary spontaneous pneumothoraxes should be evacuated by catheter aspiration by a healthcare provider most often in the Emergency Department. Tube thoracostomy is an alternative.[16]

FOLLOW-UP:

- Monitor for recurrence - most people fully recover; however, recurrence approaches 50% in the three years after initial spontaneous pneumothorax. [17]
- If the student requires the insertion of a chest tube or surgery monitor the incision sites upon return to school for signs of infection including redness, yellow or green discharge, tenderness, warmth or foul odor. [18]
- Smoking cessation referral if applicable.
- Teach student that avoidance of deep-sea diving is advised because it causes gases to expand and can lead to pneumothorax in patients with bullae and blebs.

SPONTANEOUS PNEUMOTHORAX *(continued from previous page)*

POTENTIAL COMPLICATIONS:

Recurring pneumothorax:[19]

- A recurring pneumothorax can cause considerable disability.
- Surgery can be done to prevent pneumothorax from recurring.
- Usually surgery involves repairing leaking areas of the lung, firmly attaching the inner layer of pleura to the outer layer.
- This surgery is usually done by using a video-assisted thoracoscope (a tube that allows doctors to view the pleural space).

REFERENCES

[1] Light, R. (2017). *Pneumothorax.* Merck Manual Professional Version. https://www.merckmanuals.com/professional/pulmonary-disorders/mediastinal-and-pleural-disorders/pneumothorax?query=spontaneous%20pneumothorax

[2] Children's Hospital of Philadelphia. (2018). *Spontaneous pneumothorax.* https://www.chop.edu/conditions-diseases/spontaneous-pneumothorax

[3] Light, R. (2017). *Pneumothorax*. Merck Manual Professional Version. https://www.merckmanuals.com/professional/pulmonary-disorders/mediastinal-and-pleural-disorders/pneumothorax?query=spontaneous%20pneumothorax

[4] Ibid.

[5] Children's Hospital of Philadelphia. (2018). *Spontaneous pneumothorax.* https://www.chop.edu/conditions-diseases/spontaneous-pneumothorax

[6] Light, R. (2017). *Pneumothorax*. Merck Manual Professional Version. https://www.merckmanuals.com/professional/pulmonary-disorders/mediastinal-and-pleural-disorders/pneumothorax?query=spontaneous%20pneumothorax

[7] U.S. Department of Health and Human Services, National Institute of Health. (n.d.). *Primary spontaneous pneumothorax* *https://rarediseases.info.nih.gov/diseases/4997/primary-spontaneous-pneumothorax*

[8] Light, R. (2017). *Pneumothorax.* Merck Manual Professional Version. https://www.merckmanuals.com/professional/pulmonary-disorders/mediastinal-and-pleural-disorders/pneumothorax?query=spontaneous%20pneumothorax

[9] Children's Hospital of Philadelphia. (2018). *Spontaneous pneumothorax.* https://www.chop.edu/conditions-diseases/spontaneous-pneumothorax

[10] Light, R. (2017). *Pneumothorax.* Merck Manual Professional Version. https://www.merckmanuals.com/professional/pulmonary-disorders/mediastinal-and-pleural-disorders/pneumothorax?query=spontaneous%20pneumothorax

[11] Children's Hospital of Philadelphia. (2018). *Spontaneous pneumothorax.* https://www.chop.edu/conditions-diseases/spontaneous-pneumothorax

[12] Light, R. (2017). *Pneumothorax*. Merck Manual Professional Version. https://www.merckmanuals.com/professional/pulmonary-disorders/mediastinal-and-pleural-disorders/pneumothorax?query=spontaneous%20pneumothorax

[13] Children's Hospital of Philadelphia. (2018). *Spontaneous pneumothorax.* https://www.chop.edu/conditions-diseases/spontaneous-pneumothorax

[14] Ibid.

SPONTANEOUS PNEUMOTHORAX *(continued from previous page)*

[15] Light, R. (2017). *Pneumothorax*. Merck Manual Professional Version. https://www.merckmanuals.com/professional/pulmonary-disorders/mediastinal-and-pleural-disorders/pneumothorax?query=spontaneous%20pneumothorax

[16] Ibid.

[17] Ibid.

[18] Children's Hospital of Philadelphia. (2018). *Spontaneous pneumothorax.* https://www.chop.edu/conditions-diseases/spontaneous-pneumothorax

[19] Light, R. (2017). *Pneumothorax*. Merck Manual Professional Version. https://www.merckmanuals.com/professional/pulmonary-disorders/mediastinal-and-pleural-disorders/pneumothorax?query=spontaneous%20pneumothorax

SPRAIN AND STRAINS

DEFINITION/ETIOLOGY:

A sprain is a stretched or torn ligament (fibrous tissue that connects bones to other bones). The injury can range from a stretch to a tiny tear to a complete severing of the ligament. They occur when a joint is forced to move beyond its normal range of motion and are a common athletic injury of children. Sprains are graded according to the instability that results in the joint:

- Grade 1 (mild) sprain causes pain and tenderness along the ligament without increased joint instability
- Grade 2 (moderate) sprain results in a partial tear of a ligament and moderate joint instability
- Grade 3 (severe) sprain is a complete tear or disruption of a ligament resulting in no joint stability

Of all sprains, ankle and knee sprains occur most often.

A strain results from pulling or overexerting a muscle or tendon (tough band of fibrous connective tissue that connects muscle to bone).[1]

SIGNS AND SYMPTOMS:

- History of trauma (for example, person steps down on the outside of the foot and twists the foot)
- During trauma, persons may feel a flash of heat or may describe hearing a "snap" or "pop"
- History of prior injury to same joint
- Pain/tenderness at site of injury
- Variable swelling, and/or bruising
- Limited ability to move affected part[2]

MANAGEMENT/TREATMENT:

1. Take careful detailed history of injury, including what happened, what person felt, what person heard, what others observed
2. Follow universal/standard precautions (infection prevention practices). (*Refer to STANDARD PRECAUTIONS APPENDIX).*
3. Assess and document pulse quality and capillary refill below the injured site.
4. Assess and document range of motion (ROM) and sensation (compare with corresponding area on opposite extremity).
5. Control bleeding, if necessary.
6. Avoid any movements or changes in position that cause pain.
7. Immobilize injured area.
8. Clean and bandage any open wounds.
9. Check for circulation, movement and sensation to the limb. Feel for the patient's distal pulse, skin temperature and ability to move and detect touch in the injured parts.
10. Institute RICE principle:[3]

SPRAIN AND STRAINS *(continued from previous page)*

MANAGEMENT/TREATMENT *(continued)*

Rest **of the injured area for 48 hours**	• Weight bearing may increase injury. If uncomfortable to walk, use crutches. • Review safe crutch walking technique. • Get permit to use elevator (if any). • If hall traffic is unmanageable on crutches, get permit to leave class a few minutes early. • Arrange for help to carry books.
Ice **placed on the injured area for 20 minutes every 2 -3 hours while awake for first 24 hours**	• Ice cubes or frozen wet sponges can be placed in a plastic bag, wrapped in a light cloth, and applied to the painful area. Remove compression bandage while using ice.
Compression **with elastic bandages or if authorized, splints**	• A pressure bandage may reduce swelling. Use a compression bandage, especially when the ankle is not elevated while crutch walking. • A 3" elastic ACE wrap is generally used. A more convenient material is elastic tubular bandage, a surgical dressing available from a medical or athletic supply store.
Elevate **injured part**	Keep the foot higher than the hip when not mobile at least 24 hours following injury.

WHEN TO REFER TO HEALTHCARE PROVIDER:

- All injuries associated with severe pain or immediate swelling/or injured area is misshapen (may indicate fracture)
- If there are signs that circulation beyond the injured area is impaired
- Inability to bear weight
- All suspected fractures

FOLLOW UP:

- Monitor for blood flow above and below injured area; if a splint/wrap/cast has been applied, observe fingers and toes for cyanosis and coldness.
- For mild to moderate pain, a non-steroidal anti-inflammatory analgesic (ibuprofen) taken with food to limit stomach upset may be administered (if medically approved or with parent/guardian approval and per policy). Alert parent/guardian when medication is administered and if requests are increasing in frequency.
- Range of motion (ROM) or physical therapy, as recommended by healthcare provider, to retain full use of injured part.
- Request written guidelines from healthcare provider re: return to school and activity restrictions, including recess and physical education.

SPRAIN AND STRAINS *(continued from previous page)*

FOLLOW UP *(continued)*

- Provide plan to school staff to address need for accommodations, such as use of wheelchair, elevator, crutches, etc.
- Advise student to abide by recommended physical activity restrictions for time period recommended by healthcare provider and until pain has subsided.
- If directed by healthcare provider, support joint by taping, bracing, or wearing high top sneakers when student returns to activities.[4]

POTENTIAL COMPLICATIONS:

- Swelling may decrease blood flow to area below sprain.
- Unrecognized and inappropriately managed injury can lead to more long-term functional disability.

NOTES:

Once an ankle has been sprained, it may be susceptible to recurring sprains because of instability in the joint.[5] The following are suggestions to avoid re-injury:

- Avoid activities (exercising or sports) when tired or in pain.
- Wear correctly fitted shoes and equipment.
- Warm-up and stretch before participating in exercises or sports.

REFERENCES

[1] American Academy of Pediatrics. Healthy Children.org. (2015). *Sports injuries: Acute soft-tissue injuries.* https://www.healthychildren.org/English/health-issues/injuries-emergencies/sports-injuries/Pages/Sports-Injuries-Acute-Soft-Tissue-Injuries.aspx

[2] Mayo Clinic. (2018). *Sprains.* https://www.mayoclinic.org/diseases-conditions/sprains/symptoms- causes/syc-20377938

[3] Michigan Medicine, University of Michigan. (2018). *Rest, ice, compression and elevation (RICE).* https://www.uofmhealth.org/health-library/tw4354spec

[4] Voskuio, V., & Selekman, J. (2019). Health issues related to physical activity and athletics. In J. Selekman, R. Adair Shannon, & C. F. Yonkaitis (Eds.). *School nursing: A comprehensive text* (3rd ed., pp. 388-390). F.A. Davis Company.

[5] American National Red Cross. (2017). Muscle, bone and joint injuries. *Responding to emergencies: Comprehensive first aid/CPR/AED e-Textbook.* Published online: American National Red Cross. http://pchs.psd202.org/documents/mopsal/1539703875.pdf

STOMATITIS (ORAL LESION)

DEFINITION/ETIOLOGY:

Stomatitis is an inflammation of the oral mucous membrane and may include lesions that can occur anywhere in the mouth including the cheeks, gums, soft and hard palate, and on the tongue and lips.[1] Many things can contribute to the development of oral lesions such as trauma; viral, bacterial or fungal infections; poor dental hygiene; and chewing (smokeless) tobacco. Mouth sores may also occur after dental work, with braces or from accidental biting of the inside of the mouth, sunlight, stress or other environmental irritants. Certain autoimmune diseases such as Crohn's disease can also affect the mucous membranes of the mouth. Mouth ulcers are also a common side effect of chemotherapy. In some cases, the cause is unknown.[2] May also occur from sensitivity/allergy to chemicals in oral hygiene products such as toothpaste.[3]

SIGNS AND SYMPTOMS:

Symptoms are dependent on the etiology of the oral lesion. General symptoms include:

- Oral ulcers
- Pain in the mouth

TYPE	SYMPTOMS
Aphthous Ulcer (canker sore)	• Small, oval, indurated papules with surrounding redness and a white, gray or yellow center • Often preceded by a "burning" sensation that progresses into an ulcer with surrounding redness • Usually a single lesion but may occur in a cluster of four to five • May experience enlarged lymph nodes • Lesions are painful • Lesions heal in one to two weeks without scarring [4]
Herpes simplex virus (cold sore, fever blister) [5] **Refer to HSV*	• Painful, vesicular, fluid filled lesions • Lesions are generally located on or around the outer lips • Contagion until the lesions crust over • During an episode the lesions may last seven to 10 days [6]
Oral candidiasis (thrush) – fungal (yeast) infection that occurs when there is overgrowth of *Candida.* Thrush may occur after a course of antibiotics or in immunocompromised individuals. Typically, not seen in healthy youth.	• White patches on tongue, gums and oral mucous membrane • Lesions may bleed when gently scraped • A warm environment enables growth • Person to person transmission is rare • Repeated infections may indicate a disease process [7]

STOMATITIS *(continued from previous page)*

MANAGEMENT/TREATMENT:

- Do not exclude from school since the condition is not considered contagious
- Treatment is focused on relieving symptoms; a topical anesthetic may be used
- Rinse with saltwater
- Avoid irritating foods/liquids (spicy, salty or acidic)
- Advise careful tooth brushing to avoid the lesion(s)

FOLLOW UP:

Oral lesions may be an indication of a compromised immune system.

- Refer to healthcare provider if oral lesions are not healed in two to three weeks or if lesions are severe.
- Healthcare provider may consider performing a biopsy on a lesion that does not heal properly.

POTENTIAL COMPLICATIONS:

- Dehydration – encourage non-acidic fluids
- Oral cellulitis – secondary from bacterial infection
- Oral cancer

NOTES:

- If prone to mouth sores, avoid acidic and/or spicy foods.
- Practice good oral hygiene. Brush teeth (with soft bristle toothbrush) in the morning, after meals/bedtime and floss daily; change toothbrush at least two times per year.
- Ulcers in the mouth occur with some childhood infections including:
    - Hand, foot and mouth disease (Coxsackie group A virus & enterovirus)
    - Herpangina (typically caused by Coxsackie group A virus) [8]
- Sexually Transmitted Diseases
    - Syphilis chancres may be present with primary syphilis.
    - Syphilis and Gonorrhea can also be transmitted during oral sex.

      Syphilis
        - Lesion is located at point of syphilis entry.
        - Syphilis ulcer is firm, round and painless.
        - Syphilis lesion may last three to six weeks.

      Oral gonorrhea (rare) may have redness and/or ulcerative lesions on gingiva and tongue.
        - Inquire about history of engaging in oral sex.
        - Refer to healthcare provider for appropriate treatment.[9]
        - Educate adolescent on safe sex practices.

STOMATITIS *(continued from previous page)*

REFERENCES

[1] Merck Manual. (2019). *Stomatitis.* http://www.merckmanuals.com/professional/dental disorders/symptoms of dental and oral disorders/stomatitis.html?qt=oral%20lesions&alt=sh

[2] Medline Plus, U.S. National Library of Medicine. (2019). *Mouth ulcers.* http://www.nlm.nih.gov/medlineplus/ency/article/001448.htm

[3] Minciullo, P. L., Paolino, G, Vacca, M., Gangemi, S. & Nettles, F. (2016). Unmet diagnostic needs in contact oral mucosal allergies. *Clinical & Molecular Allergy*, 14 (10), 1-8. https://doi.org/10.1186/s12948-016-0047-y

[4] Martin, B. Baumnardt, H., D'Alesia, A., & K. Woods. (2018). Oral disorders. In B. J. Zitelli, BS. McIntire, & A.J. Nowalk (Eds.), *Atlas of pediatric physical diagnosis* (7th ed., p.p. 746-747). Elsevier Inc.

[5] American Academy of Pediatrics. (2020). Herpes simplex (cold sores). In S. Aronson & T. Shope (Eds.), *Managing infectious diseases in child care and schools* (5th ed., pp. 107-108). American Academy of Pediatrics.

[6] American Academy of Dermatology. (2018). Herpes simplex. https://www.aad.org/public/diseases/contagious-skin-diseases/herpes-simplex#symptoms

[7] American Academy of Pediatrics. (2020). Thrush (candidiasis). In S. Aronson & T. Shope (Eds.), *Managing infectious diseases in child care and schools* (5th ed., pp. 171). American Academy of Pediatrics.

[8] Martin, D., B. Baumnardt, H., D'Alesia, A., & K. Woods. (2018). Oral disorders. In B. J. Zitelli, BS. McIntire, & A.J. Nowalk (Eds.), *Atlas of pediatric physical diagnosis* (7th ed., p.p. 746-747). Elsevier Inc.

[9] Centers for Disease Control and Prevention (CDC). (2017). *Syphilis – CDC fact sheet.* http://www.cdc.gov/std/syphilis/STDFact-Syphilis.htm

OTHER REFERENCES CONSULTED

Medline Plus, U.S. National Library of Medicine. (2019). *Canker sore.* http://www.nlm.nih.gov/medlineplus/ency/article/000998.htm

WebMD. (2019). *Stomatitis.* http://www.webmd.com/oral-health/guide/stomatitis-causes-treatment

STRESS DISORDER, POST-TRAUMATIC

DEFINITION/ETIOLOGY:

Stress is the body's reaction to a stressor that requires a response of adjustment that may be physical, mental, or emotional. Stress includes cognitive, emotional, behavioral, and somatic symptoms due to intense fear or feelings of helplessness. Stress can be a positive response to a situation.[1]

After a real or perceived trauma, an individual may have acute stress in the immediate period after the event. The diagnosis may be changed to post-traumatic stress disorder (PTSD) if symptoms and behavioral problems associated with acute stress disorder continue for more than one month and if these characteristics are associated with functional impairment or significant distress to the sufferer. Symptoms of PTSD typically begin within three months of the traumatic incident but may not occur until years after the event and may vary over time.[2]

The DSM-5 has a diagnostic criteria that apply to adults and children over six as well as corresponding criteria for children younger than six.[3] An individual child's response to a tragedy or disaster is related to age and development, parent or guardians' responses, separation from parent or guardian(s) or peers, and disruption of routines. The severity of anxiety is usually related to proximity to the event, significant losses, and changes in lifestyle and relationships.

<u>CAUSES</u>

PTSD can be a result of sustained or repeated traumatic incidents that can be either experienced directly, witnessed, or learning of the event that occurred to a family member or friend.[4] Some examples may include child abuse, domestic violence, a natural disaster, terrorist attacks, or exposure to chronic poverty. A person may also perceive that something was a dangerous event.[5]

Additionally, pediatric medical traumatic stress is psychological and physiological responses of children to pain, injury, serious illness, medical procedures, and invasive treatment experiences, especially in children younger than six of years of age.[6, 7]

SIGNS AND SYMPTOMS:[8]

Symptoms vary from person to person. General signs and symptoms associated with PTSD include:

- Intrusive memories – flashbacks (reliving the traumatic event); upsetting dreams about the disturbing event
- Avoidance and numbing – tries to avoid talking or thinking about the event, feels helpless or hopeless, avoids activities that they once enjoyed, avoids to the point of developing a phobia of person or place that reminds them of the traumatic incident
- Increased anxiety – easily startled or frightened, difficulty sleeping, irritability, anger, has trouble concentrating, focusing, guilt, shame surrounding the event
- Intense psychological reactions to things that symbolize the event
- Inability to remember aspects of the event
- Persistent distorted beliefs about the event or about one's self or others
- Persistent negative emotional state
- Irritable and or self-destructive behaviors

STRESS DISORDER, POST-TRAUMATIC *(continued from previous page)*

SIGNS AND SYMPTOMS *(continued)*

Common somatic symptoms often reported by those experiencing extreme stress include:[9]

- Sleep disturbances
- Muscle tension
- Headache
- Gastrointestinal disturbances
- Fatigue
- Poor concentration
- Hypervigilance

Preschoolers and young elementary children[10]

- Crying or sadness
- Confusion, regression to toddler behaviors (thumb sucking, clinging, enuresis)
- Sleep problems or nightmares
- Hyperactivity or withdrawal from everyday activities
- May act out traumatic event during play
- Reliving the event in thought or play
- Angry outbursts
- Lack of positive emotions

Adolescents:[11]

- Irritable or moody
- Difficulty sleeping
- Changes in eating patterns
- Anxiety, depression
- Acting out, behavior problems, impulse control
- Self-destructive behaviors
- Poor school performance, trouble concentrating
- Denying that the event ever happened
- Substance abuse, risk taking

MANAGEMENT/TREATMENT:

- Students suspected of having symptoms consistent with PTSD should be referred to their healthcare provider for an evaluation, diagnosis, and treatment to help mitigate possible negative consequences. The student may also benefit from an Individualized Healthcare Plan (IHP) and may be referred to the Section 504 team.

- If warranted an in-school evaluation for general safety including suicide ideation should be completed utilizing school nurses, school psychologists, and counselors who have been trained in suicide assessment. *(Refer to SUICIDE IDEATION/THREATS).*

STRESS DISORDER, POST-TRAUMATIC *(continued from previous page)*

MANAGEMENT/TREATMENT *(continued)*

General management, treatment for stress:

- Get regular exercise.
- Encourage student to share thoughts and worries.
- Encourage student to eat a healthy, balanced diet; drink less caffeine.
- Utilize relaxation techniques.
- Encourage adequate sleep.
- Help student set realistic goals.
- Encourage student to talk to parent, guardian, school nurse, teacher, friend when they are feeling stressed.

PTSD treatment includes:

1. **Medication** – antidepressants and antianxiety medications can help symptoms of depression and anxiety, help improve sleep problems, and improve concentration.[12]

2. **Psychotherapy**
   - Trauma –focused cognitive behavioral therapy is the treatment of choice for students with PTSD this includes anxiety management, skill development and gradual exposure.[13]

3. **Crisis Management**
   - Talk to the student and help assure them that the environment is safe.
   - Implement a crisis plan at school to deal with student tragedies or natural disasters; create mock drills so school will be familiar with plan.
   - After a crisis, restore contact with parent/guardian as soon as possible; for adolescents contact with close friends is equally important during a crisis.
   - Provide simple, honest, age appropriate explanations to correct distorted perceptions of what occurred.
   - Re-establish routines as soon as possible.
   - Help the child gain control of fear by choosing how to express the event in role-play, pictures, and games.
   - Facilitate group activities to help children tell their stories (disasters, school tragedy).
   - Class projects related to the event or disaster may help children take control of information (cognitive coping) and recognize that their feelings are normal and shared.
   - After disasters, include children in efforts to help others more affected; helping others assists the child in regaining a sense of normalcy.[14]

STRESS DISORDER, POST-TRAUMATIC *(continued from previous page)*

FOLLOW UP:

- Monitor students for side effects from prescribed medications.
- Educate staff on the condition as well as related signs and symptoms.
- Professional intervention with a mental healthcare provider is indicated when reactions interfere with usual daily activities:
    - Continuing sleep disturbance
    - Prolonged separation anxiety or clinging
    - Fears about stimuli that remind the child of the event
    - Acting out behaviors
    - Withdrawal and expressions of declining self-worth

RESOURCES

National Traumatic Child Stress Network. https://www.nctsn.org/

REFERENCES

[1] Cleveland Clinic. (2015). *Stress*. https://my.clevelandclinic.org/health/articles/11874-stress

[2] American Psychiatric Association. (2013). Trauma and stress related disorders. In *Diagnostic and statistical manual of mental disorders* (5th ed., pp. 267-277). American Psychiatric Association.

[3] Ibid.

[4] Ibid.

[5] Leingang, C., Shannon, R., & Mechan, J. (2019). Students with mental/behavioral health concerns and disorders. In J. Selekman, R.A. Shannon, & C. F. Younkaitis (Eds.), *School Nursing: A comprehensive text* (3rd ed., pp.779-780). F.A. Davis.

[6] National Traumatic Child Stress Network. (n.d.). *Medical trauma*. https://www.nctsn.org/what-is-child-trauma/trauma-types/medical-trauma

[7] Stanford Children's Health. (2019). *Posttraumatic stress disorder (PTSD) in children.* https://www.stanfordchildrens.org/en/topic/default?id=post-traumatic-stress-disorder-in-children-90-P02579#.XbXaTneiqf0.email

[8] American Psychiatric Association. (2013). Trauma and stress related disorders. In *Diagnostic and statistical manual of mental disorders* (5th ed., pp. 267-277). American Psychiatric Association.

[9] Ibid.

[10] Centers for Disease Control and Prevention. (2019). *Post-traumatic stress disorder in children.* https://www.cdc.gov/childrensmentalhealth/ptsd.html

[11] Ibid.

[12] Mayo Clinic. (2019). *Post-traumatic stress disorder.* https://www.mayoclinic.org/diseases-conditions/post-traumatic-stress-disorder/symptoms-causes/syc-20355967

[13] Leingang, C., Shannon, R., & Mechan, J. (2019). Students with mental/behavioral health concerns and disorders. In J. Selekman, R.A. Shannon, & C. F. Younkaitis (Eds.), *School Nursing: A comprehensive text* (3rd ed., pp.779-780). F.A. Davis.

[14] Centers for Disease Control and Prevention. (2019). *Helping children cope during emergencies.* https://www.cdc.gov/childrenindisasters/helping-children-cope.html

OTHER RESOURCES CONSULTED

Mayo Clinic. (2019). *Post-traumatic stress disorder.* https://www.mayoclinic.org/diseases-conditions/post-traumatic-stress-disorder/symptoms-causes/syc-20355967

STY or STYE (Hordeolum and Chalazion)

DEFINITION/ETIOLGY:

A **hordeolum** is a sudden onset, localized, staphylococcal infection of the eyelash follicle at the margin of the eyelid or associated sebaceous or sweat gland.[1]

A **chalazion** is an inflammatory/noninfectious nodule due to a blocked meibomian gland duct.[2] The nodule is painful and localizes to an eyelid margin. With time, a chalazion becomes a small non-tender nodule in the eyelid center.

Both conditions are diagnosed by a healthcare provider and initially cause eyelid hyperemia, edema, swelling, and pain.[3] Both improve spontaneously.

HORDEOLUM

SIGNS AND SYMPTOMS:

Hordeolum

- Tiny abscess (0.5-1.0 mm) on edge of eyelid
- Slight redness around abscess Usually filled with pus (may look like a pimple or boil)
- Local tenderness / pain over the affected area
- Eyelid swelling (this may make it difficult to see because eyelid can't open fully)
- Tearing
- Crusting around eyelids
- Photophobia[4]
- Internal styes tend to recur [5]

MANAGEMENT/TREATMENT:

- Apply warm, moist compresses approximately 15 minutes several times a day.[6]
- Improves spontaneously.
- Instill ophthalmic antibiotic drops or ointment if prescribed by healthcare provider.
- DO NOT use bacitracin or other topical ointment.
- DO NOT try to open (or squeeze) the abscess.[7]
- Refer to healthcare provider if no improvement in two-three days or if redness or swelling extends beyond eyelid into face.
- Sometimes drainage or oral antibiotics are needed.[8]
- School exclusion is not necessary; it is not spread from one person to another. Exclusion may be necessary if the eye is draining.[9]

FOLLOW UP:

- Watch for unusual spread; should heal in three to five days.
- If infection continues or a hordeolum (cyst) develops, refer to an ophthalmologist.

POTENTIAL COMPLICATIONS:

- Cross-contamination - avoid rubbing eyes. This may spread the infection to the other eye.
- Seek medical advice if vision is impaired.

STY (STYE) *(continued from previous page)*

NOTES:

Education:

- Encourage frequent hand washing
- Person should keep hands away from face
- Avoid wearing eye make-up until infection heals[10]
- Do not share cosmetics
- Discard all used and outdated eye make-up
- Wash hands thoroughly before handling, cleaning or inserting/removing contact lens

CHALAZION

SIGNS AND SYMPTOMS:

Chalazion

- Hard, non-tender nodule
- If infected, there is painfully swollen eyelid

MANAGEMENT/TREATMENT:

- Small chalazion disappears without intervention
- Apply warm, moist compresses (15-minute duration)
- Healthcare provider may order antibiotic ointment if there is secondary infection

FOLLOW UP: Recheck large chalazion in two to three weeks for resolution.

REFERENCES

[1] Children's Hospital of Philadelphia. (2018). *Chalazion.* https://www.chop.edu/conditions-diseases/chalazion

[2]The Merck Manual, Professional Edition. (2019). *Chalazion & hordeolum (stye).* https://www.merckmanuals.com/professional/eye-disorders/eyelid-and-lacrimal-disorders/chalazion-and-hordeolum-stye

[3] Ibid.

[4] Ibid.

[5] Ibid.

[6] Children's Hospital of Philadelphia. (2018). *Chalazion.* https://www.chop.edu/conditions-diseases/chalazion

[7] Children's Hospital of Philadelphia. (2018). *Stye (Hordeolum).* https://www.chop.edu/conditions-diseases/stye-hordeolum

[8] The Merck Manual, Professional Edition. (2019). *Chalazion & hordeolum (stye).* http://www.merckmanuals.com/home/eye_disorders/eyelid_and_tearing_disorders/chalazion_and_stye_hordeolum?query=stye#V954208

[9] American Academy of Pediatrics. (2020). Sty. In S. Aronson, & T. Shope (Eds.), *Managing infectious diseases in child care and schools* (5th ed., pp. 169-170). American Academy of Pediatrics.

[10] Children's Hospital of Philadelphia. (2018). *Stye (Hordeolum).* https://www.chop.edu/conditions-diseases/stye-hordeolum

OTHER REFERENCES CONSULTED

Children's Hospital of Boston. (2019). *Stye hordeolum.* http://www.childrenshospital.org/conditions-and-treatments/conditions/s/stye-hordeolum/symptoms-and-causes

SUBSTANCE ABUSE DISORDER

DEFINITION/ETIOLOGY:

Substance abuse refers to the harmful or hazardous use of psychoactive substances, including alcohol that can lead to dependence.[1] Although alcohol remains the most commonly used drug in adolescence there has been a steady decline but binge drinking among adolescents remain a major concern.[2] Substance abuse tends to be a chronic, progressive disease and can lead to devastating social and health consequences including an impact on the adolescent's developing brain.

Substance abuse among adolescents is substantial. A variety of substances can be abused and include alcohol, tobacco, marijuana, cocaine, opiates, "club drugs" (ecstasy or molly), stimulants, hallucinogens, inhalants, prescription drugs and steroids. More recently the use of E-cigarettes which are electronic devices which heat a liquid and produce an aerosol and usually contain nicotine flavorings, other chemicals or THC has become very popular among adolescents. This process is often referred to as "vaping or juuling".[3] *(Refer to VAPING).* Synthetic cannabinoids, also known as synthetic marijuana, has also increased in popularity recently. Common names are K2, spice, and Black Mamba. These can be smoked, ingested or vaped. They can contain unknown chemicals and have a high rate of abuse.

Adolescence is a time of rapid growth and development and a time when they become more independent and seek exploration. Although the majority of adolescents who use drugs do not progress to abuse or dependence, the use and abuse of substances is associated with high-risk behaviors in adolescents including sexual risk behavior, experience of violence and mental health and suicide risks.[4] While all substance use in adolescents is maladaptive, the presence of compulsive use, cravings, and substance related problems are most associated with the diagnosis of Substance Use Disorder (SUD).[5] Common comorbid conditions associated with substance abuse are depression, anxiety disorders, bipolar and attention deficit/hyperactivity disorder and compulsive disorders.[6]

The Centers for Disease Control and Prevention (CDC) reports that deaths related to opioids, both prescription and illicit, have increased steadily since 1999. Since 2016 there has been a surge in accidental deaths by overdose with opioids that contain synthetics, specifically illegally manufactured fentanyl.[7] Although heroin use among high school students has remained low, the average age of use is lowering and the impact of deaths from overdoses is affecting many students, families and communities.[8]

CAUSES:

The cause of SUD can be multifactorial and vary from person to person. While no one definitive cause exists, contributing factors can include, a genetic disposition, parental substance abuse, poor family relationships with rigid or poor supervision, negative life events, psychiatric co-morbidities and overall low self- esteem.[9]

SUBSTANCE ABUSE DISORDER *(continued from previous page)*

CAUSES *(continued)*

Risk factors and protective factors are important in understanding substance abuse among youth and adolescents. According to the National Institute of Drug Abuse (NIDA), risk factors can increase a person's chances for drug abuse while protective factors can reduce the risk.[10] Protective factors may include connectiveness to family and school, or participation in extracurricular activities while risk factors may be parental drug use or peer pressure. It is important to note that most people at risk for drug abuse never start using drugs or become addicted to drugs. Risk factors and protective factors can occur at different stages of children's lives. However, risks that occur at early stages can be mitigated by prevention interventions.[11] Assisting students to build resiliency by identifying their strengths may help students make better choices regarding substance abuse and all high-risk behaviors.

SIGNS AND SYMPTOMS:

Physiologic symptoms:[12]

- Stimulants: dilated pupils, rapid pulse, talkativeness and sometimes elevated blood pressure; very high doses may cause psychotic symptoms
- Depressants: normal to constricted pupils, drowsiness and slurred speech (in the absence of an alcohol odor)
- Runny or stuffy nose, epistaxis and perforations of the nasal septum (associated with cocaine or inhalant use)
- Needle tracks with drug use
- Red eyes associated with marijuana use
- Slurred speech
- Memory impairment, impaired coordination
- Sudden jitteriness, tremors, nervousness, and/or aggression
- Tachycardia
- Hypoventilation which could indicate pending overdose

General signs and symptoms/behaviors:[13]

- Sudden personality changes that include abrupt changes in work or school attendance, quality of work, work output, grades, discipline
- Unusual flare-ups or outbreaks of temper
- Withdrawal from responsibility
- General changes in overall attitude
- Loss of interest in what were once favorite hobbies and pursuits
- Changes in friends and reluctance to have friends visit or talk about them
- Difficulty in concentration, paying attention
- Wearing of sunglasses at inappropriate times
- Continual wearing of long-sleeved garments particularly in hot weather or reluctance to wear short-sleeved attire when appropriate
- Association with known substance abusers
- Unusual borrowing of money from friends, co-workers or parents

SUBSTANCE ABUSE DISORDER *(continued from previous page)*

General signs and symptoms/behaviors *(continued)*

- Stealing small items from employer, home or school
- Secretive behavior regarding actions and possessions; poorly concealed attempts to avoid attention and suspicion such as frequent trips to storage rooms, restroom, basement, etc.
- Change, sometimes radical, in behavior
- Weight loss or gain; change in eating habits

MANAGEMENT/TREATMENT:

School nurses are often requested to do an assessment of a student who may be impaired due to substances used in the school setting or suspected of having a substance abuse problem. It is essential that the school nurse utilize a non-judgmental, nonthreatening, matter of fact attitude. Use of broad open-ended questions is the best approach. An example would be to start by allowing the student to describe the circumstances in their own words, such as "why do you think you are here today? "Tell me about this". It would be helpful for schools to have specific protocols to assist the nurse when performing an assessment of possible substance abuse. These may include assessment of pupil size, horizontal gaze nystagmus and balance.

- As with any medical condition, a medical emergency must be quickly identified and addressed. School nurses have the training and expertise to identify an emergent situation and quickly respond. Opioids can result in respiratory depression and if not treated quickly can result in death. The use of naloxone (Narcan®) can reverse opioid toxicity and quickly revive the individual. Naloxone is available in the form of an IM or SQ injection as well as a nasal spray. Additional doses can be given every two to three minutes until emergency response arrives.[14] School nurses should work with their Boards of Education and communities to develop policies that support the use of Narcan® in the school setting. Stock naloxone in the health office can be a valuable tool in responding to an opioid overdose. School nurses should be familiar with state laws and regulations regarding its use.

- Any student who presents to the health office with a suspicion of substance abuse should undergo assessment including vital signs and screened for other signs of use. Health services staff should collaborate with administration to develop policies for health office staff to follow with students suspected of substance use. The NASN toolkit is a resource (see RESOURCES below).

- In situations when it is not an acute emergency, the school nurse can utilize the SBIRT framework (screening, brief intervention, and referral to treatment). The school nurse should be prepared to provide students with a list of local resources for students and families in need of treatment. Resources regarding SBIRT including training for the school nurse can be found at https://www.samhsa.gov/sbirt

- Smoking or vaping cessation programs can be delivered in the school setting and even be provided during the school day.
- School nurses can be instrumental in bringing evidenced-based programs into the school.

SUBSTANCE ABUSE DISORDER *(continued from previous page)*

POTENTIAL COMPLICATIONS:
The following table defines the five stages of substance abuse and serves as a guide for referral in non-acute cases.[15]

Stage 1	Stage 2	Stage 3	Stage 4	Stage 5
Experimentation • Voluntary use • Usually used with peers • Use is infrequent • Some are able to stop use by themselves, but many believe their use is solving their problems.	*Regular Use* • Use on a regular basis • Few, if any, consequences • May use in a predictable pattern • May use with peers or alone	*Problem/Risky Use* • May have legal or social consequences • Behavioral changes and poor grades, lack of interest • Increased frequency of use; use alone	*Dependence* • Continued use despite negative outcomes • Use in risky situations • Increased tolerance and dependency • Estrangement from family and "straight" friends	*Addiction* • Craving and drug seeking behaviors • Guilt, withdrawal, remorse, depression • Physical and mental deterioration • Increased risk-taking, self-destructive behavior, compulsive and out of control use

FOLLOW UP:

- Some students may require inpatient treatment for their addiction and/or substance use.
- Returning to school after an inpatient stay can be a major and stressful transition. School nurses can take the lead in planning a thoughtful and safe reentry by being a liaison between the treatment facility and the school team.
- A **transition plan** with helpful accommodations and supports should be developed with reasonable and achievable goals to help set the returning student up for success.

PREVENTION:
According to NIDA, drug abuse and addiction is preventable.[16] Prevention programs that involve family, schools, communities, and the media are effective in reducing drug abuse. Youth who experience a positive connection to school, family, and community are less likely to engage in risky behaviors, including alcohol and drug abuse. Effective prevention strategies may include the following:

- Drug and alcohol prevention should start in elementary school and enhance protective factors while reducing risk factors. Protective factors can include participating in extracurricular activities, high family cohesion, family supervision and a safe school climate.[17]
- The school nurse can provide prevention information to parents, students, and the community through the school website, bulletin boards and pamphlets.
- School nurses can help arrange evening programs to help to educate the community.
- School nurses can serve on broader community collaboratives to help design and implement comprehensive programming.

SUBSTANCE ABUSE DISORDER *(continued from previous page)*

OTHER CONCERNS:

- Drug testing in schools has been a debatable issue. Although a potential strategy to decrease use, this has not been validated or supported through research. Other potential obstacles are cost to the school district and civil rights of the student. The American Academy of Pediatrics (AAP) is opposed to this practice.[18]

- Medical marijuana is emerging as a treatment for children with conditions such as seizures and pain relief for cancer and other conditions. While legal in most states, standards and regulations of medical marijuana on school grounds or administered by the school nurse remains controversial. More research is needed in this area. School nurses need to be familiar with their individual state Nurse Practice Act regarding the nurses' role in the administration of medical marijuana as well as their school district policy.

RESOURCES:

National Association of School Nurses (NASN). (2016). **Naloxone in Schools Toolkit.** https://www.pathlms.com/nasn/courses/3353

Substance Abuse and Mental Health Services Administration (SAMSHA). (2019). **Opioid Overdose Prevention Toolkit**. https://store.samhsa.gov/system/files/sma18-4742.pdf

Substance Abuse and Mental Health Services Administration (SAMSHA). (2017). **Screening, Brief Intervention, Referral to Treatment**. https://www.samhsa.gov/sbirt

REFERENCES

---

[1] World Health Organization (2019). *Substance abuse.* https://www.who.int/topics/substance_abuse/en/

[2] Johnson, K. & Selekman, J. (2019). Students engaging in high risk behavior. In J. Selekman, R. Adair Shannon, &**C. F.** Yonkaitis (Eds.), *School nursing: A comprehensive text* (3rd ed., pp. 834-340). F.A. Davis.

[3]Center for Disease Control. (2019). Quick facts on the use of e-cigarettes for children, teens and adolescents. https://www.cdc.gov/tobacco/basic_information/e-cigarettes/Quick-Facts-on-the-Risks-of-E-cigarettes-for-Kids-Teens-and-Young-Adults.html

[4] Center for Disease Control (CDC). (2017). *Youth Risk Survey.* https://www.stanfordchildrens.org/en/topic/default?id=stages-of-substance-abuse-1-3060

[5] Garzon, D. (2017). Approaches to health management in pediatric primary care. In C. Burns, A.M. Dunn, M.A. Brady, N.B. Starr, C.G. Blosser, & D.L. Garzon (Eds.), *Pediatric primary care* (6th ed., pp. 383-385). Elsevier Inc.

[6] Ibid.

[7] Centers for Disease Control (CDC). (2018). *Understanding the epidemic.* https://www.cdc.gov/drugoverdose/epidemic/index.html

[8] Johnson, K. & Selekman, J. (2019). Students engaging in high risk behavior. In J. Selekman, R. Adair Shannon, &**C. F.** Yonkaitis (Eds.), *School nursing: A comprehensive text* (3rd ed., pp. 834-340). F.A. Davis.

[9] Garzon, D. (2017). Approaches to health management in pediatric primary care. In C. Burns, A.M. Dunn, M.A. Brady, N.B. Starr, C.G. Blosser, & D.L. Garzon (Eds.), Pediatric *primary care* (6th ed., pp. 383-385). Elsevier Inc.

SUBSTANCE ABUSE DISORDER *(continued from previous page)*

[10] National Institute of Drug Abuse (NIDA). (2016). *Protective and risk factors.* https://www.drugabuse.gov/publications/principles-substance-abuse-prevention-early-childhood/chapter-2-risk-protective-factors

[11] Ibid.

[12] Garzon, D. (2017). Approaches to health management in pediatric primary care. In C. Burns, A.M. Dunn, M.A. Brady, N.B. Starr, C.G. Blosser, & D.L. Garzon (Eds.), *Pediatric primary care* (6th ed., pp. 383-385). Elsevier Inc.

[13] National Youth Network. (2019). *Teen substance abuse and adolescent substance abuse treatment.* http://www.nationalyouth.com/substanceabuse.html

[14] Johnson, K. & Selekman, J. (2019). Students engaging in high risk behavior. In J. Selekman, R. Adair Shannon, & **C. F.** Yonkaitis (Eds.), *School nursing: A comprehensive text* (3rd ed., pp. 834-340). F.A. Davis.

[15] Stanford Children's Health. (2019). *Stages of substance abuse.* https://www.stanfordchildrens.org/en/topic/default?id=stages-of-substance-abuse-1-3060

[16] National Institute of Drug Abuse (NIDA). (2016). *Protective and risk factors.* https://www.drugabuse.gov/publications/principles-substance-abuse-prevention-early-childhood/chapter-2-risk-protective-factors

[17] Johnson, K. & Selekman, J. (2019). Students engaging in high risk behavior. In J. Selekman, R. Adair Shannon, &**C. F.** Yonkaitis (Eds.), *School nursing: A comprehensive text* (3rd ed., pp. 834-340). F.A. Davis.

[18] Ibid.

OTHER REFERENCES CONSULTED

Center for Disease Control. (2019). Quick facts on the use of e-cigarettes for children, teens and adolescents. https://www.cdc.gov/tobacco/basic_information/e-cigarettes/Quick-Facts-on-the-Risks-of-E-cigarettes-for-Kids-Teens-and-Young-Adults.html

National Association of School Nurses. (2015). *Policy statement on substance use prevention and intervention.* https://schoolnursenet.nasn.org/blogs/nasn-profile/2017/03/12/national-association-of-school-nurses-issue-policy-statements-on-substance-use-prevention-and-intervention

National Institute of Drug Abuse (NIDA). (2019). *NIDA for teens.* http://teens.drugabuse.gov

National Institute of Drug Abuse (NIDA). (2017). Naloxone for accidental overdose: life- saving science. https://www.drugabuse.gov/publications/naloxone-opioid-overdose-life-saving-science/naloxone-opioid-overdose-life-saving-science

Substance Abuse and Mental Health Service Administration (SAMSHA). (2019). *Talk – They hear you. Underage drinking prevention national media campaign.* http://www.samhsa.gov/underagedrinking/

U.S. Department of Health and Human Services. (2018). *U.S. surgeon general's advisory on naloxone and opioid use disorders.* https://www.hhs.gov/surgeongeneral/priorities/opioids-and-addiction/naloxone-advisory/index.html

U.S. Department of Health and Human Services. (2019). *Addiction report and publication.* https://www.hhs.gov/surgeongeneral/reports-and-publications/addiction/index.html

SYNCOPE (Fainting)

DEFINITION/ETIOLOGY:
Fainting or syncope is "a reversible, temporary, and acute loss of consciousness and postural tone" resulting from decreased oxygen to the brain.[1] Causes may include dehydration, problems with the autonomic nervous system, cardiac conditions, neurological problems, medications, metabolic disorders or psychogenic illness.[2]

It may be caused by low blood sugar from not eating enough, inadequate fluid intake, standing in place for a long time, being in a warm place, standing up too quickly, headache, seizure, drug or alcohol use, breath holding, stress or anxiety. However, it may be a result of a more serious situation such as head injury, neurological disorder or an underlying condition such as heart disease/complications.[3]

Children and adolescents often experience syncope from vaso-vagal (neurocardiogenic) episodes. During a vasovagal response the heart rate increases causing a rapid drop in blood pressure leading to decreased oxygen to the brain which causes the child to faint.[4] These episodes are commonly precipitated by trigger or situational events such as unpleasant sights or smells, anxiety, emotional stress, anticipated pain or fear.[5]

Orthostatic hypotension is also a common cause of syncope. This occurs when the child stands quickly and there is a transient increase in the heart rate and inadequate cerebral perfusion resulting in low blood pressure.[6]

Most syncope episodes have a benign etiology. Although rare, syncope may be due to cardiac disease such as dysrhythmias or valvular disease.[7] Syncope due to cardiac disease often occurs suddenly and may present on exertion and with generalized weakness and pallor.[8]

SIGNS AND SYMPTOMS:
- Loss of consciousness may be preceded by pale, cool or diaphoretic skin, lightheadedness, tunnel vision, nausea, frequent yawn, and/or restless feeling.[9]
- Loss of consciousness is usually brief.[10]
- As the child begins to lose consciousness, they may have a brief eye roll and/or body twitching.[11]
- Other associated symptoms include the child's sense of impeding loss of consciousness, tingling of lips and fingertips and palpitations.[12]

SEIZURES VS. FAINTING (Note: Not all symptoms may be present)[13]

Seizure specifics	Fainting specifics
• Lasts for longer than 1 minute • Loss of bladder or bowel control • Tongue biting • Convulsions • Involuntary movements • Lip smacking • Drooling • Random eye movements	• Lasts for less than 1 minute • Jerking movements • Loss of consciousness • Tunnel or blurred vision • Nausea • Cold sweats • Skin pallor • Dizziness • Dilated pupils

SYNCOPE (Fainting) *(continued from previous page)*

MANAGEMENT/TREATMENT:

1. If it is observed that the child about to faint, instruct them to lie down to prevent falling.[14]
2. Help ease the child to floor or reclining position.
3. Place the child on his/her back with no pillow and elevate feet about 12 inches to encourage blood flow to head.[15]
4. Apply a cool washcloth to forehead if diaphoretic.[16]
5. Roll child to their side if they vomit.
6. As the child awakens, do not allow them to stand immediately (be prepared to have the child resume reclining position if dizzy).[17]
7. Follow district guidelines if the child does not awaken. Prepare for possibility of CPR.[18]
8. Activate Emergency Medical Services (EMS) if sustained abnormal vital signs, acute change from baseline mental status, chest pain, neurological deficit, head trauma, severe headache with altered mental status, or seizure activity.[19]
9. If the child is known to have diabetes, proceed with diabetes Emergency Care Plan (ECP).
10. Refer to the healthcare provider to rule out serious cause of syncope.[20]
11. If the child sustained injury from fainting episode – administer first aid.[21]
12. Follow district guidelines for first time syncope with unknown etiology or known history of syncope.

FOLLOW UP:

- Determine history of fainting and if applicable, results of past medical evaluation for fainting.[22]
- If prior evaluation determined no cause or need for medical intervention, educate students who faint frequently about safety; for example, when experiencing warning symptoms, sit down in a chair, position head between knees close to floor.[23] Educate the child with postural hypotension about getting up slowly.

NOTES:

It is important to note that after medical workup the etiology of some cases of syncope remain unknown.[24]

SYNCOPE (Fainting) *(continued from previous page)*

REFERENCES

[1] Jakubowski, T. & Perron, T. (2019). Students with common health complaints. In J. Selekman, R. A. Shannon, & C. F. Yonkaitis (Eds.), *School nursing: A comprehensive text* (3rd ed., pp. 361-362). F.A. Davis Company.

[2] Ibid.

[3] Ibid.

[4] Mayo Clinic. (2019). *Vasovagal syncope*. https://www.mayoclinic.org/diseases-conditions/vasovagal-syncope/symptoms-causes/syc-20350527

[5] Ibid.

[6] Merck Manual. (2019). *Syncope*. https://www.merckmanuals.com/professional/cardiovascular-disorders/symptoms-of-cardiovascular-disorders/syncope

[7] Ibid.

[8] Ibid.

[9] Mayo Clinic. (2019). *Vasovagal syncope*. https://www.mayoclinic.org/diseases-conditions/vasovagal-syncope/symptoms-causes/syc-20350527

[10] Merck Manual. (2019). *Syncope*. https://www.merckmanuals.com/professional/cardiovascular-disorders/symptoms-of-cardiovascular-disorders/syncope

[11] Jakubowski, T. & Perron, T. (2019). Students with common health complaints. In J. Selekman, R. A. Shannon, & C. F. Yonkaitis (Eds.), *School nursing: A comprehensive text* (3rd ed., pp. 361-362). F.A. Davis Company.

[12] Merck Manual. (2019). *Syncope*. https://www.merckmanuals.com/professional/cardiovascular-disorders/symptoms-of-cardiovascular-disorders/syncope

[13] Cedars-Sinai. (2019). *Fainting vs. seizure: How to tell the difference*. https://www.cedars-sinai.org/blog/fainting-or-seizure.html

[14] Cosby, M., Lyons, E., & Prestidge, L. (2019). Students with acute illness and injury. In J. Selekman, R. A. Shannon, & C. F. Yonkaitis (Eds.), *School nursing: A comprehensive text* (3rd ed., pp. 440-441). F.A. Davis Company.

[15] Mayo Clinic. (2019). *Fainting: First aid*. https://www.mayoclinic.org/first-aid/first-aid-fainting/basics/art-20056606

[16] Jakubowski, T. & Perron, T. (2019). Students with common health complaints. In J. Selekman, R. A. Shannon, & C. F. Yonkaitis (Eds.), *School nursing: A comprehensive text* (3rd ed., pp. 361-362). F.A. Davis Company.

[17] Mayo Clinic. (2019). *Fainting: First aid*. https://www.mayoclinic.org/first-aid/first-aid-fainting/basics/art-20056606

[18] Ibid.

[19] Cosby, M., Lyons, E., & Prestidge, L. (2019). Students with acute illness and injury. In J. Selekman, R. A. Shannon, & C. F. Yonkaitis (Eds.), *School nursing: A comprehensive text* (3rd ed., pp. 440-441). F.A. Davis Company.

[20] Ibid.

[21] Mayo Clinic. (2019). *Fainting: First aid*. https://www.mayoclinic.org/first-aid/first-aid-fainting/basics/art-20056606

[22] Ibid.

[23] Mayo Clinic. (2019). *Fainting: First aid*. https://www.mayoclinic.org/first-aid/first-aid-fainting/basics/art-20056606

[24] Merck Manual. (2019). *Syncope*. https://www.merckmanuals.com/professional/cardiovascular-disorders/symptoms-of-cardiovascular-disorders/syncope

TATTOO/BODY PIERCING

DEFINITION/ETIOLOGY:
Tattoos and body piercing are forms of body art that have been practiced for years by various cultures. The English word tattoo derived from the Polynesian word *tatau* that means, "to mark".[1] Tattooing became a trendy fashion statement in the U.S. in the 1990s. Tattoos and body piercing can express individuality, rebellion or group membership. It may signify spiritual meaning or a life milestone, such as a new love or a social bonding act. Others feel it provides a sense of control or permanence, define uniqueness, and transmit personal messages.[2]

At least 45 states have laws prohibiting minors from getting tattoos, and 38 states have laws that prohibit both body piercing and tattooing on minors without parental permission.[3] While most states prohibit tattooing of minors, school nurses see students with tattoos or piercings, often done by peers and outside of commercial establishments.

Permanent tattoos are created using a needle to repeatedly inject pigmented ink into the skin. Tattoo pigments are not Food and Drug Administration (FDA) approved and there are no practice regulations for tattoo parlors. When considering a tattoo, caution should be taken to select a reputable tattooing studio that employs trained personnel and uses sterile equipment.

Body piercing has become increasingly popular for both females and males. The entire ear can be pierced, as well as the tongue, nose, lips, eyebrows, cheeks, nipples, and navel. Large gromets are also sometimes placed in the ear to enlarge the pierced openings. It is essential that piercing areas are kept clean, and students should be encouraged to leave jewelry in place until piercing is healed.[4]

SIGNS AND SYMPTOMS:
Possible complications from tattooing and piercing that may require treatment:

- Inflammation of the tattooed/pierced area
- Allergic reaction includes swelling, redness, and itching
- Severe allergic reaction can lead to anaphylactic shock
- Scars and keloid formations [5]
- Methicillin-resistant Staphylococcus aureus (MRSA) [6], and blood borne infections (Hepatitis B and C, Human immunodeficiency virus (HIV), if contaminated equipment is used [7]

MANAGEMENT/TREATMENT:

- After care instructions following receiving a tattoo should include:
  - Keep bandage on for 24 hours, then wash with soap and warm water.
  - Keep skin moist by applying antibiotic ointment or Vitamin E oil.
  - Do not use petroleum jelly, rubbing alcohol, or peroxide.[8]
- Treatment for local infection may range from warm compresses and antibacterial ointment for local infection, to a course of oral antibiotics.
- Tattoos are considered permanent; removal can be both painful and expensive. The methods of tattoo removal include the following:[9]
- Surgical removal – cutting the tattoo away

TATTOO/BODY PIERCING *(continued from previous page)*

MANAGEMENT/TREATMENT *(continued)*

- Dermabrasion – sanding the skin (epidermis and dermis)
- Salabrasion – using a salt solution to soak the tattooed skin
- Scarification – removing the tattoo with an acid solution and creating a scar in its place
- Laser therapy as regulated by the FDA may also be used as a method of tattoo removal
- Piercing sites should be washed with liquid antibacterial soap and water twice a day, and jewelry should be rotated at that time. Alcohol and hydrogen peroxide delay healing and should not be used.[10]

FOLLOW UP:

- Youth are a population at risk and influenced by media, peers, and "heroes". Most tattoos are done on a whim, so youth may not consider the long-term health risks of receiving a tattoo or the permanent marking of the skin. School personnel such as health educators and school nurses can educate students in making informed decisions about tattoos.
- When a student presents with a complication from a tattoo or body piercing, the school nurse should obtain a history and perform an assessment in a non-judgmental manner.
- Infection control may depend on certification of artists and shop inspections. If a student intends to get a tattoo or piercing, the Alliance of Professional Tattooists suggests safety measures and asking about or looking for autoclaving instruments, one-time needle and pigment use, and how the workspace is cleaned.

COMPLICATIONS:

Tattoos and body piercings may be popular but pose definite health risks.

- When proper sterilization and safety procedures are not exquisitely followed, tattooing can transmit blood- borne pathogens including Hepatitis B and C, and HIV.
- Body piercing can also present the risk of scarring (formation of granulomas or keloids).
- Skin infections.
- Allergic reactions: Tattoo dyes — especially red, green, yellow and blue dyes — can cause allergic skin reactions, such as an itchy rash at the tattoo site. This can occur even years after receiving the tattoo.

TATTOO/BODY PIERCING *(continued from previous page)*

REFERENCES

[1] McGill University: Office for Science and Society. (n.d.) https://www.mcgill.ca/oss/article/history-you-asked/what-history-tattoos

[2] Johnson, K., & Selekman, J. (2019). Students engaging in high-risk behaviors. In J. Selekman, R. Adair Shannon, & C. F. Yonkaitis (Eds.), *School nursing: A comprehensive text* (3rd ed., pp. 853-854). F.A. Davis.

[3] American Academy of Pediatrics. (2018). *Talking about tattoos to your teen: AAP report explained.* https://www.healthychildren.org/English/ages-stages/teen/Pages/Tattoos.aspx

[4] Johnson, K., & Selekman, J. (2019). Students engaging in high-risk behaviors. In J. Selekman, R. Adair Shannon, & C. F. Yonkaitis (Eds.), *School nursing: A comprehensive text* (3rd ed., pp. 853-854). F.A. Davis.

[5] American Academy of Pediatrics. (2018). *Talking about tattoos to your teen: AAP report explained.* https://www.healthychildren.org/English/ages-stages/teen/Pages/Tattoos.aspx

[6] Ross, L., & Selekman, J. (2019). Skin disorders. In J. Selekman, R. Adair Shannon, & C. F. Yonkaitis (Eds.), *School nursing: A comprehensive text* (3rd ed., p. 415). F.A. Davis.

[7] Mayo Clinic. (2018). *Tattoos: Understanding risks and precautions.* http://www.mayoclinic.com/health/tattoos-and-piercings/MC00020

[8] American Academy of Pediatrics. (2018). *Talking about tattoos to your teen: AAP report explained.* https://www.healthychildren.org/English/ages-stages/teen/Pages/Tattoos.aspx

[9] U.S. Food and Drug Administration. (2017). *Tattoo removal: Options and results.* https://www.fda.gov/consumers/consumer-updates/tattoo-removal-options-and-results

[10] Ross, L., & Selekman, J. (2019). Skin disorders. In J. Selekman, R. Adair Shannon, & C. F. Yonkaitis (Eds.), *School nursing: A comprehensive text* (3rd ed., p. 415). F.A. Davis.

OTHER REFERENCES CONSULTED

Alliance of Professional Tattooist. (n.d.). *Guidelines for getting a tattoo.* http://www.safe-tattoos.com/pamphlets/basic.html

TIC DISORDERS AND TOURETTE SYNDROME

DEFINITION/ETIOLOGY:[1]

A *tic* is a sudden, rapid, recurrent, non-rhythmic, stereotyped motor movement or vocalization. Any part of the body can be involved—face, neck, hands, legs. The person can hold a tic back for a little while, but the condition is involuntary. Many children have mild tics that disappear over time without intervention.

TICS

Tics are classified as **simple and complex** (Tourette Syndrome) and are most common during adolescence.

SIMPLE

- The essential feature of Simple Tic Disorder sometimes called Provisional Tic Disorder, is the presence of single or multiple motor tics and/or vocal tics using limited muscle groups. The tics occur many times a day, nearly every day for at least 4 weeks, but for no longer than 12 consecutive months.[2]

COMPLEX

- Last longer than 12 months and may include many simple tics. Complex tics may seem to be intentional with gestures and words that appear to have social meaning. These tics are not voluntary and do not represent bad behavior.[3]
- Tourette Syndrome is a complex tic. The full name of the disorder is Gilles de la Tourette Syndrome (GTS). *Tourette Syndrome* is an inherited, neurological disorder characterized by repeated, involuntary body movements and vocal sounds. It may be accompanied by obsessions, attention problems, learning disabilities and impulsivity. The onset is before age 18, usually between 4 and 8 years with an average onset of 6 years of age and peak in intensity in the early teen years.[4] The cause of Tourette syndrome is unknown, but research suggests that it is very complex.

The essential features of Tourette Syndrome are:

- Multiple motor tics and one or more vocal tics involving several muscle groups appear simultaneously or at different periods.
- Tics occur many times a day (usually in bouts), nearly every day or intermittently for a period of more than one year, and during this period, there is never a tic-free period of more than 3 consecutive months.[5]
- The disorder is not due to direct physiological effects of a substance (e.g., a stimulant) or a general medical condition (e.g., post-viral encephalitis).
- The type, number, frequency, complexity and severity of tics change over time. Complex sounds such as obscenities occur in only 10-15 % of cases.[6]

TIC DISORDERS AND TOURETTE SYNDROME *(continued from previous page)*

SIGNS AND SYMPTOMS:

Motor tics:[7]

Simple	*Complex*
Eye blinking	Touch and smell objects
Head jerking	Repeats observed movement
Shoulder shrugging	Stepping in a certain pattern
Eye darting	Obscene gesturing
Nose twitching	Bend and twist
Mouth movement	Hopping

Vocal tics:[8]

Simple	*Complex*
Grunting	Repeats own words/phrases
Coughing	Repeats others words/phrases
Throat clearing	Vulgar, obscene, or swear words
Barking	

Tics vary greatly between and within individuals. Some clinical features include:

- Simple motor tics with brief, sudden, and meaningless muscle movements.
- Tics may only appear when tired, stressed, or anxious.
- Complex motor tics are more purposeful and include involve several muscle groups (touching, gesturing, hopping, etc.).
- Vocal tics range from meaningless sounds to sudden utterance of words, phrases, and complete sentences (echolalia or coprolalia).
- Tic intensity can vary from barely visible and audible tics to extremely forceful and loud expressions.
- Tics may severely interfere with everyday activities including social relationships and school performance.

ANTICIPATED CONCERNS/PROBLEMS:

- Marked distress or significant impairment in occupational or other important areas of functioning
- Decreased self esteem
- Social isolation
- Victim of bullying

TIC DISORDERS AND TOURETTE SYNDROME *(continued from previous page)*

MANAGEMENT/ POTENTIAL INTERVENTIONS:[9, 10, 11]

- Identification and careful diagnosis of the disruptive effects of tics.
- Minimize stress and teach relaxation techniques.
- Educate staff and student to understand the disorder. GTS does not diminish intellect.
- Refer to support groups.
- Medication is available but pharmacological treatment is prescribed only if tics are troublesome to the child.[12]
- Medications are used when tics significantly interfere with functioning and for co-morbid conditions (e.g., ADHD, obsessive-compulsive disorder, anxiety).
- Medication side effects include tremors, depression, weight gain, decreased cognitive abilities and heart problems.
- Cognitive behavioral therapy may to reduce tics.

FOLLOW-UP:

- Communicate with parents/guardians regarding health needs and special accommodations during school (may need a Section 504 plan).[13]
- Participate as a member of the multidisciplinary team to promote health and academic success.
- Schedule the student for a break in the nurse office during the school day where he/she can allow tics to happen. This gives the student a break from trying to control the tics all day in school and this break allows the student to then return to class with fewer or less obvious tics.
- Provide information and educate school staff.
- Routinely follow up on individualized healthcare plans, emergency plans, and health goals for continuity of care in school and at home.
- Provide support and strategies to build self- esteem in student.
- Provide an emotionally and physically safe environment.
- Monitor symptoms in various situations and communicate with licensed healthcare provider.

NOTES:[14, 15]

- Co-morbidities include attention deficit/hyperactivity disorder and obsessive-compulsive disorder. migraines, learning disabilities, sleep difficulties, anxiety and mood swings may also accompany this disorder.
- Rewards and punishments are not indicated or helpful.
- Explosive-onset tics or related obsessive compulsiveness may indicate a streptococcal infection.
- Students with Tourette Syndrome require a setting that is flexible and allows them to work to their full potential.
- Untimed testing reduces stress for students with Tourette Syndrome.

TIC DISORDERS AND TOURETTE SYNDROME *(continued from previous page)*

REFERENCES

[1] Mayo Clinic. (2018). *Tourette syndrome*. https://www.mayoclinic.org/diseases-conditions/tourette-syndrome/symptoms-causes/syc-20350465

[2] Patterson, B. R., Bohnenkamp, J., Hoover, S., Bostic, J., & Selekman, J. (2019). Students with mental/behavioral health concerns and disorders. In J. Selekman, R. Adair Shannon, & C. F. Yonkaitis (Eds.), *School nursing: A comprehensive text* (3rd ed., pp. 756-789). F.A. Davis.

[3] Merck Manual. (2018). *Tic disorders and tourette's syndrome in children and adolescents.* https://www.merckmanuals.com/professional/pediatrics/neurologic-disorders-in-children/tic-disorders-and-tourette-syndrome-in-children-and-adolescents?query=tic%20disorders

[4] Ibid.

[5] Psych Central. (2018). *Tourette's disorder symptom.* https://psychcentral.com/disorders/tourettes-disorder-symptoms/

[6] Tourette Association of America. (n.d.) *What is tourette syndrome?* http://tourette.org/media/WhatisEnglish.proof_.r1.pdf

[7] Mayo Clinic. (2018). *Tourette syndrome*. https://www.mayoclinic.org/diseases-conditions/tourette-syndrome/symptoms-causes/syc-20350465

[8] Ibid.

[9] Merck Manual. (2018). *Tic disorders and tourette's syndrome in children and adolescents.* https://www.merckmanuals.com/professional/pediatrics/neurologic-disorders-in-children/tic-disorders-and-tourette-syndrome-in-children-and-adolescents?query=tic%20disorders

[10] Merck Manual. (2018). *Tic disorders and tourette's syndrome in children and adolescents.* https://www.merckmanuals.com/professional/pediatrics/neurologic-disorders-in-children/tic-disorders-and-tourette-syndrome-in-children-and-adolescents?query=tic%20disorders

[11] National Institute of Neurological Disorders and Stroke. (2014). *Tourette syndrome fact sheet.* http://www.ninds.nih.gov/disorders/tourette/detail_tourette.htm#220493231

[12] Merck Manual. (2018). *Tic disorders and tourette's syndrome in children and adolescents.* https://www.merckmanuals.com/professional/pediatrics/neurologic-disorders-in-children/tic-disorders-and-tourette-syndrome-in-children-and-adolescents?query=tic%20disorders

[13] Tourette Association of America. (n.d.) *What is tourette syndrome?* http://tourette.org/media/WhatisEnglish.proof_.r1.pdf

[14] Ibid.

[15] National Institute of Neurological Disorders and Stroke. (2014). *Tourette syndrome fact sheet.* http://www.ninds.nih.gov/disorders/tourette/detail_tourette.htm#220493231

OTHER REFERENCES CONSULTED:

National Institute of Neurological Disorders and Stroke. (2012). *Tourette syndrome fact sheet.* https://www.ninds.nih.gov/Disorders/Patient-Caregiver-Education/Fact-Sheets/Tourette-Syndrome-Fact-Sheet#3231_3

Schreiner, T. L., Yang, M. L., Martin, J.A., Messer, R., Demarest, S., & Walleigh, D. (2018). Neurologic & muscular disorders. In W.W. Hay, M.J. Levin, R. R. Deterding, & M. J. Abzug (Eds.), *Current diagnosis and treatment: Pediatrics* (24th ed., pp. 752-823). McGraw Hill Education.

TICK-BORNE DISEASES

DEFINITION/ETIOLOGY:

A tick is a small, blood-sucking, parasitic arachnid that lives in moist or humid environments, particularly in or near wooded or grassy areas. Ticks live in a variety of environments depending on the type of tick. Ticks live on the blood of large animals such as deer, but can also attach to humans. Once a tick attaches to a host, it will often move to a warm, moist location such as the armpit, groin, or hair. Ticks vary in size, can range from very large to very small that are almost impossible to see. Daily skin exams while in tick-laden environments are advised. Most tick-borne illnesses do not develop until the ticks have been attached for 24 hours.[1]

Ticks attach as the host moves by bushes, plants, or grass and in tall wooded areas or fields. Tick bites can cause a variety of health conditions ranging from harmless to serious. While most ticks are harmless and do not carry disease, some ticks can carry bacteria which can lead to diseases such as Colorado tick fever, Rocky Mountain spotted fever, and Tularemia.[2,3]

Prevalence of Tick-borne Illness in the United States[4]

Reported Tickborne Diseases, U.S.	2018
Lyme Disease (confirmed and probable)	33,666
Anaplasmosis/Ehrlichiosis	6,123
Spotted Fever Rickettsiosis	5,544
Babesiosis	2,160
Tularemia	229
Powassan virus	21
Total	**47,743**

How ticks spread disease:[5]

- Ticks transmit pathogens that cause disease through the process of feeding.
- Depending on the tick species and its stage of life, preparing to feed can take from 10 minutes to 2 hours. When the tick finds a feeding spot, it grasps the skin and cuts into the surface.
- The tick then inserts its feeding tube. Many species also secrete a cement-like substance that keeps them firmly attached during the meal. The feeding tube can have barbs which help keep the tick in place.
- Ticks also can secrete small amounts of saliva with anesthetic properties so that the animal or person can't feel that the tick has attached itself. If the tick is in a sheltered spot, it can go unnoticed.
- A tick will suck the blood slowly for several days. If the host animal has a bloodborne infection, the tick will ingest the pathogens with the blood.
- Small amounts of saliva from the tick may also enter the skin of the host animal during the feeding process. If the tick contains a pathogen, the organism may be transmitted to the host animal in this way.
- After feeding, most ticks will drop off and prepare for the next life stage. At its next feeding, it can then transmit an acquired disease to the new host.

TICK-BORNE DISEASES *(continued from previous page)*

SIGNS AND SYMPTOMS:
Initially, the tick bite is usually painless and remains that way after the tick stops the blood meal and falls off the skin. Later, the following signs and symptoms may develop at the site of the tick bite:

- Itching
- Burning
- Redness
- Localized pain in some individuals

Some individuals develop sensitivity or an allergic reaction to tick bites and may experience:[2]

- Rash
- Shortness of breath
- Swelling
- Numbness
- Paralysis
- Erythema migrans (EM)—red ring-like or homogenous expanding rash; classic rash not present in all cases.

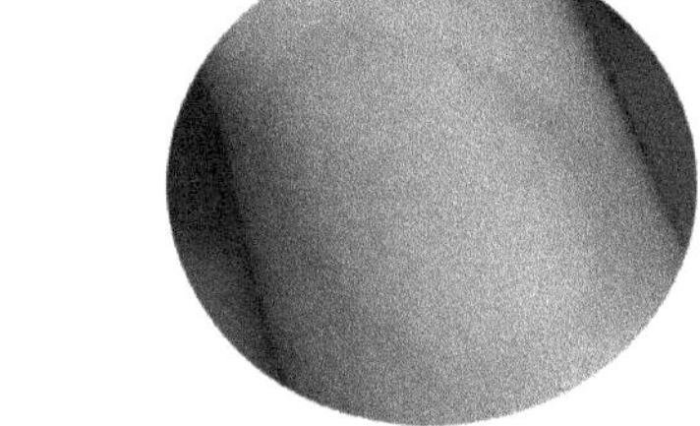

Classic EM – Lyme's disease (Photo: CDC, 2019)

- Signs and symptoms of Lymes Disease: Flu-like symptoms—malaise, headache, fever, myalgia, arthralgia and lymphadenopathy.

MANAGEMENT/TREATMENT, Tick removal:[6]

1. Try to establish source and duration of tick adherence. Be familiar with the types of ticks in the area that carry disease.
2. Cleanse the site with rubbing alcohol or soap and water and then remove the tick with a small, fine-tipped forceps or tweezers grasping the tick as close to the skin as possible, pulling upward with a firm, steady pressure to keep the tick intact. Do not twist or jerk the tick or cause the mouth part to break off and remain in the skin.

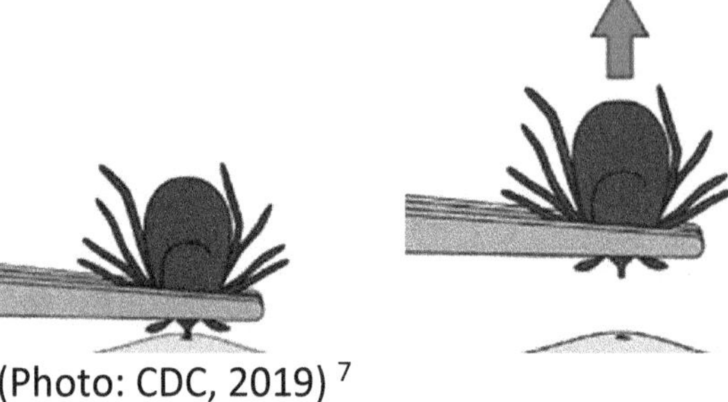

(Photo: CDC, 2019) [7]

TICK-BORNE DISEASES *(continued from previous page)*

MANAGEMENT/TREATMENT, Tick removal *(continued)*

3. Re-cleanse the site with rubbing alcohol or soap and water.
4. Dispose of a live tick by placing it in alcohol, placing it in a sealed container, wrapping it tightly in tape, or flushing it down the toilet unless local policy is different.
5. Inform parent/guardian of signs that need a healthcare provider's attention following a tick bite.
6. Monitor student for signs of illness for up to one month.

PREVENTION:

- Prevention efforts have to include recognition of the ticks and disease in your area and the types of places and seasonality/prevalence to the disease carrying ticks. It is important that children are checked for ticks after playing outside. This includes instructing the children on looking for any ticks. If ticks are found they should be removed (see tick removal instructions) and notify parents of the exposure.

- Grounds Management - use of acaricides (tick pesticides) can reduce the number of ticks in treated areas of playgrounds. Areas should be cleared of tall grasses and brush. Wood chips or gravel may help deter ticks.

FOLLOW-UP:

- Educate about tick avoidance (e.g., proper clothing, DEET repellents, and pet protection), frequent checks, and careful removal of tick.[8]
- Educate regarding the need to use long sleeve clothing and long pants when children are outside for extended periods.
- Educate regarding checking pets and service animals for ticks. Pets and farm animals may be a source of ticks.

NOTES:

- Children should be taught to seek the help of an adult for tick removal.
- If the tick must be removed using fingers, use a barrier such as a tissue or leaf to avoid contact with possible infected fluids.
- Do not pick, crush, or burn the tick as it may release infected tissues or fluids.
- Do not attempt to smother the tick with substances such as petroleum jelly or nail polish. Smothering is not an effective technique for tick removal as the tick has enough oxygen to complete the feeding (adopted from Lyme Disease Foundation, Inc.).[9]
- Check state and local health department websites for details pertinent to the occurrence and types of ticks in your school's location.

TICK-BORNE DISEASES *(continued from previous page)*

REFERENCES

[1] Science Direct. (2019). *Tick-borne disease.* https://www.sciencedirect.com/topics/medicine-and-dentistry/tick-borne-disease

[2] Ibid.

[3] Centers for Disease Control and Prevention (CDC). (2019). Stop ticks. http://www.cdc.gov/features/stopticks/

[4] Centers for Disease Control and Prevention (CDC). (2019). Tick-borne disease surveillance data summary. https://www.cdc.gov/ticks/data-summary/index.html

[5] Ibid.

[6] Centers for Disease Control and Prevention (CDC). (2019) *Tick removal.* https://www.cdc.gov/ticks/removing_a_tick.html

[7] Centers for Disease Control and Prevention (CDC). (2019). S*top ticks.* http://www.cdc.gov/features/stopticks/

[8] American Academy of Pediatrics. (2017). *Prevention of lyme disease.* https://pediatrics.aappublications.org/content/105/1/142

[9] American Lyme Disease Foundation. (2019). Lyme disease. https://www.aldf.com/

TUBERCULOSIS (PRIMARY OR CHILDHOOD)

DEFINITION/ETIOLOGY:

Tuberculosis (TB) is caused by *Mycobacterium tuberculosis*, an acid-fast bacillus (AFB). It is the most common cause of infection-related death worldwide.[1] The bacteria usually attack the lungs, but TB bacteria can attack any part of the body, such as the kidney, spine and brain. Not everyone infected with TB bacteria becomes sick.[2] In the pediatric population, children under the age of three are most susceptible, and then again at adolescence. Most cases in children and adolescents are asymptomatic.[3] Additional information related to TB definitions and etiology includes the following:[4]

- **Childhood or Primary TB** is *M. tuberculosis* infection in older infants and children, contracted from prolonged household case contact. It is usually an asymptomatic infection. The diagnosis is confirmed only by a positive tuberculin skin test (TST).
- **Tuberculin Skin Test (TST)** also known at the Mantoux test or purified protein derivative (PPD) is the standard for identifying infected persons. The Mantoux test is read 48-72 hours after being placed by the healthcare provider or a registered nurse.
- **Positive tuberculin skin test**: The classifications of reactions (measuring *induration*, not redness, of the wheal from the TST) are:
    - Induration ≥ 5mm: Positive if patient is at high risk, such as household contact with TB disease, clinical evidence of TB, abnormal chest radiograph, or HIV+.
    - Induration ≥ 10 mm: Positive if patient is at moderate risk, e.g., children younger than 4 years of age, or born in high-prevalence regions, or those who travel to these regions, children with other medical conditions (e.g. Hodgkin's disease, lymphoma, diabetes, or chronic renal failure).
    - Induration ≥ 15mm: Positive if patient is 4 years of age or older without any risk factor.[5]
- **Latent tuberculosis infection (LTBI)** is defined as TB infection in a person who has a positive TST result but no physical finding of TB disease; chest radiograph findings are normal or reveal evidence of healing infection.
- **Active tuberculosis disease** is defined as disease in a person with TB infection having symptoms, signs, or radiographic manifestations. Healthy people who are infected with tuberculosis have a 5-10% lifetime risk of developing active disease.

TRANSMISSION:

All cases of TB are passed from person to person through airborne transmission of droplets. Inhalation of droplets can occur from an adult or adolescent with contagious, cavity, pulmonary tuberculosis. When a person with TB infection coughs, sneezes, or talks, tiny droplets of saliva or mucus are expelled in the air and can be transmitted through inhalation by another person.

- The incubation period from infection to development of a positive TST is two to10 weeks. The risk of developing of TB disease is highest during the six months after infection and remains high for two years.
- Once the infectious particles are inhaled and reach the alveoli, small sac-like structures develop in the air spaces in the lungs and the macrophage cell engulfs the TB bacteria.
- The TB bacteria are then transmitted to the lymphatic system and bloodstream and the spread to other organs occurs.
- The TB bacteria begin to multiply in organs with high oxygen pressures, e.g. the upper lobes of the lungs, kidneys, bone marrow, and meninges.

TUBERCULOSIS (PRIMARY OR CHILDHOOD) *(continued from previous page)*

TRANMISSION *(continued)*

- TB disease occurs when the bacteria cause clinically detectable disease.
- Persons who have inhaled the TB bacterium but show no signs of clinically detectable disease are referred to as infected. Persons infected with TB have no symptoms of disease because the immune system has walled off the organism in an inflammatory focus known as a granuloma.
- The skin test for TB will often be positive in people infected with TB, but the disease cannot be transmitted to others while in the latent phase of TB infection.

EVIDENCE-BASED RECOMMENDATIONS FOR SCREENING FOR CHILDREN AND ADOLESCENTS[6]

- Screen for risk factors of TB and LTBI, utilizing local department of health guidelines as appropriate.
- Test with a TST only if more than one of the following risk factors is present:
  - Contact with adult with active TB disease
  - Foreign birth
  - Travel to a country with high prevalence of infection
  - Household member with latent tuberculosis infection (LTBI)

SIGNS AND SYMPTOMS:[7]

- Common symptoms of TB may include fever, cough, chest x-ray abnormalities, loss of appetite, weight loss, night sweats, nonproductive cough, failure to thrive, and difficulty gaining weight.
- Most children and adolescents with tuberculosis infection have no symptoms (asymptomatic).
- Children and adolescents with continued exposure or weakened immunity can develop symptoms such as fatigue, malaise, low-grade fever, and symptoms resulting from lymph node enlargement, especially in the center of the chest (hilar node).
- In eight to twelve weeks, the body's defenses wall off the infection with scar tissue. There are no further consequences other than positive TST. This is the typical course of childhood or primary TB.

MANAGEMENT/TREATMENT:[8]

Medical treatment of TB includes the following recommendations:

- Treatment is recommended for all children and adolescents diagnosed with LTBI, because young children are at higher risk for progression to TB disease.
- Multiple antimicrobial drugs are available for treatment of TB.
- First line drugs are isoniazide (INH), rifampin (RIF), pyrazinamide (PZA), and ethambutol (EMB).
- Children are usually treated with isoniazid (INH), daily by mouth for 9 months.
- For children less than four years of age with a close contact, INH should be initiated, even if the TST result is first negative. TST should be retested 12 weeks after the last contact. If the result is negative, INH may be discontinued.

TUBERCULOSIS (PRIMARY OR CHILDHOOD) *(continued from previous page)*

MANAGEMENT/TREATMENT *(continued)*

- Second line drugs are used with patients with drug-resistant TB ((DR-TB) or with those who do not tolerate first line medications. The most used second line drugs include both the aminoglycosides (streptomycin, kanamycin, amikacin, and capreomycin) and fluroquinolones (levofloxacin, moxifloxacin).

Management for schools of TB includes the following recommendations:

- Suspected or known tuberculosis must be reported to state and local health deaprtments immediately, because early reporting may help minimize the spread of TB.
- **With rare exception, primary TB is non-contagious; student may remain in school, even though a person at home has active TB**. Comply with healthcare provider orders, health department guidance and school policy.
- Children with LTBI can participate in all activities whether they are receiving treatment or not.
- Educate faculty and staff to understand relative risk.
- Cooperate with the state and local public health department and the school medical advisor (if available) to assist students with skin testing and/or x-rays of students and staff when these tests are recommended.
- Develop an Individualized Healthcare Plan (IHP) for student to manage care in school.

FOLLOW UP:

- Promote and monitor adherence to treatment of LTBI in all students.
- Provide education about the importance of adhering to completing treatment and the potential side effects of INH. These side effects include hepatitis, gastrointestinal disturbances, and peripheral neuropathy.
- If a student demonstrates any symptom of liver toxicity, stop treatment immediately and refer the student to the healthcare provider for assessment.

NOTES:[9]

- Exposure to an infected adult is the most common risk factor in children.
- TB is preventable through effective management and treatment. Treatment of TB in a single person prevents latent infection from becoming active disease. Treatment is also effective in controlling the spread of disease among large populations.
- The TB vaccine, bacilli Calmette-Guerin (BCG), may often be used in foreign countries to prevent the spread of disease among children. However, the vaccine does not protect against pulmonary tuberculosis and often results in a false positive TST.
- Human Immunodeficiency Virus (HIV) is an important risk factor for both development and spread of disease.

TUBERCULOSIS (PRIMARY OR CHILDHOOD) *(continued from previous page)*

REFERENCES

[1] Batra, V. (2018*). Pediatric tuberculosis*. https://emedicine.medscape.com/article/969401-overview

[2] Centers for Disease Control and prevention (CDC). (2019). *Tuberculosis: Basic TB facts.* https://www.cdc.gov/tb/topic/basics/default.htm

[3] American Academy of Pediatrics. (2018). Tuberculosis. In L. K. Pickering, C. J. Baker, D. W. Kimberlin, & S. S. Long (Eds.), *Red Book: 2018 report of the committee on infectious diseases,* (31st ed., pp. 829-853). American Academy of Pediatrics.

[4] Merck Manual. (2019). *Tuberculosis*. https://www.merckmanuals.com/professional/infectious-diseases/mycobacteria/tuberculosis-tb

[5] Centers for Disease Control and Prevention. (2016). *Tuberculosis fact sheets*. https://www.cdc.gov/tb/publications/factsheets/testing/skintesting.htm

[6] American Academy of Pediatrics. (2018). Tuberculosis. In L. K. Pickering, C. J. Baker, D. W. Kimberlin, & S. S. Long (Eds.), *Red Book: 2018 report of the committee on infectious diseases,* (31st ed., pp. 829-853). American Academy of Pediatrics.

[7] American Academy of Pediatrics. (2020). Tuberculosis. In S.S.Aronson, & T.R.Shope (Eds.), Managing infectious diseases in child care and schools: A quick reference guide, (5th ed., pp. 173-174). American Academy of Pediatrics.

[8] Merck Manual. (2019). *Tuberculosis*. https://www.merckmanuals.com/professional/infectious-diseases/mycobacteria/tuberculosis-tb

[9] Ogle, J.W., & Anderson, M.S. (2016). Infections: Bacterial & spirochetal. In W. Hay, M. Levin, R. Deterding, & M. Abzug (Eds.), *Current diagnosis and treatment pediatrics* (23rd ed., pp. 1273-1276). McGraw Hill Education, Inc.

UPPER RESPIRATORY INFECTION or "COMMON COLD"

DEFINITION/ETIOLOGY:

The common cold can be described as a viral infection of the upper respiratory tract that affects the nose, throat, ears and eyes. More than 200 viruses can cause a cold. The rhinovirus is the most common pathogen that causes upper respiratory infections (URIs) and commonly students may have four to seven upper respiratory infections in a year. The incidence will usually decrease as the student gets older.[1] The incubation period is generally two-14 days and the contagion period may be a few days before the symptoms appear and while symptoms are present. Symptoms typically last seven – 10 days although a mild cough may continue into the second week. The virus is spread by airborne droplets, hand to hand contact or by sharing contaminated objects.[2]

SIGNS AND SYMPTOMS:

- Runny nose – nasal drainage initially clear; after a few days mucous becomes whitish or yellowish in color; as the cold progresses the mucous may change to a greenish color (this is normal)
- Sneezing
- Watery eyes
- Sore (or scratchy/itchy) throat
- Cough
- Mild headache
- Mild joint pain
- Earache (may result from the URI virus or from a secondary bacterial infection)
- May have a low-grade fever although temperature is usually normal[3]

MANAGEMENT/TREATMENT:

There is no immediate cure for an URI. Most common colds resolve within 10 days. Treatment is supportive.

1. Limit exercise if cough is troublesome. Coordinate with Physical Education teacher.
2. Exclude from school if student has severe cough and is disruptive to learning.
3. Educate about hygienic use and disposal of tissues and thorough hand washing.
4. Educate to not pick at nose and to blow nose gently.
5. Encourage fluids and rest.
6. Diet as tolerated.[4]
7. Do not use aspirin under age 18. Aspirin can play a role in causing Reye's Syndrome.
8. If giving acetaminophen or ibuprofen, follow medication orders.
9. Watch for adverse side effects even with over-the-counter medicines taken at home; antihistamines can cause drowsiness; decongestants can cause excitability.
10. If symptoms last more than 10-14 days, another diagnosis may be explored by the healthcare provider.

UPPER RESPIRATORY INFECTION or "Common Cold" *(continued from previous page)*

FOLLOW UP:

- Refer to healthcare provider for persistent cough or complications: earache, rising fever or fever lasting more than a few days, vomiting, headache, loss of appetite, sore throat, wheezing, dehydration, or symptoms that fail to improve.[5]

POTENTIAL COMPLICATIONS:

Complications are rare. Potential complications include:

- Sinus infection
- Ear infection
- Bronchitis
- Wheezing – upper respiratory infections may exacerbate asthma

NOTES:

Educate parent/guardians and staff regarding the importance of:

- Good handwashing. *(Refer to HANDWASHING APPENDIX).*
- Covering nose and mouth with a tissue when coughing or sneezing, and proper disposal of tissues; wash hands or use alcohol-based hand sanitizer after blowing nose or touching nasal secretions. *(Refer to COVER YOUR COUGH APPENDIX).*
- To prevent the spread of infection, teach children to cough or sneeze into their shoulder or elbow if a tissue is not available.
- Table surfaces, desks and doorknobs should be routinely sanitized.
- Keep fingers away from eyes and nose to prevent the spread of the virus.
- Educate parent/guardian that antibiotics will not cure the common cold; a cold is caused by a virus; an antibiotic may be needed for secondary bacterial infections (ear infection, etc.).
- Exposure to cold temperature (outdoor recess, etc.) does not make a person more susceptible to an upper respiratory infection.
- It is not necessary to exclude children from school unless other exclusionary criteria exist, or the child feels otherwise unwell. Exclusion of children with signs or symptoms has no benefit in reducing the spread of common respiratory infections.[6]

REFERENCES

[1] Jakubowski, T. & Perron, T. (2019). Students with common health complaints. In J. Selekman, R. Adair Shannon, &C. F. Yonkaitis (Eds.), *School nursing: A comprehensive text* (3rd ed., pp. 347-348). F.A. Davis.

[2] American Academy of Pediatrics. (2020). Upper respiratory infection (common cold). In S. Aronson, & T. Shope (Eds.), *Managing infectious diseases in child care and schools* (5th ed., pp. 175-176). American Academy of Pediatrics.

[3] Ibid.

[4] Jakubowski, T. & Perron, T. (2019). Students with common health complaints. In J. Selekman, R. Adair Shannon, & C. F. Yonkaitis (Eds.), *School nursing: A comprehensive text* (3rd ed., pp. 347-348). F.A. Davis.

[5] Mayo Clinic. (2019). *Common cold.* https://www.mayoclinic.org/diseases-conditions/common-cold/syptoms-causes/syc-203516055

[6] American Academy of Pediatrics. (2020). Upper respiratory infection (common cold). In S. Aronson, & T. Shope (Eds.), *Managing infectious diseases in child care and schools* (5th ed., pp. 175-176). American Academy of Pediatrics.

UPPER RESPIRATORY INFECTION or "Common Cold" *(continued from previous page)*

OTHER REFERENCES CONSULTED

Centers for Disease Control and Prevention. (2017). *Common cold and runny nose*. Retrieved from http://www.cdc.gov/getsmart/antibiotic-use/URI/colds.html

Merck Manual. (2018). *Common cold.* Retrieved from http://www.merckmanuals.com/professional/infectious_diseases/respiratory_viruses/common_cold.html?qt=UpperRespiratory Infection&alt=sh

URINARY TRACT INFECTIONS (UTI)

DEFINITION/ETIOLOGY:

Urinary tract infections (UTI) are a common occurrence in childhood with approximately 8% of girls and 1% of boys having at least one UTI by age seven.[1] In addition, 30 to 50% of them will have more than one. Most UTIs are caused by the gram-negative enteric bacterium, Escherichia coli.[2] An infection can occur anywhere in the urinary tract and can be bacterial, viral or fungal. Pyelonephritis is the term that refers to the upper urinary tract involving the pelvis, ureters and renal parenchyma. Cystitis is a lower urinary tract infection and involves the urethra or bladder.[3] Pyelonephritis is the more severe type of UTI.[4]

Causes

- Urinary stasis is a common cause of a UTI.
- School-aged children commonly void infrequently leading to incomplete emptying.
- Abnormal anatomy or abnormal functioning such as a neurogenic bladder in which the nerve supply to the bladder is interrupted is also a common cause of incomplete bladder emptying.[5]
- Recurrent UTIs in children may be caused by vesicoureteral reflux where the urine travels backwards from the bladder towards the kidney.[6]
- Other causes include an irritated perineum, poor hygiene especially after bowel movements, constipation and sexual activity in the adolescent.[7]

SIGNS AND SYMPTOMS:[8]

- Fever
- Urinary incontinence "accidents"
- Painful urination
- Blood in the urine
- Sensation of the need to urinate
- Change in appearance and smell of urine
- Abdominal and flank pain, renal tenderness (especially in pyelonephritis)
- Vomiting (especially in preschool children)

MANAGEMENT/TREATMENT:[9]

- Urinalysis and culture remain the gold standard for diagnosis. In addition, a renal ultrasound may be done to rule out congenital urologic abnormalities.[10]
- Students suspected of a UTI should be referred to their healthcare provider for possible antimicrobial treatment.
- Hydration should be encouraged.
- Encourage young children to use the bathroom every 3-4 hours.
- Teach and encourage proper hygiene.
- Teach to avoid irritants such as bubble bath and perfumed soap.
- Sexually active females should be encouraged to void after intercourse.
- For recurrent UTIs or for vesicoureteral reflux, prophylactic antibiotics may be ordered.[11]

URINARY TRACT INFECTIONS (UTI) *(continued from previous page)*

MANAGEMENT/TREATMENT *(continued)*

- Treatment of constipation if present.
- Cranberry juice may be helpful in preventing UTIs caused by E. coli.[12]

FOLLOW-UP:

- Cultures are repeated 3-4 days after treatment is initiated.
- Students should be monitored for any continued or new symptoms indicative of a UTI and referred immediately.
- Blood pressure and growth may be monitored especially in students with recurrent UTIs in the event of any chronic renal disease.[13]
- An Individualized Healthcare Plan (IHP) may be indicated for a student with frequent or recurrent UTI.

POTENTIAL COMPLICATIONS:

- A complicated UTI refers to a child younger than three to six months or a child with high fever, toxicity or dehydration. This may require hospitalization with intravenous antibiotics.[14]
- Untreated chronic UTIs may lead to chronic renal disease.[15]

NOTES:

School nurses can be instrumental in providing prevention education for all students and individualized education for a student with a UTI. This education may include:[16]

- Stay well hydrated
- Use the bathroom often and avoid "holding back "urinating
- Take showers instead of baths and avoid "bubble baths"
- Avoid irritating feminine products
- Urinate after sexual intercourse
- Avoid douches and powders
- Wipe from front to back after voiding or bowel movements

REFERENCES

---

[1] Cadnapaphornchai, M.A., & Lum, G. M. (2018). Kidney & urinary tract. In W.W. Hay, M.J. Levin, R. R. Deterding, & M. J. Abzug (Eds.), *Current diagnosis and treatment: Pediatrics* (24th ed., pp. 749-751). McGraw Hill Education.

[2] Ibid.

[3] Ibid.

[4] Ball, J.W., Binder, R. C., Cowen, K. J., & Shaw, M.R. (Eds.). (2017). Alterations in genitourinary function. *Principles of pediatric nursing: Caring for children* (7th ed., pp. 701-738). Pearson Education.

[5] Cadnapaphornchai, M.A., & Lum, G. M. (2018). Kidney & urinary tract. In W.W. Hay, M.J. Levin, R. R. Deterding, & M. J. Abzug (Eds.), *Current diagnosis and treatment: Pediatrics* (24th ed., pp. 749-751). McGraw Hill Education.

[6] American Academy of Pediatrics. (2019). Kidney and other urinary problems. In E.A. Donoghue, & C.A. Kraft, *Managing chronic health needs in child care and schools* (2nd ed., p.p. 157-159). American Academy of Pediatrics.

[7] Cadnapaphornchai, M.A., & Lum, G. M. (2018). Kidney & urinary tract. In W.W. Hay, M.J. Levin, R. R. Deterding, & M. J. Abzug (Eds.), *Current diagnosis and treatment: Pediatrics* (24th ed., pp. 749-751). McGraw Hill Education.

URINARY TRACT INFECTIONS (UTI) *(continued from previous page)*

[8] American Academy of Pediatrics. (2019). Kidney and other urinary problems. In E.A. Donoghue, & C.A. Kraft, *Managing chronic health needs in child care and schools* (2nd ed., p.p. 157-159). American Academy of Pediatrics.

[9] Gaylord, N. (2017). Genitourinary disorders. In C. Burns, A.M. Dunn, M.A. Brady, N.B. Starr, C.G. Blosser, & D.L. Garzon (Eds.), *Pediatric primary care* (6th ed., pp. 915-920). Elsevier.

[10] Ibid.

[11] American Academy of Pediatrics. (2019). Kidney and other urinary problems. In E.A. Donoghue, & C.A. Kraft, *Managing chronic health needs in child care and schools* (2nd ed., p.p. 157-159). American Academy of Pediatrics.

[12] Gaylord, N. (2017). Genitourinary disorders. In C. Burns, A.M. Dunn, M.A. Brady, N.B. Starr, C.G. Blosser, & D.L. Garzon (Eds.), *Pediatric primary care* (6th ed., pp. 915-920). Elsevier.

[13] Ibid.

[14] Ibid.

[15] Ibid.

[16] Mayo Clinic. (2019). Urinary tract infections. https://www.mayoclinic.org/diseases-conditions/urinary-tract-infection/symptoms-causes/syc-20353447

URTICARIA (Hives)

DEFINITION/ETIOLOGY:

Urticaria, also known as hives, is a skin condition identified by pruritic red or skin colored wheals that vary in size, change shape, and appear and fade.[1] They can appear anywhere on the body and resemble spots, blotches or large connected bumps.[2] It may be considered angioedema (swelling of tissue under the skin) when there is swelling of the eyes, mouth, hands, feet or the throat.[3] Acute urticaria can last six weeks or less. In contrast, chronic urticaria lasts six weeks or longer.[4] Acute cases (70%) are more common than chronic (30%).[5] Urticaria affects about 20% of the population during their lifetime.[6]

CAUSES:

Urticaria is triggered by an inflammation in the skin due to mast and basophil cells releasing histamine and other chemicals into the blood stream.[7] Triggers for urticaria can be difficult to pinpoint and the underlying cause may be difficult to identify.

Below are some known causes of urticaria:[8, 9]

- Food allergens: Fruits (especially citrus fruits), milk, eggs, peanuts, tree nuts, and shellfish
- Viral and bacterial infections
- Drug hypersensitivities (antibiotics, especially penicillin and sulfa, and nonsteroidal anti-inflammatory drugs, such as aspirin and ibuprofen, are the most frequent triggers)
- Latex
- Anxiety
- Physical triggers such as, heat, cold, sun exposure and exercise
- Inhalants (e.g., pollens, dust)
- Contact substances (e.g., some plants)
- Pet dander
- Insect bites or stings
- Cold urticaria (e.g. exposure to cold water or snow)

SIGNS AND SYMPTOMS:

Characteristics of the wheals in urticaria:[10,11]

- Circular, oval or irregular varying in size from very small to the size of dinner plates
- Pale in center with surrounding redness
- Tenderness
- Pruritic
- Can intensify with heat, exercise or stress
- Characteristically short-lived but reappear often in other parts of body
- May be accompanied by swelling of lips, eyes, throat (angioedema)

URTICARIA (Hives) *(continued from previous page)*

NOTE: Anaphylaxis and respiratory distress are the most serious complication and requires immediate emergency care – activate Emergency Medical Services (EMS).[12] (*Refer to Anaphylaxis*)

MANAGEMENT/TREATMENT: [13]

1. Cool moist compresses to help control itching.
2. Avoid implicated foods or other suspect triggers.
3. Administer antihistamines if prescribed.
4. Notify parents/guardians about the occurrence of hives. Communicate any known or contributing causes of the urticaria.
5. Carefully monitor a child with hives for signs and symptoms of a progressive and serious allergic reaction (potentially anaphylaxis).

FOLLOW UP:

1. It's important that policies are in place for supporting students with allergies and allergic responses.
2. Provide appropriate training to school staff.
3. Develop individualized school emergency plan for students with known allergies.
4. Avoid triggers at school.

REFERENCES

[1] Mayo Clinic. (2018). *Chronic hives.* https://www.mayoclinic.org/diseases-conditions/chronic-hives/symptoms-causes/syc-20352719

[2] Kids Health/Nemours. (2018). *Hives (urticaria).* https://kidshealth.org/en/parents/hives.html?ref=search

[3] American College of Allergy, Asthma and Immunology. (2018). *Hives (urticaria).* https://acaai.org/allergies/types-allergies/hives-urticaria

[4] Merck Manual. (2019). *Urticaria.* https://www.merckmanuals.com/professional/dermatologic-disorders/approach-to-the-dermatologic-patient/urticaria

[5] Ibid.

[6] American College of Allergy, Asthma and Immunology. (2018). *Hives (urticaria).* https://acaai.org/allergies/types-allergies/hives-urticaria

[7] Merck Manual. (2019). *Urticaria.* https://www.merckmanuals.com/professional/dermatologic-disorders/approach-to-the-dermatologic-patient/urticaria

[8] American Academy of Dermatology. (2019). *Hives.* https://www.aad.org/public/diseases/itchy-skin/hives#overview

[9] Ibid.

[10] Kids Health/Nemours. (2018). *Hives (urticaria).* https://kidshealth.org/en/parents/hives.html?ref=search

[11] Mayo Clinic. (2018). *Chronic hives.* https://www.mayoclinic.org/diseases-conditions/chronic-hives/symptoms-causes/syc-20352719

[12] American Academy of Dermatology. (2019). *Hives.* https://www.aad.org/public/diseases/itchy-skin/hives#overview

[13] Mayo Clinic. (2018). *Chronic hives.* https://www.mayoclinic.org/diseases-conditions/chronic-hives/symptoms-causes/syc-20352719

VARICELLA (Chickenpox)

DEFINITION/ETIOLOGY:

Chickenpox (varicella) is an acute, highly contagious, generalized viral disease that is caused by the zoster virus (VZV). A person with varicella is contagious beginning one to two days before onset of rash and until all lesions have crusted. Transmission occurs through contact with respiratory droplets/secretions and inhalation of aerosols from vesicular fluid of skin lesions of acute varicella or zoster. Incubation is 14 – 16 days (range 10-21 days) from exposure to onset of symptoms.[1] It is vaccine preventable.[2] Most cases appear in children under age 10.

SIGNS AND SYMPTOMS:[3]

- A mild prodrome of fever and malaise may occur one to two days before rash onset.
- Vesicular exanthem that usually begins on the scalp or trunk.
- Sudden onset of slight fever, mild constitutional symptoms.
- Itchy, fluid filled blister like rash. Typically, a clear vesicle on an erythematous base.
- New bumps continue to appear for several days thus all stages may present simultaneously (macular rash, vesicle, scab).
- Contagious one -two days before the rash appears while experiencing symptoms of fever, malaise, decrease appetite and headache.
- Pruritis is common and sometimes severe.
- No longer contagious when all blisters have formed scabs.

MANAGEMENT/TREATMENT:

- Treatment is supportive:
  - management of itching with antihistamines administered daily, calamine lotion or oatmeal baths;
  - acetaminophen for fever; and
  - antistaphylococcal penicillin or cephalosporins for bacterial superinfections.
- Exclusion from school until all lesions are scabbed over and dry (five - seven days; longer for immunocompromised persons to assure all blisters are crusted). Incubation period averages 14-16 days for new exposures, but may range 10-21 days.
- Immunosuppressed individuals are particularly at risk and may develop life threatening disease (e.g., students with leukemia or Human Immunodeficiency Virus [HIV]).[3]
- Alert parents of students with immunity problems that their child may have been exposed to chickenpox at school.
- Alert school staff members, who may be immunocompromised or pregnant, of the outbreak of chickenpox.[4]
- Advise parent or guardian to:
- DO NOT give aspirin or products containing salicylates due to the link with Reye's Syndrome.[5]
- Oatmeal baths in lukewarm water may be comforting to the itching rash.
- Trim fingernails to reduce secondary infections from scratching.

VARICELLA (Chickenpox) *(continued from previous page)*

POTENTIAL COMPLICATIONS:

- Complications are uncommon, but may include dehydration from vomiting or diarrhea.
- Secondary bacterial infections may occur from scratching the blister. Common bacterial infections are staphylococcal and streptococcal superinfection of the skin lesions.
- Complications that are more serious include chicken pox lesions in the throat, eyes and mucous membranes, pneumonia, and encephalitis.

NOTES:

- Varicella tends to be more severe in adolescents and adults.
- Remind all parents that a vaccine (or proof of disease) is required for school entry.
- Children receive two doses of the vaccine, the first between ages 12 and 15 months and the second between ages 4 and 6 years.[6]
- Adults may get "shingles" if they have had chicken pox.[7] *(Refer to SHINGLES).*
- 95% of adults have had chickenpox (even if they do not remember it).
- After exposure to a person with shingles, someone can get chickenpox if they have not been vaccinated or have never had chickenpox.[8]
- Persons vaccinated can still get chickenpox. However, the symptoms are usually milder. They usually recover more quickly and have less than 50 pox.[9] These cases are often harder to diagnose. Someone with even a mild case can still spread the chickenpox virus.

REFERENCES

[1] Centers for Disease Control and Prevention (CDC). (2019). *Chickenpox fact sheet.* https://www.cdc.gov/vaccines/parents/diseases/varicella.html

[2] American Academy of Pediatrics. (2016). Varicella. In A. J. Mancini, & D. P. Krowchuk (Eds.), *Pediatric dermatology* (3rd ed., pp. 155-159). American Academy of Pediatrics.

[3] American Academy of Pediatrics, Committee on Infectious Diseases. (2018). Varicella-zoster virus infections. In D.W. Kimberlin, M. T. Brady, M.A. Jackson, & S.S. Long (Eds.), *Red Book: 2018-2021 report of the committee on infectious diseases* (31st ed., pp.869-883). American Academy of Pediatrics.

[4] Centers for Disease Control and Prevention (CDC). (2014). *Chickenpox and pregnancy.* http://www.cdc.gov/pregnancy/infections-chickenpox.html

[5] National Reye's Syndrome Foundation. (n.d,). *Reye's and chickenpox.* http://www.reyessyndrome.org/chickenpox.html

[6] Immunization Action Coalition. (2019). *Varicella state mandates on immunizations and vaccine-preventable diseases.* http://www.immunize.org/laws/varicella.asp

[7] Mayo Clinic. (2019). *Chickenpox.* http://www.mayoclinic.org/diseases-conditions/chickenpox/basics/definition/con-20019025

[8] Mayo Clinic. (2019). *Shingles.* http://www.mayoclinic.org/diseases-conditions/shingles/basics/causes/con-20019574

[10] Centers for Disease Control and Prevention. (2019). Varicella. Epidemiology and Prevention of Vaccine Preventable Diseases (13th ed.). https://www.cdc.gov/vaccines/pubs/pinkbook/varicella.html

[9] Centers for Disease Control and Prevention. (2019). Varicella. Epidemiology and Prevention of Vaccine Preventable Diseases (13th ed.). https://www.cdc.gov/vaccines/pubs/pinkbook/varicella.html

WARTS (VERRUCAE VULGARIS)

DEFINITION/ETIOLOGY:

Warts are non-cancerous epidermal skin growths caused by the *Human Papillomavirus* (HPV). There are over 100 different types of warts. Types include common, flat, plantar and genital. Warts affect all age groups but are more common in children and people with weakened immune systems. Most warts are asymptomatic.[1]

SIGNS AND SYPMTOMS:

Type	Location	Symptoms
Common warts [2]	Often appear on hands and/or fingers	• Small, grainy flesh-colored, white, tan or pink lesions • Often have tiny black dots in middle • Lesions may be rough to touch
Flat [3]	Appear on face or legs Appear on places where you shave	• Flat topped, slightly raised lesions, smoother than other warts • Tend to grow in clusters or several in the area but tend to stay small in size
Plantar [4]	Found on heels and other weight bearing areas of the foot	• Small, fleshy colored lesion • Callus on the bottom of foot often at base of toes or heel area • May have black "seeds" • May have mild pain when walking or standing
Genital [5]	Sexually transmitted disease; lesions grow on penis (tip or shaft), exterior female genitals, vulva, walls of vagina, anus, and cervix; genital warts can appear in the mouth after oral sex with an infected person. Transmitted during sexual intercourse or skin to skin contact. Can be transmitted by asymptomatic infected persons.	• More common in women • Itching, burning or discomfort around lesions • Small and flat (may be so small that they are not visible) • Bleeding with intercourse

MANAGEMENT/TREATMENT:

Most warts resolve spontaneously. If treatment is indicated:[6]

- Over the counter (OTC) medication (salicylic acid)
  - OTC medication is typically effective if the individual is motivated to adhere to treatment
  - Can take several weeks for the medication to be effective
- Cryotherapy (freezing) – may take several treatments and can be painful
- Excision – virus may remain in tissue even though the lesion has been removed
- Laser surgery
- See healthcare provider if wart is located on face, genitals, rectum, or on a very young child/infant. [7]
- Seek medical advice if not sure it is a wart or is bothersome, painful or other symptoms are present.[8]

Do not treat genital warts with OTC wart removers.

WARTS *(continued from previous page)*

FOLLOW UP:

- To avoid the spread of warts, educate child/youth to avoid picking at own wart (autoinoculation); avoid touching someone's wart.[9]
- Educate child/youth to avoid biting nails.[10]
- Per district policies and aligned with the health education curriculum, educate teens on higher risk behaviors including sexually transmitted infections.
- Refer diabetic students with plantar warts to a healthcare practitioner for treatment – poor healing could lead to nerve damage.[11]
- Monitor wart lesions – skin cancer may look like a wart.[12]
- Educate students and staff to wear flip-flops in public showers, locker rooms and pool decks.[13]
- Prevention – Gardasil® vaccine is available to protect from certain strains of HPV that cause genital warts and other types of warts caused by HPV.[14]

POTENTIAL COMPLICATIONS:[15]

- Secondary infection that may spread to other people
- Cervical cancer is linked to genital warts
- Difficult ambulation with plantar warts
- Emotional distress

REFERENCES

---

[1] Mayo Clinic. (2018). *Common warts.* http://www.mayoclinic.org/diseases-conditions/common warts/ symptoms-causes/syc-20371125

[2] Ibid.

[3] Medline Plus/ U.S. National Library of Medicine. (2019). *Warts.* https://www.medlineplus.gov/warts.html

[4] Mayo Clinic. (2018). *Plantar warts.* https://www.mayoclinic.org/diseases-conditions/plantar-warts/symptoms-causes/syc-20352691

[5] Mayo Clinic. (2016). *Genital warts.* https://www.mayoclinic.org/diseases-conditions/genital-warts/symptoms-causes/syc-20355234

[6] Mayo Clinic. (2018). *Common warts.* https://www.mayoclinic.org/diseases-conditions/common-warts/ symptoms-causes/syc-20371125

[7] Kids Health/Nemours. (2019). *Warts.* https://kidshealth.org/en/parents/wart.html?ref=search

[8] Ibid.

[9] Ibid.

[10] Ibid.

[11] American Academy of Dermatology. (2018). *Warts.* https://www.aad.org/public/diseases/contagious-skin-diseases/warts#overview

[12] Merck Manual. (2018). *Warts.* https://www.merckmanuals.com/professional/dermatologic-disorders/viral-skin-diseases/warts?query=warts

[13] Kids Health/Nemours. (2019). *Warts.* https://kidshealth.org/en/parents/wart.html?ref=search

[14] Merck Manual. (2018). *Warts.* https://www.merckmanuals.com/professional/dermatologic-disorders/viral-skin-diseases/warts?query=warts

[15] Medscape. (2019). *Human papillomavirus (HPV) clinical presentation.* https://emedicine.medscape.com/article/219110-clinical#b3

SECTION II

CLINICAL PROCEDURES

CATHETERIZATION, URINARY: INSERTION OR REINSERTION OF URINARY CATHETER

DEFINITION/ETIOLOGY:
Urinary catheterization requires the placement of a tube through the urinary meatus into the bladder or into a ureterostomy to drain urine from the bladder. Clean intermittent catheterization (CIC) is a clean procedure and is performed every few hours in order to eliminate urine from the bladder before bacterial growth can lead to infection.[1] The catheter is removed once the bladder is emptied.

CIC may also be performed through a stoma in the abdomen for students with a continent ureterostomy or vesicostomy.[2]

Rarely, students may have an indwelling urinary catheter, which may become dislodged during the school day and need to be replaced. The indwelling catheter is kept in place by a balloon, which is inflated after insertion, and allows for continuous drainage into a drainage bag.

PURPOSE:
To ensure emptying of the bladder for students who are unable to void independently or completely. These problems are often seen in children with spina bifida, spinal cord injuries, or some urinary tract defects.[3] Clean intermittent catheterization helps prevent urinary tract infections by preventing stagnant urine in bladder for long periods of time. CIC also eliminates overflow incontinence.[4]

EQUIPMENT:
- Gloves
- Clean or sterile catheters
- Collection bag and tubing (for indwelling catheters)
- Receptacle for collection
- Water based lubricant (do not use a petroleum lubricant such as Vaseline®)
- Disposable pad (i.e. Chux®) or disposable towel
- Soap and water or disposable wipes
- Sterile water (for indwelling catheters)
- 10 cc syringe (for indwelling catheters)

PROCEDURE:

Note: All healthcare procedures in the school should have a healthcare provider order outlining the reason/diagnosis, what procedure is to be performed during the school day, technical specifics including size of catheter, amount of fluid in balloon for indwelling catheter, whether sterile procedure or clean procedure, and if clean, the manner and duration of cleaning and storage. Potential adverse reactions for the individual student should also be addressed.

CATHETERIZATION, URINARY *(continued from previous page)*

PROCEDURE *(continued)*

Male Clean Intermittent Catheterization[5]

Position: Male students may be catheterized standing, sitting on a toilet, lying down or in a wheelchair.

1. Wash hands.
2. Put on gloves.
3. Open the catheter utilizing clean technique.
4. Hold sides of penis with non-dominant hand at a straight angle from the body.
5. Clean the urethra and the tip of penis with wipes or mild soap and water.
6. Retract the foreskin if uncircumcised.
7. Generously coat the distal end of the catheter with a water-soluble lubricant
8. Have the student take a deep breath and slowly insert the catheter into the urethra until there is a good flow of urine. Depending on the size of the student, you may advance the catheter ½ to 1 inch more.
9. If resistance is met prior to the flow of urine, have the student take another deep breath and gently advance further. Some resistance of the catheter is normal. If necessary, have the student bear down or adjust student's position or the penis may need to be repositioned.
10. If the student is experiencing pain or the catheter is not advancing, notify the parent/healthcare provider.
11. When the urine flow has ended, remove the catheter slowly, rotating the catheter, pausing if the urine flow begins.
12. When the bladder is empty pinch off the catheter and withdraw it from the urethra. Measure urine if indicated and observe urine for color, mucus or odor.
13. If the catheter can be used again, wash, rinse, dry and store in an appropriate container.
14. Wash hands.
15. Document results and time.

Female Intermittent Clean Catheterization

Position: Female students may be catheterized sitting on a toilet, lying down or in a wheelchair. When catheterizing on the toilet, have the student sit on the back of the toilet seat with legs straddled.

1. Wash hands.
2. Put on gloves.
3. Open the catheter utilizing clean technique.
4. Position the student to expose the urethral opening.
5. Clean the vulva from front to back.
6. Generously coat the distal end of the catheter with a water-soluble lubricant.

CATHETERIZATION, URINARY *(continued from previous page)*

PROCEDURE *(continued)*

7. Use your non-dominant hand to separate the labia minora to visualize the urinary meatus.
8. Have the student take a deep breath, insert the catheter until there is a good flow of urine, and advance the catheter slightly.
9. If necessary, have the student bear down or adjust position.
10. If there is no flow of urine, check for catheter placement. The catheter may be in the vagina. If it is, remove and discard the catheter and use a clean catheter.
11. When the urine flow has ended remove the catheter slowly, rotating the catheter, pausing if flow begins. When the bladder is empty pinch off the catheter and withdraw it from the urethra.
12. Measure if indicated and observe urine for color, mucus, or odor.
13. If the catheter can be used again, wash, rinse, dry, and store in an appropriate container.
14. Wash hands.
15. Document results and time.

Indwelling Catheters
Generally, indwelling catheters only require emptying of the collection bag as it accumulates and measuring the output if indicated. In the event it becomes dislodged, the nurse may be responsible for reinsertion.

Reinsertion of indwelling catheters

1. Follow procedure for insertion of clean intermittent catheterization as above.
2. When catheter is in position and urine is freely flowing, inflate the balloon with the ordered amount of sterile water.
3. If resistance is met prior to the flow of urine, have the student take another deep breath and gently advance further. Some resistance of the catheter is normal.
4. If the student is experiencing pain or the catheter is not advancing notify the parent/healthcare provider.
5. Gently pull catheter until inflation balloon is snug against bladder neck.
6. Attach the catheter to the drainage system.
7. Wash hands.
8. Document results.

CATHETERIZATION, URINARY *(continued from previous page)*

NURSING CONSIDERATIONS:

- Only a registered nurse (RN) or licensed practical nurse/ licensed vocational nurse (LPN/LVN) generally perform this procedure. Nurses should check with their state Nurse Practice Act or state rulings regarding whether catheterization can be delegated to an unlicensed staff member.
- Bladder catheterization should be done in a private location with little possibility of interruption.
- Assess area for swelling, redness, breakdown, or discharge.
- If frank bleeding or edema is present, the health care provider should be notified.
- If insertion is difficult or the decision is made that insertion is not to be done, the student should be diapered to prevent soiling.
- If the bladder does not appear to be emptying, reposition student, have student bear down, or apply gentle downward pressure just above the bladder (Crede maneuver).[6]
- Be aware of the student's medications that affect changes in his/her urine.
- Note the baseline status of the student's urine color, amount and pattern of continence and notify parent and/or health care provider of any change.
- Depending on the student's ability, promote independence and teach student how to perform the procedure.
- The facilities may need to be wheelchair accessible or have special equipment such as a raised toilet or handrails.
- Catheters come in different sizes; the same sized catheter should be inserted each time.

REFERENCES

[1] Grant, R.H., & Dunleavy, M. J. (2014). Clean intermittent catheterization. In S.M. Porter, P.A. Branowicki, & J.S. Palfrey, J.S. Paul (Eds.), *Supporting students with special health care needs: Guidelines and procedures for schools* (3rd ed., pp. 279-289). H. Brookes Publishing Co., Inc.

[2] Porter, S., Page, D., Engholm, H., & Somppi, C. (2019). Students supported by medical technology. In J. Selekman, R. Shannon, & C. Yonkaitis (Eds.), *School nursing: A comprehensive text* (3rd ed., pp. 731-732). F.A. Davis.

[3] American Academy of Pediatrics/ Healthy Children.org. (2015). *Clean intermittent catheterization*. Retrieved from https://www.healthychildren.org/English/health-issues/conditions/chronic/Pages/Clean-Intermittent-catheterization.aspx

[4] Grant, R.H., & Dunleavy, M. J. (2014). Clean intermittent catheterization. In S.M. Porter, P.A. Branowicki, & J.S. Palfrey, J.S. Paul (Eds.), *Supporting students with special health care needs: Guidelines and procedures for schools* (3rd ed., pp. 279-289). H. Brookes Publishing Co., Inc.

[5] Connecticut State Department of Education. (2019). *Clinical guidelines for Connecticut school nurses: Catheterizations.* Retrieved from https://portal.ct.gov/SDE/Publications/Clinical-Procedure-Guidelines-for-Connecticut-School-Nurses/7-Specialized-Health-Care-Procedures#catheterci

[6] Porter, S., Page, D., Engholm, H., & Somppi, C. (2019). Students supported by medical technology. In J. Selekman, R. Adair Shannon, & C. F. Yonkaitis (Eds.), *School nursing: A comprehensive text* (3rd ed., pp. 731-732). F.A. Davis Company.

DIABETES MONITORING (GLUCOSE AND KETONE TESTING)

DEFINITION/ETIOLOGY:

Blood glucose monitoring measures the amount of glucose (sugar) in a drop of blood utilizing a blood glucose meter. Alternate site testing measures interstitial fluid.

Continuous blood glucose monitoring measures the glucose in the interstitial fluid at very frequent intervals throughout the day using a device (continuous glucose monitor).

Ketone testing (urine) checking the urine for the presence of chemicals (ketones) made by the body when there is not enough insulin and the body must break down fat for energy.

Ketone testing (blood) measuring the amount of ketones in a drop of blood utilizing a specific meter and strips.

PURPOSE:

For students with diabetes measuring the blood glucose during the school day is an essential indicator of whether the student is maintaining an optimal balance of food intake, insulin and activity.[1] Whether done by fingerstick or continuous glucose monitoring (CGM), these readings will help guide insulin dosages and food intake. In addition to the current level, CGM devices indicate whether the blood glucose is rising, dropping or static. Severe low and high blood glucose levels can be a medical emergency and may require prompt treatment **(*Refer to DIABETES EMERGENCIES*).** Self-monitoring of glucose is a necessary skill that all individuals with diabetes must possess.[2]

A student's individualized health care plan (IHP), based on the Diabetes Medical Management Plan (DMMP), will provide standard times for testing, generally before meals and snacks. In addition, testing should be done whenever the student feels that they are low or high, and as needed prior to recess, times of high activity or before leaving school for the day if taking the school bus and/or participating in after school sports. The healthcare provider will also provide goals or target ranges for appropriate blood glucose levels for the student.[3]

In addition to blood glucose monitoring, when the blood glucose is elevated, in accordance with the Emergency Care Plan for Hyperglycemia, the student's urine or blood should be checked for ketones, the chemicals the body makes when there is not enough insulin in the blood and the body must break down fat for energy.[4] Left unchecked, ketones can build up and result in diabetic ketoacidosis (DKA). Research suggests that even a single episode of moderate/severe DKA in very young children with type 1 diabetes can potentially have long-term effects.[5]

DIABETES MONITORING (GLUCOSE AND KETONE TESTING) (continued from previous page)

FINGER STICK BLOOD GLUCOSE MONITORING EQUIPMENT

Blood glucose meter and testing strips
A lancet, automatic lancet or lancet pen
Alcohol swab or pad
Cotton swabs or 2x2 gauze pads
Sharps container

PROCEDURE:
Recommended Steps for Blood Glucose Monitoring[6,7,8,9]

1. Gather supplies.
2. Wash hands with warm soapy water.
3. If the student is NOT able to perform this task independently, the school nurse or trained diabetes personnel should also perform hand hygiene and apply clean gloves.
4. Load device with lancet.
5. Wipe finger or other target area with warm soapy water. Let dry. Use alcohol swabs only if warm water is not available.
    - If the student in unable to perform this task independently, select finger or alternate site to be used for testing and clean with an alcohol swab/pad for 5-10 seconds.
    - Allow finger/alternate site to dry completely.
    - Fingertip/alternate sites should be rotated.
    - *Meters, capable of testing a small volume of blood, can use an alternate site (forearm, thigh, or palm). It must be understood that the readings obtained from the small volume of blood may not be as accurate as readings from blood samples from the fingertips.*
6. Hold lancet device to the side of the fingertip or other area and press button to puncture skin.
7. Gently squeeze the finger or alternate site, as needed, to obtain a first drop of blood.
8. Use gauze pad to wipe away the first drop of blood.
9. Test the second drop of blood. Touch and hold the testing strip to the drop of blood. The test strip will wick the blood sample into the strip. The meter will signal when an adequate blood volume sample has been collected. Do not scrape blood onto the test strip as this may result in an inaccurate test measurement. Refer to the specific meter manufacturer's instructions to assure an adequate blood volume is collected for testing.
10. Record the reading in the student's personal blood glucose log and the student's health record.
11. Dispose of the lancet using proper guidelines for disposal.

Adapted and provided for general information only. Students should follow the instructions of their individual healthcare providers.

DIABETES MONITORING (GLUCOSE AND KETONE TESTING) (continued from previous page)

CONTINUOUS BLOOD GLUCOSE MONITORING

Many students use a CGM, a device that measure blood glucose levels and trends throughout the day. The CGM uses a sensor inserted under the skin to measure interstitial glucose levels at regular intervals (every one to five minutes) and sends the current glucose equivalent wirelessly to a receiver. The receiver may be part of the insulin pump, a separate device or an app on a smartphone. The data may be shared via a WiFi network with multiple recipients including parents. Due to recent improvement in accuracy, some devices have been approved by the FDA for dosing and treatment.[10] The benefits of CGM's include the ability to predict impending hypoglycemia, availability of data on trend patterns for dose adjustments, a decrease in finger sticks and remote monitoring capability.[11] The DMMP should indicate specific action to take for alarms that may alert the student to impending hypoglycemia or hyperglycemia and specific treatment based on trend arrows.[12,13]

Safety Measures for CGM:

- Calibrate per manufacturer's instructions
- Avoid the use of acetaminophen
- Assess when a sensor was inserted (CGM is less accurate the first day)
- Confirm blood glucose with a fingerstick when results are erratic
- Ensure display shows both the glucose level and the directional arrow
- Consider rate of change and lag time if glucose levels are changing quickly
- Assess insulin on board to avoid overdosing
- Determine if symptoms match the glucose level, if not, do a finger stick

KETONE MONITORING

Measuring ketones is very important during hyperglycemia or illness. Ketones should be checked if the blood glucose is greater that 250 or 300 mg/dl or when the student is experiencing nausea, vomiting, abdominal pain, drowsiness, or rapid breathing as directed in the DMMP.
The IHP should include who will perform the ketone testing, when to check for ketones and the actions to be taken when ketones are detected. Both urine and blood can be check for ketones.

URINE KETONE TESTING

URINE KETONE TESTING EQUIPMENT

- Disposable paper or plastic cup
- Urine ketone test strips (Bottles of urine ketone strips expire six months after opening. Date the bottle when opened. Individually foil-wrapped ketone strips expire as per manufacturer date.
- Gloves
- Watch or clock with second hand
- Protected testing area (waterproof plastic pad)

DIABETES MONITORING (GLUCOSE AND KETONE TESTING) (continued from previous page)

URINE KETONE TESTING *(continued)*

PROCEDURE:

1. Gather equipment and supplies.
2. Wash hands and put on gloves.
3. Saturate the test strip with urine by one of the following:
   a. Pupil to hold test strip in urine flow.
   b. Pupil to urinate in cup, then strip is dipped into urine.
4. Wait for test strip to develop per manufacturer's directions on test strip bottle. Count the number of seconds from the time the strip is dipped in the urine until it is read.
5. Compare color of strip to chart on bottle or chart in box. Results will be read as negative, trace, small, moderate, or large.
6. Empty cup and then dispose of cup and ketone test strip in lined wastebasket.
7. Remove and dispose of gloves. Wash hands.
8. Record results per school policy.
9. Refer to student's IHP for management of urine ketone results.

BLOOD KETONE TESTING

BLOOD KETONE TESTING EQUIPMENT

- Ketone meter
- A lancet, automatic lancet or lancet pen
- Alcohol swab or pad
- Testing strips specifically for ketone testing
- Cotton swabs or 2x2 gauze pads
- Sharps container

PROCEDURE:

Recommended Steps for Blood Ketone Monitoring[14]

1. Gather supplies.
2. Wash hands with warm soapy water.
3. If the student is NOT able to perform this task independently, the school nurse or trained diabetes personnel should also perform hand hygiene and apply clean gloves.
4. Load device with lancet.
5. Wipe finger or other target area with warm soapy water. Let dry. Use alcohol swabs only if warm water is not available.
6. Hold lancet device to the side of the fingertip or other area, and press button to puncture skin.
7. Turn finger or area of punctured skin down to get a full drop of blood. If a larger drop is necessary, squeeze the area around the puncture.
8. Put full drop of blood on strip pad.
9. Follow directions for use of monitor.
10. Record results on log sheets provided by parent/guardian or school nurse.

Adapted and provided for general information only. Students should follow the instructions of their individual healthcare providers.

DIABETES MONITORING (GLUCOSE AND KETONE TESTING) *(continued from previous page)*

NURSING CONSIDERATIONS:

- These procedures may be performed by the school nurse or may be delegated to unlicensed personnel (if permitted by state and local regulations) who have been properly trained and are supervised.
- All students with diabetes should have an IHP based on their DMMP to address their needs. This plan may be part of a Section 504 plan.
- Blood glucose self- monitoring should be encouraged for students when developmentally appropriate, allowing them to spend less time out of class. The IHP should include a plan for communication between the student and the school nurse that enables a response to blood glucose levels out of the normal range for that student.
- Blood glucose testing may be done in the health office, in a classroom, or other area of the school. There are significant advantages of checking blood glucose levels any time and any place.[15]
- Schools must adhere to standard precautions to reduce the transmission of blood borne pathogens.
- Fingerstick devices should never be shared. Meters and test strips should not be shared. This is an infection control issue.
- Meters that can test blood samples from alternate site must be able to test small volume blood samples.

REFERENCES

---

[1] Mayo Clinic. (2018). *Blood sugar testing: Why, when and how.* http://www.mayoclinic.org/diseases-conditions/diabetes/in-depth/blood-sugar/art-20046628?pg=1

[2] American Association of Diabetes Educators. (2016). Management of children with diabetes in the school setting (Position Statement). The Diabetes Educator, *34*(3), 439-443. https://www.diabeteseducator.org/docs/default-source/practice/practice-resources/positionstatements/diabetes-in-the-school-setting-position-statement_final.pdf

[3] U.S. Department of Health and Human Services. (2016). *Helping the student with diabetes succeed A guide for school personnel.* https://www.niddk.nih.gov/health-information/communication-programs/ndep/health-professionals/helping-student-diabetes-succeed-guide-school-personnel

[4] Ibid.

[5] Aye, T., Mazaika, P.K., Mauras, N., Marzelli M. J., Hanyang S., Hershey, T., Cato, A., Weinzimer, S.A., White, N.H., Tsalikian,E., Jo, B., Reiss, A.L. for the Diabetes Research in Children Network (DirecNet) Study Group. (2019). Impact of early diabetic ketoacidosis on the developing brain. *Diabetes Care, 42* (3), 443-449. https://doi.org/10.2337/dc18-1405

[6] American Diabetes Association. (2018) *Checking your blood glucose.* http://www.diabetes.org/living-with-diabetes/treatment-and-care/blood-glucose-control/checking-your-blood-glucose.html

[7] Connecticut State Department of Education. (2019). *Clinical guidelines for Connecticut school nurses: Guidelines for self-blood glucose monitoring.* https://portal.ct.gov/SDE/Publications/Blood-Glucose-Self-Monitoring

[8] Ibid.

DIABETES MONITORING (GLUCOSE AND KETONE TESTING) (continued from previous page)

[9] U.S. Food and Drug Administration. (2015). *Blood glucose monitoring devices.* http://www.fda.gov/medicaldevices/productsandmedicalprocedures/InVitroDiagnostics/GlucoseTestingDevices/default.htm

[10] U.S. Food and Drug Administration. (2016, December 20). *FDA expands indication for continuous glucose monitoring system, first to replace fingerstick testing for diabetes treatment decisions.* https://www.fda.gov/news-events/press-announcements/fda-expands-indication-continuous-glucose-monitoring-system-first-replace-fingerstick-testing

[11] Wyckoff, L. (2019). Students with diabetes in J. Selekman, R.A. Shannon, & C. F. Younkaitis (Eds.), *School Nursing: A comprehensive text* (3rd ed., pp. 575-602). F.A.Davis.

[12] Forlenza, G., Argento, N., & Laffel, L. (2017). Practical considerations on the use of continuous glucose monitoring in pediatrics and older adults and non-adjunctive use. *Diabetes Technology & Therapeutics, 19*(Suppl. 3), S13–S20. https://doi.org/10.1089/dia.2017.0034

[13] Wyckoff, L. (2019). Students with diabetes in J. Selekman, R.A. Shannon, & C. F. Younkaitis (Eds.), *School Nursing: A comprehensive text* (3rd ed., pp. 575-602). F.A.Davis.

[14] Connecticut State Department of Education. (2019.) *Guidelines for blood glucose self-monitoring in Connecticut schools.* https://portal.ct.gov/-/media/SDE/School-Nursing/Publications/CSDE_DPH_Diabetes_Guidance_June-_2019.

[15] National Diabetes Education Program. (2016). *Helping the student with diabetes succeed: A guide for school personnel.* https://www.niddk.nih.gov/health-information/communication-programs/ndep/health-professionals/helping-student-diabetes-succeed-guide-school-personnel

ENTERAL TUBE FEEDINGS

DEFINITION/ETIOLOGY:

Enteral Nutrition: Nutrition administered directly in the stomach or small intestine.[1]

Bolus Feedings: The administration of liquid into a feeding tube usually through a syringe using gravity.[2]

Tube Feeding Pump: A mechanical pump that administers a designated amount of liquid over a prescribed amount of time. A tube feeding bag and tubing is also utilized.

Nasogastric Tubes (NGT): Tubes inserted through the nose and into the stomach. They can be inserted and removed for each feeding or can stay in place for a predetermined amount of time. Some tubes can be weighted for additional security for staying in place.[3]

Gastrostomy Tube (GT): The most common type of tube in children and utilized in the school setting. A surgically implanted tube is placed through the stomach wall with one end accessible on the abdomen. The "mic-key" is a common type utilized. It may also be referred to as a "button". The tube remains in place at all times and is capped between feedings to prevent leakage of stomach contents. It stays flush with the abdomen and tubing is connected for feeding or medication administration.[4]

Gastro-jejunostomy Tube (G-JT): Inserted surgically through the stomach wall, it passes through the pylorus and ends in the jejunal segment of the small intestine. They may be double lumened with one lumen that ends in the stomach and the other lumen that ends in the jejunum. These are placed in students who cannot tolerate food or liquid in their stomachs. The lumen in the stomach is often utilized for medication administration.[5]

Jejunostomy Tube (JT): Inserted surgically through the abdominal wall and into the jejunal section of the small intestine.[6] Utilized for students who cannot tolerate food or liquid in their stomachs.

PURPOSE:
To deliver a liquid formula/medication directly to the duodenum, jejunum or stomach. Generally, the purpose of such a feeding method is to provide nutrition to a student who is unable to eat orally or to supplement oral feedings to provide nutrients and calories.

EQUIPMENT:
- Prescribed formula (room temperature)
- Tube feeding bag and tubing (as indicated by order)
- Syringe (generally 30 or 60 cc)
- Feeding pump (as indicated by order)

ENTERAL TUBE FEEDINGS *(continued from previous page)*

PROCEDURE:

Note: All healthcare procedures in the school should have a healthcare provider order outlining the reason/diagnosis, what procedure is to be performed during the school day, and potential adverse reactions.

Nasogastric Tube (NGT)[7]

- Wash hands.
- Prepare feeding. Ensure the NGT is in the stomach. Using a previously measured NGT, check that the position of a black mark on the tube is the same length from the nose for each use. You may also inject 5cc of air into the NGT while listening with a stethoscope over the stomach for the sound of air entering the stomach. Check with the healthcare provider's orders to ascertain if this is necessary.
- Don gloves.
- Position student (to prevent aspiration):
  - On right side with head elevated minimum of 30 degrees, OR
  - Lying on back with head elevated 45 degrees OR
  - In a sitting position.

  > The student should remain in an elevated or upright position for 30 minutes after the feeding (avoid lying flat).

- Check for residuals, if ordered. Slowly withdraw the gastric juice, formula or medication from the stomach with a syringe, assess, return the fluid and document. Follow healthcare provider's orders as to parameters and guidance regarding residual amount and when to hold feedings.
- Attach syringe and administer the feeding via gravity or feeding pump as ordered. If performing a bolus feeding, hold the syringe 4-6 inches above abdomen or per orders. Raising or lowering the height of the syringe will help control the rate of intake.
- When feeding is complete, detach the syringe and flush with water utilizing a syringe.
- Disconnect and cap the tube.
- Wash syringe and other reusable equipment with soapy water and store in a clean area.
- Document.

ENTERAL TUBE FEEDINGS *(continued from previous page)*

PROCEDURE *(continued)*

Gastrostomy and Jujenal (GJ) Tube Feeding[8]

- Wash hands.
- Prepare feeding.
- Don gloves.
- Ensure tube placement is appropriate. Mic-key tubes should be parallel with the skin and not leaking. They should be able to rotate 360 degrees.
- Fill the extension tubing with water or formula, clamp and attach to the mic-key button by connecting and locking it into place by positioning the mark, rotate clockwise and feel the "click". If using a pump, prime the pump before connecting tubing to G-JT and attaching to the mic-key.
- Insert the syringe into the open end of the extension set.
- Pour the feeding into the syringe until it is half-full. Unclamp the extension set to begin feeding. Hold the tip to the syringe no higher than the child's shoulders. If the food is not flowing, squeeze the tube in downward strokes to bring the food down.
- When feeding is complete, flush with water. Pinch the tubing and detach the syringe. Cap and disconnect tubing.
- Wash syringe and other reusable equipment with soapy water and store in a clean area.
- Document.

Medication Administration[9]

- Wash hands and don gloves.
- Prepare the medication as prescribed.
- The medicine should be liquid, or finely crushed and dissolved in water, so that the tube does not get blocked.
- Medication is more effective if given before feeding. Medication should never be mixed in the formula. Always flush before and after giving medication to make sure all medication goes in the stomach and is not left in the feeding tube.
- If more than one medication is to be given, give separately and flush between medications. Never mix medications together in one syringe.
- Clamp or pinch off the tube prior to opening to air to avoid reflux of gastric secretions.
- Attach syringe and administer medications by unclamping the tube.
- Flush after feeding is complete.

ENTERAL TUBE FEEDINGS *(continued from previous page)*

NURSING CONSIDERATIONS:

If the student begins to cough, choke or have a color change, stop the feeding and re-check tube placement. Perform a respiratory assessment including respiratory status and color. Aspirating for stomach contents is a good way to ascertain tube placement.

- A registered nurse (RN) or a licensed practical nurse/licensed vocational nurse (LPN/LVN) generally initiates tube feedings. School nurses should check with their individual state nurse practice act and any delegation laws/rulings regarding whether GT feedings can be delegated to an unlicensed staff member. If so, competency-based training should be done with the appropriate level of supervision including protocols as to when to contact the RN or LPN/LVN.
- Tube feedings in school require a healthcare provider's order or treatment authorization which would include the type of formula, infusion type, rate and frequency, as well as flushing instructions.
- Consider securing the GT/NGT for young or special needs students. Secure by placing a piece of tape around the tube and pinning to clothing or putting the tube under the student's clothing.
- Administer a bolus feeding over 15-30 minutes unless otherwise specified. A slow drip feeding is delivered continuously over a set number of hours.
- Assess the insertion site for skin integrity with each use, as rashes tend to occur with leaking around the stoma site. A barrier ointment or use of a dry dressing may be utilized.
- Aspiration of feeding into the lungs is a risk with enteral feedings. Ensuring and securing proper placement of the tubing is essential.
- If there is any nausea, vomiting or cramping the feeding rate may need to be slowed or the formula may be too cold.
- A healthcare provider's order may include venting the GT (open the cap to air). This procedure allows the release of air and makes the student comfortable.
- Open formula should be labeled with the student's name and date and may be stored in the refrigerator for 24 hours and then discarded.
- If a mic-key button dislodges, nurses should be trained in insertion of a new tube. Keep an additional mic-key at school. Insertion involves filling an internal balloon with 5cc of water for securing the tube to the side of the stoma.
- Before attempting to dislodge a blockage try rolling the tube between fingers in a milking motion towards the site of insertion. If unsuccessful in removing the blockage, warm water seems to work best. Fill a syringe with warm water and try to slightly move the plunger slightly back and forth. If the blockage remains, contact the parent.

ENTERAL TUBE FEEDINGS *(continued from previous page)*

NURSING CONSIDERATIONS *(continued)*

- If the student does not receive any food by mouth, consider oral stimulation with a toothette or similar option during the feeding.
- Students with tube feedings can be fed anywhere and as long as the setting is appropriate to the student's desire for privacy or the desire to be with their peers. The cafeteria can be used or if the student prefers, the health room. If frequent feedings are needed the student may be fed in the classroom.
- Students with tube feedings should have an Individualized Healthcare Plan (IHP) tailored to the individual student's needs.
- Depending on the age and capabilities of the student, have him or her assist with the feeding by holding the syringe or pouring fluid into it.

REFERENCES

[1] Mayo Clinic. (2018). *Home enteral nutrition*. https://www.mayoclinic.org/tests-procedures/home-enteral-nutrition/about/pac-20384955

[2] Memorial Sloan Kettering Cancer Center. (2017). *Tube feeding using the bolus method*. https://www.mskcc.org/cancer-care/patient-education/tube-feeding-using-bolus-method

[3] [3] Mayo Clinic. (2018). *Home enteral nutrition*. https://www.mayoclinic.org/tests-procedures/home-enteral-nutrition/about/pac-20384955

[4] Ibid.

[5] Cardiovascular and Interventional radiologist Society of Europe. (n.d.). *Gastrojunostomy.* https://www.cirse.org/patients/ir-procedures/gastrojejunostomy/

[6] Medline Plus. (2018). *Jejunostomy feeding tube*. https://medlineplus.gov/ency/patientinstructions/000181.htm

[7] Children's Minnesota (2019). Nasogastric tube feeding. https://www.childrensmn.org/educationmaterials/childrensmn/article/15553/nasogastric-tube-feeding/

[8] Medline. (2018). *Gastrostomy feeding tubes.* https://medlineplus.gov/ency/patientinstructions/000165.htm

[9] Connecticut State Department of Education. (2019). *Clinical procedure guidelines for Connecticut school nurses.* https://portal.ct.gov/SDE/Publications/Clinical-Procedure-Guidelines-for-Connecticut-School-Nurses/Introduction

OTHER REFERENCES CONSULTED

Avanos (2018). Mic-key GJ Feeding tube quick start guide. https://www.mic-key.com/patient-resources/patientdischargeguides/

MEDICATION ADMINISTRATION

DEFINITION/ETIOLOGY:

Medication administration is an important component of the role of the school nurse. Schools will need to fulfill their legal obligation to provide health related services to all children, which may include medication administration. Under section 504 of the Rehabilitation Act and the Individuals with Education Improvement Act 2004, all children with health care needs will be provided these services.[1] Needed medications may stabilize a chronic condition or improve a student's overall health therefore improving school attendance and educational outcome. The school nurse is critical to the safe and effective administration of medications.

In addition to properly and safely administering medications themselves, school nurses as the health leader in the school should be involved in developing evidenced-based policies and procedures that help to decrease errors and ensure safety. When allowed by state law, training and supervision of unlicensed assistive personnel (UAP) in the proper techniques for medication administration when the school nurse is unavailable is also an essential component of the role.

PROCEDURE (General):
Prior to administering any medication by any route, the six rights of medication administration should be followed. This includes the following:[2]

- Right medication
- Right dose
- Right student
- Right route
- Right time
- Right documentation

In addition, a medication authorization signed by the prescribing provider and parent/guardian should be reviewed. A complete medical order includes the student's name, the date and time of the order, the name of the medication, the ordered dosage and form of the medication, the route of administration, the time and frequency of the medication and signature of the authorized healthcare provider. The medication order should be reviewed prior to administration. In some states the use of a standing order may be allowed for certain medications, usually including over the counter medications and emergency medications.

After administration of any medication, the administrations should be documented utilizing a consistent and accurate method. District policies and procedures should be developed and utilized to guide all aspects of medication administration.

MEDICATION ADMINISTRATION *(continued from previous page)*

PROCEDURE (General) *(continued)*

Oral Medication Administration[3]

DEFINITION	EQUIPMENT	PROCEDURE
Placing medication in a student's mouth to be swallowed	• A precise measuring device for a liquid medication such as a dose marked medication syringe or cup • A crushing or cutting device such as a pill cutter or mortar and pestle for crushing • A food substance for mixing such as applesauce if indicated **Note that not all medications are meant to be crushed due to the coating. School nurses should read instructions carefully or check with pharmacist or manufacturer prior to crushing or mixing.**	1. Give the student the oral medication. 2. Stay with the student until you can assure the medication was swallowed.

Injectables: Intramuscular, Subcutaneous [4]

DEFINITION	EQUIPMENT	PROCEDURE [5]
Injecting a medication into a muscle or subcutaneous tissue directly below the dermis and epidermis	• Sterile needle (appropriate size) • Syringe or autoinjector • Gloves • Alcohol swab	**(Subcutaneous)** 1. Select the site (generally the abdomen, upper arms or front of the thighs). 2. Don gloves. 3. Clean the injection site with an alcohol swab in an outward, 2-inch circular pattern. 4. Gently pinch the site so 1 inch of fat appears. 5. Position the needle at a 45-degree angle with the bevel up and insert. 6. Release the skin pinch. 7. Pull the plunger back to check for blood. If blood fills the plunger withdraw and start again. 8. Slowly inject the medication. 9. Withdraw and wipe with an alcohol swab. 10. Dispose of syringe in an appropriate sharps container.
		(Intramuscular) 1. Select the site (generally the gluteus maximus, the deltoid muscle, the vastus lateralis, the rectus femoris and the ventrogluteal muscle). 2. Don gloves. 3. Clean the injection site with an alcohol swab in an outward, 2-inch circular pattern. 4. Position the needle at a 90-degree angle with the bevel up and insert. 5. Pull the plunger back to check for blood. If blood fills the plunger withdraw and start again. 6. Slowly inject the medication. 7. Withdraw and wipe with an alcohol swab. 8. Dispose of the syringe in an appropriate sharps container.

MEDICATION ADMINISTRATION *(continued from previous page)*

PROCEDURE (General) *(continued)*

Intravenous Medication Therapy [6]

DEFINITION	EQUIPMENT	PROCEDURE
Administration of prescribed medication via an intravenous route using a pump infusion method * Not a common method of medication administration in the school setting*	• Gloves • IV pole • Alcohol wipes • IV setup (disposable) • Infusion pump	1. Don gloves. 2. Hang the secondary IV set. 3. Clean the port with alcohol wipe. 4. Expel all air from the tubing by flushing the fluid through. 5. Follow orders for flow rate. 6. When finished, disconnect bag and discard appropriately.

Buccal and Sublingual Medication Administration[7]

DEFINITION	EQUIPMENT	PROCEDURE [8]
Administration of the medication between the gum and cheek or under the tongue where it dissolves and is absorbed in the blood stream	• Gloves	1. Don gloves. 2. Place the medications between the gum and the inner lining of the cheek for buccal administration and below the tongue for sublingual. 3. Allow the medication to dissolve. 4. Educate the student to avoid swallowing while the medication is being dissolved and to avoid drinking for at least 15 minutes after administration.

Transdermal Medication Administration[9]

DEFINITION	EQUIPMENT	PROCEDURE[10]
Medication administration through a skin patch which delivers the medication through the skin and into the bloodstream	• Gloves • Soap and water	1. Don gloves. 2. Remove the old patch if there is one. 3. Cleanse site to remove any remaining medication left on skin. 4. Measure the ordered dose on the patch if needed. Avoid having the medication touch your own skin. 5. Apply the medication/patch on the skin and lightly spread it out. 6. Do not rub the medication into the skin 7. Secure as needed.

MEDICATION ADMINISTRATION *(continued from previous page)*

PROCEDURE (General) *(continued)*

Ophthalmic Medication Administration

DEFINITION	EQUIPMENT	PROCEDURE [11]
Medication administered in the eye	• Gloves	1. Don gloves. 2. Position the student in a sitting position. 3. Have the student tilt their head back towards the eye getting the drops or ointment. 4. Have the student look up and away. 5. Rest your hand on the forehead to steady it. 6. To administer drops, pull down the lower lid and instill the ordered number of drops into the conjunctival space. 7. To administer an ointment, pull down the lower lid and squeeze the ointment into the conjunctival space. 8. Do not allow the tip of tube to touch the eye.

Rectal Medication Administration

DEFINITION	EQUIPMENT	PROCEDURE [12]
Medication administered through the rectum	• Gloves • Drape or cover	1. Position the student on the left side with the top leg flexed. 2. Don gloves. 3. Cover the student with a drape or blanket to expose only the buttocks. 4. Lift the upper buttocks with the non-dominant hand and insert the medication into the rectal sphincter (have the student take deep breaths to help relax the sphincter).

Intranasal Administration

DEFINITION	EQUIPMENT	PROCEDURE [13]
Medication administered through the nasal cavity	• Gloves • I cc luer lock syringe • Facial tissue	1. Don gloves. 2. Position the student with the head back 3. Put the tip of the device in the nostril pointing up and outward. 4. Briskly compress the plunger or device delivering medication to the nostrils based on directions or prescriber's order.

MEDICATION ADMINISTRATION *(continued from previous page)*

NURSING CONSIDERATIONS:

- All incomplete, illegible or questionable medication orders should be clarified using critical thinking and professional judgement.
- Medication administration should be part of the student's Individualized Healthcare Plan (IHP) or Emergency Care Plan (ECP).
- The decision to delegate medication administration is a nursing judgement that carefully considers state laws, state nurse practice act, district policy and benefits and risks to students.
- Student confidentiality should be addressed in all medication administration.
- Medication should not be pre-poured or prepared for someone else to administer.
- The temperature for all refrigerators storing medications should be monitored.
- All medications, except emergency rescue medication should be in a locked cabinet or locked drawer.
- Emergency rescue medication should be locked/stored securely at the end of the school day to prevent theft.
- A system of tracking medication should be utilized.
- Control substances should be counted when received, each time given, and at least weekly with 2 persons.
- Medications should be delivered to the school by a responsible adult in original containers and properly labeled.
- During medication administration students should be educated on the goal of the medication and other important components of the medical condition with the overall goal of increasing knowledge and independence.
- The first dose of any medication should be given at home.
- All medications should be given within 30 minutes of the prescribed time.

REFERENCES

---

[1] Halbert, L., Yonkaitis, C. (2019). Federal laws protecting students with disabilities. In J. Selekman, R. Adair Shannon, & **C.** F. Yonkaitis (Eds.), *School nursing: A comprehensive text* (3rd ed., pp. 156-159). F.A. Davis.

[2] Oregon Department of Human Services. (2013). The six rights of medication administration. https://www.oregon.gov/DHS/PROVIDERS-PARTNERS/LICENSING/SafeMedDocs/poster-1.pdf

[3] Ibid.

[4] Ibid.

[5] Registered Nursing.org. (n.d.). *Medication administration: NCLEX-RN*. https://www.registerednursing.org/nclex/medication-administration/

MEDICATION ADMINISTRATION *(continued from previous page)*

[6] Connecticut State Department of Education (2019). *Clinical procedure guidelines for Connecticut school nurses.* Retrieved from: https://portal.ct.gov/SDE/Publications/Clinical-Procedure-Guidelines-for-Connecticut-School-Nurses/Introduction

[7] Healthline. (2019). *When sublingual and buccal medications are given.* Retrieved from: https://www.healthline.com/health/sublingual-and-buccal-medication-administration#advantages

[8] Khan, A., Kinsley. T., & Preeta, C., (2017). *Sublingual tablets and the benefits of administration.* http://journalofpharmaceuticalresearch.org/index.php/kpc/article/viewFile/118766/81984

[9] Lippincott Nursing Center. (2019). *Do's and don't's applying a transdermal patch.* https://www.nursingcenter.com/journalarticle?Article_ID=789127&Journal_ID=54016&Issue_ID=789113

[10] Registered Nursing.org. (n.d.). *Medication administration: NCLEX-RN.* https://www.registerednursing.org/nclex/medication-administration/

[11] Ibid.

[12] Khan, A., Kinsley. T., & Preeta, C., (2017). *Sublingual tablets and the benefits of administration.* http://journalofpharmaceuticalresearch.org/index.php/kpc/article/viewFile/118766/81984

[13] Evidenced Informed Practice Tools. (2015). *Intranasal medication administration.* http://www.wrha.mb.ca/extranet/eipt/files/EIPT-055.pdf

TRACHEOSTOMY CARE (Tracheostomy Suctioning and Tracheostomy Tube Change)

DEFINITION/ETIOLOGY:

A tracheostomy is a surgical opening in the neck into the trachea. It is often referred to as a "trach". The opening is called a stoma and a tracheostomy tube is inserted into the stoma. The trach allows breathing and removal of secretions by suctioning or coughing. The trach tubes are primarily made of specialized plastic and come in a variety of brands and sizes. Tracheostomies may be temporary or long term. Common indications for tracheostomies include:[1]

- chronic lung disease (CLD)/bronchopulmonary dysplasia (BPD), which can be a sequela of severe prematurity
- central hypoventilation syndrome
- chronic pulmonary diseases
- congenital anomalies
- degenerative neuromuscular diseases, such as Muscular Dystrophy
- spinal cord injuries

Many children with tracheostomies also require support from a ventilator, either all of the time or for parts of the day. There must always be a trained person with the student who can identify an emergency, suction a tracheostomy and replace a tracheostomy tube that is blocked with secretions or has fallen out. There should be persons capable and certified in cardiopulmonary resuscitation (CPR) available including a registered nurse to assess for breathing difficulty.[2] Accidental deaths in patients with tracheostomies account for 27.5% of deaths. The primary causes of these preventable deaths are inadequate training, improper response to emergencies, and lack of vigilance by care givers. Mechanical ventilation is a high-stake, high risk intervention.[3]

PURPOSE:

The primary goal of tracheostomy care is airway maintenance. It will allow long-term access to a ventilator and provides access to clear the trachea of secretions. Tracheostomy tube change is not a routine procedure in the health office but may be needed if the tube is blocked with secretions and is impeding respiration or has fallen out.

EQUIPMENT:[4]

It is recommended that all supplies be stored together in an "emergency travel bag" or "go bag" that is easily transported with the student during transportation and throughout the school day.

Tracheostomy Change

- Extra trach tube, with obturator placed inside
- Additional extra trach tube, one size smaller than normal, with obturator placed inside
- Clean trach ties
- Blunt Scissors
- Water-soluble jelly or lubricant (never use an oil-based lubricant, such as Vaseline®)
- Suction equipment with correct size catheters
- Ambu bag and mask
- Oxygen (if part of student's individualized healthcare plan)
- Gloves

TRACHEOSTOMY CARE *(continued from the previous page)*

Tracheostomy Change *(continued)*
- Trach dressing
- DuLee mucus trap
- Bulb syringe

Tracheostomy Suctioning
- Tracheostomy suctioning machine
- Suction catheter of prescribed size
- Disposable clean gloves
- Ambu bag and mask
- Tracheostomy adapter and mask
- Saline ampules

MANAGEMENT/TREATMENT:[5]

The school nurse should develop an Individualized Healthcare Plan (IHP) outlining the procedure, along with emergency interventions based on healthcare provider orders.
NOTE: All procedures in the school setting should have a prescriber's order annually.

I. **RESPIRATORY ASSESSMENT. Tracheostomy may need to be suctioned if the school nurse or health paraprofessional observes the following after checking the placement of trach tube:**
   - Increased respiratory rate
   - Trouble breathing
   - Noisy respirations
   - Visible mucus
   - Restlessness
   - "Wet" sounding breathing
   - Color change, particularly blue or pale around the mucous membranes and nail beds
   - Increased heart rate
   - Skin feels moist or "clammy" to the touch
   - Eyes watering
   - Flushed face
   - Difficulty with oral feeding

II. **SUCTIONING:[6]**
   - Clean technique is recommended for home and school.
   - Suctioning should be done in a clean, private area.
   - Shallow suctioning: this method is used when mucus is visible at the opening of the trach. This may occur after the child coughs. A Yankauer catheter or even a bulb syringe may be used to remove the mucus.

TRACHEOSTOMY CARE *(continued from the previous page)*

SUCTIONING *(continued)*

- Premeasured depth suctioning: Measure the length of the trach tube and add ¼ inch. Make a note of this on the child's IHP. When suctioning, only advance the catheter as far as the premeasured length. It is beneficial to use pre-marked suction catheters when available.
- Deep suctioning: The catheter is advanced beyond the tip of the tracheal tube until resistance is felt. After resistance is felt, pull back slightly before applying suction. This procedure usually is not needed in the school setting and requires specific orders from the licensed healthcare provider. If deep suctioning necessary, it should be performed by a licensed nurse.
- Depending on the student's age, he or she may be able to request suctioning when needed or assist with the procedure.[7]
- Suctioning should last no more than five to 10 seconds to prevent hypoxia. The routine use of normal saline into the tracheostomy tube before suctioning is NOT supported by research and is not recommended unless specifically ordered.

TRACHEOSTOMY SUCTIONING PROCEDURE[8]

1. Wash hands.
2. Glove.
3. Set up equipment.
4. Position student as is recommended. Most students are suctioned while seated.
5. Explain the procedure to the student using developmentally appropriate language.
6. Encourage the student to cough to loosen secretions.
7. If ordered, insert several drops of saline into the tracheostomy and use the Ambu bag to disperse the saline.
8. Turn on the suction machine. Check the suction by dipping the tip of catheter into a cup of normal saline or water.
9. Advance the catheter to pre-measured length into the trach tube.
10. Cover the air vent with your thumb to apply suction, gently twirl the catheter as you withdraw the catheter from the trach tube. This should take 5 seconds or less.
11. Allow the student to rest for approximately 30 seconds between suctioning.
12. After each suction pass, rinse the tip and inside of the catheter using normal saline or water.
13. Notify the parent/guardian if:
    - increased need for suctioning
    - a color change in the mucus, such as green or yellow
    - bleeding from the tracheostomy

Note: If oral suctioning is also required, the oral cavity may be suctioned with the trach catheter; but a catheter used in the oral cavity cannot be used to suction the trach.

TRACHEOSTOMY CARE *(continued from previous page)*

III. TRACHEOSTOMY TUBE CHANGE:

- Indications for trach change or replacement should be written into the IHP. Note trach tube type and size in IHP.
- Maintain a "go bag" containing emergency supplies for trach change. This bag should travel with the student and must be checked daily upon arrival at school.
- A checklist should be developed and utilized for documentation of "go bag" supplies.
- Activate the Emergency Medical Services (EMS) for any situations that are emergent based on clinical assessment findings and the student's medical history.
- Always notify the parent/guardian and the healthcare provider when a student requires a tracheostomy tube change.[9]
- If student experiences frequent plugging of tracheostomy tube, cough assist device may be considered a preventative intervention

TRACHEOSTOMY TUBE CHANGE PROCEDURE[10]

1. Wash hands.
2. Assemble equipment.
3. Glove.
4. Explain the procedure to the student utilizing appropriate developmental language.
5. Position the child. Small children may be positioned on their backs with a blanket under their shoulders.
6. Open tracheostomy tube package and insert obturator.
7. Attach holders to tube (some students may have Velcro® or fabric ties).
8. Lubricate the end of the tracheostomy tube with water-soluble lubricant or sterile saline.
9. Suction nose and mouth if needed.
10. Give two to four breaths with the Ambu bag as needed.
11. Have a second person hold the tracheostomy tube in place while removing the ties.
12. With the new tube in hand, have the second person remove the tube.
13. Insert the new tube at a right angle rotating it downward.
14. Immediately remove the obturator.
15. Observe the student for signs of respiratory distress.
16. Secure the tracheostomy tube holder.
17. Assess breath sounds and chest movement.

TRACHEOSTOMY CARE *(continued from the previous page)*

NURSING CONSIDERATIONS:

- Assessment of the stoma site:[11]
    - Assessment of the site may be done during routine tracheostomy care.
    - Incorporate the type of care recommended by the provider (i.e. cleaning with soap and water vs. half-strength hydrogen peroxide) into the school health plan.
    - The area around the stoma should be kept clean and dry. Many students use a trach dressing and the dressing should be changed when it becomes moist.
    - Notify parent/guardian if there is an increased need for dressing changes secondary to increased drainage, redness or "crusting" at the stoma site, or any type of skin breakdown, including signs of infection.
- Emergency "go bag" should always be kept with the student (during recess, field trips, school bus rides). This bag should be checked at the start of each day to ensure all appropriate supplies are present.
- The tracheostomy holders and ties should be loose enough to slip one finger between the tracheostomy tube holder and the neck.
- A small amount of bleeding may occur around the stoma, if persistent or unusual notify parent/guardian.
- Document tracheostomy tube insert, ties secure, respiratory status, assessment of stoma site, and any airway maintenance interventions (suctioning, trach tube).

REFERENCES

---

[1] Selekman, J., Bochenek, J., & Lukens, M. (2013). Children with chronic conditions. In J. Selekman (Ed.), *School nursing: A comprehensive text* 2nd ed., pp. 700-783. F.A. Davis.

[2] Ibid.

[3] Thrasher, J., Baker, J., Ventre, K., Martin, S., Dawson, J., Cox, R., Moore, H., Brethouer, S., Sables-Baus, Baker, C. (2018). Hospital to Home: A Quality Improvement Initiative to Implement High-fidelity Simulation Training for Caregivers of Children Requiring Long-term Mechanical Ventilation. *Journal of Pediatric Nursing: Nursing Care of Children and Families*, 38, 114 – 121.

[4] American Academy of Pediatrics. (2019). Tracheostomy. In Donoghue, E.A., & Kraft, C.A. (Eds.), *Managing chronic health needs in child care and schools (2nd ed.,* pp. 193-194). American Academy of Pediatrics.

[5] Porter, S.M., Page, D., Engholm, H., & Somppi, C. (2019). Students supported by medical technology. In J. Selekman, R. Adair Shannon, & C. F. Yonkaitis (Eds.), *School nursing: A comprehensive text* (3rd ed., pp. 732-736). F.A. Davis.

[6] Selekman, J., Bochenek, J., & Lukens, M. (2013). Children with chronic conditions. In J. Selekman (Ed.), *School nursing: A comprehensive text* (2nd ed., pp. 700-783). F.A. Davis.

[7] American Academy of Pediatrics. (2019). Tracheostomy. In Donoghue, E.A., & Kraft, C.A. (Eds.), *Managing chronic health needs in child care and schools (2nd ed.,* pp. 193-194). American Academy of Pediatrics.

[8] Selekman, J., Bochenek, J., & Lukens, M. (2013). Children with chronic conditions. In J. Selekman (Ed.), *School nursing: A comprehensive text* (2nd ed., pp. 700-783). F.A. Davis.

[9] Connecticut State Department of Education. (2019). *Clinical guidelines for Connecticut school nurses: Tracheostomy care and suctioning*. http://www.sde.ct.gov/sde/cwp/view.asp?a=2663&q=334188

[10] American Academy of Pediatrics. (2019). Tracheostomy. In Donoghue, E.A., & Kraft, C.A. (Eds.), *Managing chronic health needs in child care and schools (2nd ed.,* pp. 193-194). American Academy of Pediatrics.

[11] Ibid.

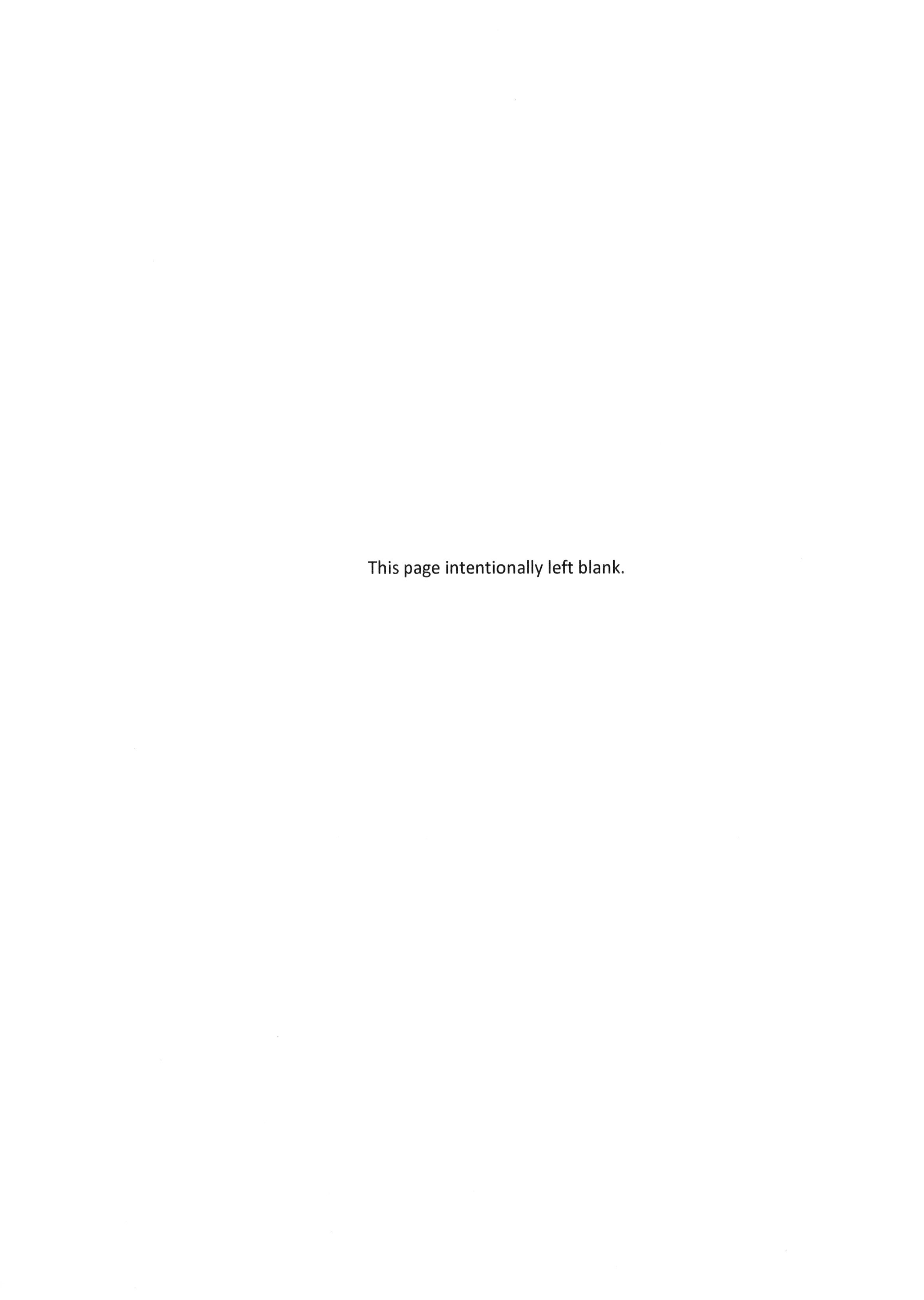

This page intentionally left blank.

SECTION III

SCHOOL NURSE MANAGEMENT

DISASTER PREPAREDNESS

OVERVIEW/DEFINITION:[1]
Disaster preparedness is the ongoing and continuous cycle of planning, preparing, training and evaluating in order to effectively respond to any disaster or emergency within the school or community. Disasters in the school setting can be the result of natural disasters, such as a hurricane, blizzard, flood or tornado, or human-generated disasters, such as accidents, school shootings, hazardous explosions, or fire. Disasters and emergencies can involve individual students, staff and visitors or large numbers of persons within the school community. By definition, a disaster is any event that causes human suffering and requires resources beyond the normal amount and outside assistance to recover.

ANTICIPATED CONCERNS/PROBLEMS:
- Physical Injuries – immediate and long-term
- Psychological Conditions – immediate and long-term
- Socioeconomic shifts – loss of resources, employment, homes, food and water sources

MANAGEMENT/POTENTIAL INTERVENTIONS:[2,3]
Planning: the purpose of planning is to prevent and mitigate problems resulting from any disaster. The creation of a school or district-wide disaster plan, based on input from all stakeholders (i.e., school officials, agencies involved in emergency responses as well as community members), is essential to effective preparation and response. The school nurse has a critical role in planning and responding to disasters and as such is an essential member of the planning and response team.[4]

The key elements of a disaster plan are:
- Establish lines of authority during the event.
- Establish communication methods both internally and externally.
- Determine where or how resources and equipment needed will be obtained based on student/staff needs and existing building resources.
- Identify access to human resources that may be needed during or after a disaster.
- Identify of roles and responsibilities of team members (by title and not person to avoid changing the plan when persons leave or change positions within the organization).
- Establish transportation patterns to evacuate or control access and gridlock at the site
- Determine documentation procedures and how records will be managed (health and resources).
- Designate evacuation routes (within the building and away from the site).
- Plan for evacuation of students with special needs (in wheelchairs, visually or hearing impaired, developmental or emotional disabilities, etc.).
- Establish search and rescue plans with local emergency responders.
- Plan for provision of acute care including collection site, triage plans, and roles of healthcare providers and laypersons.
- Consider shelter management in the event that the staff and students remain on site for more than a few hours (e.g., food, water, medications, etc.).

DISASTER PREPAREDNESS *(continued from previous page)*

Planning *(continued)*

- Establish a secure and confidential file that contains staff's health information that is generated upon hire and updated annually.
- Determine any special considerations needed for any children or staff with special healthcare needs or chronic conditions.
- Establish debriefing plans during the recovery phase.
- Evaluate the plan routinely through disaster drills and review of response in any actual events.

Note: Disaster plans should be based on routine procedures whenever possible to avoid confusion (e.g., evacuation of the building may be designed in a way that is similar to evacuations during fires so the route is familiar to staff and students).

Preparedness requires conducting regular disaster drills based on the school disaster plan, evaluating the outcomes of the drill or an actual event, reviewing and revising the plan using information gathered during the drill or an actual event, training of school personnel for specific responsibilities (e.g., triage training for the school nurse or media training for the designated spokesperson), and a review of the current evidence on effective disaster management.

Response requires an immediate and organized approach to the disaster based on the established disaster plan. The school nurse may be involved in the acute management of victims including assessment of the situation, triage, establishing the collection area for victims if they can be moved, administering first aid and nursing care, directing others to assist in the management of care, determining resources and equipment needed, establishing and providing psychological care and counseling to indirect victims, such as witnesses to the event, family members, and community members. During the event, the school nurse may also need to respond to or delegate any routine health care needs of the students.

Recovery is the process of returning to optimal functioning after an event. It is suggested that even for the most well-prepared person, the results of a disaster can be devastating and have long-term effects. How individuals and communities affected by the disaster recover are impacted by many factors: duration of the event, degree of injury, witnessing graphic scenes, disruption of social and economic structures within the community, and the characteristics of the group (s) impacted. The school nurse along with mental health professionals will need to address the psychological needs of the community and intervene to assist the transition back to pre-disaster functioning. The school nurse may also be involved in managing any new acute or chronic physical health needs as a result of the disaster.

DISASTER PREPAREDNESS *(continued from previous page)*

FOLLOW-UP:
As noted in the preparedness phase of disaster response, reviewing and revising the disaster plan is an important follow-up to any actual disaster. Debriefing is key to helping the first responders and disaster team members recover from the event too.[5] Recognizing event and occupational stressors is a necessary step for nurses to identify what care and assistance they may need to recover. It is also important for the nurse to assist in the mitigation review process in an effort to indicate how the incident occurred and what measures might be taken to minimize any problems that occurred while responding to the incident.

NOTES: Disaster preparedness is not a one-time activity; being prepared requires ongoing assessment and collaboration regarding student and faculty needs, resources, staffing, equipment and clear lines of communication with the community- wide response team.

Children affected by disasters do not have the same coping skills as adults and may need additional support and intervention. Common concerns in children following a disaster are new fears, phobias, sleep disturbances, fear of being alone, increased dependency, hypersensitivity to noise and weather, and developmental regressions.[6]

RESOURCES
Caring for Children in Disasters. http://www.cdc.gov/childrenindisasters/schools.html

Centers for Disease Control and Prevention. (2018). Emergency preparedness. http://emergency.cdc.gov/index.asp

REFERENCES

[1] Stanhope, M., & Lancaster, J. (2018). *Foundations of nursing in the community* (5th ed.). Elsevier/Mosby.

[2] The Center for Health and Health Care in Schools. (2016). Emergency preparedness: A quick guide for school staff. http://healthinschools.org/issue-areas/other-school-health-issues/school-health-issues/emergency-preparedness/emergency-preparedness-a-quick-guide-for-school-staff/#sthash.E16q56K8.dpbs

[3] U.S. Department of Education. (2016). Practical Information on Crisis Planning Brochure Practical Information on Crisis Planning Brochure. https://www2.ed.gov/admins/lead/safety/crisisplanning.html

[4] National Association of School Nurses. (2019). *Emergency preparedness* (Position Statement). https://www.nasn.org/advocacy/professional-practice-documents/position-statements/ps-emergency-preparedness

[5] Centers for Disease Control and Prevention. (2018). *Response resources for leaders* https://emergency.cdc.gov/coping/leaders.asp

[6] Centers for Disease Control and Prevention. (2019). *Before, during and after an emergency.* https://www.cdc.gov/childrenindisasters/before-during-after.html

DISASTER PREPAREDNESS *(continued from previous page)*

OTHER REFERENCES CONSULTED

American Academy of Pediatrics. (2019). *Children and disasters: Disaster preparedness to meet children's needs.* https://www.aap.org/en-us/advocacy-and-policy/aap-health-initiatives/Children-and-Disasters/Pages/default.aspx

Emergency and Safety Alliance. (2019). *School emergency response plan and management guide.* https://esa.dc.gov/sites/default/files/dc/sites/esa/publication/attachments/school_emergency_response_plan-1-5-10.pdf

Centers for Disease Control and Prevention. (2019). *Helping children cope with emergencies.* https://www.cdc.gov/childrenindisasters/helping_children_cope.html

DO NOT ATTEMPT RESUSCITATION (DNAR)

OVERVIEW/DEFINITION:

Due to medical advances along with federal laws such as Individuals with Disabilities Education Improvement Act, an increased number of children with life-threatening, complex and chronic medical conditions attend school.[1] Chronic conditions include terminal and irreversible illnesses, congenital diseases and anomalies, malignancies and injuries. There are developmental, psychosocial, and emotional benefits for the child to continue to attend school. School attendance maintains a sense of community and normalcy for the student and family.

Parents/guardians, in collaboration with schools and healthcare providers, make difficult end of life decisions about steps to be taken in the event that respiratory/cardiac arrest occurs at school. Schools may receive *Do Not Attempt Resuscitation* (DNAR) orders from the healthcare provider and parents/guardians requesting that life support procedures be withheld in the event respirations and heartbeat have ceased and that the student be allowed to die without emergency intervention. This also may be referred to as *Do Not Resuscitate* (DNR), *Allow Natural Death* (AND) or Medical or Physician Orders for Life Sustaining Treatment (MOLST) that offer a broad Palliative or Comfort Care. It is important to note that a DNAR order is not an order to stand by and not intervene, but rather to provide supportive and comfort measures that are integrated into the plan of care. Spiritual and emotional needs also should be addressed in the plan.[2]

ANTICIPATED CONCERNS/PROBLEMS:

- Schools face difficult decisions in the presence of DNAR directives that are framed by medical, emotional, legal, and ethical issues for the educational setting. These directives reflect the need of school districts to have local, school-based policies and guidelines.
- Acceptance of the DNAR order vary according to state.
- Staff's attitudes and cultural beliefs concerning dying.

MANAGEMENT/INTERVENTIONS:[3, 4, 5, 6]

- Identification of federal, state, and local laws related to DNAR directives in the educational setting and the care of medically fragile children at school. General counsel at the state Department of Education is a good resource to define federal, state, and local laws and the ability of schools to comply with "do not attempt resuscitation" directives in the school district).
- Local policy development and the development of guidelines that support policy should include both members of the school community (i.e. attorney for the school board of education, school administrator, the school nurse, other members of the school services team), and members of the medical community (e.g., Emergency Medical Services [EMS], healthcare providers and funeral directors).
- Obtain release of information and DNAR order.
- Organize team meeting including school staff, parents/guardians, and palliative care team. Other community members that may be considered: clergy, local EMS, funeral home director, healthcare provider.

DO NOT ATTEMPT RESUSCITATION (DNAR) *(continued from previous page)*

MANAGEMENT/INTERVENTIONS *(continued)*

- Conduct student assessment and assessment of staffing needs.
- Develop an Individualized Healthcare Plan. Components to consider:
    - Disease-directed treatment
    - Symptom control
    - Copy of the DNAR order
    - Specific explanation of what actions may be taken by staff members
    - Specific comfort measures such as holding the child, providing oxygen, keeping student warm
    - Address spiritual needs
    - Clear instructions on classroom management should child's health status change, i.e. a code that elicits quick staff response, privacy considerations for student
    - Education of identified school staff to include defining staff roles and accommodations for bus transportation
- Develop a plan to provide and support staff and student's peers.

FOLLOW-UP:

- Re-evaluate the plan annually, at minimum.
- Implement the plan to provide support to school staff and student's peers.

NOTES:

- A comprehensive planning checklist for a DNAR order for a child at school can be found in an article, *Do Not Attempt Resuscitation (DNAR) Orders in School Setting* (NASN School Nurse, March 2013) and also in *School Nursing: A Comprehensive Text*. See reference list for complete information.

REFERENCES

[1] American Academy of Pediatrics. (2010). Policy statement: Honoring do-not-attempt resuscitation requests in schools. *Pediatrics, 125*, 1073-1077. https://doi/org/10.1542/peds.2010-0452

[2] Selekman, J., & Ness, M. (2019). Students with chronic conditions. In J. Selekman, R. Adair Shannon, & C. F. Yonkaitis (Eds.), *School nursing: A comprehensive text* (3rd ed., pp. 480-499). F.A. Davis.

[3] Putman, S. (2017). Do not attempt to resuscitate (DNAR) in the school setting. In C.A. Resha & V. L. Taliaferro (Eds.). *Legal resource for school health services* (pp. 243-252). SchoolNurse.com.

[4] American Academy of Pediatrics. (2020). Sample documents and forms. In S. Aronson, & T. Shope (Eds.), *Managing infectious diseases in child care and schools* (5th ed., p. 217). American Academy of Pediatrics.

[5] Selekman, J., & Ness, M. (2019). Students with chronic conditions. In J. Selekman, R. Adair Shannon, & C. F. Yonkaitis (Eds.), *School nursing: A comprehensive text* (3rd ed., pp. 480-499). F.A. Davis.

[6] Deutch, J.M., Martin, L. G., & Mueller, J. A. (2015). *Managing students with health issues: Section 504 plans, DNR orders and contagious disease.* National School Boards Association. https://cdn-files.nsba.org/s3fs-public/file/16_PPT_Deutch_Martin_Managing_Students_with_Health_Issues.pdf?GxZmlwOOHmj1_ZgbVBGYakhaT0Fzbwt5pdf?GxZmlw00Hmj_ZgbVBGYakhaTOF-zbtw5

DO NOT ATTEMPT RESUSCITATION (DNAR) *(continued from previous page)*

OTHER REFERENCES CONSULTED

Adelman, J. (2010). *The school-based do-not-resuscitate-order.* Retrieved from https://via.library.depaul.edu/jhcl/vol13/iss2/3

National Association of School Nurses. (2018). *Do not attempt resuscitation—The role of the school nurse* (Position Statement). https://www.nasn.org/advocacy/professional-practice-documents/position-statements/ps-dnar?CLK=b3c89bea-2183-4e10-b9a2-7a25d3c6bb5c

Weise, K. L. (2010). Do-not-attempt-resuscitation orders in public schools. *American Medical Association Journal of Ethics, 12*(7), 569-572. http://virtualmentor.ama-assn.org/2010/07/pfor1-1007.html

Zacharski, S., Minchella, L., Gomez, S., Grogan, S., Porter, S., & Robarge, D. (2013). Do not attempt resuscitation (DNAR) orders in school settings: Special needs nurses review current research and issues. *NASN School Nurse, 28*(2), 71-75. https://doi.org/10.1177/1942602X12472540

DO NOT ATTEMPT RESUSCITATION (DNAR) *(continued from previous page)*

Do Not Attempt to Resuscitation (DNAR): Planning for the Child in School

PRE-DNAR ORDER

- Hold team meeting, including family
- Obtain assessment data
- Obtain Current Medical Summary
- Acquire equipment
- Order/obtain supplies
- Determine schedule

DNAR ORDER

- Obtain releases of information for EMS and appropriate agencies
- Write DNAR plan congruent with state laws and district policies
- Obtain DNAR (original order if required)
- Obtain out of hospital DNAR bracelet (if required)
- Note DNAR order expiration date
- Obtain student permission for DNAR if 18 years old
- Determine need for full time or 1:1 nurse in school
- Contact emergency Medical Services
- Contact medical examiner
- Determine emergency contacts
- Involve palliative care or hospice
- Include Comfort Care orders, POLST/ MOLST as appropriate
- Determine protocol for calling in case of emergency:
- family, physician, prearranged EMS
- Communicate plan between school nurse and
  - palliative care team
  - local EMS
  - funeral director
  - involved local agencies, others as needed
  - all members of student's health care team
- Develop a code that everyone will recognize
- Determine which staff members should be informed and receive training/education
- Train designated staff
- Address staff: moral, cultural, and ethical issues
- Conduct student population assessment for education and needs if DNAR is implemented
- Plan transportation
  - to and from school
  - field trips
  - after school activities
  - door to door, curb to curb
  - special bus (air conditioning, seating)
  - bus aide (UAP, health care aide, RN)

IMMINENT DEATH

- Clarify end of life issues vs. acute issues
- Designate an area for care to be delivered
- Direct Comfort Care orders, POLST/ MOLST if appropriate
- Plan for comfort care, including
  - holding
  - positioning
  - oxygen
  - pain management
  - bleeding control
- Outline what may and may not be performed by staff that requires treatment/management vs. comfort care
- Determine plan if no risk of imminent death:
  - EMS consultation
  - consultation with parent
  - transport to hospital (hospital of choice vs. nearest hospital needs to be discussed)

DEATH

- Determine where student will be moved
  - for serious distress event or death
  - to provide privacy for student and family
- Plan for other students and staff
- Determine who can pronounce death (per state regulations)
  - physician
  - nurse practitioner
  - physician assistant
- Determine when student will be moved from school
- EMS may not be able to move the body once death has occurred

TRANSPORTATION AND MORTUARY ARRANGEMENTS

- Determine plans for
  - funeral home
  - type of vehicle and where it will be parked
  - how student will be transported (stretcher, etc.)
  - who will clear the hallways
  - which doors to use

ROLE OF THE CRISIS TEAM

- Utilize bereavement team for staff and students
- Determine who will call parent(s)
- Determine a plan if sibling in same building
- Review and update plan whenever student's condition changes, at least annually

Source: Zacharski, et al. (2013). Used with permission.

EMERGING AND REEMERGING INFECTIOUS DISEASES IN SCHOOLS

OVERVIEW/DEFINITION:

"Emerging infectious diseases can be defined as infectious diseases that have newly appeared in a population or have existed but are rapidly increasing in incidence or geographic range".[1] Reemerging infectious diseases are those that have been well controlled but are now reappearing.[2,3] Several factors contribute to the development of emerging and reemerging infectious diseases including:[4]

- New infections resulting from changes or evolution of existing organisms
- Known infections spreading to new geographic areas or populations
- Previously unrecognized infections appearing in areas undergoing ecologic transformation
- Old infections reemerging as a result of antimicrobial resistance in known agents or breakdowns in public health measures

The presence of infectious diseases, including those that are emerging or reemerging, at a rate above that which is expected, is referred to as an outbreak or epidemic.[5] Recent emerging infectious diseases include HIV infections, severe acute respiratory syndrome (SARS) fever, West Nile virus, Middle East respiratory syndrome (MERS), and Zika virus. Recent reemerging infectious diseases include malaria, tuberculosis, cholera, pertussis, influenza, pneumococcal disease, measles, and gonorrhea.[6]

The school environment provides a unique opportunity for the spread of disease and the potential for an outbreak. The close proximity of large numbers of students and staff in both school and on school buses allow for easy transmission of many infectious diseases. Use of shared equipment in the classroom and lab setting, including technology, may also contribute to the transmission of infectious diseases. In addition, children are one of our most vulnerable populations due to their limited immune systems. Developmental stage and understanding of infection control contribute to this vulnerability. School nurses are a vital link in the healthcare system and are essential for mitigating the risk of an outbreak through screening, monitoring, communication and educational efforts. They are the bridge between health care and education by serving as leaders in the development of policies, advocating for students and communities, providing case management and care coordination, and integrating the principles of community/public health into clinical practice, such as health promotion, surveillance, and immunization administration and monitoring.[7]

ANTICIPATED CONCERNS/PROBLEMS:

"Infectious diseases are a leading cause of death worldwide, particularly in low income countries, especially in young children".[8] Outbreaks may occur due to new infections, changes in characteristics of pathogens (virulence, infectivity), or route of transmission. For example, genetic changes in influenza type A resulted in a new, stronger strain (subtype) of influenza A known as H1N1.[9] Recent trends in withholding of vaccinations, increase the potential for reemerging diseases, such as measles and pertussis.[10, 11] Outbreaks may negatively impact academics due to absenteeism. Reduced socialization may occur in ill children and those who are immunocompromised and are unable to attend school or participate in social activities. Children, parents, guardians, and families may require additional support from school nurses, staff, and administration during times of long-term illness

EMERGING AND REEMERGING INFECTIOUS DISEASES IN SCHOOLS *(continued from previous page)*

ANTICIPATED CONCERNS/PROBLEMS *(continued)*

and/or complications, including death. Although statistics on infectious disease mortality rates among school-age children are not readily available, school nurses must recognize that death due to serious infectious diseases is a possibility. They need to be prepared to support and counsel parents, families, and community members, as well as, students, staff, and administrators.

MANAGEMENT/INTERVENTIONS:

A collaborative approach to preventing and managing infectious diseases is critical for achieving the best outcomes. Coordinated efforts between the school nurse(s), local and state health departments, the superintendent and other administrators of the school district, and medical director of the district, to develop emergency plans and protocols for preventing and responding to outbreaks are essential. The school nurse's role related to all infectious diseases, applies to emerging and reemerging infectious diseases. Responsibilities include surveillance, monitoring/assessment, education, communication, collaboration, and advocacy. Interventions focus on primary, secondary, and tertiary prevention.[12]

Primary Prevention: Prior to the Outbreak

1. Establish partnerships and collaborate with key stakeholders (state and local health departments; local healthcare providers) to:
   - Develop templates of letters or informational blasts for distribution to community members in the event of an outbreak.
   - Establish communication about outbreaks, school closures, and other pertinent information, that is consistent, accurate and clear.
2. Understand laws related to reportable/notifiable diseases and associated processes for reporting.
3. Establish protocols and policies to address infectious disease prevention.
4. Understand the Family Educational Rights and Privacy Act (FERPA) and the Health Insurance Portability and Accountability Act (HIPAA) as they apply to student health.[13, 14, 14]
5. Provide education on infection control and prevention for students, staff, and parents/guardians, including hand hygiene, signs and symptoms of illness, and action to take.
   - Assure that information (oral and written) is available for non-English speaking individuals and families.
6. Provide education on the importance of vaccines, particularly for high risk individuals; being prepared for thoughtful discussions with parents/guardians who devalue the importance of vaccines.
7. Participate in community programs to increase awareness of risk for and control of infectious diseases.
8. Maintain adequate supplies for infection control, e.g. personal protective supplies (soap, masks, gowns, gloves).
9. Collect data on illness and absenteeism at different times of the year to provide a framework for comparison of future spikes in illness.

EMERGING AND REEMERGING INFECTIOUS DISEASES IN SCHOOLS *(continued from previous page)*

Primary Prevention: Prior to the Outbreak *(continued)*

10. Identify at risk populations (e.g. immunocompromised) in the district and specific schools. Inform these individuals, parents, families, or guardians of any potential outbreak or exposure and advise them to consult with their healthcare provider.

Secondary Prevention: Early Identification of an Outbreak and Prompt Intervention

1. Monitor and report symptom patterns that may reflect a possible outbreak (for example, several children presenting to the health office with a measles-like rash).
2. Identify clusters of ill children who share common workspaces or supplies in the classroom/lab, ride the same school bus, or participate in the same extracurricular programs.
3. Notify students, parents/guardians of immunocompromised students or unvaccinated students if the disease is vaccine preventable.
4. Monitor threshold absenteeism rates that alert a potential outbreak and report to the local health department.
5. Inquire about travel history of students and families.
6. Follow district, local, and state policies to report suspected outbreaks.

Tertiary Prevention: Decreasing Impact of the Outbreak and Preventing Complications

1. Coordinate communications with families and the school community with the local health department.
2. Update school websites regularly with clear, accurate information to minimize misinformation and anxiety.
3. Intentionally re-educate students, staff, parents, guardians, and the community when an outbreak or increase in illness is either strongly suspected or confirmed.
    - Make certain that information (oral and written) is available for non-English speaking individuals and families.
4. Emphasize that all students and staff who become ill/develop a fever should stay home until fever free for 24 hours and all symptoms have resolved.
5. Students with chronic health concerns such as asthma should work with their healthcare provider to ensure optimal health during an outbreak.
6. Consider the use of a public information officer for press releases, media alerts and other public service announcements.
7. Refer to FERPA and HIPAA guidelines for specific information regarding outbreaks.[15,16,17]
8. It is generally sufficient to report that a child in a particular school or class has been diagnosed rather than identifying the child.

FOLLOW-UP:

School nurses must continually familiarize themselves with the most current information regarding emerging diseases and be prepared to act when it presents. Early planning is essential in the event of an outbreak and the same strategies and principles discussed above will help address whatever emerging disease is on the horizon.

EMERGING INFECTIOUS DISEASES IN SCHOOLS *(continued from previous page)*

REFERENCES

[1] National Institute of Allergy and Infectious Diseases. (2018). *NIAID emerging infectious diseases/pathogens.* https://www.niaid.nih.gov/research/emerging-infectious-diseases-pathogens

[2] Centers for Disease Control and Prevention. (2014). *EID journal background: What are emerging infectious diseases?* https://wwwnc.cdc.gov/eid/page/background-goals

[3] World Health Organization. (2018). *Disease outbreaks.* https://www.who.int/environmental_health_emergencies/disease_outbreaks/en/

[4] Centers for Disease Control and Prevention. (2014). *EID journal background: What are emerging infectious diseases?* https://wwwnc.cdc.gov/eid/page/background-goals

[5] World Health Organization. (2018). *Disease outbreaks.* https://www.who.int/environmental_health_emergencies/disease_outbreaks/en/

[6] Johns Hopkins Medicine. (2019). *Emerging infectious diseases.* https://www.hopkinsmedicine.org/health/conditions-and-diseases/emerging-infectious-diseases

[7] National Association of School Nurses. (2018). *The role of the school nurse in the 21st century* (Position Statement). https://www.nasn.org/advocacy/professional-practice-documents/position-statements/ps-role

[8] Baylor College. (2019). *Introduction to infectious diseases. Para. 2.* https://www.bcm.edu/departments/molecular-virology-and-microbiology/emerging-infections-and-biodefense/introduction-to-infectious-diseases

[9] Centers for Disease Control and Prevention. (2019). Types of influenza viruses. https://www.cdc.gov/flu/about/viruses/types.htm

[10] Centers for Disease Control and Prevention. (2019). Morbidity and Mortality Weekly Report: Increase in Measles Cases – United States, January 1 – April 26, 2019. https://www.cdc.gov/mmwr/volumes/68/wr/mm6817e1.htm

[11] Centers for Disease Control and Prevention. (2019). *Pertussis (whooping cough).* https://www.cdc.gov/pertussis/index.html

[12] Centers for Disease Control (2019). *Picture of America. Prevention.* https://www.cdc.gov/pictureofamerica/pdfs/picture_of_america_prevention.pdf

[13] U.S. Department of Education. (n.d.). *Protecting student privacy. FERPA regulations.* https://studentprivacy.ed.gov/node/548/

[14] Ibid.

[15] U.S. Department of Education. (2019). *Student privacy and policy office.* https://www2.ed.gov/policy/gen/guid/fpco/index.html

[16] U.S. Department of Education. (n.d.). *Protecting student privacy. FERPA regulations.* https://studentprivacy.ed.gov/node/548/

[17] U.S. Department of Education and US Department of Health and Human Services. (2019). *Joint guidance on the application of the Family Educational Rights and Privacy Act (FERPA) and the Health Insurance Portability and Accountability Act of 1996 (HIPAA) to student health records- update December 2019.* https://www.hhs.gov/sites/default/files/2019-hipaa-ferpa-joint-guidance-508.pdf

ENVIRONMENTAL HEALTH

OVERVIEW/DEFINITION:

Environmental health, a division of public health, is "the science and practice of preventing human injury and illness and promoting well-being by identifying and evaluating environmental sources and hazardous agents and limiting exposures to hazardous physical, chemical, and biological agents in air, water, soil, food, and other environmental media or settings that may adversely affect human health".[1]

Unhealthy school environments can lead to issues with attendance, concentration, cognitive functioning, and performance, of both students and educators.[2, 3]

Examples of environmental exposures that a child might encounter in the school setting include poor indoor air quality, chemical exposure (secondary to pest management, cleaning products, building materials, science lab materials, art room supplies, etc.), injuries/death due to building code violations, playground injuries, air pollutants (such as exhaust fumes, radon), heating and cooling ventilation, etc.

Environment-related diseases, disorders, and other health problems that affect a child's current and future health and potentially the child's academic success including:

- Unsafe equipment inside the school and on the playground
- Weather related hazards which may result in injury (ice, slippery floors)
- Climate related risks such as floods, fires, extreme temperatures (hot and cold)
- Exposure to infectious diseases

ANTICIPATED CONCERNS/PROBLEMS:

Children are more vulnerable to environmental exposures and usually suffer more harm from exposure to these toxic substances than adults due to physiological, metabolic and behavioral differences.[4]

Environmental toxin exposure has been linked to the following:[5, 6]

- Asthma (from allergens/pesticides/pollutants/poor indoor air quality/ventilation, etc.)
- Lead poisoning leading to cognitive deficits, aggressive behaviors, learning disabilities, hearing problems, headaches, ADHD symptoms
- Birth defects secondary to mother's exposure to environmental toxicants (mercury, PCBs, pesticides)
- Childhood cancer (linked to pesticides, radon)

ENVIRONMENTAL HEALTH *(continued from previous page)*

SIGNS AND SYMPTOMS:
Signs and symptoms that children/youth may present with after exposure to environmental toxins (e.g. molds, pesticides, exhaust, cleaning solutions, etc.):[7, 8]

- Shortness of breath
- Cough
- Chest tightness
- Dizziness
- Irritation of eyes, nose and throat
- Irritation to skin (burning, itching, or rash)
- Wheezing
- Headache
- Fatigue

MANAGEMENT/POTENTIAL INTERVENTIONS:

Create a healthier environment:[9, 10, 11, 12]

1. Implement and enforce "no idling" of bus and car engines while waiting to pick up children.
2. Maintain school grounds (e.g., cutting grass) after school hours.
3. Clean school buildings with "green cleaners".
    a. Clean outside of school hours.
    b. Heavy cleaning done during summer or vacation breaks.
4. Inspect air and water quality routinely.
    a. Change furnace filters every three months.
    b. Test water sources for lead.
    c. Test and observe for mold.
5. Maintain adequate lighting and ventilation in classrooms/buildings.
6. Minimize the use of fragrances (perfumes/air fresheners).
7. Reduce indoor allergens.
    a. Minimally, vacuum classroom carpets weekly with vacuum cleaner equipped with high-efficiency particulate air (HEPA) filter.
    b. Steam clean carpets every eight weeks.
8. Avoid classroom pets.
9. Inspect and maintain playground structures to promote safety and minimize injuries.
10. Consider using organic lawn products.
11. Pest prevention – improve school sanitary conditions to avoid insect infestation.
12. Integrated pest management (IPM) to reduce risks to health and environment
    a. Use pesticide application as a last resort; use least toxic pesticide.
    b. Notify parents/guardians prior parents/guardians pesticide application. This is required by law in some states.
    c. Post signs notifying parents/guardians of upcoming pesticide application.
    d. Follow product health warning.

ENVIRONMENTAL HEALTH *(continued from previous page)*

MANAGEMENT/POTENTIAL INTERVENTIONS *(continued)*

e. Follow state regulations and/or school policies to determine when students and staff may re-enter the building (a minimum of two-hours).

f. Re-entry to building by students/staff should not be allowed into the building within a minimum two hours of pest extermination; follow product health warnings. State regulations and school policy may impact when students and staff can re-enter building

13. Monitor outdoor air quality including pollution levels near road and areas surrounding school.

FOLLOW-UP:

Role of the school nurse[13, 14]

- Facilitate annual comprehensive environmental assessments.
- Be alert to maintenance (building and playground) concerns that could be contributing to environmental health issues; notify appropriate staff regarding potential issues.
- Track and identify trends in health problems that may be linked to environmental toxins.
- Participate in school committees that advocate for reducing exposures to environmental contaminants.
- Advocate for moderation in the use of fragrances; may need to intervene if odors become too strong.
- Educate staff about sources of exposure, safeguards to avoid exposure, reporting policy for exposures, and action to take in the event of an exposure.
- Educate students about the importance of healthy environments and what they can do to create and maintain healthy environments.
- Comply with environmental health protection policies.

POTENTIAL COMPLICATIONS:

- Lead poisoning resulting in cognitive impairment
- Asthma/allergies: respiratory distress, or death
- Cancer: extensive treatment, or death

NOTES:

Children living in poverty are especially vulnerable to environmental toxic exposures. Pollutants, such as lead (paint chips, lead dust, etc.), molds, pollution (commerce, diesel exhaust, etc.) are more prevalent in lower socioeconomic communities. Parents may lack the resources and finances needed to reduce their child's exposure to the toxins. The school nurse may need to act as a liaison between the school, community, and healthcare provider to meet the health needs of the most vulnerable.

School nurses should be knowledgeable about climate change its impact on the environment and weather patterns which increase potential health risks for children (air and water quality). Storm related damage to natural and man-made structures may result in environmental hazards such as contaminated water, the influx of toxic chemicals into the air, smoke from fires, and unsafe buildings, bridges, etc. Advocacy to establish policies addressing primary, secondary, and tertiary prevention related to climate change is an important role for the school nurse. In addition, providing education for staff, students, and parents is essential to reduce exposure and injury.

ENVIRONMENTAL HEALTH *(continued from previous page)*

RESOURCES

- Environmental Protection Agency (n.d.) **How does indoor air quality impact student health and academic performance?** https://www.epa.gov/iaq-schools/how-does-indoor-air-quality-impact-student-health-and-academic-performance

- Children's Environmental Health Network
110 Maryland Avenue NE Suite 404
Washington, D.C. 20002
Phone: (202) 543-4033, Email: cehn@cehn.org
Resources for Parents, Families, and Other Child Health Advocates
https://cehn.org/resources/for-parents-families-and-other-child-health-advocates/childrens-environmental-health-101/

- American Nurses Association and National Association of School Nurses (2017). **School nursing: Scope and standards of practice (3rd ed.)**. American Nurses Association.

- Children's environmental health 101. https://cehn.org/resources/for-parents-families-and-other-child-health-advocates/childrens-environmental-health-101/

REFERENCES

[1] National Environmental Health Association. (n.d.). *Definition of environmental health,* para. 1. https://www.neha.org/about-neha/definitions-environmental-health

[2] World Health Organization. (2019). *Children's environmental health.* www.who.int/ceh/risks/en/

[3] *Children's environmental health.* https://www.who.int/ceh/risks/en/

[4] Ibid.

[5] Ibid.

[6] U. S. Department of Health and Human Services, Office of Disease Prevention and Health Promotion. (2019). *Healthy People 2020. Environmental health.* https://www.healthypeople.gov/2020/topics-objectives/topic/environmental-health

[7] Environmental Protection Agency. (2019). Indoor air quality and problem-solving tool. https://www.epa.gov/iaq-schools/indoor-air-quality-problem-solving-tool

[8] American Academy of Pediatrics. (2018). *AAP environmental health ECHO.* https://www.aap.org/en-us/professional-resources/practice-transformation/echo/Pages/AAP-EnvironmentalHealth-ECHO.aspx

[9] Environmental Protection Agency. (2019). Indoor air quality and problem-solving tool. https://www.epa.gov/iaq-schools/indoor-air-quality-problem-solving-tool

[10] Environmental Protection Agency. (2019). *Clean school bus idle reduction*. https://www.epa.gov/cleandiesel/clean-school-bus-idle-reduction

[11] Environmental Protection Agency. (2017). EPA *programs supporting schools.* http://www2.epa.gov/iaq-schools/epa-programs-supporting-schools

[12] Environmental Protection Agency. (2019). *State school environmental health guidelines.* https://www.epa.gov/schools/read-state-school-environmental-health-guidelines

[13] Ibid.

[14] National Association of School Nurses. (2015). *Environmental health in the school setting: The role of the school nurse* (Position Statement). Author. https://www.nasn.org/nasn/advocacy/professional-practice-documents/position-statements/ps-environmental-health

FOODBORNE ILLNESS

DEFINITION/ETIOLOGY:

Foodborne Illness (food poisoning) is an illness that results from consuming or handling contaminated food or beverages. Foodborne illnesses are associated with the lack of adequate knowledge regarding food preparation, storage, and hygiene; and increasing amounts and types of imported foods. Children are more prone to severe illness and death from food and water contamination because of their immature gastrointestinal and immune systems. Children who are immunocompromised are at greater risk.[1] Foodborne illness is suspected when clusters of unrelated sick people who ate at the same restaurant, shopped at the same grocery store, or attended the same event become ill.[2]

NOTIFICATION:

It is important to have established criteria with the local or state health department about when and how they are to be involved if a foodborne illness is known or suspected. Many such illnesses are reportable to the local or state department of health by the school nurse. Health department authorities will determine if the outbreak should be followed by the Centers for Disease Control and Prevention (CDC). It is important to involve the health department almost immediately because of the actions they can take to identify whether the illness is indeed foodborne and to prevent further spread of the outbreak.

CAUSE:

Foodborne illness arises from the ingestion of food that is contaminated with bacteria, viruses, parasites, or chemicals both natural and manufactured. Outbreaks have been associated with consumption of cold foods, including salads, sandwiches and bakery products. Liquid items (e.g., salad dressings or cake icing) that allow a virus to mix evenly have also been implicated in outbreaks. Food can be contaminated at its source (e.g., oysters harvested from contaminated waters have been associated with widespread outbreaks). Rough, wet, uncooked foods (such as ready-to-eat produce) and contaminated produce are at highest risk of transmission of norovirus. Most foodborne outbreaks of norovirus illness arise from direct contamination of food by a food handler immediately before the food is eaten.

Top Pathogens Causing Foodborne Illness	Top Pathogens Causing Hospitalization
Norovirus	Clostridium botulinum
Salmonella	Listeria
Clostridium perfringens	Escherichia coli
Campylobacter	Vibrio
Staphylococcus aureus	[3]

FOODBORNE ILLNESS *(continued from previous page)*

SIGNS AND SYMPTOMS:

- Frequent vomiting
- Abdominal pain and cramps
- Watery or bloody diarrhea
- Fever
- Chills
- Dehydration
- Depend on the type and amount of the source
- Last for a few hours to several days
- Range from mild to severe and death

Signs and symptoms may start within hours after eating the contaminated food, or they may begin days or even weeks later. Sickness caused by food poisoning generally lasts from a few hours to several days.[4]

MANAGEMENT/TREATMENT:

1. Report cluster of cases to health department; they will usually:
    a. Investigate food source (possible cultures)
    b. Interview individuals (possible stool cultures)
    c. Inspect food preparation area and handlers
2. Refer individuals to healthcare provider or emergency room (some students may require hospitalization; others merely antibiotics for treatment).
3. Replace fluids and electrolytes.

FOLLOW UP:

- Obtain results of any cultures taken and determine from treating healthcare provider if any student returning to school might pose a threat to others (e.g., carrier state of Salmonella).
- Monitor student's state of hydration, temperature and general status.
- Report relapses and new cases to health department.

POTENTIAL COMPLICATIONS:

- Dehydration (in severe cases, dehydration can be deadly)
- Hemolytic uremic syndrome (rare - affects children under 10 years old)
- Thrombotic purpura

NOTES:

- Children are at greatest risk for diarrhea and dehydration when exposed to foodborne illness.
- The food handler is the most common source of food contamination (this includes volunteers who conduct food events at school).
- Antibiotic resistance has become an increasing problem in foodborne illness. The germs that contaminate food can be resistant because of the use of antibiotics in people and in food animals.[5]
- Sometimes food suppliers are the source of contamination (eggs, poultry, ground meat, instant mashed potatoes).

FOODBORNE ILLNESS *(continued from previous page)*

PREVENTION

Educate school personnel, families and youth about the following:

- Hand washing by food handlers is the single most effective means of minimizing foodborne illness transmission. (*Refer to HANDWASHING APPENDIX*).
- Follow recommended or required techniques for food storage, preparation, and holding (hot or cold, covered, etc.), such as USDA *Be Food Safe*.[6]
- Sanitize food preparation and serving areas and of items used to prepare and serve food.
- Most food if properly cooked/heated is rendered harmless (temperature depends on the type of food).
- Avoid cross contamination by separating foods.
- Refrigerate food promptly.
- Uncooked foods such as salads require the greatest care with preparation because *E. coli*, norovirus and hepatitis A can be transmitted.

REFERENCES

[1] Ball, J., Bindler, R., & Cowen, K. & Shaw, M. (Eds.). (2017). Child and adolescent nutrition. *Principles of Pediatric Nursing: Caring for Children* (7th ed., pp. 295-296). Pearson Education, Inc.

[2] Centers for Disease Control and Prevention. (2019). *Foodborne outbreaks.* https://www.cdc.gov/foodsafety/outbreaks/investigating-outbreaks/investigations/contamination.html

[3] Centers for Disease Control and Prevention. (2015). *Foodborne germs and illness.* http://www.cdc.gov/foodsafety/foodborne-germs.html

[4] Mayo Clinic. (2017). *Food poisoning.* https://www.mayoclinic.org/diseases-conditions/food-poisoning/symptoms-causes/syc-20356230

[5] Centers for Disease Control and Prevention. (2018.) *Antibiotic resistance and food safety.* https://www.cdc.gov/foodsafety/challenges/antibiotic-resistance.html#connection

[6] U.S. Department of Agriculture (USDA). (2017). *Be food safe.* https://www.fsis.usda.gov/wps/portal/fsis/topics/food-safety-education/teach-others/fsis-educational-campaigns/be-food-safe/be-food-safe

OTHER REFERENCES CONSULTED

Centers for Disease Control and Prevention. (2014). *CDC estimates of foodborne illness in the United States.* http://www.cdc.gov/foodborneburden/

Centers for Disease Control and Prevention (2018). *CDC and food safety.* https://www.cdc.gov/foodsafety/cdc-and-food-safety.html

Partnership for Food Safety Education: Fight Bac.org (n.d.). *Food Safety Basics.* http://www.fightbac.org/food-safety-basics/the-core-four-practices/

U.S. Department of Health and Human Services. (2019). *Your gateway to food safety information.* https://www.foodsafety.gov

U.S. Department of Health and Human Services. (2019). *Food poisoning.* http://www.foodsafety.gov/poisoning/index.html

IMMUNIZATIONS

OVERVIEW/DEFINITION:

One of the greatest public health achievements of the 20th century has been the reduction and elimination of vaccine-preventable disease. Immunizations reduce disease morbidity and mortality in students and their families, as well as school staff and the community.[1] When school immunization rates are high, herd immunity protects those who are unable to be vaccinated because of pre-existing medical conditions or immunosuppression. Herd immunity, also known as community immunity, is defined as protection from contagious disease that benefits an individual as a result of living in a community where a critical number of people are vaccinated.[2]

The school nurse plays a critical role in monitoring and promoting vaccine compliance; educating parents, students and staff about the importance of vaccines in disease prevention; and assisting families to access vaccines either through their medical home, community healthcare providers or school located vaccine clinics. The school nurse should be familiar with laws protecting students in special circumstances such as provisions for homeless students and those in the foster care system; this should also include identification of resources for special populations such as undocumented students.

School nurses should be familiar with current Advisory Committee on Immunization Practices (ACIP) recommendations for mandated vaccines,[3] as well as state regulations and district policies related to exclusion and exemptions. As a trusted source of health information, school nurses can influence vaccine uptake through education of the role of children in vaccine-preventable disease transmission and dispelling myths that parents may have heard or read.[4]

Types of Vaccines

1. **Live attenuated vaccines** are vaccines in which live virus is weakened (attenuated) through chemical or physical processes in order to produce an immune response without causing the severe effects of the disease. Live vaccines currently licensed in the United States include measles, mumps, rubella, varicella, rotavirus, yellow fever, smallpox, and some formulations of influenza, shingles, and typhoid vaccines. Healthcare providers may defer administration of a live attenuated vaccine to students who are immunocompromised, as they may be at increased risk of contracting the actual disease.
2. **Inactivated vaccines** are vaccines made from viruses and bacteria that have been killed through physical or chemical processes. These killed organisms cannot cause disease. Hepatitis A, injectable influenza vaccine, and injectable polio are inactivated vaccines.
3. **Polysaccharide vaccines** are composed of long chains of sugar molecules that resemble the surface of certain types of bacteria. Polysaccharide vaccines are available for pneumococcal disease, meningococcal disease and *Haemophilus Influenzae* type b.
4. **Recombinant vaccines** are developed from new combinations of genetic material or cells; the genetic material produced when segments of DNA from different sources are joined to produce recombinant DNA.[5] Hepatitis B (HBV) and Human Papillomavirus vaccine (HPV) are examples of currently licensed recombinant vaccines.

IMMUNIZATIONS *(continued from previous page)*

ANTICIPATED CONCERNS/PROBLEMS:

- The success of vaccines in disease prevention and eradication has resulted in a shift in public focus from the risk of diseases to the risk of vaccines.[6]
- An increase of international travel and migration from countries with endemic infections has increased the need to assure high rates of immunizations in schools and communities.[7]
- Access to accurate, recordable, and retrievable vaccine information has become more challenging as families become more mobile.
- The increase of natural disasters such as fires, hurricanes and floods has led to the loss of immunization records.
- Expansion of recommended types and number of vaccines has led to parent reluctance to complete all vaccine series.
- Social media and celebrity efforts to link vaccines to conditions such as autism have misled the public and resulted in vaccine hesitancy and refusal by some parents.
- Many healthcare providers are unfamiliar with the Health Information and Portability and Accountability Act (HIPAA) which allows immunization records to be shared between healthcare providers for the purpose of protecting public health.[8] This lack of understanding of the laws may lead to delay in transmission of immunization data to schools and delay in student school entry.

MANAGEMENT/POTENTIAL INTERVENTIONS:

School nurses have a multifaceted role in maintaining immunization compliance in schools that includes: [9]

- Record review to assess compliance
- Referral to provider for needed vaccines
- Educating families, students, and staff about vaccines and vaccine safety
- Collaborating with school or district administrators to educate on state regulations related to immunization compliance
- Assisting families and students with their decision to vaccinate and/or locating resources
- Advocating for and championing efforts to improve immunization compliance

School Located Vaccine Clinics

In some cases, vaccines may be administered in school by either the school nurse or an outside agency through School Located Vaccine Clinics (SLVC).

- Clinics may be held during school day and allow students to receive needed vaccines with written consent from parents.
- Clinics may also be held after school for students, families, and community members. These after-school clinics are an efficient method to increase influenza vaccine uptake.

IMMUNIZATIONS *(continued from previous page)*

MANAGEMENT/POTENTIAL INTERVENTIONS *(continued)*

When students receive immunizations at school, the school nurse should be aware of and have protocols in place to respond to possible vaccine adverse reactions:

- **Local reactions** are common, and consist of redness, discomfort, and swelling at injection site and usually resolve within 48 hours. An ice pack may help the discomfort.
- **Systemic reactions** may include headache, body aches, fever, and lack of appetite and resolve on their own. Systemic reactions to live attenuated vaccines such as MMR and varicella may occur three to 21 days following administration of vaccine.
- **Allergic reactions** are rare but may be serious, resulting in anaphylaxis (hives, swelling of mouth and throat, difficulty breathing, wheezing, hypotension and shock). Epinephrine should always be kept on site during a vaccine clinic.[10] (*Refer to ANAPHYLAXIS*).

FOLLOW-UP:

In order to protect students, staff, families, and communities from vaccine-preventable disease, school nurses should:

- Understand how vaccines work and the diseases they prevent.
- Be aware of current ACIP recommendations for vaccine types, number of doses, age range dose should be given, and minimal intervals between doses.
- Know and follow state regulations and district policies regarding exemptions and exclusions.
- Access state immunization information systems (formerly known as immunization registries) to obtain student immunization data.
- Collect immunization data for each student and monitor compliance with regulations.
- Communicate with parents and healthcare providers to obtain missing immunization data.
- Work with administrators to enforce state and school district policy for immunization compliance.
- Maintain accurate records regarding student immunizations.
- Conduct communicable disease surveillance.
- Be aware of students who are exempt so that in the case of an outbreak, they are prepared to collaborate with local or state health officials to determine if there is a need to exclude non-vaccinated students and the length of time they should be excluded.
- Educate staff on recommended vaccines and on exclusion policies for staff in the event of outbreaks.

IMMUNIZATIONS *(continued from previous page)*

NOTES:

- There are rare but serious contraindications to administer vaccines to children (known allergy to a component of the vaccine; immunosuppression or pregnancy for live vaccines). Mild illness should not prevent vaccine administration. Moderate or severe illness is a reason to temporarily delay vaccine administration.
- Live attenuated vaccines may be given on the same day or must wait and be given at least 28 days apart to minimize potential risk of interference.
- A four day grace period is generally accepted practice when considering minimum age for a vaccine to be given.[11]

REFERENCES

[1] Boyer-Chu, L., & Yonkatis, C. (2019). Disease prevention in schools. In J. Selekman, R. Shannon, & C. Yonkaitis (Eds.), *School nursing: A comprehensive text* (*3rd ed.,* pp. 320-334). F.A. Davis.

[2] Centers for Disease Control and Prevention. (2016). *Vaccines and immunizations: Glossary*. https://www.cdc.gov/ /terms vaccines /glossary.html

[3] Centers for Disease Control and Prevention. (2019). *Immunization schedules*. https://www.cdc.gov/vaccines/schedules/hcp/imz/child-adolescent.html

[4] National Association of School Nurses. (2015). *Immunizations* (Position Statement). Author.

[5] Centers for Disease Control and Prevention. (2016). *Vaccines and immunizations: Glossary*. https://www.cdc.gov/ /terms vaccines /glossary.html

[6] Ibid.

[7] Boyer-Chu, L., & Yonkatis, C. (2019). Disease prevention in schools. In J. Selekman, R. Shannon, & C. Yonkaitis (Eds.), *School nursing: A comprehensive text* (3rd ed., pp. 320-334). F.A. Davis.

[8] U.S. Department of Health and Human Services (HHS). (2013). *Does the HIPAA Privacy Rule allow a health care provider to disclose protected health information (PHI) about a student to a school nurse or physician?* https://www.hhs.gov/hipaa/for-professionals/faq/517/does-hipaa-allow-a-health-care-provider-to-disclose-information-to-a-school-nurse/index.html

[9] National Association of School Nurses. (2015). *Immunizations* (Position Statement). Author.

[10] Boyer-Chu, L., & Yonkatis, C. (2019). Disease prevention in schools. In J. Selekman, R. Shannon, & C. Yonkaitis (Eds.), *School nursing: A comprehensive text* (3rd ed., pp. 320-334). F.A. Davis.

[11] Center for Disease Control and Prevention. (2019). *Vaccine recommendations and guidelines of the ACIP: Timing and spacing of immunobiologics*. https://www.cdc.gov/vaccines/hcp/acip-recs/general-recs/timing.html

MEDICAL DEVICES (visible and implanted), Management of

OVERVIEW/DEFINITION:

Approximately 19.4 % of children have chronic health conditions in the United States and are entering schools each year who might be aided by a medical device that is wearable or implanted to help manage their health care needs.[1] Some examples of wearable devices and implanted devices are:[2]

- Insulin pumps and continuous glucose monitors (CGM's)
- Holter monitors
- Ventilators
- Oxygen level monitors
- Cardiac monitors
- Internal defibrillators, pacemakers
- Intrathecal baclofen pumps
- Cochlear implants
- Hearing aids
- Vagal nerve stimulators

ANTICIPATED CONCERNS/PROBLEMS:

- Malfunction of the device.
- Device becomes damaged due to being dropped.
- Lack of/or intermittent Wi-Fi in the school building.
- Lack of training regarding medical device.
- Lack of information and contact numbers for Durable Medical Equipment company, or device specific serial number.

MANAGEMENT/POTENTIAL INTERVENTIONS:

The school nurse should:

- Be involved with the development of written policies and procedures that define the ability and limits of schools and school personnel to monitor and respond to medical devices data.[3]
- Develop an Individualized Healthcare Plan (IHP) and Emergency Care Plan (ECP) for the student with the device.[4]
- Train school personnel regarding the specific medical device, safety precautions, and signs and symptoms of malfunction, and what action to take if there is a malfunction.[5]
- Refer the student to the Section 504 or Individualized Education Program (IEP) team as appropriate.[6]
- Stay updated on technology changes.[7]
- Follow the Family Educational Rights and Privacy Act (FERPA) and the Health Insurance Portability and Accountability Act (HIPAA) policies regarding confidentiality and privacy needs in the school setting.[8]
- Be sure not to use a personal cell phone or iPad®/tablet. All monitoring devices should be school owned and encrypted using a secure server.
- Assess the student's ability and competency for self-management of their device according to their healthcare provider orders and parental input.

MEDICAL DEVICES (visible and implanted), Management of *(continued from previous page)*

MANAGEMENT/POTENTIAL INTERVENTIONS *(continued)*

- Plan for all school sponsored activities and any extra training or accommodations that would be required to keep the student safe outside the school setting.
- Be knowledgeable of the specific device and the user manual, which should cover battery life, safety concerns, beeps, flashing lights, etc.

FOLLOW-UP:

- Be aware and knowledgeable of state and federal laws regarding downloading of applications or communications which contain medical information.[9]
- Know if the device is U.S. Food and Drug Administration (FDA) approved for the age of the student.

NOTES: Advances in technology are rapidly changing and it is important for the school nurse to be aware of the advances that are being used and understand the impact on the student as well as the management of the student in the school setting.

REFERENCES

[1] Child and Adolescent Health Measurement Initiative: Data Resource Center for Child and Adolescent Health. (2016). 2016 National Survey of Children's Health (NSCH) data query. http://childhealthdata.org/browse/survey/results?q=4562&r=1

[2] National Association of School Nurses. (2018). *Wearable medical technology in schools-The role of the school nurse* (Position Brief). National Association of School Nurses. https://www.nasn.org/advocacy/professional-practice-documents/positionbriefs/pb-wearable

[3] Obst, B., & Roesler, M. (2017). Hidden devices in the school setting: What the nurses needs to know about shunts. NASN School Nurse, 32(3). 154-158. http://doi.org/10.1177/1942602x17697026

[4] Ibid.

[5] Ibid.

[6] Ibid.

[7] Ibid.

[8] Ibid.

[9] National School Boards Association Council of School Attorneys. (2017*). 50 years of school technology lessons learned from past and legally defendable practices of the future*. https://cdn-files.nsba.org/s3fs-public/FINAL%20Gilsbach%2050%20Years%20of%20Technology%20Paper.pdf

ORGAN TRANSPLANT, MANAGEMENT OF STUDENTS WITH SOLID

DEFINITION/ETIOLOGY:

Solid organ transplant has become routine practice for management of numerous disease processes and the number of children undergoing solid organ transplants has increased over the last ten years with one-year survival rates passing 95% in heart, lung, liver and kidney recipients with five-year survivals being not far behind.[1] With increased survival rates and desired outcomes for this population, a primary goal is for these children to return to school with their peers. Special considerations for this population exists.

The student will undergo an extensive medical evaluation to ensure that transplant is an appropriate and safe option for them. They will then be listed on the transplant waiting list. Depending on their diseases process and the organ that they need,[2] there are medical requirements and ongoing testing to remain active on the list. While waiting for a transplant, the student may miss school due to illness or medical appointments. This is a stressful time for the family as often the child will become very ill before an organ offer is received with potential for mortality. Given the organ offer can be received 24 hours a day, the family should have a plan in place to pick up the child, if not at home, and bring them immediately to the hospital. There are times a child may be brought in for a transplant but the surgery is cancelled due to the organ being unsuitable for transplantation. For kidney and liver recipients, the family may be considering living donation.

ANTICIPATED CONCERNS/PROBLEMS:

Medication Regimes

Long term survivals in this population is in part a result of the transplant community gaining a better understanding of immunosuppression. Protocols have been developed which utilize a combination of drug therapy; organ specific planned tapering of medication and doses; and diligent monitoring for viral infections and evidence of over immunosuppression.[3] The pediatric population requires different management as metabolism, pharmacokinetics, immune-responsiveness and long-term effects due to longer exposure of immunosuppression differ in this population.[4]

Corticosteroids

Most immunosuppression protocols in the pediatric patient include rapid reduction of steroids given the potential for: impaired growth, increased infection rates, osteoporosis, glucose intolerance and hyperglycemia, weight gain and psychiatric disturbances.

ORGAN TRANSPLANT, MANAGEMENT OF STUDENTS WITH SOLID *(continued from previous page)*

ANTICIPATED CONCERNS/PROBLEMS *(continued)*

Calcineurin Inhibitors (CIs)
Tacrolimus and Cyclosporine are the main immunosuppressant medications for these students which they will require for the rest of their lives. l. Side effects include:[5]

- nephrotoxicity
- neurotoxicity, infections
- hypertension
- hyperlipidemia
- gastrointestinal disturbances
- hyperglycemia (associated with tacrolimus)

As a result of these side effects, trough levels are checked periodically to ensure appropriate immunosuppression level and compliance.

Mycophenolate Mofetil
Used as an adjunct to CIs so lower levels of CIs can be tolerated. If using two immunosuppressants instead of just one, the trough level of the CI can be run lower with the goal of less long-term side effects.

Side effects are mostly gastrointestinal including cramping, vomiting and diarrhea as well as pancytopenia. Mycophenolate Mofetil may also contribute to the development of ulcers.

Vaccines
Vaccination of solid organ transplant recipients prior to transplant is the goal of treatment to protect the patient prior to the onset of immunosuppression. However, sometimes vaccinations are delayed as a result of age, disease status and urgency of transplant.[6] The current trend of vaccine hesitancy or refusal has led to outbreaks of vaccine preventable diseases such as measles and varicella which potentially puts solid organ transplant patients at risk. These diseases, specifically Measles and Varicella cause significant morbidity and mortality in transplant recipients including disseminations, respiratory failure, end organ involvement, organ rejection and mortality.[7]

Educational Considerations
Similar to other children with chronic illness, cognitive and developmental delays are prevalent. Specific to end organ failure and patients undergoing transplant evaluation, research highlights the importance of intervention and long-term monitoring for this population.[8] Post-transplant, these delays and impaired function can persist with students requiring support to catch up to their peers.[9] Referral for and implementation of Individualized Education Plans (IEPs)s and Section 504 Plans should be completed for these students. The need for early evaluation, intensive intervention including speech, occupational, and physical therapy and ongoing monitoring and intervention for these patients' neurodevelopmental/neuropsychological functioning over time is essential for their long term academic success.[10]

ORGAN TRANSPLANT, MANAGEMENT OF STUDENTS WITH SOLID *(continued from previous page)*

ANTICIPATED CONCERNS/PROBLEMS *(continued)*

Psychological Considerations and Quality of Life

While solid organ transplant provides increased quantity and quality of life, children and their families experience numerous burdens and stressors including the stress of waiting for an organ, financial struggles, stress on siblings, pressure of implementing complex medical regimens and scarcity of time for office visits and hospitalizations.[11] Post- transplant, patients and their parents fear morbidity, rejection of the transplanted organ, stress of medication compliance and need for frequent follow ups with potential medical procedures.[12] Family function is assessed ahead of the transplant and interventions are provided by the transplant team; however, increased stress, mental health issues and even post-traumatic stress disorder (PTSD) can persist. Support to the student should be provided as well as continued assessment of the functioning of the family unit. Siblings of the transplant recipient could also benefit from support.

MANAGEMENT/POTENTIAL INTERVENTIONS:

In addition to their IEP or Section 504 Plan, students, both pre- and post-transplant should have an Individualized Healthcare Plan (IHP) developed in collaboration with the parents and transplant team. It may include (but not limited to) the following:

Infectious/Communicable Disease Control

As with all students, the transplant recipient will experience the common colds and viruses. The duration of illness likely will be longer for these patients given immunosuppression.

- Encouraging the student to use hand sanitizer often in the classroom, and always after bathroom use and before eating. (*Refer to HANDWASHING APPENDIX*).
- Any outbreak or exposure to communicable diseases in the school requires immediate notification of the parents and transplant team. The child may require treatment for the exposure with possible hospitalization.

Routine Care

Students will also present with other common complaints such as fever, headache and abdominal pain. During the school nurse assessment, it is important to be mindful if this is a "routine" complaint or possible symptom of transplant complication. Establishing a collaborative relationship with the transplant team early on will be important to foster good two-way communication.

Fevers

All fevers should be reported to the parent and transplant team. Fever is defined in the immunosuppressed transplant patient as 100.5 F or higher as they may not mount a response for a higher temperature.

ORGAN TRANSPLANT, MANAGEMENT OF STUDENTS WITH SOLID *(continued from previous page)*

MANAGEMENT/POTENTIAL INTERVENTIONS *(continued)*

Medication Management

Some medication administration may be required at school. Collaboration with the transplant team should occur to ensure appropriate and timely administration.

For the student who presents with common complaints to the school nurses office, such as headache, abdominal pain, GI upset etc., close attention should be made in the assessment of these chief complaints to assess whether or not they are related to side effects of medication that can occur at any time. It would include assessment for hypertension, signs of ulcers, signs of hyperglycemia, tremors or other neurocognitive side effects.

Full assessment should be done with medication side effects and potential long-term surgical complications in collaboration with the transplant team.

Diet and Physical Activity

Any physical and dietary limitations in these students should be defined by the transplant team prior to the child returning to school post-transplant. Prior to transplant, more physical and dietary limitations will be expected:

- No contact sports for the liver failure patient with a large spleen.
- Post-transplant, any limitations will be based specifically to the status of the student and should be defined by the transplant team.
- Some foods such as grapefruit and pomegranate are not advised due to medication interaction.
- Post-transplant, raw foods should be washed well, sushi is not advised.
- Parents should have a clearly defined plan from the transplant nutritionist and share that with the school nurse.
- Some physical activities may be restricted due to infection prevention as well, such as swimming in lakes. Some contact sports may be limited. Depending on the opinion of the transplant program winter sports such as skiing, and snowboarding may be restricted post-transplant as well.

ORGAN TRANSPLANT, MANAGEMENT OF STUDENTS WITH SOLID *(continued from previous page)*

FOLLOW-UP:

- Frequency of visits prior to and post-transplant depends on the organ and is transplant program specific. Post-transplant the child will be seen in the clinic twice a week for the first month or so. Visits are then spread out if the child is well. Blood work still may be done frequently while appropriately titrating medication levels and monitoring for signs of rejection and infection. Long term goal is for blood work to be done about three to four times a year with yearly visits. Depending on the type of organ received, follow up biopsies may be needed routinely, most especially in heart transplants. Office visits, medical interventions and blood work may differ for each child based on their post-transplant status and comorbidities.
- Depending on length of time absent from school, homebound education should be considered intermittently based on federal Individuals with Disabilities Education Act (IDEA) and state regulations.
- Revise IHP as needed throughout transplant process.

NOTES:

As noted above, it is important to provide support to the siblings of the transplant recipient as well. This may include a referral to the school mental health team or simply having an identified staff member to support them.

REFERENCES

---

[1] U.S. Department of Health and Human Services. (n.d.). Organ procurement and transplantation network. https://optn.transplant.hrsa.gov/

[2] Ibid.

[3] Blondet, N., Healey, P. & Hsu, E. (2017). Immunosuppression in the pediatric transplant recipient. *Seminars in Pediatric Surgery,* 26 (193-198). https://doi.org/10.1053/j.sempedsurg.2017.07.009

[4] Ibid.

[5] U.S. Department of Health and Human Services. (n.d.). Organ procurement and transplantation network. https://optn.transplant.hrsa.gov/

[6] Suresh, S., Upton, J., Green, M., Pham-Huy, A., Posfay-Barbe, K., Michaels, M, Top, K.A., Avitzur, Y., Burton,C., Chong, P.P., Danziger-Isakov, L., Dipchand, A., Hébert, D., Kumar, D., Morris, S.K., Nalli. N., Ng, V.L., Nicholas, S.K., Robinson, J.L., Allen, U.D. (2019). Live vaccines after pediatric solid organ transplant: Proceedings of a consensus meeting, 2018. *Pediatric Transplant*, oo:e13572, 1-18. https://doi.org/ 10.1111/petr.13571

[7] Ibid.

[8] Antonini, T.N., Beer, S.S., Miloh, T., Dreyer, W.J., & Caudle, S.E. (2017). Neuropsychological functioning in preschool-aged children undergoing evaluation for organ transplant. *Clinical Neuropsychology, 31*(2), 352-370. https://doi.org/ 10.1080/13854046.2016.1211245

[9] Ohnemus, D., Neighbors, K., Rychlik, K., Venick, R.S., Bucuvalas, J.C., Sundaram, S.S., Ng V.L., Andrews, W.S., Turmelle, Y., Mazariegos, G.V., Sorensen, L.G., Alonso, E.M. (2019). Studies of Pediatric Liver Transplantation (SPLIT). Health-Related Quality of Life and Cognitive Functioning in Pediatric Liver Transplant Recipients. *Liver Transplant*. 2019 Sep 11. https://doi.org/10.1002/lt.25634 [Epub ahead of print]

ORGAN TRANSPLANT, MANAGEMENT OF STUDENTS WITH SOLID *(continued from previous page)*

[10] Antonini, T.N., Dreyer, W.J., & Caudle, S.E. (2018). Neurodevelopmental functioning in children being evaluated for heart transplant prior to 2 years of age. *Child Neuropsychology 24*(1),46-60. https://doi.org/10.1080/09297049.2016

[11] Cousino, M., Rea, Kelly., Schumacher, K., Magee, J., & Fredericks, E. (2017). A systemic review of parent and family functioning in pediatric solid organ transplant populations. *Pediatric Transplantation*, *21*(3), 1-13. https://doi.org/10.1111/petr.12900

[12] Ibid.

RECESS: PROMOTING SAFE PHYSICAL ACTIVITY DURING THE SCHOOL DAY

DEFINITION/OVERVIEW:
Recess is regularly scheduled periods of supervised physical activity and play during the school day.[1] Physical activity involves movement of the body that uses energy.

Benefits of physical activity for children and adolescents include: improved bone health, improved cardiovascular health and muscle fitness, decreased body fat, and reduced symptoms of depression.[2] Brain health benefits for school-aged children include improved cognition, as well as improved cognitive processes of memory, executive function, processing, attention, and overall academic performance.[3,4] Recess activities and school health programs that promote active lifestyles among children and adolescents have also been shown to improve health-related quality of life in primary school children.[5,6]

In contrast, children who are not physically active are at risk for being overweight and/or obese, putting them at risk for the development of serious chronic health problems including type 2 diabetes, hypertension, and heart disease. The existence of inequities in access to safe outdoor spaces for racial and ethnic minorities places children in these groups at greater risk for weight-related health problems. [7]

Regularly scheduled recess is supported by the National Association of School Nurses,[8] the American Academy of Pediatrics,[9] and the Centers for Disease Control and Prevention (CDC).[10]

ANTICIPATED PROBLEMS/CONCERNS:
As important as recess is to promote health and wellness in children and adolescents, there are risks for injury and exposures for which the school nurse needs to be prepared. Examples include injuries from playground equipment, unintentional head injuries, traumatic brain injuries and concussions, insect bites, sprains, bumps and bruises, burns, and broken bones. Pesticide exposure may also be a concern.[11]

PROMOTION OF RECESS:
The nurse's role in promoting recess is threefold:

1. Encouraging physical activity to improve overall health and well-being
2. Facilitating the establishment of safe environments and policies for recess
3. Provision of prompt and efficient care to children with injuries occurring during recess

RECESS: PROMOTING SAFE PHYSICAL ACTIVITY DURING THE SCHOOL DAY *(continued from previous page)*

PROMOTION OF RECESS *(continued)*

Strategies to Promote Physical Activity

1. Advocate for regularly scheduled outdoor recess during the school day (weather permitting; available safe environment).
2. Incorporate short breaks during classroom time for students to move around (e.g., jumping jacks).
3. Establish policies for indoor recess activities that promote physical activity when outdoor recess is not feasible (e.g. indoor basketball, structured walking throughout the building, or relay races in the gymnasium).
4. Encourage adults (teachers, administrators, and others) to engage in physical activity with the students.
5. Educate students on the benefits of physical activity to promote health and wellness, as well as academic success.
6. Establish structured recess programs to engage students with lower levels of physical activity (such as sitting on a swing or talking in a small group).
7. Incorporate national guidelines for recess established by the CDC in collaboration with the Society of Health and Physical Educators (SHAPE).[12] Some states have legislation in place with required minimum time allotments for physical activity.
    a. Provide all students K–12 with at least 20 minutes of recess daily.
    b. Prohibit the replacement of physical education with recess.
    c. Provide schools and students with adequate spaces, facilities, equipment, and supplies for recess.
    d. Establish spaces and facilities for recess that meet or exceed recommended safety standards.
    e. Prohibit the exclusion of students from recess for disciplinary reasons or academic performance in the classroom.
    f. Prohibit the use of physical activity during recess as punishment.
    g. Provide recess before lunch.
    h. Provide staff members who lead or supervise recess with ongoing professional development.

Strategies to Promote Safe Environments and Policies for Recess

1. Collaborate with school maintenance/engineering staff to ensure that playgrounds and playground equipment are inspected for safety hazards (scheduled and unscheduled).
2. Facilitate the development and updating of playground safety policies.
3. Monitor for playground injury trends that may require establishment of new policies, revision of current policies, or inspection of equipment or playground environment.

RECESS: PROMOTING SAFE PHYSICAL ACTIVITY DURING THE SCHOOL DAY *(continued from previous page)*

PROMOTION OF RECESS *(continued)*

Interventions to Prevent and Treat Recess Related Injuries

1. Educate students regarding safe use of playground equipment.
2. Facilitate proper supervision of recess activity by teachers, staff, and administrators.
3. Educate teachers, staff, and administrators regarding action to take when an injury occurs.
4. Establish protocols outlining action to take when an injury is observed.
5. Make supplies needed to treat recess related injuries readily available (bandages, soap and water, tape, ace bandages, ice packs, and other first aid items as needed).
6. Notify parents of pesticide application.
7. Participate in professional development activities focused on evidence-based practice for common recess-related injuries.

RESOURCES

- United States Consumer Product Safety Commission. (2015). ***Public safety handbook***. https://www.cpsc.gov/s3fs-public/325.pdf
- United States Consumer Product Safety Commission. ***Safety education resources***. https://www.cpsc.gov/safety-education/safety-guides

REFERENCES

[1] Institute of Medicine. (2013). *Educating the student body: Taking physical activity and physical education to school.* The National Academies Press: 2013. https://www.nap.edu/catalog/18314/educating-the-student-body-taking-physical-activity-and-physical-education

[2] Healthy People 2020. (2019). *Physical activity.* U.S. Department of Health and Human Services, Office of Disease Prevention and Health Promotion. https://www.healthypeople.gov/2020/topics-objectives/topic/physical-activity

[3] U.S. Department of Health and Human Services. (2018). *Physical activity for Americans* (2nd edition). U.S. Department of Health and Human Services. https://health.gov/paguidelines/second-edition/pdf/Physical_Activity_Guidelines_2nd_edition.pdf

[4] Michael, S.L., Merlo, C. L., Basch, C.E., Wentzel, K.R., & Weschler, H. (2015). *Critical connections: Health and academics.* Journal of School Health, 58 (11), 740-758. https://doi.org/10.1111/josh.12309

[5] Hyndman, B., Benson, A.C., Lester, L., & Telford, A. (2017). *Is there a relationship between primary school children's enjoyment of recess physical activities and health related quality of life? A cross-sectional exploratory study.* Health Promotion Journal of Australia, *28*(1), 37-43. https://doi.org/10.1071/HE15128

[6] Wu, X.Y., Han, L. H, Zhang, J.H., Luo, S., Hu, J.W., & Sun, K. (2017). *The influence of physical activity, sedentary behavior on health-related quality of life among the general population of children and adolescents: A systematic review.* PLoS One, 12(11). https://www.ncbi.nlm.nih.gov/pmc/articles/PMC5679623/

[7] Isong, I.A., Sowmya, R.R., Bind, M., Avendano, M., Kawachi, I., & Richmond, R.K. (2018). *Racial and ethnic disparities in early childhood obesity.* Pediatrics, *141*(1), 2-10. https://doi.org/10.1542/peds.2017-0865

RECESS: PROMOTING SAFE PHYSICAL ACTIVITY DURING THE SCHOOL DAY *(continued from previous page)*

[8] National Association of School Nurses. (2019). *Supporting scheduled recess.* (Position Statement). National Association of School Nurses. https://www.nasn.org/advocacy/professional-practice-documents/position-statements/ps-recess

[9] American Academy of Pediatrics. (2013). *The crucial role of recess in school.* (Policy Statement). Pediatrics, *131*(1), 183-188. https://www.aappublications.org/new

[10] Centers for Disease Control and Prevention. (2019). *Healthy schools: Recess.* https://www.cdc.gov/healthyschools/physicalactivity/recess.htm

[11] Centers for Disease Control and Prevention. (2019). *Child safety and injury prevention: Playground safety.* https://www.cdc.gov/safechild/playground/index.html

[12] Centers for Disease Control and Prevention and Society of Health and Physical Educators (n.d.) *Physical activity during school: Providing recess to all students.* U.S. Department of Health and Human Services. https://www.cdc.gov/healthyschools/physicalactivity/pdf/Recess_All_Students.pdf

SCHOOL REFUSAL

OVERVIEW/DEFINITION:

The umbrella term of school refusal refers to a student who refuses to come to school or to stay in school. It is emotionally based and has often been associated with other conditions such as anxiety disorder, depression, oppositional defiant disorder and post- traumatic stress disorder.[1] School nurses encounter numerous children and adolescents that have trouble attending school or difficulty remaining in school for the entire day. This can be for a myriad of reasons and the school nurse can be an integral part of the school team in addressing these issues:[2]

- Prevalence is greater than many childhood behavioral disorders
- Similar incidence between boys and girls
- Affects approximately 2-5% of all school-aged children
- Most common in children between the ages of five to six and 10-11-year old
- Common during school transitions

Every Student Succeeds Act (ESSA) law requires the reporting of chronic absenteeism and provides some federal funds for preventive measures.[3, 4] Students experiencing school refusal generally fall into these reporting requirements.

<u>Definitions</u>

<u>School Phobia</u> (outdated term): Fear-based, intense anxiety about being in school.[5]

<u>Separation Anxiety</u>: Excessive worry and difficulty separating from parent on the part of a child and possibly a parent. Seen especially at the start of the school year. Concerns are excessive and interfere with academic functioning.[6]

<u>Truancy</u>: Absence from school without permission or good reason with or without parental permission.[7]

<u>Chronic Absenteeism</u>: Legitimate or illegitimate absence from school or class and missing 10% of school or more for any reason.[8]

ANTICIPATED CONCERNS/PROBLEMS:

Students with chronic school refusal are at a high risk for never finishing school. If poor attendance is allowed to persist, the impact undermines academic achievement and social emotional skills. Students who are chronically absent in kindergarten and first grade are much less likely to read proficiently by third grade.[9] Students with anxiety-based refusal have high rates of somatic complaints including stomachaches, headaches, shortness of breath, crying and general feelings of "I don't feel good".[10] School nurses can be instrumental is helping to determine whether these are a result of a true medical condition or attempts at school avoidance.

SCHOOL REFUSAL *(continued from previous page)*

ANTICIPATED CONCERNS/PROBLEMS *(continued)*

Warning Signs[11]

- Frequent unexcused or excused absences
- Post- holiday absences
- Frequent tardiness
- Absence on significant days
- Frequent requests to call home
- Worrying about a parent while at school
- Parent who frequently calls to "check on" child during school
- Frequent requests to go to the nurse's office
- Somatic complaints such as headache, nausea, "not feeling well"
- Crying in school or when school is brought up
- Unsubstantiated issues with peers or teachers

MANAGEMENT/INTERVENTIONS:

- Educate all families on the importance of school attendance and attendance policies in school.
- Use data to develop or contribute to the development of a surveillance system to monitor and notify parents/guardians of students at risk for poor attendance to provide early intervention.
- Notify school administrators of students with excessive visits to the health office or high absenteeism rates.
- Meet with parents/guardians early in the process when attendance issues arise.
- Connect struggling students with positive and engaging supports.
- Work with educational colleagues to regularly discuss students with attendance issues.
- Provide parent and student education about appropriate health reasons for staying home from school.
- Support and assist parents as needed, to get students into the school building.
- Assist parents in setting up consistent morning routines and ignoring pleas to stay home and inappropriate behaviors.
- Consider home visits from a team of educators when students are refusing to come to school.
- Assist families of students with anxiety and depression to seek counseling to learn cognitive behavioral strategies to manage their feelings.
- Encourage school connectedness.
- Collaborate with outside providers such as healthcare provider and therapist as needed.
- Develop an Individualized Healthcare Plan (IHP) or refer to the Section 504 Accommodation Team as appropriate.

SCHOOL REFUSAL *(continued from previous page)*

NOTES:

Early identification and intervention are key. Once students get too far behind in school and feel they have missed too much school it becomes more difficult to get them back in school. Often the longer they are out of school the more difficult it is to return. Homebound tutoring should be discouraged as an effective approach. Sometimes partial days or slow reintroduction back into school may be utilized as a tool for re-entry.

REFERENCES

[1] Kawsar MDS, & Marwaha R. (2019). *School refusal.* In StatPearls [Internet]. StatPearls Publishing. https://www.ncbi.nlm.nih.gov/books/NBK534195/

[2] Ibid.

[3] Lara, J., Noble, K., Palecka, S., & Coons, A. (2018). *Chronic absenteeism.* National Education Association. http://www.nea.org/assets/docs/Chronic%20Absenteeism%20NBI%2057-2017.pdf

[4] Elementary and Secondary Education Act of 1965. (2018, Amended). https://legcounsel.house.gov/Comps/Elementary%20And%20Secondary%20Education%20Act%20Of%201965.pdf

[5] Brook Road Academy. (2018). *What is school phobia?* https://www.brookroadacademy.com/news/how-to-overcome-school-phobia/

[6] Leingang, C., Shannon, R., & Mechan, J. (2019). Students with mental/behavioral health concerns and disorders. In J. Selekman, R. Adair Shannon, & C. F. Yonkaitis (Eds.), *School nursing: A comprehensive text* (3rd ed., pp.767-769). F.A. Davis Company.

[7] U.S. Legal. (2019). *Truancy law and legal definition.* https://definitions.uslegal.com/t/truancy/

[8] Connecticut Department of Education. (2017). All students in school and engaged. https://portal.ct.gov/-/media/SDE/Chronic-Absence/webinarpresentation53117final.pdf?la=en

[9] Ibid.

[10] Leingang, C., Shannon, R., & Mechan, J. (2019). Students with mental/behavioral health concerns and disorders. In J. Selekman, R. Adair Shannon, & C. F. Yonkaitis (Eds.), *School nursing: A comprehensive text* (3rd ed., pp.767-769). F.A. Davis Company.

[11] Partners in School Based Mental Wellness. (2018). *Tackling school refusal.* https://www.sagethrivetoday.com/taking-charge-of-school-refusal-10-warning-signs-and-8-interventions/

SCHOOL-SPONSORED TRIPS

OVERVIEW/DEFINITION:

School-sponsored trips, also known as field trips, should be designed to support the school curricula, enhance a student's education outside of the school-day or school-site and are approved by the local board of education. Students may be off the school grounds for a few hours, overnight, days and may be out-of-state or the country. Section 504 of the Rehabilitation Act of 1973, Individuals with Disabilities Education Act and the Americans with Disabilities Act are federal laws that require individuals to have equal access to school-sponsored activities with accommodation for their disability and the exclusion of students based on disability is not permissible.[1, 2]

Since there is no universal definition for field trips, each local district needs to develop a policy for school-sponsored trips that meet the requirements of the federal laws.

NURSING LICENSURE and PRACTICE POINTS

- Implementation of the enhanced Nursing Licensure Compact (eNLC) began on January 19, 2018, with goals to increase access to healthcare, provide for the protection of the patient safety, to reduce costs and support the provision of care across state lines.[3]
  - It allows registered nurses (RNs) and licensed practical/vocational nurses (LPN/LVNs) to have one multistate license that allows them to practice in their home state and other eNLC states without obtaining additional licenses outside their home state.
  - Currently there are 33 member states per the Nurse Licensure Compact in 2019.
- The National Council of State Boards of Nursing (NCSBN) has a links to each state's nurse practice act at https://www.ncsbn.org/npa.htm.[4]
- The U.S. Embassy can provide contact information for specific considerations pertaining to out-of-country field trips.[5] Since United States nursing licenses are not recognized outside the country, school nurses are not permitted to practice nursing in other countries.
- It is necessary to identify and understand school district policy, in state, out of state and out of country scope of practice issues, rules and regulations and nursing responsibilities related to school health services, as applicable.[6,7,8] Even in those states with eNLC agreements, rules for delegation, medication administration, emergency care and procedures can vary from state to state.
  - "The abilities to delegate, assign and supervise are critical competencies for every RN. It is important to note that states/jurisdictions have different laws and rules/regulations about delegation, and it is the responsibility of all licensed nurses to know what is permitted in their jurisdiction." [9]
  - The American Nurses Association (ANA) and NCSBN Joint National Guidelines for Nursing Delegation (2019) defines assistive personnel (AP) (formerly called unlicensed assistive personnel [UAP]) as those trained to function in a supportive role, regardless of title, to whom a nursing responsibility may be delegated.[10]
  - According to the (ANA) and NCSBN (2019) Joint National Guidelines for Nursing Delegation, policies and procedures must be developed that outline what may and may not be delegated that are consistent with current nursing practice and the state's Nurse Practice Act.[11] The Five Rights of Delegation, student health needs, safety, assistive personnel competence and school health capacity are factors to consider when delegating for school-sponsored trips.[12,13]

SCHOOL-SPONSORED TRIPS *(continued from previous page)*

ASSESSMENT:

- Student healthcare needs:
  Healthcare needs of the students on school-sponsored trips are coordinated by the school nurse.[14] Individualized Healthcare Plans (IHP), Section 504 Plans and Emergency Care Plans (ECP), also known as Emergency Action Plans (EAPs) are developed through a collaborative process and should include accommodations that are necessary for all school-sponsored functions.[15] This includes but is not limited to management of chronic medical conditions, medication administration and storage, special dietary needs, health and emergency procedures.

- The needs assessment includes some of the following questions: What are the staffing needs? Are any students independent with self- management of their medical condition? Will delegation be needed? Will a nurse be required? What are the delegation and medication administration regulations in the state/country where the care will take place? Are there any restrictions to delegation in the other states/countries?[16]
  Note: This may need to include states/countries that you are travelling through while going to/from your final destination.

- Medication: When transporting medication, the following questions should be considered:
  - The preparation for medication distribution should be addressed in the school health services/school nursing policy on medication with the procedure developed with the board of pharmacy input, i.e., does it need to be in the labeled pharmacy medication container, or can one dose be put in a labeled envelope?
  - How will the medication be stored and carried during the trip in keeping with district policy?
  - How will medication administration be documented and by whom per the school nursing/school health services policy?
  - Does it need refrigeration?
  - Is there privacy for treatments and medications?
- Evaluate overall student safety while away from the school campus.

PLANNING:

1. Field Trip Planning: It is important to educate administrators about the legal implications of the nurse practice act and licensure for the provision for care to students when travelling out of state so that they are knowledgeable about the time frame and processes required to provide safe care to the students. School nurses should be involved in all phases of the approval and planning process of the proposed trip before the final administrative approval is obtained. This involvement allows the school nurse to determine:
   - student health needs
   - feasibility of providing needed care
   - staffing needs
   - accessibility of proposed experience for all students (i.e., accommodating students with special health care needs)

SCHOOL-SPONSORED TRIPS *(continued from previous page)*

PLANNING *(continued)*

- unique needs based on location
- training needs
- nursing licensure procedures in the destination state/country

2. Emergency Planning:
   - Emergency plans established prior to the school-sponsored trip allows for effective communication and management of an emergent situation to increase the potential for a positive resolution
   - Emergency plans should include lines of authority among the staff present, and communication between the staff present and the school administration at the school building or district level
   - Communication with school medical personnel as needed
   - Communication with families
   - Plans for emergency transportation of student (s) as needed, such as Emergency Medical Services (EMS) or use of a local emergency department
   - Emergency equipment/supplies for the staff on the trip; and
   - Training needs, such as first aid or CPR training prior to the trip

3. Training and Supervision: In the absence of the school nurse or other nursing personnel on school-sponsored trips, the training and assessment of the AP's ability by the delegating nurse to provide safe and competent nursing tasks are essential components of delegation based on the Rights of Delegation and state nurse practice acts.
   Supervision and evaluation of the APs needs to be established prior to the trip.
   - What is the communication plan and emergency plan for the trip?

   NOTE: The scope of practice for LPN/LVNs varies greatly from state to state.

EVALUATION:

Upon return from a school-sponsored trip, a brief discussion between the school nurse, staff participating on the trip and school administration is useful to evaluate what worked well as well as suggestions for improvement on subsequent trips. If an unanticipated event or emergency occurred while away, a more in-depth discussion may be needed.

SCHOOL-SPONSORED TRIPS *(continued from previous page)*

REFERENCES

[1] U.S. Department of Education: Office of Civil Rights. (2014). *Resolution Agreement: Triton Regional School District.* https://www2.ed.gov/about/offices/list/ocr/docs/investigations/more/01131248-b.html

[2] Americans with Disabilities Act Amendments. (2010). 42 U.S.C. § 12102. http://www.ada.gov/pubs/adastatute08.htm#12101

[3] Kappel, D.M. (2018). Unlocking access to nursing care across the nation. *NASN School Nurse, 33*(3), 186–188. https://doi.org/10.1177/1942602X18765241

[4] National Council of State Boards of Nursing. (2019). *Find your nurse practice act.* https://www.ncsbn.org/npa.htm

[5] New York State Center for School Health. (2018). *Field trip/FAQs.* https://www.schoolhealthny.com/site/default.aspx?PageType=3&ModuleInstanceID=189&ViewID=7b97f7ed-8e5e-4120-848f-a8b4987d588f&RenderLoc=0&FlexDataID=485&PageID=140

[6] Ibid.

[7] National Association of School Nurses. (2019). *Nursing delegation in the school setting* (Position Statement). https://www.nasn.org/nasn/advocacy/professional-practice-documents/position-statements/ps-delegation

[8] National Association of School Nurses. (2018). *School-sponsored trips -The role of the school nurse* (Position Statement). Amended June 2019. https://www.nasn.org/nasn/advocacy/professional-practice-documents/position-statements/ps-trips

[9] American Nurses Association & National Council of State Boards of Nursing. (2019). *National guidelines for nursing delegation*. Page 1, Introduction, para 1. https://www.ncsbn.org/NGND-PosPaper_06.pdf

[10] American Nurses Association & National Council of State Boards of Nursing. (2019). *National guidelines for nursing delegation*. https://www.ncsbn.org/NGND-PosPaper_06.pdf

[11] Ibid.

[12] National Association of School Nurses. (2019). *Nursing delegation in the school setting* (Position Statement). https://www.nasn.org/nasn/advocacy/professional-practice-documents/position-statements/ps-delegation

[13] National Association of School Nurses. (2018). *School-sponsored trips -The role of the school nurse* (Position Statement). Amended June 2019. https://www.nasn.org/nasn/advocacy/professional-practice-documents/position-statements/ps-trips

[14] National Association of School Nurses. (2018). *School-sponsored trips -The role of the school nurse* (Position Statement). Amended June 2019. https://www.nasn.org/nasn/advocacy/professional-practice-documents/position-statements/ps-trips

[15] Ibid.

[16] Ibid.

OTHER REFERENCES CONSULTED

Connecticut State Department of Education. (2014). *Field trips: Guidance for school nurses.* https://portal.ct.gov/SDE/Publications/Field-Trips-Guidance-for-School-Nurses

Erwin, K. & Clark, S. (2017). School-sponsored field trips. In C.A. Resha & V. L. Taliaferro (Eds.). *Legal resource for school health services* (pp.621- 629). Nashville, TN: Schoolnurse.com.

Massachusetts Field Trip Toolkit. (2015). *ESHS CQI Project.* https://neushi.org/student/programs/attachments/FieldTrip.pdf

National Council of State Boards of Nursing. (2019). *Nurse licensure compact.* https://www.nursecompact.com/about.htm

Wisconsin Department of Public Instruction. (2019). *Meeting student health needs while on field trips toolkit.* https://dpi.wi.gov/sites/default/files/imce/sspw/pdf/Meeting_Student_Health_Needs_While_on_Field_Trips_Tool_Kit.pdf

SCHOOL-SPONSORED TRIPS *(continued from previous page)*

TWO COMPACTS COMPARED

A Driver's License Compact vs. a Nurse License Compact

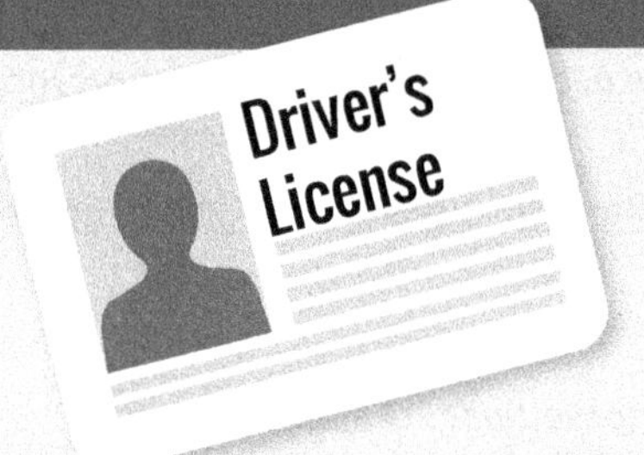

- Issued in your primary state of residence.
- When driving in other states, you must know and obey that state's laws (rules of the road).
- While driving in other states, if you violate the state's law, the state can remove your driving privileges in that state.
- When you change your primary state of residence (move) to another compact state, you need to apply for that state's driver's license. You can drive on your former license for a certain number of days (depending on the state). The former license then becomes invalid.
- While driving in other states, if you violate the state's laws and the state takes action (discipline), it is reported to the state that issued your license (where you reside). Most home states can take the same action as if you committed the violation in your home state.

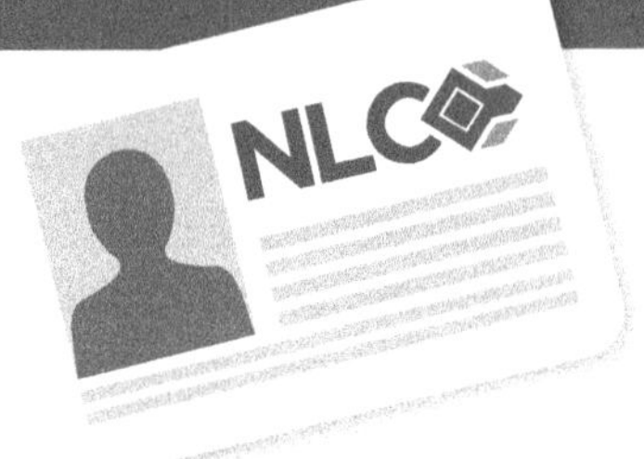

- Issued in your primary state of residence
- When practicing in other states, you must know and obey that state's laws (Nurse Practice Act).
- While practicing in other states, if you violate the state's laws, the state can remove your practice privileges in that state.
- When you change your primary state of residence (move) to another compact state, you need to apply for that state's nursing license. You can practice on your former license for 90 days. The former license then becomes invalid.
- While practicing in other states, if you violate the state's laws, and the state takes action (discipline), it is reported to the state that issued your license (where you reside). Most home states can take the same action as if you committed the violation in your home state

NCSBN, May 2016
https://www.ncsbn.org/Drivers-License-Comparison-and-Supporting-Organizations.pdf

APPENDIX B:

SCHOOL NURSE FIELD TRIP CHECKLIST

Trip Destination:____________________ Date of Field Trip: ________________

Field Trip Coordinator: ________________

_____1) Review school district policy and follow plan accordingly.
_____2) Review district/school filed trip request form and develop list of all attending students.

_____3) Identify all health-related issues and concerns, including students with food allergies and accessibility for attending students.

_____4) Review Individualized Healthcare Plans, Individualized Education Plans, Section 504 Accommodation Plans and Emergency Care Plans (ECP) for attending students.

_____5) Evaluate to determine whether student parent/guardian with medical need plans to accompany field trip.

_____6) Review nursing scope of practice and applicable state laws and regulations for in-state, out-of-state, and out-of-country field trips; including whether delegation to UAP and who may delegate (RN, LPN)? Is the destination state a MLS state?

_____7) Notify Field Trip Coordinator if a nurse is required for the field trip.

_____8) Prepare any necessary forms for documentation of medication administration, special healthcare procedures/treatments, copies of ECP's, licensed prescribed orders, parent and healthcare provider contact information is to be included.

_____9) Prepare necessary equipment, medications and first aid supplies, including medications to be refrigerated, care plans, and treatment plans.

_____10) Review medical concerns, medication administration, treatment plans and emergency protocols with the nurse or staff member attending field trip.

_____11) Provide current cell phone number to attending nurse/staff/chaperone for on-going consultation for student health concerns if needed.

_____12) If a nurse is **NOT** accompanying field trip:

- Notify parent/guardian the name of staff personnel who will be administering students' medications and or/treatments. Obtain parenteral/guardian written consent.

- Train staff members in medication administration, epinephrine and glucagon medication administration (as state practice act allows), Cardio-Pulmonary Resuscitation and necessary health care treatments as indicated and document all trainings.

_____13) When the field trip is completed assure all medications, equipment, care plans, first aid supplies and other confidential information/forms are returned to the school nurse.

CHECKLIST COMPLETED:
School Nurse: ____________________ DATE: __________________

(2017). School-sponsored field trips. In C.A. Resha & V. L. Taliaferro (Eds.). *Legal resource for school health services* (p629). Nashville, TN: schoolnurse.com. Permission to use granted by author, Karen Erwin, 2020.

VAPING

OVERVIEW/DEFINITION:

Vaping, also called JUULing, is the act of using a battery powered electronic nicotine delivery system (ENDS) also known as e-cigarettes, e-cigs, e-hookahs, pod mods or vape pens.[1, 2, 3] These e-cigarettes might look like regular cigarettes, pipes, flash drives, pens, dew drops, pens, hookahs and other common items.[4] The products used in vaping, commonly called cigarette or vape juice, are often are flavored.[5, 6, 7] E-cigarettes have also been used to vape marijuana or other chemicals.[8]

According to the Centers for Disease Control and Prevention (CDC) and U.S. Food and Drug Administration (FDA) study, in 2018 more than 3.6 million youth (1 in 5 high school students and 1 in 20 middle school students) had vaped within the month of the survey.[9] Vaping has become a six-billion-dollar industry.[10] Manufactures deny marketing to youth, yet many of the designs of the e-cigarettes and the flavors appeal to youth. Much of the marketing for e-cigarettes is through social media, although it is not illegal to advertise e-cigarettes on other media.[11, 12] Many states are looking at passing laws to limit vaping use, even to the point of making vaping products illegal.

ANTICIPATED CONCERNS/PROBLEMS:

- Nicotine is extremely addictive.[13] As the brain continues to develop until around 25 years old, nicotine can harm brain development especially the areas of attention control, learning, mood, and impulse control.[14, 15]
- Youth who vape are very likely to continue to smoke nicotine.[16,17, 18, 19]
- Non-cigarette smoking youth are more likely to try vaping than smoking cigarettes believing it is safer.[20, 21, 22, 23]
- The 2019 National Youth Tobacco Survey indicates a dramatic increase of vaping in youth. At the same time, an increase in cigarette smoking has not increased, but remained been stable at less than 6% of youth smoking cigarettes.[24]
- Flavored tobacco is appealing to many youth. Examples of flavors include Candy Crush, Cotton Candy, Bubble Gum, etc. Some of the flavorings are safe to eat, but not to inhale.[25] Children and adults have been poisoned by eating, inhaling or exposing skin to e-cigarette juice.[26, 27]
- Other harmful substances could be in the e-cigarette juice including marijuana, ultra-fine particles, cancer-causing agents, heavy metals, volatile organic compounds, and other chemicals.[28, 29]
- The CDC, the FDA, state and local health departments, and other clinical and public health partners are investigating a national outbreak of e-cigarette, or vaping, product use-associated lung injury (EVALI).[30] While the cause is not known at this point, vitamin E acetate is strongly linked to the EVALI outbreak.[31] Most hospitalized individuals report vaping marijuana products in their e-cigarettes.[32]
- People who vape frequently complain of mouth and throat irritation and dry cough.[33]
- Defective e-cigarette batteries have exploded causing fires and injuries.[34, 35]

VAPING *(continued from previous page)*

ANTICIPATED CONCERNS/PROBLEMS *(continued)*

- Secondhand smoke occurs when others inhale what the person vaping exhales.[36] This could cause significant health risks for infants, children, and people with compromised respiratory conditions, such as asthma and Chronic Obstructive Pulmonary Disease (COPD).

MANAGEMENT/INTERVENTIONS:

- Serve as a role model by not smoking, or if a smoker, quit.[37, 38]
- Educate students with a tobacco prevention curriculum that includes e-cigarettes and the potential risks of vaping.[39, 40] Dispel the "myth" that vaping is risk free or safer than smoking cigarettes.[41]
- Enforce tobacco free school grounds, which includes vaping.
- Review and revise school policies and procedures to include vaping products (e-cigarettes and vaping juice).[42]
- Refer students to cessation programs for those students who regularly use.
- Refer anyone for evaluation if suspected of severe lung disease.[43]

PREVENTION:

The FDA recommends a three-pronged approach to prevention of vaping by youth.

1. Preventing access of vaping products to youth. Strictly enforce current rules on sales of tobacco products to youth.
2. Curb marketing of vaping products to youth. Warn companies to restrict advertising to entice youth to explore vaping, including appealing flavorings.
3. Educate youth on the dangers of tobacco use including vaping. Promote the "Real Cost" Campaign. https://www.fda.gov/tobacco-products/real-cost-campaign [44]

FOLLOW UP:

- Collaborate on developing and implementing school policies and procedures regarding vaping on school property, installation of vaping detectors, and discovery of vaping products students bring into the school.
- Follow up with the student after a vaping incident or discovery of vaping products to clarify school policies, make referrals, and educate on the risks of vaping.
- Contribute to education of students on vaping individually and in classes.
- Advocate for laws to eliminate vaping juice flavors that appeal to youth, increase the age selling tobacco products, and eliminate advertising of vaping or any tobacco delivery products.

VAPING *(continued from previous page)*

ROLE OF THE SCHOL NURSE:

- School nurses are in a critical position to address the vaping issue by promoting healthy choices, preventing vaping promotion and access, and educating students and staff on the dangers of vaping.[45,46]
- As leaders in schools, school nurses can use motivational interviewing to promote positive healthy behavior choices of not vaping.[47]
- Working with students and families, school nurses can create a treatment plan to focus on strategies to prevent vaping, to educate students who are vaping, and to refer students to stop vaping.[48]
- With the outbreak of the severe lung disease caused by vaping, school nurses need to be aware of the symptoms of EVALI in order to refer students and staff for rapid medical treatment. Potential symptoms could include respiratory (cough, chest pain, shortness of breath) and gastrointestinal (nausea, vomiting, diarrhea, abdominal pain) along with tachycardia, tachypnea and O^2 saturation <95%. Lung auscultation may be unremarkable. If individuals with these symptoms acknowledge a vaping use, they should be referred for further medical evaluation.[49]

RESOURCES

Stanford Medicine, CDC, and many states' Departments of Health have curriculum to educate students on e-cigarettes.[50, 51]

REFERENCES

[1] Centers for Disease Control and Prevention (CDC). (2019). *Electronic cigarettes.* https://www.cdc.gov/tobacco/basic_information/e-cigarettes/index.htm

[2] Centers for Disease Control and Prevention (CDC). (2019). *Quick facts on the risks of e-cigarettes for kids, teens, and young adults.* https://www.cdc.gov/tobacco/basic_information/e-cigarettes/Quick-Facts-on-the-Risks-of-E-cigarettes-for-Kids-Teens-and-Young-Adults.html

[3] Perikleous, E. P., Steiropoulos, P., Paraskakis, E., Constantinidis, T. C., & Nena, E. (2018). E-cigarette use among adolescents: An overview of the literature and future perspectives. *Front Public Health,6,* 86. https://doi.org/10.3389/fpubh.2018.00086

[4] Centers for Disease Control and Prevention (CDC). (2019). *Electronic cigarettes.* https://www.cdc.gov/tobacco/basic_information/e-cigarettes/index.htm

[5] Budney, A. J., Sargent, J. D., & Lee, D. C. (2015). Vaping cannabis (marijuana): Parallel concerns to e-cigs? *Addiction, 110*(11), 1699-1704. https://doi.org/10.1111/add.13036

[6] Centers for Disease Control and Prevention (CDC). (2019). *Quick facts on the risks of e-cigarettes for kids, teens, and young adults.* https://www.cdc.gov/tobacco/basic_information/e-cigarettes/Quick-Facts-on-the-Risks-of-E-cigarettes-for-Kids-Teens-and-Young-Adults.html

[7] Centers for Disease Control and Prevention (CDC). (n.d.). *E-cigarettes and youth: What parents need to know.* https://www.cdc.gov/tobacco/basic_information/e-cigarettes/pdfs/OSH-E-Cigarettes-and-Youth-What-Parents-Need-to-Know-20190327-508.pdf

VAPING *(continued from previous page)*

[8] Budney, A. J., Sargent, J. D., & Lee, D. C. (2015). Vaping cannabis (marijuana): Parallel concerns to e-cigs? *Addiction, 110*(11), 1699-1704. https://doi.org/10.1111/add.13036

[9] Centers for Disease Control and Prevention (CDC). (2019). *Electronic cigarettes.* https://www.cdc.gov/tobacco/basic_information/e-cigarettes/index.htm

[10] U.S. Food and Drug Administration. (2019). *Youth tobacco use: Results from the National Youth Tobacco Survey.* https://www.fda.gov/tobacco-products/youth-and-tobacco/youth-tobacco-use-results-national-youth-tobacco-survey

[11] Budney, A. J., Sargent, J. D., & Lee, D. C. (2015). Vaping cannabis (marijuana): Parallel concerns to e-cigs? *Addiction, 110*(11), 1699-1704. https://doi.org/10.1111/add.13036

[12] Perikleous, E. P., Steiropoulos, P., Paraskakis, E., Constantinidis, T. C., & Nena, E. (2018). E-cigarette use among adolescents: An overview of the literature and future perspectives. *Front Public Health, 6*, 86. https://doi.org/10.3389/fpubh.2018.00086

[13] Ibid.

[14] Ibid.

[15] Centers for Disease Control and Prevention (CDC). (n.d.). *E-cigarettes and youth: What parents need to know.* https://www.cdc.gov/tobacco/basic_information/e-cigarettes/pdfs/OSH-E-Cigarettes-and-Youth-What-Parents-Need-to-Know-20190327-508.pdf

[16] Budney, A. J., Sargent, J. D., & Lee, D. C. (2015). Vaping cannabis (marijuana): Parallel concerns to e-cigs? *Addiction, 110*(11), 1699-1704. https://doi.org/10.1111/add.13036

[17] Centers for Disease Control and Prevention (CDC). (2019). *Quick facts on the risks of e-cigarettes for kids, teens, and young adults.* https://www.cdc.gov/tobacco/basic_information/e-cigarettes/Quick-Facts-on-the-Risks-of-E-cigarettes-for-Kids-Teens-and-Young-Adults.html

[18] Centers for Disease Control and Prevention (CDC). (n.d.). *E-cigarettes and youth: What parents need to know.* https://www.cdc.gov/tobacco/basic_information/e-cigarettes/pdfs/OSH-E-Cigarettes-and-Youth-What-Parents-Need-to-Know-20190327-508.pdf

[19] Levy, D. T., Warner, K. E., Cummings, K. M., Hammonds, D., Kuo, C., Fong, G.T., Thrasher, J.F., Goniewicz, M.L., & Borland, R. (2018). Examining the relationship of vaping to smoking initiation among US youth and young adults: A reality check. *Tobacco Control.* http://dx.doi.org/10.1136/tobaccocontrol-2018-054446

[20] Budney, A. J., Sargent, J. D., & Lee, D. C. (2015). Vaping cannabis (marijuana): Parallel concerns to e-cigs? *Addiction, 110*(11), 1699-1704. https://doi.org/10.1111/add.13036

[21] Cummings, K. M., Morris, P. B., & Benowitz, N. L. (2018). *Another article about e-cigarettes: Why should I care?* Journal of the American Heart Association. https://doi.org/10.1161/JAHA.118.009944

[22] Levy, D. T., Warner, K. E., Cummings, K. M., Hammonds, D., Kuo, C., Fong, G.T., ...& Borland, R. (2018). Examining the relationship of vaping to smoking initiation among US youth and young adults: A reality check. *Tobacco Control.* http://dx.doi.org/10.1136/tobaccocontrol-2018-054446

[23] U.S. Food and Drug Administration. (2019). *Youth tobacco use: Results from the National Youth Tobacco Survey.* https://www.fda.gov/tobacco-products/youth-and-tobacco/youth-tobacco-use-results-national-youth-tobacco-survey

[24] Ibid.

[25] Centers for Disease Control and Prevention (CDC). (2019). *Quick facts on the risks of e-cigarettes for kids, teens, and young adults.* https://www.cdc.gov/tobacco/basic_information/e-cigarettes/Quick-Facts-on-the-Risks-of-E-cigarettes-for-Kids-Teens-and-Young-Adults.html

[26] Ibid.

[27] Cummings, K. M., Morris, P. B., & Benowitz, N. L. (2018). *Another article about e-cigarettes: Why should I care?* Journal of the American Heart Association. https://doi.org/10.1161/JAHA.118.009944

VAPING *(continued from previous page)*

[28] Centers for Disease Control and Prevention (CDC). (2019). *Quick facts on the risks of e-cigarettes for kids, teens, and young adults.* https://www.cdc.gov/tobacco/basic_information/e-cigarettes/Quick-Facts-on-the-Risks-of-E-cigarettes-for-Kids-Teens-and-Young-Adults.html

[29] Centers for Disease Control and Prevention (CDC). (n.d.). *E-cigarettes and youth: What parents need to know.* https://www.cdc.gov/tobacco/basic_information/e-cigarettes/pdfs/OSH-E-Cigarettes-and-Youth-What-Parents-Need-to-Know-20190327-508.pdf

[30] Centers for Disease Control and Prevention (CDC). (2020). *Outbreak of lung injury associated with the use of e-cigarette, or vaping, products.* https://www.cdc.gov/tobacco/basic_information/e-cigarettes/severe-lung-disease.html

[31] Ibid.

[32] Ibid.

[33] Cummings, K. M., Morris, P. B., & Benowitz, N. L. (2018). *Another article about e-cigarettes: Why should I care?* Journal of the American Heart Association. https://doi.org/10.1161/JAHA.118.009944

[34] Ibid.

[35] Centers for Disease Control and Prevention (CDC). (2019). *Quick facts on the risks of e-cigarettes for kids, teens, and young adults.* https://www.cdc.gov/tobacco/basic_information/e-cigarettes/Quick-Facts-on-the-Risks-of-E-cigarettes-for-Kids-Teens-and-Young-Adults.html

[36] Ibid.

[37] Centers for Disease Control and Prevention (CDC). (2019). *Quick facts on the risks of e-cigarettes for kids, teens, and young adults.* https://www.cdc.gov/tobacco/basic_information/e-cigarettes/Quick-Facts-on-the-Risks-of-E-cigarettes-for-Kids-Teens-and-Young-Adults.html

[38] Centers for Disease Control and Prevention (CDC). (n.d.). *E-cigarettes and youth: What parents need to know.* https://www.cdc.gov/tobacco/basic_information/e-cigarettes/pdfs/OSH-E-Cigarettes-and-Youth-What-Parents-Need-to-Know-20190327-508.pdf

[39] Ibid.

[40] Centers for Disease Control and Prevention (CDC). (2019). *Quick facts on the risks of e-cigarettes for kids, teens, and young adults.* https://www.cdc.gov/tobacco/basic_information/e-cigarettes/Quick-Facts-on-the-Risks-of-E-cigarettes-for-Kids-Teens-and-Young-Adults.html

[41] Perikleous, E. P., Steiropoulos, P., Paraskakis, E., Constantinidis, T. C., & Nena, E. (2018). E-cigarette use among adolescents: An overview of the literature and future perspectives. *Front Public Health*, *6*, 86. https://doi.org/10.3389/fpubh.2018.00086

[42] Centers for Disease Control and Prevention (CDC). (2019). *Quick facts on the risks of e-cigarettes for kids, teens, and young adults.* https://www.cdc.gov/tobacco/basic_information/e-cigarettes/Quick-Facts-on-the-Risks-of-E-cigarettes-for-Kids-Teens-and-Young-Adults.html

[43] Siegel, D. A., Jatlaoui, T. C., Koumans, E. H., Kiernan, E. A., Layer, M., Cates, J. E, Kimball, A., Weissman, D.N., Petersen, E.E., Reagan-Steiner, S., Godfred-Cato, S., Moulia, D., Moritz, E., Lehnert, J.D., Mitchko, J., London, J., Zaki, S.R., King, B.A., Jones, C.M., ... Lung Injury Response Epidemiology/Surveillance Group. (2019). Update: Interim guidance for health care providers evaluating and caring for patients with suspected e-cigarette, or vaping, product use associated lung injury. https://www.cdc.gov/mmwr/volumes/68/wr/mm6841e3.htm?s_cid=mm6841e3_e&deliveryName=USCDC_921-DM10905

[44] U.S. Food and Drug Administration. (2019). *Youth tobacco use: Results from the National Youth Tobacco Survey.* https://www.fda.gov/tobacco-products/youth-and-tobacco/youth-tobacco-use-results-national-youth-tobacco-survey

[45] Leingang, C. H, Shannon, R. A., & Mecham, J. (2019), Student behavior assessment and management. In J. Selekman, R. A. Shannon, & C. F. Yonkatais (Eds.), *School nursing: A comprehensive text* (3rd ed., pp. 742-755). F. A. Davis.

VAPING *(continued from previous page)*

[46] National Association of School Nurses. (2018). *The school nurse's role in behavioral/mental health of students* (Position Paper). https://www.nasn.org/nasn/advocacy/professional-practice-documents/position-statements/ps-behavioral-health

[47] Leingang, C. H, Shannon, R. A., & Mecham, J. (2019), Student behavior assessment and management. In J. Selekman, R. A. Shannon, & C. F. Yonkatais (Eds.), *School nursing: A comprehensive text* (3rd ed., pp. 742-755). F. A. Davis.

[48] Paterson, B. R, Bohnenekamp, J., Hoover, S., Bostic, J., & Selekman, J. (2019). Students with mental/behavioral health concerns and disorders. In J. Selekman, R. A. Shannon, & C. F. Yonkatais (Eds.), *School nursing: A comprehensive text* (3rd ed., pp. 757- 789. F. A. Davis.

[49] Siegel, D. A., Jatlaoui, T. C., Koumans, E. H., Kiernan, E. A., Layer, M., Cates, J. E, Kimball, A., Weissman, D.N., Petersen, E.E., Reagan-Steiner, S., Godfred-Cato, S., Moulia, D., Moritz, E., Lehnert, J.D., Mitchko, J., London, J., Zaki, S.R., King, B.A., Jones, C.M., ... Lung Injury Response Epidemiology/Surveillance Group. (2019). Update: Interim guidance for health care providers evaluating and caring for patients with suspected e-cigarette, or vaping, product use associated lung injury. https://www.cdc.gov/mmwr/volumes/68/wr/mm6841e3.htm?s_cid=mm6841e3_e&deliveryName=USCDC_921-DM10905

[50] Centers for Disease Control and Prevention (CDC). (2019). *Presentation for youth. Know the risks: A youth guide to e-cigarettes.* https://www.cdc.gov/tobacco/basic_information/e-cigarettes/youth-guide-to-e-cigarettes-presentation.html

[51] Stanford Medicine. (2019). *Tobacco prevention toolkit.* https://med.stanford.edu/tobaccopreventiontoolkit/E-Cigs.html

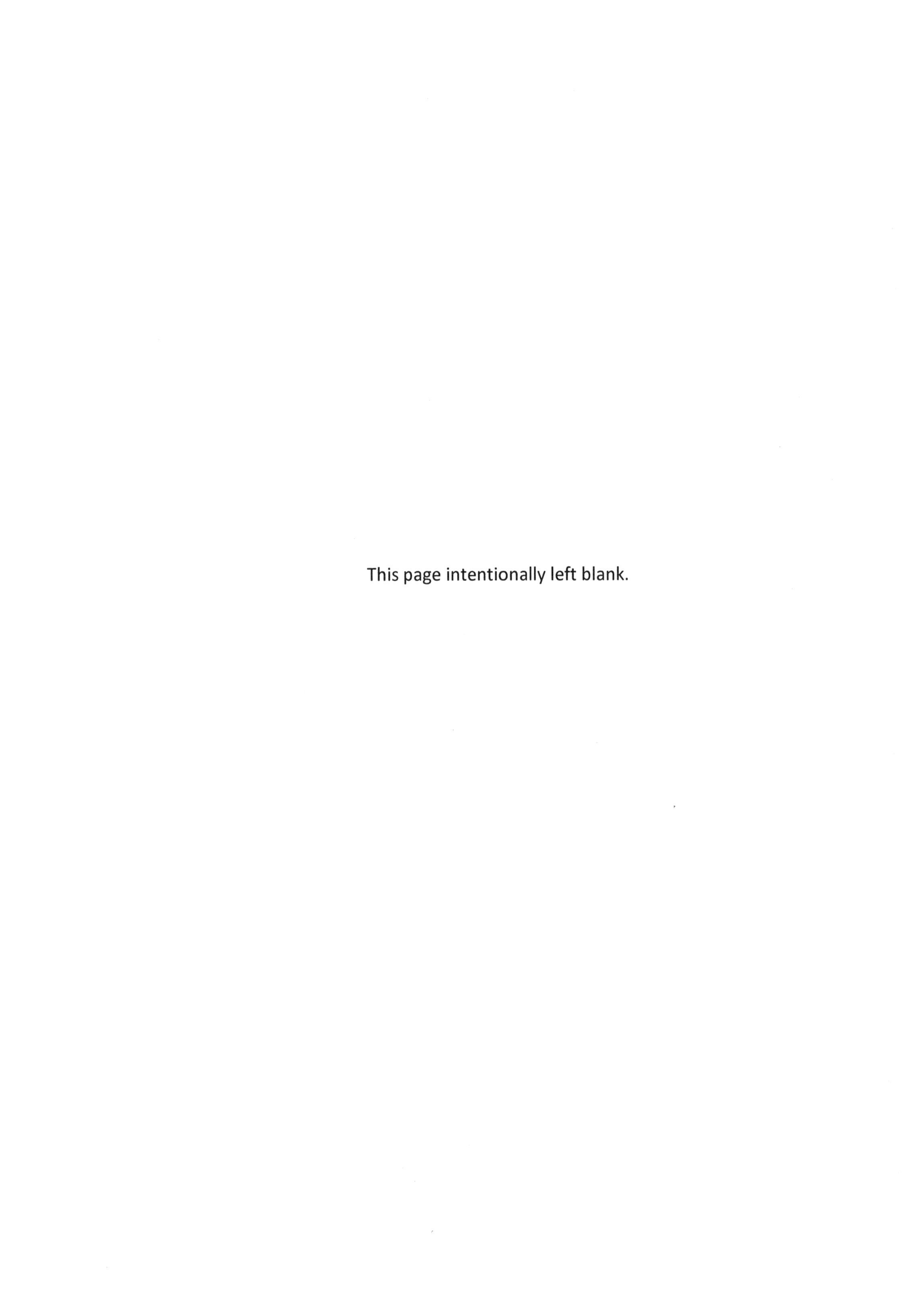
This page intentionally left blank.

SECTION IV

MANAGEMENT OF VULNERABLE POPULATIONS

SOCIAL DETERMINANTS OF HEALTH (SDOH)

This section of the manual discusses vulnerable populations, i.e. those populations with special considerations and needs due to a multitude of factors that influence their health and well-being. When developing policies and practices for these populations, attention must be paid to the social determinants of health (SDOH) in order to fully understand and affect change at the individual and community level.

DEFINITION:
According to Healthy People 2020, SODH are "conditions in the environments in which people are born, live, learn, work, play, worship, and age that affect a wide range of health, functioning, and quality-of-life outcomes and risks".[1]

The *place-based* social determinants of health framework include the following categories: economic stability, neighborhood and built environment, health and health care, social and community context, and education. Each of these areas of influence represents many of the issues that can impact the health of persons, families, and communities.[2] The following figure from the Kaiser Family Foundation is a clear depiction of the many factors in each domain.[3]

Figure 1

Social Determinants of Health

Economic Stability	Neighborhood and Physical Environment	Education	Food	Community and Social Context	Health Care System
Employment Income Expenses Debt Medical bills Support	Housing Transportation Safety Parks Playgrounds Walkability Zip code / geography	Literacy Language Early childhood education Vocational training Higher education	Hunger Access to healthy options	Social integration Support systems Community engagement Discrimination Stress	Health coverage Provider availability Provider linguistic and cultural competency Quality of care

Health Outcomes
Mortality, Morbidity, Life Expectancy, Health Care Expenditures, Health Status, Functional Limitations

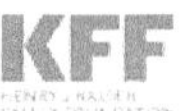

SOCIAL DETERMINANTS OF HEALTH (SDOH) *(continued from previous page)*

Within these domains, school nurses may witness many indicators that influence the health and well-being of their students, families, and communities. They include, but are not limited to, food insecurity, poverty, housing instability, access to healthcare, health literacy, green space availability, safe neighborhoods, early childhood education, and high school graduation rates.[4]

School nurses play a vital role in the health of their respective communities. According the National Association of School Nurses (NASN), "school nurses are public health's eyes and ears for the nation's children and families".[5] As part of the public health system, school nurses understand the needs of their students and families and are ideally situated to collaborate with others to strengthen the positive attributes and mitigate the negative impact of the SDOH on children and their communities.

Using the ten essential components for public health practice (as seen in the figure below), school nurses can focus on SDOH by assessing need, developing interventions and resources, and continually evaluating outcomes and risks.[6, 7]

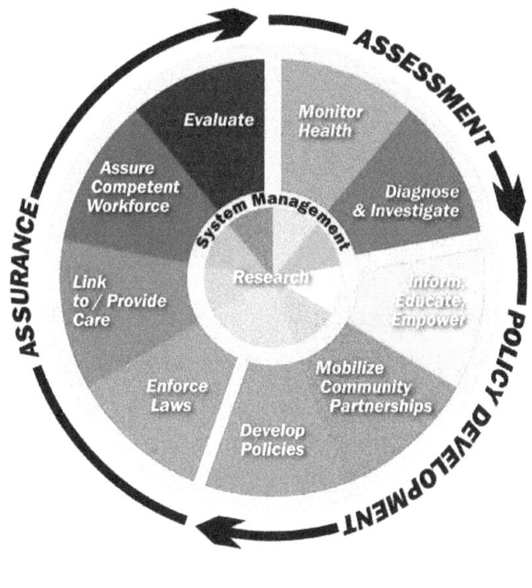

CDC (2018)

For example, in one study, adolescent males were more likely to receive sexual health services after school nurses simply provided information about sexual and reproductive health to the adolescent males during routine visits to the health office (no matter what the reason for the visit).[8] Clearly, this is an example how a school nurse's assessment and intervention regarding a social need (access to care) can have a significant impact.

SOCIAL DETERMINANTS OF HEALTH (SDOH) *(continued from previous page)*

POTENTIAL IMPLICATIONS:

Emerging research related to SDOH and health outcomes suggests that these conditions impact health equity and health disparities. Data from the Centers for Disease Control and Prevention (CDC) and World Health Organization indicate that those experiencing greater negative social conditions have more inequities related to access and care as well as higher incidences of diseases/infections.[9,10] An extensive systematic review conducted in 2018 used civil rights (i.e., housing, education, employment and health) as a framework for examining SDOH and the evidence suggests that improvement in civil rights in turn improves population health. [11] This review further supports the impact of social disparities on health equity and access and calls upon the public health sector to consider these conditions in efforts to improve the health of populations.

STRATEGIES TO ADDRESS SDOH:

The Whole School, Whole Community, Whole Child (WSCC), developed by ASCD and CDC, is a national model that can engage the whole community to help these vulnerable children and their families overcome social conditions. According to CDC, "the education, public health, and school health sectors have each called for greater alignment that includes, integration and collaboration between education leaders and health sectors to improve each child's cognitive, physical, social, and emotional development…the WSCC model focuses on the child to align the common goals of both sectors to put into action a whole child approach to education". [12] This whole child approach provides a structure for the school nurse to collaborate with partners in the school and community to work together to address the SDOH.

According to the NASN (2017), the role of the school nurse in community engagement and collaboration within the WCSS approach is fully appreciated when school nurses employ the principles of the Framework for 21st Century School Nursing. This framework calls for the school nurse to practice under five tenets: Standards of Practice, Care Coordination, Leadership, Quality Improvement, and Community/Public Health. Using this framework to guide practice, school nurses can positively affect student health and achievement. [13]

The following activities can be employed by the nurses:

1. Inform decision makers on the need to develop policies that address social and physical environments where students and their families live, work, learn, and play.
2. Develop resources for families regarding health insurance, health care, and access to health care, such as referrals to healthcare providers, promoting use of school-based health centers or telehealth, and engaging in wellness programs in the school and community.
3. Serve as a leader in the promotion of the WSCC approach to engage partners within and outside of the school to assist in meeting the social and health needs of children and their families.

SOCIAL DETERMINANTS OF HEALTH (SDOH) *(continued from previous page)*

STRATEGIES TO ADDRESS SDOH *(continued)*

4. Support the implementation of school meal programs that include addressing food insecurity during non-school time, such as school vacations and weekends.
5. Promote the development of social programs, such as before- and after-school programs for all-aged youth and adult education programs for young adults and parents.
6. Engage in school climate initiatives that encourage healthy relationships, civility, and anti-bullying efforts.
7. Assess and recommend strategies to improve the physical environments for children and their families, such as indoor air quality in schools, safe housing and playgrounds, and green spaces for outside activities.
8. Partner with health educators within the school to promote health literacy and enable students to develop positive health behaviors and wellness skills.
9. Support the increased physical activity and physical education opportunities both within and outside school.
10. Strategize with school team members to address chronic absenteeism.

RESOURCES

- **Centers for Disease Control and Prevention**. (2018). *Ten Essential Public Health Services and How They Can Include Addressing Social Determinants of Health Inequities.* https://www.cdc.gov/publichealthgateway/publichealthservices/pdf/ten_essential_services_and_sdoh.pdf
- **Centers for Disease Control and Prevention.** (2018). Tools for Putting Social Determinants of Health into Action [webpage]. https://www.cdc.gov/socialdeterminants/tools/index.htm

REFERENCES

[1] U.S. Department of Health and Human Services. (2019). *Social determinants of health*. p. 5. https://www.healthypeople.gov/2020/topics-objectives/topic/social-determinants-of-health

[2] Ibid.

[3] Artiga, S. & Hinton, E. (2018). *Beyond health care: The role of social determinants in promoting health and health equity. Kaiser Family Foundation* [Issue Brief]. p. 2. https://www.kff.org/disparities-policy/issue-brief/beyond-health-care-the-role-of-social-determinants-in-promoting-health-and-health-equity/

[4] U.S. Department of Health and Human Services. (2019). *Social determinants of health*. https://www.healthypeople.gov/2020/topics-objectives/topic/social-determinants-of-health

[5] ASTHO, APHN, NACCHO, & NASN. (2016). *Public health and school nursing: Collaborating to promote health* (White Paper). https://higherlogicdownload.s3.amazonaws.com/NASN/3870c72d-fff9-4ed7-833f-215de278d256/UploadedImages/PDFs/Advocacy/2016PHandSN.pdf

[6] Ibid.

SOCIAL DETERMINANTS OF HEALTH (SDOH) *(continued from previous page)*

[7] Centers for Disease Control and Prevention. (2018). *Ten essential public health services and how they can include addressing social determinants of health inequities.* https://www.cdc.gov/publichealthgateway/publichealthservices/pdf/ten_essential_services_and_sdoh.pdf

[8] Dittus, P., Harper, C., Becasen, J., Donatello, R., & Etheir, K. (2018). Structural intervention with school nurses increases sexual health care among male high school students. *Journal of Adolescent Health*, 62 (1), 52-58. doi: 10.1016/j.jadohealth.2017.07.017

[9] Centers for Disease Control and Prevention. (2018). *CDC research on SDOH.* https://www.cdc.gov/socialdeterminants/index.htm

[10] World Health Organization. (2019). *World conference on social determinants of health.* https://www.who.int/sdhconference/resources/case_studies/en/

[11] Hahn, R., Truman, B., & Williams, D. (2018). Civil rights as determinants of public health and racial and ethnic health equity: Health care, education, employment and housing in the United States. *Social Science & Medicine -Population Health*, 4, 17-24. doi: 10.1016/j.ssmph.2017.10.006

[12] Centers for Disease Control and Prevention, Healthy Schools. (2019). *Whole School, Whole Community, Whole Child (WSCC).* p. 1. https://www.cdc.gov/healthyschools/wscc/index.htm

[13] National Association of School Nurses. (2017). *Whole School, Whole Community, Whole Child: Implications for 21st century school nurses* (Position Statement). Silver Springs, MD: author. p. 2. https://www.nasn.org/nasn/advocacy/professional-practice-documents/position-statements/ps-wscc

BULLYING IN THE SCHOOL SETTING

OVERVIEW/DEFINITION:

In 2017, approximately 20% of students reported being bullied during the school year.[1] Definitions of bullying may vary but can generally be described as unwanted, aggressive behavior that involves a real or perceived power imbalance. The behavior is repeated or has the potential to be repeated over time. It can include physical, social or verbal bullying.[2] It has become increasingly common that student's may be bullied on-line with platforms such as Facebook, Twitter, Snapchat or by a text. This is referred to as cyberbullying.[3] Bullying in the school setting can happen to any student but vulnerable populations such as students with disabilities or lesbian, gay, bisexual or transgender students are more likely to be subject to all types of bullying.[4] The incidence of bullying peaks in middle school around ages 11 to 14 years and decreases somewhat in high school.[5] Most states have laws that require districts and schools to have a bullying policy and procedures and to investigate and respond to bullying when it occurs.[6] **School nurses are a crucial part of the school team. Preventing bullying as well as identifying students who may be or have been bullied is an essential component of the school nurse role.**

ANTICIPATED CONCERNS:

- The negative effects of bullying can be seen not only in the student that is the perceived subject of the bullying behavior but also in those that have witnessed the bullying, or the student who is the aggressor.[7]
- Short- and long-term consequences can include increased school absenteeism, diminished educational achievement, sleep deprivation, low self-esteem, depression and anxiety as well as an increase in physical symptoms such as stomachaches and headaches, some of which can continue into adulthood.[8]
- The targets of bullying are at three times higher risk for depression, anxiety, intentional non-suicidal self- injury and suicide ideation.[9]
- An increased use of alcohol and drug use is also associated with students who bully.[10]
- There have also been many high-profile cases which include suicide or violence in schools that involve allegations of bullying impacting school safety.

MANAGEMENT/POTENTIAL INTERVENTIONS:

Prevention:

- Work with school administrators, staff and the community to develop anti-bullying policies that should be widely distributed and woven into the school environment.
- Educate students on the why sometimes the intent on "teasing" can be interpreted as hurtful.
- Model respect, kindness and appropriate language when interacting with students and staff.
- Develop a sense of community in the school.
- Identify students at risk for bullying and help develop protective factors such as connectedness with the school, increased self -esteem, having a friend and having at least one adult the student trusts in the school.
- Share observations of students at risk and any suspicion of bullying with school teams.
- Assure that the health office is a safe place where students can share concerns openly.

BULLYING IN THE SCHOOL SETTING *(continued from previous page)*

MANAGEMENT/POTENTIAL INTERVENTIONS *(continued)*

- Be alert to the possibility of bullying for students with frequent somatic complaints.
- Be an advocate for social-emotional learning in the classroom.
- Advocate for and become involved in school wide prevention programs.
- Be knowledgeable about you state laws and school policies regarding bullying.

Intervention:

- Address all incidences of mean-spirited behavior in the health office with consistency.
- Report all incidences of perceived bullying to school administration.
- Reassure all students involved in the perceived bullying that school is a safe place.
- Educate students who demonstrated tendencies to bully or to exhibit aggressive behavior of what specific behaviors were problematic.[11]
- Reassure and educate students who have witnessed bullying on what they can do in the future to help stop the bullying behavior.[12]
- Address the medical and mental health needs of students involved in perceived bullying, both the aggressor and the recipient of any behavior.

FOLLOW-UP:

Incidences of bullying should be monitored to note trends and assess effectiveness of school wide interventions. Individual incidences of bullying should be addressed quickly and calmly. This gives the message to all students that bullying is taken seriously in the school. Notifying parents/guardians of all students involved is essential as well as providing evidenced based interventions that can be supported at home.

NOTES:

Bullying is a complex problem that involves families and communities as well as schools. Education of all school staff including cafeteria workers, custodians and bus drivers is essential to make improvements in school climate throughout the school community. This may happen through in-service programs to help raise awareness and provide them with prevention and intervention strategies. As bullying often happens on the bus ride or in the cafeteria or hallways, all staff should be prepared to intervene and bring it to the attention of administration. Zero tolerance policies or policies that involve suspension or exclusion have not been found to be effective because they do not address behavior change or the address the root of the problem.[13]

BULLYING IN THE SCHOOL SETTING *(continued from previous page)*

REFERENCES

[1] National Center for Educational Statistics. (2019). https://nces.ed.gov/fastfacts/display.asp?id=719

[2] Stop Bullying. (2018). *What is bullying?* https://www.stopbullying.gov/what-is-bullying/index.html

[3] Stop bullying. (2018). *What is cyberbullying?* https://www.stopbullying.gov/cyberbullying/what-is-it/index.html#frequencyofcyberbullying

[4] National Association of School Nurses. (2018). *Bullying and cyberbullying-prevention in school* (Position Statement). https://www.nasn.org/nasn/advocacy/professional-practice-documents/position-statements/ps-bullying

[5] Gordon, S., & Selekman, J. (2019). Student victimization. In J. Selekman, R. Adair Shannon, & C. F. Yonkaitis (Eds.), *School nursing: A comprehensive text* (3rd ed., pp. 738-804). F.A. Davis.

[6] Stop Bullying. (2018). *Laws, policies and regulations.* https://www.stopbullying.gov/laws/index.html

[7] Bradshaw, C. (2015). Translating research to practice in bullying prevention. *American Psychologist,70* (4,) 322–332. https://www.apa.org/pubs/journals/releases/amp-a0039114.pdf

[8] National Association of School Nurses. (2018). *Bullying and cyberbullying-prevention in school* (Position Statement). https://www.nasn.org/nasn/advocacy/professional-practice-documents/position-statements/ps-bullying

[9] Gordon, S., & Selekman, J. (2019). Student Victimization. In J. Selekman, R. Adair Shannon, & C. F. Yonkaitis (Eds.), *School nursing: A comprehensive text* (3rd ed., pp. 738-804). F.A. Davis.

[10] National Association of School Nurses. (2018). *Bullying and cyberbullying-prevention in school* (Position Statement). https://www.nasn.org/nasn/advocacy/professional-practice-documents/position-statements/ps-bullying

[11] Gordon, S., & Selekman, J. (2019). Student victimization. In J. Selekman, R. Adair Shannon, & C. F. Yonkaitis (Eds.), *School nursing: A comprehensive text* (3rd ed., pp. 738-804). F.A. Davis.

[12] Ibid.

[13] Ibid.

CHILD MALTREATMENT

DEFINITION/ETIOLOGY:

Child abuse and neglect is defined in federal legislation as "any recent act or failure to act on the part of a parent or caretaker which results in death, serious injury or emotional harm, sexual abuse or exploitation, or an act or failure to act which presents an imminent risk of serious harm".[1] At least one in seven children have experienced child abuse or neglect in the past year.[2] Children with disabilities are nearly four times more likely to be physically abused or neglected and three times more likely to be sexually abused than children without disabilities.[3]

ANTICIPATED CONCERNS/PROBLEMS:

School nurses need to be skilled at recognizing, assessing and responding to the signs of child abuse and neglect in addition to understanding and complying with school policies and state laws. School nurses often work with a large population of students that includes providing care to youth who have been reported to state child protection agencies, removed from their biological parents or have been returned to their biological parents. Providing school nursing services to children that were maltreated requires ongoing assessment and monitoring to ensure their safety and that adequate growth and development is occurring. Impaired academic functioning, growth failure, obesity, eating disorders, and unmet oral health needs are examples of some of the areas of concern for children with a history of maltreatment.[4]

Research has shown there are long term and intergenerational consequences from child maltreatment. Individuals who experienced abuse, neglect, or other forms of childhood adversity are more likely than nonexposed individuals to have children who go on to have similar adverse childhood experiences.[5] Adverse Childhood Experiences (ACEs) is the term used to describe all types of abuse, neglect, and other potentially traumatic experiences that occur to people under the age of 18. The adverse experiences have been linked to risky health behaviors, chronic health conditions, low life potential and early death.[6]

RISKS FOR CHILD ABUSE:

Some risk factors can make a child more vulnerable to abuse. Examples can be found in the background of parents, environmental situations and attributes of the child.[7]

Parental Factors:

- Parent who has already abused a child
- Pregnancy was not wanted
- Parent has a background of abuse when growing up
- Young, unsupported mother often with low education
- Parents have unrealistic expectations of the child and lack parenting knowledge
- Parent is isolated and has few supports
- Parent has a mental illness or is abusing drugs or alcohol

CHILD MALTREATMENT *(continued from previous page)*

RISKS FOR CHILD ABUSE *(continued)*

Environmental Factors:

- Overcrowding in the house
- Poverty or lack of opportunity to improve the family's resources
- Family violence is present
- A non-biological adult living in the house
- Family is experiencing multiple stresses

Child Factors:

- Baby is sickly, colicky or unwanted
- Child has a physical or developmental disability
- Child is the product of an abusive relationship
- Lack of attachment between child and parent

SIGNS AND SYMPTOMS:

Physical Signs of Child Maltreatment:[8,9]

- Any injury (bruise, burn, fracture, abdominal or head injury) that cannot be explained or is inconsistent with the injury
- Failure to gain weight (especially in infants) or a sudden dramatic weight gain
- Genital pain or bleeding
- A sexually transmitted disease or pregnancy

Other Changes/Signs that Should Raise Concern:[10,11]

- Fearful behavior
- Abdominal pain
- Bed wetting after they have learned to stay dry
- Attempts to run away
- Extreme sexual behavior that seems inappropriate for the child's age
- Sudden change in self-confidence
- Headaches or stomachaches with no medical cause
- Abnormal fears, increased nightmares
- School failure or poor school attendance
- Extremely passive or aggressive behavior
- Desperately affectionate behavior or social withdrawal
- Big appetite or stealing food
- Statements that he or she was sexually abused
- Lack of appropriate attention for medical, dental or psychological problems or lack of necessary follow-up care

CHILD MALTREATMENT *(continued from previous page)*

MANAGEMENT/POTENTIAL INTERVENTIONS:

- Utilize a trauma-informed approach as an effective strategy for working with victims of child maltreatment.[12]
- Identify safety concerns and determine if there any urgent or life-threatening medical conditions that need to be addressed.
- Follow state law and school district/fiduciary policies and procedures for reporting child maltreatment.
- Follow school district/fiduciary guidelines for retaining records of child abuse reporting and documentation.
- Use a body diagram noting all cutaneous lesions by size, location and color.[13]
- Understand that it is not the healthcare provider's responsibility to conduct the investigation and determine whether abuse exists. It is the responsibility of the provider to report any suspicion of child maltreatment.
- Maintain confidentiality.
- Document subjective and objective findings, interventions and follow-up plan.
- Ensure that any screening for child sexual abuse is completed by an individual/team that has appropriate training and credentials.

FOLLOW UP:

- Monitor the child to ensure safety, food security, academic growth and ongoing health care (may require more frequent visits to healthcare provider, dental care).
- Refer children and families to evidence-based therapeutic treatment such as, cognitive behavioral therapy, which includes parent and child education; teaching safety skills and coping techniques; facilitating a coherent narrative of the traumatic event and emotional and cognitive processing.[14]
- Support the victims of child maltreatment by encouraging them to form relationships with caring adults.
- Consider routinely utilizing risk assessment and depression screening tools to identify children and youth at risk for adverse outcomes due to maltreatment.
- Provide community resources to victims and families and encourage the family to follow through with recommendations from Children's Protection Services.
- Consider a referral to Family Voices which provides resources and support to families of children with special needs (http://familyvoices.org/) or other appropriate organizations.[15]

SCHOOL AND COMMUNITY COLLABORATION:

- Educate school staff about the signs and symptoms of child maltreatment and the process for reporting child maltreatment.
- Support universal school-based programs that strengthen youth skills.
- Initiate working relationships with the local Child Protection Agency and other community agencies that provide resources and support to families.
- Collaborate with local agencies to use evidence-based strategies to prevent childhood maltreatment.[16]

CHILD MALTREATMENT *(continued from previous page)*

POTENTIAL COMPLICATIONS:

Complications are long term for victims of child maltreatment and can include:

- Aggressive behaviors, sexually reactive behaviors, depression and difficulty sustaining attention[17]
- Poor health in general as adults related to trauma (unintended pregnancy, poor pregnancy outcomes, HIV, STDs, cancer, diabetes, substance abuse)[18]
- Mental health problems as adults (depression, suicide, PTSD, anxiety)[19]

NOTES:

Each state provides its own definitions of child abuse and neglect based on minimum standards set by federal law.

REFERENCES

[1] Child Welfare Information Gateway (2019). Child abuse & neglect. https://www.childwelfare.gov/topics/can/

[2] Centers for Disease Control and Prevention (2019). Preventing child abuse and neglect. https://www.cdc.gov/violenceprevention/childabuseandneglect/fastfact.html

[3] Brodie, N., McColgan, M.D., Spector, N.D., & Turchi, R.M. (2017). Child abuse in children and youth with special health care needs. *Pediatrics in Review, 38*(10), 463-470. https://doi.org/10.1542/pir.2016-0098

[4] Flaherty, E., Legano, L., & Idzerda, S. (2019). Ongoing pediatric health care for the child who has been maltreated. *Pediatrics, 143*(4), 1-16. https://doi.org/10.1542/peds.2019-0284

[5] Merreck, M.T. & Guinn, A.S. (2018). Child abuse and neglect: Breaking the intergenerational link. *American Journal of Public Health, 108*(8), 1117 – 1118. https://doi.org/10.2105/AJPH.2018.304636

[6] Centers for Disease Control and Prevention (2019). About adverse childhood experiences. : https://www.cdc.gov/violenceprevention/childabuseandneglect/acestudy/aboutace.html

[7] Child Matters. (n.d.). *Risk factors of child abuse*. http://www.childmatters.org.nz/57/learn-about-child-abuse/risk-factors

[8] Glick, J.C., Lorand, M.A., & Bilka, K.R. (2016). Physical abuse of children. *Pediatrics in Review, 37*(4), 146-158. https://doi.org/ 1542/pir.2015-001

[9] Sege, R.D. & Amaya-Jackson, L. (2017). Clinical considerations related to the behavioral manifestations of child maltreatment. *Pediatrics, 139*(4), e1-e13. https://doi.org/10.1542/peds.2017-0100

[10] Glick, J.C., Lorand, M.A., & Bilka, K.R. (2016). Physical abuse of children. *Pediatrics in Review, 37*(4), 146-158. https://doi.org/1542/pir.2015-001

[11] Sege, R.D. & Amaya-Jackson, L. (2017). Clinical considerations related to the behavioral manifestations of child maltreatment. *Pediatrics, 139*(4), e1-e13. https://doi.org/10.1542/peds.2017-0100

[12] SAMHSA (2014). Concept of trauma and guidance for a trauma-Informed approach. https://store.samhsa.gov/system/files/sma14-4884.pdf

[13] Glick, J.C., Lorand, M.A., & Bilka, K.R. (2016). Physical abuse of children. *Pediatrics in Review, 37*(4), 146-158. https://doi.org/1542/pir.2015-001

CHILD MALTREATMENT *(continued from previous page)*

[14] Sege, R.D. & Amaya-Jackson, L. (2017). Clinical considerations related to the behavioral manifestations of child maltreatment. *Pediatrics, 139*(4), e1-e13. https://doi.org/10.1542/peds.2017-0100

[15] Brodie, N., McColgan, M.D., Spector, N.D., & Turchi, R.M. (2017). Child abuse in children and youth with special health care needs. *Pediatrics in Review, 38*(10), 463-470. https://doi.org/10.1542/pir.2016-0098

[16] Centers for Disease Control and Prevention (2016). Preventing child abuse and neglect: A technical package for policy, norm, and programmatic activities. https://www.cdc.gov/violenceprevention/pdf/CAN-Prevention-Technical-Package.pdf

[17] Sege, R.D. & Amaya-Jackson, L. (2017). Clinical considerations related to the behavioral manifestations of child maltreatment. *Pediatrics, 139*(4), e1-e13. https://doi.org/10.1542/peds.2017-0100

[18] Centers for Disease Control and Prevention (2019). About adverse childhood experiences. https://www.cdc.gov/violenceprevention/childabuseandneglect/acestudy/aboutace.html

[19] Ibid.

DEVELOPMENTAL DISABILITIES

OVERVIEW/DEFINITION:

Developmental disabilities (DD) are a diverse group of physical, cognitive, psychological, sensory, and speech impairments that are identified prenatally up to 18 years of age. They are most likely to continue throughout life.[1] The DD result in considerable limitations in three or more of the following areas. Comprehension and language skills (receptive and expressive language), learning, and self-direction, are areas of limitation. Self-care mobility and the ability to function independently without coordinated services, which is the capacity for independent living and economic self-sufficiency is another area of limitation.

Type	Description/Characteristics
Autism Spectrum Disorders[2]	• Significantly affects verbal and nonverbal communication and social interaction
Attention Deficit Hyperactivity Disorder (ADHD)[3]	• There are 3 main symptoms: o the inability to focus, o hyperactivity, and o impulsivity • May be managed with medication and /or a behavior plan
Cerebral Palsy[4]	• The inability to control muscle responses and/or a weakness of the muscle • Ankle Foot Orthotics [AFOs] (braces) and splints help support the feet and legs for walking and for use of hands
Intellectual Development Disabilities (IDD)[5]	• Considered a condition, but actually a symptom of numerous different conditions • The person with IDD has a below average intelligence (I.Q.>55-70 range) with deficits in adaptive behavior and manifested during a developmental period • Common IDD are Fragile X syndrome, Fetal Alcohol syndrome, Down syndrome, Angelman syndrome, Prader Willie syndrome and toxoplasmosis • IDD can be diagnosed during pregnancy through blood tests (amniocentesis or chorionic villus) • After birth, intelligence quotient (I.Q.) test determine diagnosis in addition to observing behavior and assessing adaptive skills • Children with intellectual disabilities may become functional adults; they are able to learn, but do so slowly, and with difficulty
Learning Disabilities[6]	Specific types of learning problems include dyscalcula (math), dysgrahia (writing), and dyslexia (reading)
Hearing	• Unable to process communication through hearing with or without implication • May be permanent or fluctuate
Vision Impairment	• Depends on what part of the eye is affected and how much correction is possible through glasses, contacts, surgery or medicine • Senses of smell, touch, taste, and hearing are heightened
Vision and Hearing Impaired	• Causes severe developmental, communication and educational needs which may require a specific program to accommodate blind and deaf students.

DEVELOPMENTAL DISABILITIES *(continued from previous page)*

OVERVIEW/DEFINITION *(continued)*

Developmental disabilities may be caused by:[7]

- Traumatic Brain Injury (TBI) and other child maltreatment manifestations (shaken baby syndrome or head trauma)
- Prenatal or after birth nutrition or growth problems
- Prenatal or after birth infections
- Chromosome abnormalities
- Poor maternal diet, lack of prenatal care, substance abuse or OTC drugs
- Prematurity
- Environmental toxins (lead poisoning, infections)

ANTICIPATED CONCERNS:

- Vary depending on condition and severity
- Delay in developmental milestones (walking, talking, etc.)
- Speaking difficulty or talking later, difficulty with memory
- Unable to follow or understand rules of social behavior
- Difficulty solving problems or understanding outcomes of action
- IDDs that show up sooner may indicate a more severe disability

MANAGEMENT/POTENTIAL INTERVENTIONS:

- No cure is available for Developmental Disabilities (DD)
- Treatment specific to disability
- Access educational related services resources- physical therapy, occupational therapy, therapeutic speech therapy or nursing services
- Early intervention for children birth-3 years of age
- Development of an Individualized Family Service Plan (IFSP)
- Special education services 3-21 of age (a few states extend services beyond 21 years of age)
- Development of an Individualized Educational Plan (IEP)
- Transitional planning from school to community
- Communication devices and computer technology
- Special equipment depending on condition (e.g., standers, bikes, braces, wheelchairs, adaptive seating, eating utensils, sensory stimulation etc.)

DEVELOPMENTAL DISABILITIES *(continued from previous page)*

FOLLOW UP:[8]

- Develop an Individualized Healthcare Plan (IHP) if needed
- Investigate instructional and classroom accommodations
- Provide interventions based on needs of the student and evaluate the impact of the outcomes
- Hearing and vision screening (minimize sensory deficits)
- Dental care (prevent periodontal disease)
- Use multi-sensory approach
- Promote good nutrition
- Along with parents, monitor for signs of infection (e.g., ear and upper respiratory infections)
- Assist with transition planning from school to the community (IEP planning for transitioning must begin before the age of 16)

NOTES:

- The average I.Q. is 100, IDD can range from mild – IQ 55-70, moderate - IQ 40-54, severe – IQ 25-39, and profound- IQ less than 25

Laws:

- The Individuals with Disabilities Education Improvement Act (IDEIA) directs how educational services available through the state, school district and public agencies are provided to infants, toddlers, children and youth with disabilities https://sites.ed.gov/idea/

- Section 504 of the Rehabilitation Law prohibits educational discrimination on the basis of disability providing students with disabilities services who do not qualify for IDEIA https://www.wrightslaw.com/info/sec504.index.htm

- The American Disabilities Act (ADA) provides equality for people with disabilities (education, employment, transportation, access to buildings, etc.) http://www.ada.gov/

RESOURCES

- **Administration of Community Living, Administration of Intellectual Developmental Disabilities**. (2017). *AoD Programs.* http://www.acl.gov/Programs/AIDD/Index.aspx
- **Early Childhood Technical Assistance Center**. (2019). *State Part C Coordinators.* http://www.ectacenter.org/contact/ptccoord.asp
- **Center for Parent Information and Resources**. (2017). *Overview of Early Intervention.* http://www.parentcenterhub.org/repository/ei-overview/
- **National Dissemination Center for Children with Disabilities**. (2019). https://www.washington.edu/doit/national-dissemination-center-children-disabilities-nichcy
- **The HSC Foundation.** *Partnering with Your Child's School: A Guide for Parents.* https://hschealth.org/sites/default/files/partnering-with-schools-guide-english.pdf

DEVELOPMENTAL DISABILITIES *(continued from previous page)*

REFERENCES

[1] American Psychiatric Association (APA). (2013). *Diagnostic and statistical manual of mental disorders (DSM-V)* (5th ed.) https://doi.org/10.1176/appi.books.9780890425596

[2] Autism Science Foundation. (2018). *How common is autism?* https://autismsciencefoundation.org/what-is-autism/how-common-is-autism/

[3] Ball, J., Binder, R., & Cowen, K. (Eds.). (2017). Alterations in mental health and cognitive function. *Principles of pediatric nursing: Caring for children* (7th ed., pp. 790-821). Pearson Education.

[4] CDC. (2019). *Cerebral palsy*. https://www.cdc.gov/ncbddd/cp/facts.html

[5] The U.S. Equal Employment Opportunity Commission. (n.d.). *Questions & answers about persons with intellectual disabilities in the workplace and the Americans with Disabilities Act (ADA).* http://www.eeoc.gov/laws/types/intellectual_disabilities.cfm

[6] American Psychiatric Association (APA). (2013). *Diagnostic and statistical manual of mental disorders (DSM-V)* (5th ed.) https://doi.org/10.1176/appi.books.9780890425596

[7] Ball, J., Binder, R., & Cowen, K. (Eds.). (2017). Alterations in mental health and cognitive function. *Principles of pediatric nursing: Caring for children* (7th ed., pp. 790-821). Pearson Education.

[8] Crawford, L.J.R., & Whitehead, S. E. (2019). Students with neurodevelopmental disorders: Intellectual disabilities and autism. In J. Selekman, R.A. Shannon, & C. F. Younkaitis (Eds.), *School Nursing: A comprehensive text* (3rd ed., pp. 603-627). F.A. Davis.

OTHER REFERENCES CONSULTED

Centers for Disease Control. (2017). *Developmental disabilities.* http://www.cdc.gov/ncbddd/developmentaldisabilities/index.html

MedlinePlus. (2019). *Developmental disabilities*. http://www.nlm.nih.gov/medlineplus/developmentaldisabilities.html

National Dissemination Center for Children with Disabilities. (2017). *Disabilities.* http://nichcy.org/disability

National Dissemination Center for Children with Disabilities. (2019). Explore DO-IT programs and resources. https://www.washington.edu/doit/national-dissemination-center-children-disabilities-nichcy

Selekman, J., & Ness, M. (2019). Students with chronic conditions. In J. Selekman, R.A. Shannon, & C. F. Younkaitis (Eds.), *School Nursing: A comprehensive text* (3rd ed., pp.480-500). F.A. Davis.

U.S. Department of Education. (2018). *OSEP's annual reports to Congress on the implementation of the Individuals with Disabilities Education Act (IDEA)*. Washington, DC: Author. http://www2.ed.gov/about/reports/annual/osep/index.html

DOWN SYNDROME (TRISOMY 21)

OVERVIEW/DEFINITION:[1, 2, 3, 4]

Down syndrome is a relatively common birth defect with an anomaly of chromosome 21 that can cause intellectual disability, microcephaly, short stature, and characteristic facies. Diagnosis is usually based on the physical anomalies, abnormal development and confirmed by cytogenic analysis.

About six thousand children with Down syndrome are born in the United States each year or in about one out of seven hundred babies. Females of any age can have a child with Down syndrome, but the risk increases in women older than thirty-five years.

There are two basic types of tests available to detect Down syndrome during pregnancy: screening tests and diagnostic tests. Screening tests do not provide definitive diagnosis but are safer for the mother and developing baby. Diagnostic tests pose more risk for the mother and developing baby, but the tests are not definitive of the full impact of Down syndrome on the baby.

There are three types of Down syndrome. People often can't tell the difference between each type without looking at the chromosomes because the physical features and behaviors are similar.

- **Trisomy 21:** About 95% of people with Down syndrome have trisomy 21. With this type of Down syndrome, each cell in the body has three separate copies of chromosome 21 instead of the usual 2 copies.[5]
- **Translocation Down syndrome:** This type accounts for a small percentage of people with Down syndrome (about 3%). This occurs when an extra part or a whole extra chromosome 21 is present, but it is attached or trans-located to a different chromosome rather than being a separate chromosome 21.[6]
- **Mosaic Down syndrome:** This type affects about 2% of the people with Down syndrome. Mosaic means mixture or combination. For children with mosaic Down syndrome, some of their cells have 3 copies of chromosome 21, but other cells have the typical two copies of chromosome 21. Children with mosaic Down syndrome may have the same features as other children with Down syndrome; however, they may have fewer features of the condition due to the presence of some, or many, cells with a typical number of chromosomes.[7]

SIGNS AND SYMPTOMS/COMMON CHARACTERISTICS:[8]

Down syndrome presents with many individual differences at varying levels as many genetic, epigenetic, and environmental factors play a role in how the Down syndrome phenotype expresses itself.[9] Down syndrome may include the following:

- Flat facial profile/flattening of nasal bridge
- Flattened occiput
- Microcephaly
- Almond shaped eyes that slant up (palpebral fissures)
- Epicanthal folds

DOWN SYNDROME (TRISOMY 21) *(continued from previous page)*

SIGNS AND SYMPTOMS/COMMON CHARACTERISTICS *(continued)*

- Midface hypoplasia
- Short neck with extra skin
- Small dysplastic ears (pinnae)
- Small hands and feet
- Short fingers
- Small pinky fingers that may curve toward the thumb
- Furrowed tongue lacking a central fissure that extends out of the mouth
- Tiny white spots on the iris of the eye (Brushfield spots)
- Palmar crease (single line across the palm of the hand)
- Minor limb abnormalities
- Shorter in height
- Atlantoaxial instability
- Propensity for obesity/overweight
- Wide gap between 1st and 2nd toes (sandal-gap toes)
- Plantar furrow
- Skin disorders (e.g., decreased skin tone, dry skin, alopecia areata, vitiligo, folliculitis)
- Umbilical hernia
- Congenital heart defects (e.g., atrioventricular or ventricular septal defects, Tetralogy of Fallot, isolated patent ductus arteriosus, murmurs, heart failure)
- Propensity for low muscle tone or loose joints
- Motor delays/development
- Feeding difficulties
- Placid, rarely cries (infant)
- Hearing loss
- Intellectual disability (IQs ranging from 20-85 with mean approximately 50)
- Behavior/psychiatric disorders
- Hirschsprung disease (absence of stools)
- Duodenal atresia or stenosis (resulting in nausea, vomiting)
- Sleep/obstructive apnea with snoring, restlessness during sleep and difficulty waking
- Thyroid disease
- Prone to dental and gum diseases
- More susceptible to or may develop more complications to respiratory tract infections (e.g., colds, ear infections)
- Diastasis recti

DOWN SYNDROME (TRISOMY 21) *(continued from previous page)*

MANAGEMENT/TREATMENT: [10]

- Genetic counseling
- Auditory brain stem response (ABR) or brainstem auditory evoked response (BAER) testing
- Standard immunizations and well-childcare
- Visits with specialists for associated conditions (e.g., endocrine, infectious, cardiac, respiratory, neurologic, psychiatric, dermatologic, and dental disorders)
- Ophthalmologic evaluations
- Frequent ear exams and auditory evaluations (annually after early infancy) due to increased risk for otitis media and secondary hearing loss
- Timely surgical treatment of cardiac and gastrointestinal anomalies
- Surgical intervention of cervical spine if neurological deficits clinically significant (atlantoaxial instability)
- Extraction of congenital cataracts soon after birth with correction (glasses, contact lenses)
- Careful anesthetic airway management with associated risk of cervical spine instability
- Early intervention programs (e.g., social, cognitive, physical therapy, early education)
- Children thirty-six (36) months and older may receive special education available through public school along with related services (e.g., occupational therapy, physical therapy, speech language therapy, nursing services, behavioral/mental health, counseling) to ensure the child can safely access and succeed in the educational environment
- Sleep study by age 4 years for possible sleep apnea
- Adenotonsillectomy may be performed to manage obstructive sleep apnea

POSSIBLE COMPLICATIONS:[11]

Complications of Down syndrome can involve almost every organ system of the body; yet, the overall outlook for individuals with Down syndrome has dramatically improved.

- Behavioral changes or school problems due to sleep apnea with difficulty waking, daytime somnolence, etc.
- Otitis media, alveolar hypoventilation, arterial hypoxemia, cerebral hypoxia, and pulmonary arterial hypertension with resulting cor pulmonale and heart failure secondary to airway obstruction in addition to pre-existing congenital heart defects
- Fainting episodes, palpitations, irregular pulse rate & rhythm, chest pain due to heart/valvular issues
- Absence of stools/defecation issues possibly due to Hirschsprung disease
- Duodenal atresia
- Esophageal atresia
- Social isolation due to low social competence
- Delay in language development, specifically expressive skills
- High risk for bullying, physical, and sexual abuse due to delays in cognitive abilities, motor development, language development, and social competence as well as physical appearance
- Mobility issues (joint dislocations, genu valgus, overpronation of the ankle, flat feet due to ligamentous laxity and hypotonia)

DOWN SYNDROME (TRISOMY 21) *(continued from previous page)*

POSSIBLE COMPLICATIONS *(continued)*

- Congenital heart disease associated issues (e.g., arrythmias, valvular)
- Leukemia (acute lymphoblastic leukemia (ALL), acute myeloid leukemia (AML)) especially in the first few years of life with a 20-fold increased risk for ALL[12]
- Thyroid diseases (e.g., hypothyroidism)
- Autoimmune disorders
- Epilepsy
- Recurrent respiratory infections
- Irreversible spinal-cord damage (if atlantoaxial instability not addressed)
- Attention-deficit/hyperactivity disorder, oppositional defiant disorder, autism spectrum disorder features, depression, obsessive-compulsive disorder
- Insulin dependent diabetes mellitus type 1
- Dental caries and periodontal disease
- Premature aging
- Alzheimer-like dementia (progressive by age 40 years due to extra copy of the APP gene which codes for the amyloid precursor protein) Would include a reference

FOLLOW UP:[13, 14]

- Highly recommended that students have an Individualized Healthcare Plan (IHP), Emergency Care Plan(s) (ECP), or if indicated, a Section 504 Plan or Individualized Education Plan (IEP) to ensure they receive appropriate school-based health related services in school
- Early intervention programs for preschool aged
- Continued annual audiologic and ophthalmologic evaluations in adolescence as well as hearing aid maintenance, if required
- Sleep studies/apnea monitoring
- Thyroid function testing annually due to the high risk for acquired hypothyroidism
- Monitoring of gastroesophageal reflux and swallowing difficulties as well as the development of celiac disease (gluten allergy)
- In addition to a primary medical home pediatrician/healthcare provider, referrals/consultations and follow-up should continue with clinical geneticist, developmental pediatrician, cardiologist, pulmonologist, ophthalmologist, dentist, neurologist/neurosurgeon, orthopedic specialist, child psychiatrist, physical and occupational therapist, speech-language pathologist, and audiologist
- Monitoring for the development of heart failure and pulmonary hypertension as well as acquired heart valve disease for those with congenital heart disease
- Monitoring for signs and symptoms of myelopathy
- Bone marrow examination to rule out leukemia
- Medication management which may include medication administration during school hours with training for unlicensed assistive personnel, if delegation is permissible and appropriate

DOWN SYNDROME (TRISOMY 21) *(continued from previous page)*

FOLLOW UP *(continued)*

- Review of the child's educational programming with possible adaptations to include the school health and related services (e.g., medication administration, physical therapy, speech-language therapy)
- Teacher and caregiver training on how to adapt daily lessons and schedules to accommodate child's educational and health needs
- Specific training on special needs conditions (e.g., seizures, diabetes mellitus, asthma)
- Parent/caregiver counseling on increased risk for physical, and sexual abuse due to delays in cognitive abilities, motor development, language development, and social competence
- Transition to adulthood issues for adolescents
    - educational progression
    - vocational training
    - pediatric to adult medical/health providers (including gynecologic for women)
    - sexual health and socialization (degree of supervision)
    - well-balanced diet and exercise routine
    - living arrangements
    - estate planning & custody arrangements
    - social and recreational program referrals with friends
    - respite care/supportive care or counseling for family
    - parent counseling on increased risk for sexual abuse of individuals with Down syndrome
- Papanicolaou smears every one to three years in sexually active women
- Regular screening for institutionalized older adults to diagnose early onset dementia, epilepsy, hypothyroidism, and early loss of visual acuity and hearing

NOTES:[15]

- Many with Down syndrome talk out loud to themselves as a way of understanding and processing information
- Strong visual learners learn best via pictures, objects or demonstration
- Many with Down syndrome can participate in regular classrooms (i.e., inclusion) though they may need extra help or modifications

RESOURCES

- **Down Syndrome Resource Foundation**. (2016). https://www.dsrf.org

DOWN SYNDROME (TRISOMY 21) *(continued from previous page)*

REFERENCES

[1] Merck Manual Professional Version. (2019). *Down syndrome (Trisomy 21).* https://www.merckmanuals.com/professional/pediatrics/chromosome-and-gene-anomalies/down-syndrome-trisomy-21#v1098913

[2] Centers for Disease Control and Prevention (CDC). (2018). *Down syndrome.* https://www.cdc.gov/ncbddd/birthdefects/downsyndrome.html

[3] Centers for Disease Control and Prevention (CDC). (2018). *Down syndrome: Data and statistics.* https://www.cdc.gov/ncbddd/birthdefects/downsyndrome/data.html

[4] Donoghue, E.A., & Kraft, C.A. (Eds.) (2019). *Managing chronic health needs in child care and schools: A quick reference guide* (2nd ed., pp. 115-116). American Academy of Pediatrics.

[5] Centers for Disease Control and Prevention (CDC). (2018). *Down syndrome.* https://www.cdc.gov/ncbddd/birthdefects/downsyndrome.html

[6] Ibid.

[7] Ibid.

[8] Donoghue, E.A., & Kraft, C.A. (Eds.) (2019). *Managing chronic health needs in child care and schools: A quick reference guide* (2nd ed., pp. 115-116). American Academy of Pediatrics.

[9] Karmiloff-Smith, A., Al-Janabi, T., D'Souza, H., Groet, J., Massand, E., Mok, K., Startin, C., Fisher, E., Hardy, J., Dean Nizetic, D., Tybulewicz, V., & Strydom, A. (2016). The importance of understanding individual differences in down syndrome. *F1000Research 2016*, 5(F1000 Faculty Rev), 389. https://www.ncbi.nlm.nih.gov/pmc/articles/PMC4806704/

[10] Mundakel, G.T. (2018). *Down syndrome.* https://emedicine.medscape.com/article/943216-overview

[11] Ibid.

[12] Brown, A.L., de Smith, A.J., Gant, V.U., Yang, W., Scheurer, M.E., Walsh, K.M., Chernus, J.M., Kallsen, N.A., Peyton, S.A., Davies, G.E., Ehli, E.A., Winick, N., Heerema, N.A., Carroll ,A.J., Borowitz, M.J., Wood, B.L., Carroll, W.L., Raetz, E.A., Feingold, E.,. ... Rabin, K.R. (2019). Inherited genetic susceptibility to acute lymphoblastic leukemia in Down syndrome. *Blood*, 134(15):1227-1237. https://doi.org/10.1182/blood.2018890764

[13] Donoghue, E.A., & Kraft, C.A. (Eds.) (2019). *Managing chronic health needs in child care and schools: A quick reference guide* (2nd ed., pp. 115-116). American Academy of Pediatrics.

[14] Mundakel, G.T. (2018). *Down syndrome.* https://emedicine.medscape.com/article/943216-overview

[15] Boston Children's Hospital. (2019). *Down syndrome.* http://www.childrenshospital.org/conditions-and-treatments/conditions/d/down-syndrome/symptoms-and-causes

OTHER REFERENCES CONSULTED

Ball, J.W., Bindler, R.C., Cowen, K., & Shaw, M.R. (2017). *Principles of pediatric nursing: Caring for children (7th ed.).* Pearson.

Crawford, L.J.R., & Whitehead, S.E. (2019). Students with neurodevelopmental disorders: Intellectual disabilities and autism. In J. Suleman, R.A. Shannon, & C. F. Younkaitis (Eds.), *School Nursing: A comprehensive text* (3rd ed., pp.603-626). F.A. Davis.

Selekman, J., & Ness, M. (2019). Students with chronic conditions. In J. Selekman, R.A. Shannon, & C.F. Younkaitis (Eds.), *School Nursing: A comprehensive text* (3rd ed., pp.480-500). F.A. Davis.

HOMELESSNESS

OVERVIEW/DEFINITION:
Emerging as a significant social problem in the U.S. in 1980, the number of homeless families with children has continued to steadily increase.[1] In 2018, families with children accounted for 33% of the overall homeless population in the U.S. with 60% of people in homeless families under the age of 18 years.[2]

Two and a half million children in America are homeless each year.[3] The most recent data from the U.S. Department of Education's count of homeless children in U.S. public schools and 2013 U.S. Census data reflects that 2,483,539 children experienced homelessness in the U.S. in 2013. This represents one in every 30 children in the U.S.[4]

The McKinney-Vento Homeless Assistance Act of 1987 marks the establishment of laws to define and track the number of homeless children in the U.S.[5] Despite efforts, unified definition of homelessness in the U.S. has not been established. The U.S. Department of Education and other governmental agencies definitions of homelessness vary, although they are similar to the McKinney-Vento definition and include these key components:[6]

- A lack of a fixed, regular, and adequate nighttime residence
- Living in a public or private place not designed for human beings (e.g., car, park, abandoned buildings)
- Living in a shelter providing temporary living arrangements (including hotels and motels), congregate shelters and transitional housing
- Residing in a makeshift shelter or other place not meant for human habitation
- Unaccompanied youth and homeless families with children and youth

Impact on Health[7, 8]
In general, homeless people are more likely to experience barriers to physical and mental health. In comparison to low-income and homeless families, homeless children experience

- higher levels of emotional and behavioral problems;
- increased risk of serious health problems;
- substance abuse; and
- a greater chance of being separated from their families.

Many homeless women are victims of domestic or sexual abuse. Homeless children have high rates of emotional and behavioral problems, often from having witnessed abuse. They may be exposed to communicable diseases/conditions as a result of living in congregate housing situations, shelters, and other locations where living conditions and sanitation may be questionable. Homeless youth are at greater risk for substance abuse and alcohol addiction.

HOMELESSNESS *(continued from previous page)*

OVERVIEW/DEFINITION *(continued)*

Impact on Education [9, 10]

Homeless children experience more school mobility than low-income and homeless families which negatively impacts their learning and progression through the education system and puts them at greater risk to repeat a grade, be expelled from or drop out of school, have lower academic performance, and slower growth in reading and math skills. The impact of educational barriers on their future should not be underestimated.

The McKinney-Vento Act also ensures that homeless children receive free transportation to and from their home school (including outside the school district) and requires schools to enroll homeless children even if they lack normally required documents, such as immunization records or proof of residence.[11]

Causes of Homelessness in Families

- Lack of affordable housing
- Poverty
- Unemployment
- Domestic violence

ANTICIPATED CONCERNS/PROBLEMS:

- Chronic health conditions (asthma, chronic otitis media, anemia, etc.)
- Behavioral problems
- Developmental delay
- Early initiation of substance abuse
- Social isolation
- Mental health problems (anxiety, depression, and withdrawal)
- Tuberculosis

MANAGEMENT/POTENTIAL INTERVENTIONS:

- Advocate to reduce and eliminate barriers to education, including implementing federal requirements under McKinney-Vento Act.
- Create a welcoming and trusting environment for homeless children and youth
- Facilitate access to special education, individualized education plans, and Section 504 accommodations as needed.
- Assist with identification of homeless children and youth.
- Ensure enforcement of laws and policies to support homeless children and youth
- Make referrals to social services, youth services bureaus, and supportive housing organizations.
- Facilitate access to health care including dental, mental health, and specialty care.
- Connect students and families with resources to meet basic needs including food, personal hygiene, clean clothing, and shelter.
- Assess for undiagnosed and untreated health conditions including anxiety, depression and refer for appropriate follow-up.

HOMELESSNESS *(continued from previous page)*

FOLLOW-UP

- Work with housing authority and homeless shelters in community to have seamless services to school.
- Facilitate timely transfer of health records if students find secure housing in new community.
- Pay particular attention to homeless youth on their own, in particular lesbian, gay, bisexual, transgender, and questioning (LGBTQ) youth.

RESOURCES

- **Childtrends.org** (n.d.) Children and youth experiencing homelessness. https://www.childtrends.org/indicators/homeless-children-and-youth
- **National Clearing House on Homeless Youth and Families**. (n.d.). U.S. Department of Education. https://rhyclearinghouse.acf.hhs.gov/partners/doe
- **National Clearing House on Homeless Youth and Families**. (n.d.) The health needs of homeless youth. https://rhyclearinghouse.acf.hhs.gov/news/2018/10/health-needs-homeless-youth
- **U.S. Department of Education**. (2018). Education for Homeless Children and Youths Grants for State and Local Activities. https://www2.ed.gov/programs/homeless/legislation.html

REFERENCES

[1] Bassuk, E. L., DeCandia, C.J., Beach, C.A., and Berman, F. (2014). *America's youngest outcasts: A report card on child homelessness.* (2014). The National Center on Family Homelessness at American Institutes for Research.

[2] U.S. Department of Housing and Urban Development. (2018). *The 2018 annual homeless assessment report.* https://files.hudexchange.info/resources/documents/2018-AHAR-Part-1.pdf

[3] Bassuk, E. L., DeCandia, C.J., Beach, C.A., and Berman, F. (2014). *America's youngest outcasts: A report card on child homelessness.* (2014). The National Center on Family Homelessness at American Institutes for Research.

[4] Ibid.

[5] U.S. Department of Education. (2001) McKinney Vento Homeless Assistance Act. https://www2.ed.gov/policy/elsec/leg/esea02/pg116.html

[6] 42 USC CHAPTER 119, SUBCHAPTER VI, Part B: Education for Homeless Children and Youths. https://uscode.house.gov/view.xhtml?path=/prelim@title42/chapter119/subchapter6/partB&edition=prelim

[7] U.S. National Library of Medicine, Medline Plus. (2019). *Homeless health concerns.* https://medlineplus.gov/homelesshealthconcerns.html

[8] Centers for Disease Control and Prevention. (2017). *Homelessness as a public health issue: Selected resources.* https://www.cdc.gov/phlp/publications/topic/resources/resources-homelessness.html

[9] National Alliance to End Homelessness. (n.d.). *Children and families.* https://endhomelessness.org/homelessness-in-america/who-experiences-homelessness/children-and-families/

[10] U.S. Department of Education. (2016). Supporting the success of homeless children and youths. https://www2.ed.gov/policy/elsec/leg/essa/160315ehcyfactsheet072716.pdf

[11] Ibid.

HUMAN TRAFFICKING

OVERVIEW/DEFINITION:

Human trafficking is a global health issue. It is also known as modern slavery and it is child abuse. It occurs in urban, suburban and rural communities, in all 50 states and Washington, DC, in all genders, socioeconomic, educational and demographic groups. It has been reported in children as young as eight,[1] and according to the U.S. State Department report (2019), 72% of known trafficked individuals were U.S. citizens and foreign nationals.[2]

Traffickers may be family members, recruiters, employers or strangers.[3] Vulnerable youth (see risk factors) are at greater risk to be victims of human trafficking and traffickers are adept at exploiting those vulnerabilities. While the exact prevalence of human trafficking is unknown due to its hidden nature, the 2018 Statistics from the National Human Trafficking Hotline reports a 25% increase in the number of calls and texts from trafficked individuals from the previous year.[4]

The Trafficking Victims Protection Act (TVPA) of 2000 and its reauthorizations is a comprehensive federal law addressing "severe forms of trafficking in persons" that includes labor and sex trafficking. This was the first federal legislation that protected victims, prosecuted traffickers and included prevention measures for education and increased public awareness.

A. Sex trafficking is the **recruitment, harboring, transportation, provision, obtaining, patronizing, or soliciting of a person** for the purposes of a commercial sex act, in which the commercial sex act is **induced by force, fraud, or coercion, or in which the person induced to perform such an act has not attained 18 years of age .**

B. Labor trafficking is the **recruitment, harboring, transportation, provision, or obtaining of a person for labor or services, through the use of force, fraud, or coercion** for the purposes of subjection to involuntary servitude, peonage, debt bondage, or slavery.[5]

The Palmero Protocol is an international instrument used to establish the parameters for the crime of "trafficking in persons"; it requires a trafficker's **actions**, the **means** of force, fraud or coercion and the **purpose** of exploitation and does not require that the person be moved from one location to another.[6] As of 2019, 168 countries have passed human trafficking legislation using the Palmero Protocol framework; it provides standard language on trafficking in persons that has promoted cooperation among countries.[7]

Due to their anonymity, the internet and social media play roles in the recruitment of victims and in the advertisement of sexual commercial businesses. The demand for cheap labor, services and commercial sex fuel human trafficking.[8] In some cases, sex and labor trafficking occur together. Child victims can be found in "brothels, strip clubs, street prostitution, truck stops, online, illicit drug trade (couriers), farms, ranches, fisheries, domestic service, nannies, manufacturing, factories, construction, landscaping, restaurants, other food services, hotels, hospitality industry, tourism, sales crews, peddling and begging rings (p.2)."[9] Human trafficking is often hidden in plain sight where the victims live, attend school and work in our communities.[10]

HUMAN TRAFFICKING *(continued from previous page)*

OVERVIEW/DEFINITION *(continued)*

Human trafficking has long term physical, emotional and mental health impacts on victims and survivors. It is important to be knowledgeable about human trafficking to identify victims/ survivors who attend school. Over 87% of trafficked victims have had contact with a healthcare professional while being trafficked but very few disclosed.[11] School nurses interact with students daily and have opportunities to develop trusting relationships that may lead to disclosure by a victim or survivor. Therefore, it is important to be knowledgeable about the school nurse role in supporting such students. The needs of the survivors/victims are complex and require a multidisciplinary approach to make referrals to support their needs. School nurses must have the support of the community to aid them in this work.

ANTICIPATED CONCERNS/PROBLEMS:

Risk Factors

Understanding the risk factors for human trafficking can help school nurses identify children and youth who may be in danger of becoming involved or currently involved in this complex crime. Many of the risk factors are connected to the Centers for Disease Control and Prevention social determinants of health.[12] *(Refer to SOCIAL DETERMINANTS OF HEALTH).* Children and youth vulnerable to human trafficking may have the following risk factors: [13, 14, 15, 16, 17]

- Gender (girls more likely to be victims than boys)
- Minority ethnicity (black women between the ages of 16 and 18 are at the greatest risk)
- Poor communities that have minimal capacity to respond to criminal networks
- Familial trafficking or having a family member involved in trafficking
- Lack of a caring adult within their family
- Children in the care of social services, for example, foster care
- History or physical or sexual abuse
- Youth who identify as lesbian, gay, bisexual, transgender or questioning
- Living in a neighborhood where poverty, high crime rates and violence exist
- History of running away
- Homeless youth
- Children with disabilities
- Youth in the juvenile justice system
- Refugees/immigrants/ethnically marginalized children, especially those that don't speak English
- Family dysfunction, domestic violence and financial troubles
- Gang involvement
- Child or parent is an immigrant and working in agriculture, construction, manufacturing, hospitality, food service, sales crews, health and elder care, salon services, or domestic services

HUMAN TRAFFICKING *(continued from previous page)*

Red Flags and Indicators of Human Trafficking [18, 19, 20, 21, 22]

This is not an all-inclusive list and may be different due to the individual circumstances of the trafficked victims. Many of these indicators result in long term physical and behavioral health consequences			
Physical	**Behavioral**	**Social**	**Academic**
• Physical abuse and neglect • Unexplained external and internal injuries and attempts to hide bruises, tattoos, scars and branding • Dental injuries • Poor general hygiene and dental hygiene • Broken bones • Sexually transmitted diseases and other infections • Pregnancies and abortions- vague answers about the father's identity • Malnutrition, dehydration, exhaustion • Substance Use disorder • Untreated chronic medical conditions • Somatic complaints associated with stress • Chronic pain • Delays in seeking medical attention • Complex trauma	• Post-traumatic stress disorder • Anxiety • Depression • Self -harming behaviors • May be withdrawn, fearful, irritable, submissive, tense, or nervous and paranoid • Attachment to the trafficker • Avoidance to being touched • Lack of eye contact	• Difficulty engaging in social interactions • Inappropriate dress based on weather • Controlling older boyfriend or girlfriend • Sudden change in attire, behavior, relationships, material possessions • Doesn't have possession of their identification documents • Sexual promiscuity, or knowledge of sexual situations/terminology outside of age appropriate norms • Allows others to speak for them when dealing with school authorities • Large amounts of cash, multiple cell phones or hotel keys	• Irregular school attendance/frequent unexplained absences, truancy • Frequently running away • Attends many schools, frequently transferring or with large gaps in attendance • May speak of unreasonable work or chore expectations at home • Indicates meals are limited or controlled • Lack of basic necessities: clothing, shelter • Daydreaming, falling asleep in class. • Forgetfulness • Sudden changes in academic performance • Inconsistencies in their story about life outside of school • Inability to clarify home address or where he/she stays or lives • Hungry with no money for food or lunch

HUMAN TRAFFICKING *(continued from previous page)*

ANTICIPATED CONCERNS/PROBLEMS *(continued)*

Identifying Victims of Human Trafficking

School nurses' frequent opportunities to interact with young people over time make it possible for them to identify red flags and possible indicators of human trafficking (see chart). It is important for school nurses to understand that many victims may not see themselves as victims, and neither know that what is being done to them is wrong nor seek help. Reasons victims may not seek help include being monitored, fear/shame, distrust of service providers, forced engagement in illegal activities and living in the normalization of exploitation.[23] Utilizing a trauma-informed approach (promoting a sense of safety; maintaining trust with clients; peer support; collaboration and mutuality; empowerment and moving past cultural stereotypes and biases) can be an effective strategy for school nurses working with victims of human trafficking and help to develop trust which is the first step in providing the needed assistance.[24, 25] (*Refer to CHILD MALTREATMENT and TRAUMA INFORMED CARE*).

MANAGEMENT/POTENTIAL INTERVENTIONS:

Children and youth involved in human trafficking need a comprehensive approach to provide necessary support and services before, during and after exploitation.[26] Utilizing a trauma-informed approach can be the most effective strategy for school nurses when intervening with possible/actual victims of human trafficking.[27, 28] <u>One of the most important steps school nurses can take to promote safety for victims of human trafficking is to collaborate with school officials and school staff to ensure there are policies and procedures for identifying, intervening and reporting students who may be at risk for human trafficking.</u>

Prevention in Schools

- Support primary prevention in the schools through education of staff, children and parents about risks, recruitment strategies and adverse effect.[29]
- Develop a list of service providers, such as, churches, shelters, nonprofit organizations that offer services within the community to help homeless and runaway youth.[30]
- Collaborate with local agencies to use evidence-based strategies to prevent childhood maltreatment.[31]

Immediate Care

- Review minor rights and confidentiality state laws with the minor.[32]
- Follow federal, state and local laws, rules and regulations pertinent to nursing practice including reporting child abuse and neglect.[33]
- Determine if the youth has a place to live.[34]
- Prioritize/identify immediate health needs of the student, such as, a physical exam, dental care, nutritional assistance, gynecological and infectious disease intervention.[35]
- Refer to community providers/agencies as appropriate.
- Refer/collaborate to develop a safety plan and a mental health plan.

HUMAN TRAFFICKING *(continued from previous page)*

MANAGEMENT/POTENTIAL INTERVENTIONS *(continued)*

- Utilize the National Trafficking Resource Center hotline (888-373-7888) for assistance and guidance as needed.[36] Victims of human trafficking who are not U.S. citizens can receive help including immigration assistance to obtain benefits through the U.S. Department of Human Services. [37]
- Document subjective and objective findings, intervention and follow-up plan.

After Care

- Continue to monitor for a multidisciplinary coordination of efforts that ensures medical, psychosocial, safety and basic needs are being met for the child/youth that has experienced human trafficking.
- Long term individualized support will be required for the victims and survivors.

COMPLICATIONS:

Research has identified long term and intergenerational consequences from child maltreatment which includes human trafficking. Individuals who experienced abuse, neglect, or other forms of childhood adversity are more likely than nonexposed individuals to have children who go on to have similar adverse childhood experiences.[38] Adverse Childhood Experiences (ACEs) is the term used to describe all types of abuse, neglect, and other potentially traumatic experiences that occur to people under the age of 18. The ACEs have been linked to risky health behaviors, chronic health conditions, low life potential and early death.[39] The numerous short and long-term consequences of human trafficking have been included in the chart above.

NOTES:

- Human trafficking is child abuse and nurses are mandated reporters. In some states, human trafficking is incorporated into the laws to improve healthcare provider education, understanding of trauma informed care and access to resources to support the victims.[40] (*Refer to CHILD MALTREATMENT and TRAUMA INFORMED CARE*).
- Know your district policy and procedures around human trafficking.
- It will require time to develop the victim's trust and the details about their circumstances may change over time.[41]
- It is important not to press them to answer questions until they are ready.[42]

REFERENCES

[1] Polaris Project (n.d.) *2018 Statistics from the National Human Trafficking Statistics Fact Sheet.* *https://polarisproject.org/sites/default/files/Polaris_National_Hotline_2018_Statistics_Fact_Sheet.pdf*

[2] United States Department of State. (2019). *Trafficking in persons report.* www.state.gov/j/tip

[3] Ibid.

[4] Polaris Project (n.d.) *2018 Statistics from the National Human Trafficking Statistics Fact Sheet.* *https://polarisproject.org/sites/default/files/Polaris_National_Hotline_2018_Statistics_Fact_Sheet.pdf*

HUMAN TRAFFICKING *(continued from previous page)*

[5] United States Congress. (2000). *Victims of Trafficking and Violence Protection Act of 2000: Public Law 106-386, 114 Stat 1470.* https://www.congress.gov/106/plaws/publ386/PLAW-106publ386.pdf

[6] United States Department of State. (2019). *Trafficking in persons report.* https://www.state.gov/wp-content/uploads/2019/06/2019-TIP-Introduction-Section-FINAL.pdf

[7] Ibid.

[8] Polaris Project, National Human Trafficking Resource Center. (n.d.) *Human trafficking.* https://humantraffickinghotline.org/type-trafficking/human-trafficking

[9] United States Department of Health and Human Services, Administration for Children and Families. (2016). *Human trafficking: Look beneath the surface, child exploitation brochure.* https://www.acf.hhs.gov/sites/default/files/endtrafficking/child_brochure_dec2016.pdf

[10] Ibid.

[11] Stoklosa, H., Grace, A., Littenberg, N., (2015). Medical education in human trafficking. *American Medical Association Journal of Ethics,17*(10), 914-921.https://doi.org/10.1001/journalofethics.2015.17.10.medu1-1510

[12] Centers for Disease Control and Prevention. (2018). *Social determinants of health.* https://www.cdc.gov/socialdeterminants/faqs/index.htm

[13] Sanchez, R.V. & Pacquiao, D.F. (2018). An ecological approach toward prevention and care of victims of domestic minor sex trafficking. *Journal of Forensic Nursing, 14*(2), 98 – 105. https://doi.org/101097/JFN0000000000000205

[14] National Center for Missing and Exploited Children (2019). *Child sex trafficking in America, A guide for child welfare professionals.* www.missingkids.com/content/dam/missingkids/pdfs/CSTinAmerica_Professionals.pdf

[15] Avila, P. (2016). A multidisciplinary response to commercial sexual exploitation of children. *The Nurse Practitioner, 41*(11), 34-40. https://doi.org/10.1097/01.NPR.0000502788.20243.0a

[16] Nierengarten, M.B. (2018). Identify, screen, treat, and advocate for child victims of sex trafficking. *Contemporary Pediatrics, 35*(12), 8-10. https://www.contemporarypediatrics.com/adolescent-medicine/identify-screen-treat-and-advocate-child-victims-sex-trafficking

[17] Greenbaum, J. (2016). Identifying victims of human trafficking in the emergency department. Clinical Pediatric Emergency Medicine, 17(4), 241 – 248. https://doi.org/10.1016/j.cpem.2016.09.006

[18] Nierengarten, M.B. (2018). Identify, screen, treat, and advocate for child victims of sex trafficking. Contemporary Pediatrics, 35(12), 8-10. https://www.contemporarypediatrics.com/adolescent-medicine/identify-screen-treat-and-advocate-child-victims-sex-trafficking

[19] United States Department of Education, Office of Safe and Healthy Students. (2015). *Human trafficking in America's schools.* https://safesupportivelearning.ed.gov/sites/default/files/HumanTraffickinginAmericasSchools.pdf

[20] Child Information Gateway. (2017). *Human trafficking and child welfare: A guide for child welfare agencies.* https://www.childwelfare.gov/pubPDFs/trafficking_agencies.pdf

[21] Sinay, K. (2017). Human trafficking – An introduction to what the Texas nurse needs to know. *Texas Board of Nursing Bulletin,* 48(3), 4-6. https://www.bon.texas.gov/pdfs/newsletter_pdfs/2017/July2017.pdf

[22] National Center for Missing and Exploited Children (2019). *Child sex trafficking in America, A guide for child welfare professionals.* www.missingkids.com/content/dam/missingkids/pdfs/CSTinAmerica_Professionals.pdf

[23] United States Department of Health and Human Services, Administration for Children and Families. (2016). *Human trafficking: look beneath the surface, child exploitation brochure.* https://www.acf.hhs.gov/sites/default/files/endtrafficking/child_brochure_dec2016.pdf

HUMAN TRAFFICKING *(continued from previous page)*

[24] Ibid.

[25] U.S. Department of Health & Human Services, Substance Abuse and Mental Health Services Administration (SAMHSA). (2014). *Concept of trauma and guidance for a trauma-informed approach.* https://store.samhsa.gov/system/files/sma14-4884.pdf

[26] Sanchez, R.V. & Pacquiao, D.F. (2018). An ecological approach toward prevention and care of victims of domestic minor sex trafficking. *Journal of Forensic Nursing, 14*(2), 98 –105. https://www.researchgate.net/publication/325212524_An_Ecological_Approach_Toward_Prevention_and_Care_of_Victims_of_Domestic_Minor_Sex_Trafficking

[27] U.S. Department of Health & Human Services, Substance Abuse and Mental Health Services Administration (SAMHSA). (2014). *Concept of trauma and guidance for a trauma-informed approach.* https://store.samhsa.gov/system/files/sma14-4884.pdf

[28] Greenbaum, J. (2016). Identifying victims of human trafficking in the emergency department. *Clinical Pediatric Emergency Medicine, 17*(4), 241 – 248. https://doi.org/10.1016/j.cpem.2016.09.006

[29] Ibid.

[30] Sanchez, R.V. & Pacquiao, D.F. (2018). An ecological approach toward prevention and care of victims of domestic minor sex trafficking. *Journal of Forensic Nursing, 14*(2), 98 – 105. https://www.researchgate.net/publication/325212524_An_Ecological_Approach_Toward_Prevention_and_Care_of_Victims_of_Domestic_Minor_Sex_Trafficking

[31] Centers for Disease Control and Prevention. (2016). *Preventing child abuse and neglect: A technical package for policy, norm, and programmatic activities.* https://www.cdc.gov/violenceprevention/pdf/CAN-Prevention-Technical-Package.pdf

[32] Avila, P. (2016). A multidisciplinary response to commercial sexual exploitation of children. *The Nurse Practitioner, 41*(11), 34-40. https://doi.org/ 10.1097/01.NPR.0000502788.20243.0a

[33] Sinay, K. (2017). Human trafficking – An introduction to what the Texas nurse needs to know. *Texas Board of Nursing Bulletin, 48*(3), 4-6. https://www.bon.texas.gov/pdfs/newsletter_pdfs/2017/July2017.pdf

[34] Ibid.

[35] Sanchez, R.V. & Pacquiao, D.F. (2018). An ecological approach toward prevention and care of victims of domestic minor sex trafficking. *Journal of Forensic Nursing, 14*(2), 98 – 105. https://www.researchgate.net/publication/325212524_An_Ecological_Approach_Toward_Prevention_and_Care_of_Victims_of_Domestic_Minor_Sex_Trafficking

[36] Nierengarten, M.B. (2018). Identify, screen, treat, and advocate for child victims of sex trafficking. *Contemporary Pediatrics, 35*(12), 8-10. https://www.contemporarypediatrics.com/adolescent-medicine/identify-screen-treat-and-advocate-child-victims-sex-trafficking

[37] United States Department of Health and Human Services, Administration for Children and Families. (2016). *Human trafficking: Look beneath the surface, child exploitation brochure.* https://www.acf.hhs.gov/sites/default/files/endtrafficking/child_brochure_dec2016.pdf

[38] Merreck, M.T. & Guinn, A.S. (2018). Child abuse and neglect: Breaking the intergenerational link. *American Journal of Public Health, 108*(8), 1117 – 1118. https://doi.org/10.2105/AJPH.2018.304636

[39] Centers for Disease Control and Prevention. (2019). *About adverse childhood experiences.* : https://www.cdc.gov/violenceprevention/childabuseandneglect/acestudy/aboutace.html

HUMAN TRAFFICKING *(continued from previous page)*

[40] English, A. (2017). *Mandatory reporting of human trafficking: Potential benefits and risks of harm. American Medical Association Journal of Ethics,19(1), 54-62.* https://journalofethics.ama-assn/article/mandatory-reporting-human-trafficking-potential-benefits-and-risks-harm/2017-01

[41] United States Department of Health and Human Services, Administration for Children and Families. (2016). *Human trafficking: Look beneath the surface, child exploitation brochure*. https://www.acf.hhs.gov/sites/default/files/endtrafficking/child_brochure_dec2016.pdf

[42] Ibid.

OTHER REFERENCES CONSULTED

National Human Trafficking Resource Center. (2016). *Identifying victims of human trafficking: What to look for in a healthcare setting.* https://humantraffickinghotline.org/sites/default/files/What%20to%20Look%20for%20during%20a%20Medical%20Exam%20-%20FINAL%20-%202-16-16_0.pdf

National Human Trafficking Resource Center. (2016). *Framework for human trafficking protocol in the healthcare setting.* https://humantraffickinghotline.org/resources/framework-human-trafficking-protocol-healthcare-settings

National Human Trafficking Resource Center. (2010). *Educators and human trafficking: In depth review.* https://humantraffickinghotline.org/sites/default/files/In%20Depth%20Review%20for%20Educators.pdf

National Human Trafficking Resource Center. (2011). *Tools for educators. https://humantraffickinghotline.org/sites/default/files/Educator%20Assessment%20Tool.pdf*

National Human Trafficking Resource Center. (2010). *Human Trafficking power and control wheel.* https://humantraffickinghotline.org/sites/default/files/HT%20Power%26Control%20Wheel%20NEW.pdf

United States Department of Health and Human Services, Administration for Children and Families. (2017). *Fact Sheet: Human Trafficking.* https://www.acf.hhs.gov/sites/default/files/otip/fact_sheet_human_trafficking_fy18.pdf

MENTAL HEALTH MANAGEMENT

OVERVIEW/DEFINITION:

Mental health conditions can be acute or chronic. They often occur or begin in childhood or adolescence. Though the symptoms of these conditions may be apparent enough to warrant proper evaluation and treatment, there are also many children who remain undiagnosed despite a severe manifestation of symptoms. The American Academy of Pediatrics reports that only approximately 10-40% of children who need mental health services actually receive them.[1, 2] There are also children whose serious difficulties do not rise to the level of a diagnosis but cause great psychological distress. Students may visit the school nurse for matters seemingly unrelated to a mental health concern, however, they may present with physical symptoms that are actually manifestations of an emotional illness. Headaches and abdominal pain are extremely common somatic presentations. The school nurse will often be the first point of entry into mental health services, playing an essential role for the child with mental, emotional, or behavioral health issues.[3]

Providing statistics about the scope of these challenges, the Youth Risk Behavior Surveillance System (YRBSS) is a school-based questionnaire administered yearly to students in 9th through 12th grade asking about psychosocial concerns among students.[4] The YRBSS is administered across the United States, including American Indian/Native American tribal regions, and has thus a good representative sample of students across the country. Students from all socioeconomic communities express a range of frequent and intense concerns. For example, the 2018 YRBSS, reporting survey results from 2017, showed that:[5]

- 31.5% felt sad or hopeless for at least two weeks in the last 12 months (females > males)
- 17.2% considered attempting suicide
- 13.6% planned suicide
- 17.2% considered attempting suicide
- 13.6% had a suicide plan
- 7.4% attempted suicide one or more times in the last 12 months
- 2.4% sought medical attention after an injury or poisoning for suidical behavior

Of particular note, in 2017 the suicide rate in adolescents (ages 15 –19) and young adults (ages 20 – 24) increased to the highest point in the past two decades, especially in adolescent males.[6]

Other YRBSS survey responses include:[7]

- 19% were bullied on school property in the last 12 months
- 29.8% reported using alcohol currently
- 19.8% reported using marijuana currently
- 8.8% smoked a cigarette, 13.8% vaped in the past month
- 14% took a prescription pain medication witout indication at least once in their life
- 16.5% rode in a car with someone who had drunk alcohol in the past month
- 15.7% carried a weapon in the past month (3.8% on school property)
- 4.8% carried a gun in the last 12 months (not for hunting or sport)
- 9.7% were forced to do sexual things they did not want to do in the last 12 months (kissing, touching, intercourse)
- 53.8% used a condom in their last sexual encounter

MENTAL HEALTH MANAGEMENT *(continued from previous page)*

OVERVIEW/DEFINITION *(continued)*

Another common situation for the school nurse is the management of symptoms of chronic illnesses, often are accompanied by an increased risk for mental health concerns. These include, but are not limited to:

- diabetes
- asthma
- headache
- migraine and
- abdominal pain

For example, compared with the general child populaton, the risk of psychiatric morbidity in children with a new diagnosis of Type 1 diabetes is tripled within the first six months of onset, and there is an increased risk of suicide attempts.[8]

In summary, students frequently experience risk, and although students may not present to the school nurse's office with emotional issues as the main concern, these issues hover in the background. The school nurse should provide an environment that is:

- welcoming
- warm/nurturing
- safe, and
- supportive to students in a way that goes beyond the mere encounter at hand.

He or she can also serve as an advocate, referral source, and facilitator of mental health care within the school and community settings.

ANTICIPATED CONCERNS/PROBLEMS:

At times, school nurses will be called upon to engage in the social-emotional and behavioral health treatment of a child through such tasks as administering psychiatric medications or managing acute presentations of psychiatric illness. It is important for school nurses to be competent in recognizing the onset of acute exacerbations of mental health symptoms, in order to determine the appropriate interventions required for improvement or stabilization of the child's condition within the school setting. At times this will require the nurse to make a professional judgment to intervene medically, such as administering a PRN medication, or referring the child to external emergency services. Examples may include a child who self-injures on school grounds, or who has recently been discharged from a psychiatric inpatient hospitalization and may still be experiencing acute symptoms of a mental health disorder.

School nurses also play an integral role in identifying and managing suicidal ideation or behaviors in youth. These may be elicited through reports from peers, parents, or teachers, or may be expressed (vaguely or directly) from students during routine or acute care assessments by the school nurse. It is essential that the school nurse recognize these expressions and provide prompt referral to the appropriate staff member and/or agency (typically, the emergency room or a mobile crisis service).

MENTAL HEALTH MANAGEMENT *(continued from previous page)*

ANTICIPATED CONCERNS/PROBLEMS *(continued)*

Students presenting with somatic complaints may in fact be experiencing high levels of stress and symptomatology that may or may not be part of a psychiatric diagnosis. Given the school nurse's close proximity to these students while assessing and providing direct care for these complaints, he or she is in a unique position to assess the need for further diagnostic clarification, treatment, or referral to the appropriate mental health treatment.

MANAGEMENT/POTENTIAL INTERVENTIONS:

Regardless of the nature of the interventions that may be required of the school nurse, it is essential that the nurse determine the mental health history of the child in question, as well as the ongoing treatment plan as outlined by the child's school- or community-based providers and parents. Establishing and maintaining regular contact with the student, school and community resources, and the student's parent(s) or guardian(s), allows the school nurse to provide ongoing assessment, management, and reporting of the child's mental health status, with the goal of improving mental and behavioral health outcomes for the child.[9,10]

The school nurse also has an **integral role** for the child who returns to school after psychiatric hospitalization. Your school should have a protocol for such situations. The most commonly identified elements for reintegration are:

- establishing communication with the hospital to determine care needs and contingencies
- meeting or speaking with caregivers prior to the student's return
- developing an individualized re-entry plan [11]

Other elements for re-entry might include:

- obtaining a treatment plan from the clinic or hospital
- using appropriate screening tools

Clinics and hospitals increasingly use suicidal screening tools and it is appropriate for the school nurse and other appropriate staff to be trained to use such tools. One common instrument, which can be used by school nurses, is the *Ask Suicide-Screening Screening Questions Toolkit* available from the National Institue of Mental Health.[9]

School systems may use additonal comprehensive methods to assess mental health that are beyond the scope of the school nurse alone. An example is the Signs of Suicide (SOS) program.[10] Individual screening instruments that can be used by the school nurse include:

- ASQ Suicide Risk Screening Tool
- Patient Health Questionnaire Screeners for anxiety and depression (phqscreeners.com)

MENTAL HEALTH MANAGEMENT *(continued from previous page)*

FOLLOW-UP:

- This chapter stresses the importance of being aware that mental health concerns loom large for children and adolescents, whether they are obvious or not. Therefore a warm, supportive, and respectful stance should be taken at all times with students to ensure that the visit to the school nurse is a particularly positive one.
- If there are any mental health concerns noted in any encounter, it is important that the school nurse inform the school counselor, the mental health team, the parent, or all three about any concerns, depending on issues of confidentiality or safety

NOTES:

Students with significant psychosocial distress often do not report their concerns to anyone, peers, parents or other adults. The school nurse may be the only (perhaps first rather than only) professional with whom they have an encounter. This provides the possibility for the beginnings of intervention, and this chance to intervene should not be underestimated.

REFERENCES

[1] Kann, L., McManus, T., Harris, W.A., Shanklin, S.L., Flint, K.H., Queen, B., Lowry, R., Chyen,D.,Whittle, L., Thornton, J., Lim, C., Bradford, D., Yamakawa, Y., Leon, M., Brener, N.,& Ethier, K.A. (2018, June 15). *Youth Risk Behavior Surveillance - United States, 2017 | Morbidity and Mortality Weekly Report*. https://www.cdc.gov/mmwr/volumes/67/ss/ss6708a1.htm

[2] American Academy of Pediatrics, Council on School Health. (2016). Role of the school nurse in providing school health services. *Pediatrics, 137*(6), 1-6. https://doi.org/10.1542/peds.2016-0852

[3] National Association of School Nurses. (2018). *The school nurse's role in behavioral/mental health of students* (Position Statement). https://www.nasn.org/advocacy/professional-practice-documents/position-statements/ps-behavioral-health

[4] Kann, L., McManus, T., Harris, W.A., Shanklin, S.L., Flint, K.H., Queen, B., Lowry, R., Chyen,D.,Whittle, L., Thornton, J., Lim, C., Bradford, D., Yamakawa, Y., Leon, M., Brener, N.,& Ethier, K.A. (2018, June 15). *Youth Risk Behavior Surveillance - United States, 2017 | Morbidity and Mortality Weekly Report*. https://www.cdc.gov/mmwr/volumes/67/ss/ss6708a1.htm

[5] Ibid.

[6] Ibid.

[7] Ibid.

[8] Butwicka, A., Frisén, L., Almqvist, C., Zethelius, B., & Lichtenstein, P. (2015). Risks of Psychiatric Disorders and Suicide Attempts in Children and Adolescents With Type 1 Diabetes: A Population-Based Cohort Study. Diabetes Care, 38(3), 453–459. https://doi.org/10.2337/dc14-0262

[9] Kann, L., McManus, T., Harris, W.A., Shanklin, S.L., Flint, K.H., Queen, B., Lowry, R., Chyen,D., Whittle, L., Thornton, J., Lim, C., Bradford, D., Yamakawa, Y., Leon, M., Brener, N.,& Ethier, K.A. (2018, June 15). *Youth Risk Behavior Surveillance - United States, 2017 | Morbidity and Mortality Weekly Report*. https://www.cdc.gov/mmwr/volumes/67/ss/ss6708a1.htm

[10] American Academy of Pediatrics, Council on School Health. (2016). Role of the school nurse in providing school health services. *Pediatrics, 137*(6), 1-6. https://doi.org/10.1542/peds.2016-0852

[11] Marraccini, M. E., Lee, S., & Chin, A. J. (2019). School reintegration post-psychiatric hospitalization: Protocols and procedures across the nation. *School Mental Health*, First online: 09 January 2019, 1-14. https://doi.org/10.1007/s12310-019-09310-8 doi:10.1007/s12310-019-09310-8

[9] National Institute of Mental Health. (n.d.). *Ask suicide-screening questions (ASQ) toolkit* https://www.nimh.nih.gov/research/research-conducted-at-nimh/asq-toolkit-materials/index.shtml

[10] Sheftall, A. H., Asti, L., Horowitz, L. M., Felts, A., Fontanella, C. A., Campo, J. V., & Bridge, J. A. (2016, October 1). *Suicide in elementary school-aged children and early adolescents.* https://pediatrics.aappublications.org/content/138/4/e20160436

REFUGEE AND ASYLEE CHILDREN AND ADOLESCENTS

OVERVIEW/DEFINITION:

According to the United Nations High Commission for Refugees (UNHCR), in 2017, there were 68.5 million persons displaced globally with 25.4 million designated as refugees.[1] Prior to 2018, the U.S. had led the world in accepting refugees for resettlement.[2]

Refugee and Asylees

Refugees and asylees are individuals who are unable or unwilling to return to their country of origin or nationality because of persecution or a well-founded fear of persecution. Refugees and asylees are eligible for protection in large part based on race, religion, nationality, membership in a particular social group, or political opinion. The 1996 Illegal Immigration Reform and Immigrant Responsibility Act expanded this definition to include persons forced to abort a pregnancy or undergo forced sterilization or have been prosecuted for their resistance to coercive population controls.

In the United States, the major difference between refugees and asylees is the location of the person at the time of application. Refugees are usually outside the United States when they are screened for resettlement, whereas asylum seekers submit their application while they are physically present in the United States or at a U.S. port of entry. Refugees and asylees also differ in admissions process used and agency responsible for reviewing their application.[3]

Unaccompanied alien children (UAC), according to the United States law, lack legal immigration status, are under 18 years old, and are either without a parent or legal guardian in the U.S. or without a parent or legal guardian in the U.S. who is available to provide care and physical custody.[4] UAC are referred to the Office of Refugee Resettlement (ORR) and are placed in the least restrictive setting until suitable guardians or sponsors are identified to provide care and custody.[5]

The U.S. has decreased the number of refugees that are accepted to 30, 000 in 2019 and has increased the vetting process creating a backlog in processing applications.[6] As of 2017, the U.S. granted asylum to 26,568 persons.[7] Approximately 15,000 refugees entered the U.S, as of April 2019, from the Democratic Republic of the Congo (DRC), Burma (also known as Myanmar), Ukraine, Eritrea, Afghanistan, Syria, Iraq, Sudan, Burundi and Colombia.[8] The DRC and Burma account for 64% of the refugees admitted to the U.S. due to war in the DRC and persecution in Burma.[9] Fifty-two percent of the 2019 refugees, initially settled in Texas, New York, California, Washington, North Carolina, Ohio, Kentucky, Georgia, Michigan and Arizona.[10]

Many families migrate from Central America, especially from El Salvador, Guatemala and Honduras, to the U.S.[11] They make up a large portion of the those seeking asylum at the United States-Mexico border. Those that wish to claim asylum must do so at the border to a Customs and Border Protection (CBP) officer or when apprehended by a CBP officer between ports of entry to the United States.[12] Some factors that contribute to the increased migration from their countries of origin are corrupt government official and weak institutions, poverty, crime, illicit drug trade that contribute to insecurity and lack of confidence in the government.[13]

REFUGEE AND ASYLEE CHILDREN AND ADOLESCENTS *(continued from previous page)*

OVERVIEW/DEFINITION *(continued)*

Refugees and asylees, which may be family units or unaccompanied youth, are often exposed to violence, wars, torture, trafficking, poverty, loss of family and famine during displacement and awaiting approval of their refugee/asylee status.[14] They may have fled their country of origin and spent time in a host country refugee camp.[15] The problems associated with these vulnerable populations are complex. They have been exposed to multiple adverse childhood experiences that need to be addressed on an individual level and require a combination of trauma informed care, cultural congruence and self-awareness.[16]

ANTICIPATED CONCERNS/PROBLEMS:

Refugees and asylees are exposed to multiple stressors during the time from displacement to resettlement which place them at greater risk for poor physical, mental health and social outcomes.[16] Culture, poverty, lack of access to health care, and language barriers are social determinants of health that can contribute to cognitive and developmental delays and lead to mental health and behavioral problems.[17, 18] *(Refer to SOCIAL DETERMINANTS OF HEALTH).* Many children are resilient and do not experience these symptoms, while symptoms in others, improve as their lives become more settled.[19]

It is also important to be aware of the impact that the stressors have on parents and how it may affect their ability to parent. The time parents spend in detention centers can undermine their ability to parent and care for their children which impacts ongoing mental health of the family.[20, 21]

Common symptoms [22, 23, 24, 25, 26]

- Somatic complaints of headaches, stomachaches, generalized pains
- Poor oral health, lack of appetite, malnutrition, chronic diseases
- Sleep disturbances, such as nightmares, trouble falling asleep, sleeping too much
- Post-Traumatic Stress Disorder (PTSD), anxiety, depression, hopelessness, suicidal ideation, self-harm
- Behavioral problems, conduct disorders, difficulty concentrating, difficulty with relationships, feeling isolated, aggression

REFUGEE AND ASYLEE CHILDREN AND ADOLESCENTS *(continued from previous page)*

AGE SPECIFIC EXAMPLES OF TRAUMA[27]

Preschool children	Elementary school children	Middle and high school-aged youth
• Bed wetting • Thumb sucking • Acting younger than their age • Trouble separating from their parents • Temper tantrums • Aggressive behavior like hitting, kicking, throwing things, or biting • Not playing with other kids their age • Repetitive playing out of events related to trauma exposure	• Changes in behavior such as aggression, anger, irritability, withdrawal from others, and sadness • Trouble at school • Trouble with peers • Fear of separation from parents • Fear of something bad happening	• A sense of responsibility or guilt for the bad things that have happened • Feelings of shame or embarrassment • Feelings of helplessness • Changes in how they think abou the world

MANAGEMENT/POTENTIAL INTERVENTIONS:
Refugees/asylees generally undergo medical examinations that include a physical and mental health assessment and screening of vaccination status. Other components may include exams for sexually transmitted diseases and Human Immunodeficiency Virus screenings, tuberculosis screening, and evaluation for hepatitis B, malaria and intestinal infections, lead screenings, and evaluation of nutritional and growth status.[28] Many refugees/asylees have not had access to a medical home or primary surveillance in their country of origin or host country, often have chronic medical conditions and been exposed to poor sanitation, toxic chemicals, etc. [29] It is important to assist with referral to a medical home to support access to comprehensive services.[30]

Refugees and asylees, often have not had access to regular education in their country of origin or host country; the 1982 Supreme Court decision in Plyler v Doe ruled that the State may not deny a basic education to children whether they are legally in the U.S. or not.[31, 32] Education and schools provide a start to a period of stability and help integrate these students into an American life. These refugees/asylees are also beginning the process of learning about and living in an American culture and society which contribute stressors.

REFUGEE AND ASYLEE CHILDREN AND ADOLESCENTS *(continued from previous page)*

MANAGEMENT/POTENTIAL INTERVENTIONS *(continued)*

> Indeed, schools are a key protective factor, influencing such outcomes by acting as a stable social support, which helps develop children's resilience by enhancing their individual competencies, in turn adding to their inclusiveness, acceptance, respect, self-worth and sense of control over their environment. For children needing to recover from loss and trauma secondary to experiences as a refugee, school offers a developmentally appropriate space to mobilise and enhance recovery, both at a simple level and as part of more specialized secondary and tertiary level care. [33]

Trauma informed care is needed to address the complex needs of these immigrant families and individuals that have been exposed to multiple trauma and toxic stress during their journey from the country of origin to resettlement in the United States. Many families will need medical, dental and behavioral health, social service and legal supports. (*Refer to Trauma Informed Care*)

FOLLOW-UP:

- School nurses can utilize a trauma informed approach to establish a confidential, safe, open and respectful setting to help develop a trusting relationship with the student and families, over time.
- A professional translator is needed to communicate effectively; it is not acceptable to use the child as a translator.
- It is important for school nurses to understand the cultural norms, family roles and dynamics and to seek professional development opportunities about cultural congruence and how culture impacts students, families and the community.[34]
- Students and families may disclose over time a history of abuse, abandonment, persecution, human trafficking or violence that will require referral to legal services.[35]
- School nurses can provide information about the interface between the health care and educational systems.
- School nurses can help identify undiagnosed or untreated health, behavioral and academic problems and assist in securing necessary services for the students.[36]
- School nurses work collaboratively with the school psychologists, social workers and other mental health professionals to identify barriers to learning and identify the need for additional services.
- These students are at increased risk of bullying in school and over-nutrition during resettlement.[37]
- The school team can promote cultural awareness and acceptance within the school setting.
- The school team needs to be knowledgeable about the resources in the community that can provide resources for medical and behavioral health, social services and legal services, and in particular refugee resettlement agencies that can assist the populations within the school community.

Addressing the needs of refugee students helps promote educational success that can lead to good health and well- being.

REFUGEE AND ASYLEE CHILDREN AND ADOLESCENTS *(continued from previous page)*

NOTES:

- School districts cannot ask a student or family about their immigration status and cannot deny enrollment for lack of a social security number or lack of a birth certificate.[38]
- Students who are homeless do not have to provide proof of residency and must be enrolled by the school district.[39]
- School nurses are mandatory reporters of child abuse. It is important to be aware that refugee families may not be aware of the cultural norms for child-rearing in the United States. It requires balancing the cultural differences with the safety of the child.[40] School personnel need to follow the local laws and school policies for reporting child abuse.
- State laws vary regarding the ages of children guaranteed schooling.[41]
- School personnel need to advocate for parents, guardians, and sponsors to request and have school meetings in their preferred language.[42]
- Many refugees and asylees relocate to other areas after their initial settlement in the United States which presents challenges for their immunization records since this information is not shared from state to state. It is recommended to provide the transferring guardian with a copy of the immunization records that will be needed with future enrollments.
- Refugees/asylees entering through northern and southern borders (Canada and Mexico) are screened for human trafficking. Those immigrants that are victims of a crime in the U.S. may qualify for the U visa program while human trafficking victims may qualify for the T visa program if they cooperate with the authorities.[43, 44] *(Refer to HUMAN TRAFFICKING).*

RESOURCES

- **American Academy of Pediatrics**, (2013) Immigration Child Health Toolkit. https://www.aap.org/en-us/advocacy-and-policy/aap-health-initiatives/Immigrant-Child-Health-Toolkit/Pages/Immigrant-Child-Health-Toolkit.aspx

- **American Federation of Teachers** (n.d.). Protecting Our Students: What you need to know about the Rights of Immigrants and the threat of deportation. https://www.aft.org/sites/default/files/fl_im_yourrightsfactsheet_020817.pdf

- **Cultural Orientation Resource Center** has information on different immigrant populations that contain information about the conditions and circumstance associated with their status. http://www.culturalorientation.net/library/publications

- **Education of the States. (2013). 50 State Analysis: School Attendance Age Limits.** https://www.ecs.org/clearinghouse/01/07/04/10704.pdf

- **National Child Traumatic Stress Network**. (2019.) *Understanding Refugee Trauma: For Child Welfare.* https://www.nctsn.org/sites/default/files/resources/fact-sheet/understanding_refugee_trauma_for_child_welfare_workers.pdf

REFUGEE AND ASYLEE CHILDREN AND ADOLESCENTS *(continued from previous page)*

RESOURCES *(continued)*

- **National Child Traumatic Stress Network**. (2018.) *Understanding Refugee Trauma: For School Personnel.* https://www.nctsn.org/sites/default/files/resources/fact-sheet/understanding_refugee_trauma_for_school_personnel.pdf

- **Office of Refugee Resettlement** has a link to states resources and contacts that may be helpful for students and families. https://www.acf.hhs.gov/orr/state-programs-annual-overview

REFERENCES

[1] Blizzard, B. & Batalova, J. (2019). *Refugees and asylees in the United States*. Migration Policy Institute: Washington, DC. https://www.migrationpolicy.org/article/refugees-and-asylees-united-states

[2] Ibid.

[3] Ibid., Definitions.

[4] Administration for Children & Families. (2019). *Unaccompanied alien children fact sheet.* https://www.hhs.gov/sites/default/files/Unaccompanied-Alien-Children-Program-Fact-Sheet.pdf

[5] Ibid.

[6] Blizzard, B. & Batalova, J. (June 13, 2019). *Refugees and asylees in the United States*. Migration Policy Institute: Washington, DC. https://www.migrationpolicy.org/article/refugees-and-asylees-united-states

[7] Ibid.

[8] Ibid.

[9] Ibid.

[10] Ibid.

[11] Congressional Research Services. (2019). *Recent migration to the United States from Central America: Frequently asked questions.* https://crsreports.congress.gov/product/pdf/R/R45489

[12]Ibid.

[13] Ibid.

[14] Musliu, E., Snezana, V., Clausson, E.K., & Pernilla, G. (2019). School nurses' experiences working with unaccompanied refugee children and adolescents: A qualitative study. *The Journal of School Nursing. Vol.5,* 1-8. https://journals.sagepub.com/doi/pdf/10.1177/2377960819843713

[15] Ibid.

[16]Ibid.

[16] Moreau, AM., Hennous, F., Dabbagh, B. & Ferraz dos Santos, B. (2019). Oral health status of refugee children in Montreal. *Journal of Immigrant and Minority Health* 21,693- 698. https://doi.org/10.1007/s10903-018-0835-1

[17] Ibid.

[18] Cleary, M., West, S., Foong, A., McLean, L. & Kornhaber, R. (2019). Mental health of refugee children: A discursive look at causes, considerations and interventions. *Issues in Mental Health Nursing, 40:8*, 665-671. https://doi.org/10.1080/01612840.2019.1585494

[19] Ibid.

[20] Ibid.

[21] American Academy of Pediatrics Council on Community Health. (2017). Detention of immigrant children. *Pediatrics. 139(4): 1-15.* https://doi.org./*10.1542/peds.2017-0483.* https://pediatrics.aappublications.org/content/pediatrics/139/5/e20170483.full.pdf

REFUGEE AND ASYLEE CHILDREN AND ADOLESCENTS *(continued from previous page)*

[22] Moreau, AM., Hennous, F., Dabbagh, B. & Ferraz dos Santos, B. (2019). Oral health status of refugee children in Montreal. *Journal of Immigrant and Minority Health* 21, 693- 698. https://doi.org/10.1007/s10903-018-0835-1

[23] Johnson, J.L., Beard, J., & Evans, D. (2017). Caring for refugee youth in the school setting. *NASN School Nurse*. 32(2), 122-128. https://doi.org/10.1177/1942602X16672310

[24] Musliu, E., Snezana, V., Clausson, E.K., & Pernilla, G. (2019). School nurses' experiences working with unaccompanied refugee children and adolescents: A qualitative study. *The Journal of School Nursing, Vol.5,* 1-8. https://journals.sagepub.com/doi/pdf/10.1177/2377960819843713

[25] Cleary, M., West, S., Foong, A., McLean, L. & Kornhaber, R. (2019). Mental health of refugee children: A discursive look at causes, considerations and interventions. *Issues in Mental Health Nursing, 40(8)*, 665-671. https://doi.org/10.1080/01612840.2019.1585494

[26] National Child Traumatic Stress Network (n.d.) *Refugee trauma effects.* https://www.nctsn.org/what-is-child-trauma/trauma-types/refugee-trauma/effects

[27] Ibid.

[28] Centers for Disease Control and Prevention (CDC). (2019). *Guidelines for U.S. domestic medical screening newly arriving refugees.* https://www.cdc.gov/immigrantrefugeehealth/guidelines/domestic/domestic-guidelines.html

[29] American Academy of Pediatrics Council on Community Health. (2017). Detention of immigrant children. *Pediatrics. 139(4): 1-15.* https://doi.org/10.1542/peds.2017-0483https://pediatrics.aappublications.org/content/pediatrics/139/5/e20170483.full.pdf

[30] Ibid.

[31] Ibid.

[32] Plyler v. Doe, 457 U.S. 202 (1982). https://supreme.justia.com/cases/federal/us/457/202/

[33] Cleary, M., West, S., Foong, A., McLean, L. & Kornhaber, R. (2019). Mental health of refugee children: A discursive look at causes, considerations and interventions. *Issues in Mental Health Nursing, 40*(8), p.670. https://doi.org/10.1080/01612840.2019.1585494

[34] Musliu, E., Snezana, V., Clausson, E.K., & Pernilla, G. (2019). School Nurses' experiences working with unaccompanied refugee children and adolescents: A qualitative study. *The Journal of School Nursing, Vol.5,* 1-8. https://journals.sagepub.com/doi/pdf/10.1177/2377960819843713

[35] American Academy of Pediatrics Council on Community Health. (2017). Detention of immigrant children. *Pediatrics. 139(4): 1-15. DOI: 10.1542/peds.2017-0483.* https://pediatrics.aappublications.org/content/pediatrics/139/5/e20170483.full.pdf

[36] Johnson, J.L., Beard, J., & Evans, D. (2017). Caring for refugee youth in the school setting. *NASN School Nurse*. 32(2),122-128. https://doi.org/10.1177/1942602X16672310

[37] Ibid.

[38] United States Department of Education, United States Department of Justice and United States Department of Health and Human Services. (2015) *Fact sheet: Information on the rights of unaccompanied children to enroll in school and participate meaningfully and equally in educational programs.* https://www2.ed.gov/about/overview/focus/rights-unaccompanied-children-enroll-school.pdf

[39] Ibid.

[40] Bridging Refugee Youth and Children Services. (2018). *Refugee children in U.S. Schools: A toolkit for teachers and school personnel.* https://brycs.org/toolkit/refugee-children-in-u-s-schools-a-toolkit-for-teachers-and-school-personnel/

[41] Ibid.

[42] Ibid.

[43] American Academy of Pediatrics Council on Community Health. (2017). Detention of immigrant children. *Pediatrics. 139(4): 1-15.* https://doi.org/*10.1542/peds.2017-0483.* https://pediatrics.aappublications.org/content/pediatrics/139/5/e20170483.full.pdf

[44] U.S. Citizenship and Immigration Services. (2017). *Victims of human trafficking & other crimes.* https://www.uscis.gov/humanitarian/victims-human-trafficking-other-crimes

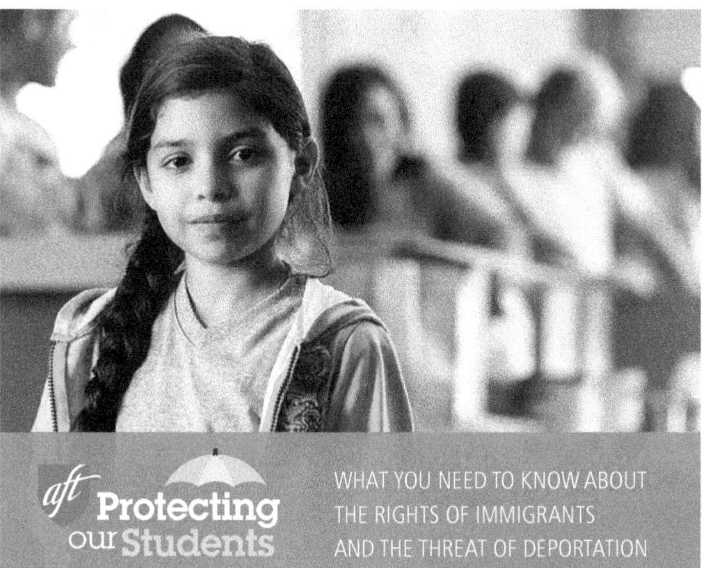

All children have a right to a public education

Under federal law, all children, regardless of their citizenship or residency status, are entitled to a K-12 education, including college counseling services. School districts that either prohibit or discourage children from enrolling in schools because they or their parents are undocumented immigrants may be in violation of federal law.

What the law says about deportation and schools

ICE officers and agents are to refrain from enforcement actions at least at the following locations and events:

- schools (including preschools, primary schools, secondary schools, colleges and universities, and other institutions of learning, such as vocational and trade schools);
- hospitals;
- churches, synagogues, mosques and other institutions of worship, such as buildings rented for the purpose of religious services;
- during funerals, weddings and other public religious ceremonies; and
- during public demonstrations, such as a march, rally or parade.

What the law says about sharing student information with immigration authorities

Under the Family Educational Rights and Privacy Act (FERPA), schools are prohibited, without parental consent, from providing information from a student's file to federal immigration agents if the information would potentially expose a student's immigration status. For more on FERPA, see **familypolicy.ed.gov/ferpa-parents-students**.

Schools must be safe havens, welcoming places of learning, and free from racism, discrimination, and the threat of deportation.

School districts are responsible for ensuring the safety and well-being of all their students. Educators and school support staff can work with community allies to reaffirm that their school and campus is a safe zone.

American Federation of Teachers, AFL-CIO
555 New Jersey Ave. N.W. • Washington, DC 20001 • 202-879-4400

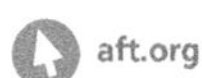 aft.org 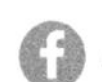 AFTunion  @AFTunion  AFTunion

Do's and Don'ts for students and their families if ICE authorities come to their homes

- **Do not open the door.** ICE authorities cannot come in without a signed warrant. Tell them to pass the warrant under the door before you open it.
- **Remain silent.** ICE can use anything you say against you in your immigration case, so claim your right to remain silent! Say **"I plead the Fifth and choose to remain silent."**
- **Do not sign.** Don't sign anything ICE gives you without talking to an attorney.
- **Report the raid immediately to the United We Dream hotline: 844-363-1423**
  Take pictures, video and notes: Write down badge numbers, the number of agents, and exactly what happened!
- **Fight back!** Get a trustworthy attorney, contact a local immigrant rights organization and explore all options to fight your case. If detained, you may be able to get bail—don't give up hope!

For more resources and information, contact:

- **American Federation of Teachers**
  www.aft.org/immigration
- **Share My Lesson**
  www.sharemylesson.com/immigration
- **Colorín Colorado**
  www.colorincolorado.org/immigration
- **National Immigration Law Center**
  www.nilc.org
- **United We Dream**
  www.unitedwedream.org
- **First Focus**
  www.firstfocus.org

SEXUAL MINORITY YOUTH

OVERVIEW/DEFINITION:
Gender identity and sexual orientation are separate concepts.[1, 2]

- Gender identity is a person's internal sense of being a man/male, woman/female, both, neither, or other.
- Sexual orientation is how an individual categorizes their emotional and sexual attraction to others. The term refers to an enduring pattern of emotional, romantic, and sexual attractions to men, women, or both sexes.
- Questioning: A term used to describe people who are in the process of exploring their sexual orientation or gender identity.
- Genderqueer or gender fluid: Describes people who have a non-binary gender identity. That is, they do not identify as either male or female, and may see themselves as a combination of the two, or some other gender.

There are three dimensions to sexual orientation, identity, behavior, and attraction:[3]

- Identity – What does the person consider themselves? (gay, lesbian, bisexual, straight, queer, or something else)
- Behavior – What gender(s) does the person have sex with?
- Attraction – What gender(s) is the person attracted to?

Terminology to describe identity has evolved from homosexual, heterosexual, transvestite or transgendered, sexual preference, and lifestyle choice and replaced by more contemporary terms:[4]

Outdated Terminology	Preferred Terminology	Definition
Homosexual	1. Gay 2. Lesbian	1. Persons who are emotionally and sexually attracted to people of their own gender. Most commonly used to describe men. 2. Women who are emotionally and sexually attracted to other women.
Heterosexual	1. Heterosexual 2. Non-binary 3. Queer	1. Women who are emotionally and sexually attracted to men, and men who are emotionally and sexually attracted to women. 2. Persons who do not identify exclusively as men or women. 3. Persons who do not identify as a specific gender, often referred to as gender fluid or LGBT.
Transvestite, transgendered	Transgender	Person whose identity does not correspond with their assigned sex at birth.
Sexual preference, lifestyle choice	Sexual orientation	How a person characterizes their emotional and sexual attractions to others.

SEXUAL MINORITY YOUTH *(continued from previous page)*

DEFINITION:

The American Psychiatric Association removed homosexuality from the Diagnostic and Statistics Manual 2nd Edition in 1973, discontinuing its classification as a psychiatric disorder.[5] In the United States, "an estimated 3.2 million youth (ages eight to 18) are lesbian, gay, bisexual, transgender, and questioning (LGBTQ). Among older youth, approximately 8% or 1.6 million youth (in grades nine to 12) identify as LGB, and nearly 1% or 150,000 youth (ages 13-17) identify as transgender".[6] Data from 2017 Youth Behavior Risk Survey (YBRS)[7] indicated that of those surveyed 2.4% identified as gay or lesbian, 8% as bisexual, and 4.2% were not sure, noting that transgender data were not available for the report.[8]

LGBT youth are more likely to think about, plan for, and attempt suicide compared to their peers who identify as heterosexual. They are also at greater risk for bullying (electronic and on school campuses), being physically forced to have sexual intercourse, and to experience sexual violence in general.[9] Additionally, the 2018 Human Rights Campaign LGBTQ Youth report indicated that those surveyed reported depression (75%), sleep disturbances (95%), and feeling worthless and hopeless (70%).[10] Stress levels were higher among youth of color and those who identified as transgender. Only 26% reported feeling safe in schools.[11] These data are congruent with the 2017 YBRS.

All youth, including the LGBT population have the right to receive an education in a safe school environment, as well as, support for their emotional, physical, and mental health and psychosocial needs. Adults in schools serve as role models and share the responsibility to help all youth develop into well-adjusted adults. Creating a safe school and community environment that respects individual difference is essential to the well-being of all youth. Tolerance and acceptance of diversity in the school is a critical component of the school's health education curricula.

POTENTIAL CONCERNS:

- Lesbians and bisexual women are at greater risk for anxiety, depression and suicide compared to other women.[12,13]
- Higher incidence of teen pregnancy among sexual minority women due to child maltreatment, bullying and gender nonconformity.[14]
- Men who have sex with men (MSM) are at increased risk of sexually transmitted infections, particularly syphilis, and major depression.[15]
- High school students who identify as lesbian, gay, or bisexual are almost five times as likely to attempt suicide compared to their heterosexual peers.[16]
- Transgender women are at increased risk for mental health issues, HIV, and sexually transmitted infections.[17]
- Bullying of lesbian, gay, bisexual, and transgender youth is associated with high risk coping behaviors leading to increased incidence of HIV.[18]

SEXUAL MINORITY YOUTH *(continued from previous page)*

POTENTIAL CONCERNS *(continued)*

- Other potential complications:
    - Human Immunodeficiency Virus/Acquired Immunodeficiency Syndrome (HIV/AIDS)
    - Human Papilloma Virus (HPV)
    - Stigma
    - Suicide
    - Sexually transmitted diseases (STDs)
    - Substance abuse (club drugs)
    - Body image and disordered eating
    - Homelessness
    - Domestic violence and victimization

MANAGEMENT/POTENTIAL INTERVENTIONS:[19, 20]

1. Use gender neutral, non-judgmental language. Avoid the term "sexual preference" as this suggests choice (which current research does not support); the preferred term is sexual orientation.
2. Ensure confidentiality; all students, including transgender, gay and lesbian students have a right to privacy; this includes keeping a student's transgender/sexual orientation private.
3. Educate students to avoid higher risk behaviors (e.g., early sexual activity, unprotected sex, alcohol abuse, driving while intoxicated, etc.) while accepting the person who views him or herself as gay, lesbian or bisexual.
4. Suggest keeping a private journal to write about stresses and challenges, personal strengths, and possible solutions or ambitions. Journaling helps separate minor from major issues.
5. Be non-judgmental when asking questions about sexual activity or orientation in order to be effective in encouraging the student to share concerns and behaviors.
6. Offer to help or refer those who need help telling parents or who are having trouble in school or with peers.
7. Provide training for all staff on establishing and maintaining a supportive and safe environment for all students regardless of sexual orientation or gender identity.
8. Emphasize that school personnel use the name/pronoun appropriate to the student's gender identity as well as the name/pronoun preferred by the student regardless of the student's assigned birth sex.
9. Encourage Gay, Straight Alliance school-based support groups and youth led groups or clubs.
10. Develop a network of community resources for youth and their parents for social and emotional support.

SEXUAL MINORITY YOUTH *(continued from previous page)*

MANAGEMENT/POTENTIAL INTERVENTIONS *(continued)*

11. Advocate for the development of district policies that allow students to have access to the restroom/locker room that corresponds to their gender identity.[21] Students may also be offered a private, non-stigmatizing alternative such as the use of the health room bathroom.
12. Provide training for all staff on establishing and maintaining a supportive and safe environment for all students regardless of sexual orientation or gender identity.
13. Develop a network of community resources for youth and their parents for social and emotional support.

FOLLOW UP:

- Observe for depression and suicidal ideation.
- Observe for and support a safe environment.
- Provide support to ensure health education curricula are implemented.

NOTES:

Guidelines for health education include:

- Integrate education on preventing sexually transmitted infections and HIV into curricula without categorizing LGBT students as different from non-LGBT students.
- Avoid "sexualizing" or defining LGBT persons only by sexual activity; non-LGBT persons do not define themselves by their sex lives.
- In HIV and AIDS prevention education, all students need to recognize risk-taking behaviors; worldwide, heterosexual transmission is significant.
- Reduce "them" versus "us" thinking and behavior. In-service and professional development can help educators reflect on their own biases, deal with their feelings, and recognize actions that covertly reinforce stereotypical ideas about LGBT youth.
- Encourage vaccination which can offer protection from hepatitis A and hepatitis B, serious liver infections that can spread through sexual contact. The HPV vaccine is available to women and men up to age 26.

Characteristics of successful school programs include:

- Keep disclosure in confidence.
- Use inclusive language, e.g., "parent" (not mother, father), "seeing anyone" or "date" (not boy or girlfriend), that conveys acceptance.
- Include LGBT issues in discussing multicultural issues.
- Establish and enforce policies that protect students from harassment, violence and discriminatory jokes or slurs by adults or students.
- Support students whose families include people in the LGBT community.

SEXUAL MINORITY YOUTH *(continued from previous page)*

RESOURCES

- **American Psychological Association (APA)**
  http://www.apa.org/

- **The Fenway Institute**
  1340 Boylston Street
  Boston, MA 02215
  https://fenwayhealth.org/the-fenway-institute/

- **Lesbian, Gay, Bisexual, and Transgender Concerns Office (LGBTCO)**
  750 First Street N.E.
  Washington, DC 20002
  http://www.apa.org/pi/lgbt/index.aspx

- **LGBT Youth Resources**
  http://www.cdc.gov/lgbthealth/youth-resources.htm

- **National Gay and Lesbian Task Force**
  1325 Massachusetts Ave NW, Suite 600
  Washington, DC 20005
  Phone: (202) 393-5177
  TTY: (202) 393-2284
  Fax: (202 393-2241
  http://www.ngltf.org/

- **National School Safety Center**
  141 Duesenberg Drive, Suite 7B
  Westlake Village, California 91362
  Phone: 805-373-9977
  Email: info@schoolsafety.us
  http://www.schoolsafety.us/

- **Centers for Disease Control and Prevention**
  LGBTQ Youth Resources | Lesbian, Gay, Bisexual, and Transgender Health
  https://www.cdc.gov/lgbthealth/youth-resources.htm/

SEXUAL MINORITY YOUTH *(continued from previous page)*

REFERENCES

[1] American Psychological Association. (2019). *Sexual orientation and homosexuality.* http://www.apa.org/helpcenter/sexual-orientation.aspx

[2] National LGBT Health Education Training Center. (n.d.). *Providing quality care to lesbian, gay, bisexual, and transgender patients: An introduction for staff training.* Boston: The Fenway Institute. https://www.lgbthealtheducation.org/lgbt-education/learning-modules/

[3] Ibid.

[4] Ibid.

[5] Drescher J. (2015). Out of DSM: Depathologizing homosexuality. *Behavioral sciences (Basel, Switzerland)*, *5*(4), 565–575. https://doi.org/10.3390/bs5040565

[6] Kann, L., McManus, T., Harris W.A., Shanklin, S.L., Flint, K.H., Queen, B. Lowry, R., Chyen, D., Whittle, L., Thornton, J., Lim, C., Bradford, D., Yamakawa, Y., Leon, M., Brener, N., & Ethier, K.A. (2018). Youth Risk Behavior Surveillance — United States, 2017. *MMWR Surveillance Summary, 67*(No. SS-8), p. 565. http://dx.doi.org/10.15585/mmwr.ss6708a1external icon

[7] Kann, L., McManus, T., Harris W.A., Shanklin, S.L., Flint, K.H., Queen, B. Lowry, R., Chyen, D., Whittle, L., Thornton, J., Lim, C., Bradford, D., Yamakawa, Y., Leon, M., Brener, N., & Ethier, K.A. (2018). Youth Risk Behavior Surveillance — United States, 2017. *MMWR Surveillance Summary, 67*(SS-8), 1–114. http://dx.doi.org/10.15585/mmwr.ss6708a1external icon

[8] Ibid.

[9] Human Rights Campaign. (2018). *LGBTQ youth report.* https://www.hrc.org/resources/2018-lgbtq-youth-report

[10] Ibid.

[11] Ibid.

[12] Mayo Clinic. (2018). *Teen depression.* https://www.mayoclinic.org/diseases-conditions/teen-depression/symptoms-causes/syc-20350985

[13] Centers for Disease Control and Prevention. (2017). *Lesbian, gay, bisexual, and transgender health: About LGBT health.* http://www.cdc.gov/lgbthealth/about.htm

[14] Charlton, B. M., Roberts, A.L., Rosario, M., Katz-Wise, S.L., Calzo, J.P., Spiegelman, D., & Bryn Austin, S. (2018). Teen pregnancy risk factors among young women of diverse sexual orientations. Pediatrics, 141 (4). https://pediatrics.aappublications.org/content/141/4/e20172278

[15] Centers for Disease Control and Prevention. (2017). *Lesbian, gay, bisexual, and transgender health: About LGBT health.* http://www.cdc.gov/lgbthealth/about.htm

[16] Kann, L., McManus, T., Harris W.A., Shanklin, S.L., Flint, K.H., Queen, B. Lowry, R., Chyen, D., Whittle, L., Thornton, J., Lim, C., Bradford, D., Yamakawa, Y., Leon, M., Brener, N., & Ethier, K.A. (2018). Youth Risk Behavior Surveillance — United States, 2017. *MMWR Surveillance Summary, 67*(SS-8), 1–114. http://dx.doi.org/10.15585/mmwr.ss6708a1external icon

[17] U.S. Department of Health and Human Services, Office on Women's Health. (2019). Recognizing the needs of lesbian, bisexual, and transgender women. https://www.womenshealth.gov/30-achievements/29

[18] GLESN and AIDS United. (2015). *Get the facts: Improve school climate to increase LGBT students' well-being and reduce HIV/AIDS risk+.* https://www.glsen.org/sites/default/files/GLSEN%20Get%20the%20Facts.pdf

[19] American College of Physicians, Makadon, H., Potter, J., Mayer, K., & Goldhammer, H. (Eds.). (2015). The Fenway guide to lesbian, gay, bisexual, and transgender health (2nd ed.). Fenway Institute, Fenway Health.

[20] Cianciotto, J., & Cahill, S. (2012). LGBT youth in America's schools. Ann Arbor, MI: University of Michigan Press. https://doi.org/10.3998/mpub.4656286

SEXUAL MINORITY YOUTH *(continued from previous page)*

[21] National Center for Transgender Equality. (n.d.). *Fact sheet on U.S. Department of Education policy letter on transgender students.* http://www.transequality.org/sites/default/files/ED-DCL-Fact-Sheet.pdf

OTHER REFERENCES CONSULTED

Bradley, B., Kelts, S., Robarge, D., Davis, C., Delger, S., & Compton, L. (2013). National Association of School Nurses (NASN) position statement: Sexual orientation and gender identity/expression (sexual minority students: School nurse practice. *NASN School Nurse, 28*(2),112-3. https://doi.org/10.1177/1942602X12473950

Institute of Medicine and the Committee on Lesbian, Gay, Bisexual, and Transgender Health Issues and Research Gaps and Opportunities. (2011). *The health of lesbian, gay, bisexual, and transgender people: Building a foundation for better understanding.* Washington, DC: The National Academy Press. http://www.ncbi.nlm.nih.gov/books/NBK64806

Makadon, H.J., Mayer, K.H., Potter, J., & Goldhammer, H. (2015). *The Fenway guide to lesbian, gay, bisexual, and transgender health*, 2nd ed. American College of Physicians.

National Center for Transgender Equality. (n.d.). *Fact sheet on U.S. Department of Education policy letter on transgender students.* http://www.transequality.org/sites/default/files/ED-DCL-Fact-Sheet.pdf

National Center for Transgender Equality. (n.d.) *Know your rights: Schools.* https://transequality.org/know-your-rights/schools

SUICIDE IDEATION/THREATS

OVERVIEW/DEFINITION:

Suicidal ideation (SI) is reoccurring thoughts of completing suicide. Suicide is the second leading cause of death for youths aged 10-24.[1] Globally, approximately 800,000 people die from completing suicide each year, or one person every 40 seconds.[2] The top three methods used in suicides of young people include firearm (45%), suffocation (40%), and poisoning (8%).[3] Many people who commit suicide have had at least one previous attempt,[4] and nine out of 10 had a mental health condition that contributed to their death.[5]

Risk factors for childhood suicide include depression, sexual abuse, prior suicide ideas or plans, being bullied, substance abuse, impulsive or aggressive behavior, and access to firearms.[6] Culture and family factors influence the possibility that youth consider suicide as an option for handling distress, depression or hopeless feelings. There are many contributing factors linked to suicidal ideation. Aggravating factors may include:

- History of mental disorder, including depression
- Chronic medical condition such as seizure disorder or diabetes
- Fewer social and personal supports than peers
- Youth who attempt suicide report more negative life events (disappointments and losses)
- May have experienced a significant loss: relationship breakup, death of someone close, physical disability, or loss of status/perceived humiliation (losing a competitive event or admission to a group/school)
- Family history of psychiatric disorder or suicide

Other risk factors for suicide include:

- Higher risk in the first month post psychiatric hospitalization[7]
- Presence of psychotic symptoms, especially psychotic depression[8]
- Gender – males are more likely than females to complete suicide, while females may be more likely to attempt, though typically use less lethal means[9]
- Substance abuse
- Physical illness[10]
- Recent initiation of an anti-depressant[11]

SUICIDE IDEATION/THREATS *(continued from previous page)*

WARNING SIGNS OF SUICIDE:[12]

- Changed eating and sleeping habits
- Withdrawal from friends, family and everyday routine personality changes
- Acting out, rebellion, running away
- Violent behavior/explosive rage
- Substance/alcohol use
- Difficulty focusing/concentrating
- Hinting that "nothing matters" and "I won't be a problem much longer"
- Preoccupation with death/dying
- Throwing or giving personal items away
- Sense of hopelessness or dramatically upbeat following a period of depression
- Talking about suicide ("I wish I was never born." and "I wish I was dead")
- Existence of specific suicide plan

MANAGEMENT/POTENTIAL INTERVENTIONS:

Emergency situations (ex. active suicidal ideation, plan, attempt)

- **Refer immediately for crisis intervention**.
- Suicidal attempts necessitate an immediate psychological evaluation.
- Assure a safe environment (this may mean psychiatric hospitalization).
- Medical treatment for underlying mental health conditions (depression, bipolar disease, schizophrenia).

Nonemergency situations (passive SI, hopelessness, reporting previous ideation or attempt)

- Recommend/refer for psychotherapy (counseling).
- Recommend/refer for medication management – antidepressants, antipsychotic medications, anti-anxiety medications, etc.
- Recommend treatment for underlying mental health and/or physical conditions.
- Identify signs of substance abuse and provide support for cessation where applicable.
- Provide numbers and names for emergency services should condition worsen, or suicide helplines for ongoing support.

General guidelines

When the child/adolescent expresses feelings of sadness, hopelessness, and despair or grief, it is important to assess for possible risk of physical harm to themselves. Begin the assessment with more general questions; if you hear affirmative answers, continue with more specific probing questions such as the following:

- Have you ever felt so blue you thought of killing yourself?
- Do you feel like hurting yourself now?*
- Do you have a plan to hurt yourself?*

SUICIDE IDEATION/THREATS *(continued from previous page)*

MANAGEMENT/POTENTIAL INTERVENTIONS *(continued)*

- If yes, how would you do it? If present plan, act immediately; provide constant supervision, set a contract, and call for local crisis assistance, notify parent/guardian(s)
- What would happen if you were dead?
- How would other people react if you were dead?
- Recognize and approach the student directly - *talking about suicide does not increase the risk.*
- Encourage verbalizing feelings (rather than internalizing); provide support.
- Suspend judgments, arguments and moral views of suicide; and listen for immediate risk.
- Be aware of others likely to identify with a student who is known to have attempted suicide and who may imitate the action; assure that a trained school person checks their well-being.

**Affirmative answers to these questions would warrant initiation of emergency action by the school RN, including, but not limited to, constantly observing student, notifying parents, and enacting emergency services*

FOLLOW UP:

- Participate in interdisciplinary team to assure that student has a plan for support and successful return to school.
- Review crisis plan with healthcare/mental health care provider to address the needs of any student who indicates intent to commit suicide.
- Provide general health education for all students about mental health, including depression and related risk and protective factors for suicide, as well as stress management programs.[13]
- Educate staff/parents on the warning signs of suicide.
- Providing at-risk, non-emergent students with the telephone number for:
  - National Suicide Prevention Lifeline—1-800-273-TALK (8255)
  - Crisis Text Line (text HOME to 741741)
  - The American Foundation for Suicide Prevention (afsp.org)

Concerns:

- Recognize that student may be consumed by suicidal thoughts and not be able to function in daily activities
- Unsuccessful suicide attempt may leave person with permanent and/or debilitating injuries such as organ failure or brain damage
- Death

RESOURCES

Printable Checklist: Do Teachers at Your School Know the Warning Signs of Student Suicide?
https://schoolleadersnow.weareteachers.com/suicide-warning-signs/

SUICIDE IDEATION/THREATS *(continued from previous page)*

REFERENCES

[1] Center for Disease Control and Prevention. (2018). *Preventing suicide*. https://www.cdc.gov/violenceprevention/suicide/fastfact.html

[2] World Health Organization. (2019). *Suicide Data.* https://www.who.int/mental_health/prevention/suicide/suicideprevent/en/

[3] Students Against Destructive Decisions (SADD). (2019). *Teen suicide and self-harm.* https://www.sadd.org/initiatives/personal-health/suicide-and-self-harm

[4] Bilsen J. (2018). Suicide and youth: Risk factors. *Frontiers in psychiatry*, *9*, 540. https://doi.org/10.3389/fpsyt.2018.00540

[5] American Foundation for Suicide Prevention (AFSP). (2019). *Talk Saves Lives*™*: An introduction to suicide prevention.* https://afsp.org/our-work/education/talk-saves-lives-introduction-suicide-prevention/?gclid=Cj0KCQjws7TqBRDgARIsAAHLHP62PpmGE_ASHxOGqXRPmmXK_CaolqakNHcsfq0yPMVntiYTqIwqB70aApKqEALw_wcB

[6] Varcarolis, E. (2018). *Essentials of psychiatric mental health nursing: A clinical approach*, (8th ed). Elsevier.

[7] Chung, D., Hadzi-Pavlovic, D., Wang, M., Swaraj, S., Olfson, M., & Large, M. (2019). Meta-analysis of suicide rates in the first week and the first month after psychiatric hospitalization. *BMJ Open*, *9*(e023883). http://dx.doi.org/10.1136/bmjopen-2018-023883

[8] Gournellis, R., Tournikioti, K., Touloumi, G., Thomadakis, C., Michalopoulou, P. G., Michopoulos, I., ... Douzenis, A. (2018). Psychotic (delusional) depression and completed suicide: A systematic review and meta-analysis. *Annals of general psychiatry*,17(39). https://doi.org/10.1186/s12991-018-0207-1

[9] Miranda-Mendizabel, A. et al. (2019). Gender differences in suicidal behavior in adolescents and young adults: Systematic review and meta-analysis of longitudinal studies. *International Journal of Public Health, 64*(2), 265-283. https://doi.org/10.1007/s00038-018-1196-1

[10] Mayo Clinic. (n.d.). *Suicide and suicidal thoughts.* https://www.mayoclinic.org/diseases-conditions/suicide/symptoms-causes/syc-20378048

[11] Ibid.

[12] Ibid.

[13] Centers for Disease Control (CDC). (2018). *Suicide factsheet.* https://www.cdc.gov/violenceprevention/pdf/suicide-factsheet.pdf

OTHER REFERENCES CONSULTED

American Psychiatric Association. (2017). *Diagnostic and statistical manual of mental disorders (DSM-V)* (5th ed.). American Psychiatric Association.

Patterson, B.R., Bohnenkamp, J., Hoover, S., Bostic, J. & Selekman, J., (2019). Students with mental health/behavioral health concerns and disorders. In J. Selekman, R. Adair Shannon, & C. F. Yonkaitis (Eds.), School nursing: A comprehensive text (3rd ed., pp. 709-711). F.A. Davis.

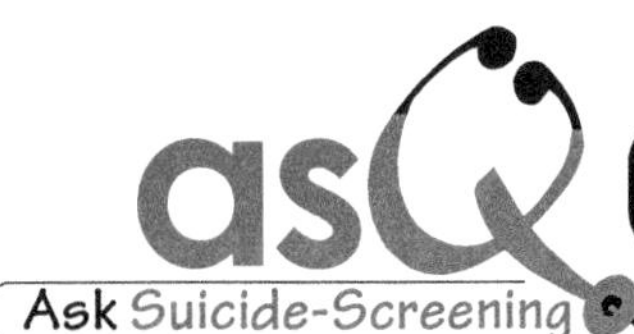

NIMH TOOLKIT

Suicide Risk Screening Tool

Ask the patient:

1. **In the past few weeks, have you wished you were dead?** ❍ Yes ❍ No
2. **In the past few weeks, have you felt that you or your family would be better off if you were dead?** ❍ Yes ❍ No
3. **In the past week, have you been having thoughts about killing yourself?** ❍ Yes ❍ No
4. **Have you ever tried to kill yourself?** ❍ Yes ❍ No

   If yes, how? ______________________________

   ____

   ____

   When? ______________________________

   ____

If the patient answers Yes *to any of the above, ask the following acuity question:*

5. **Are you having thoughts of killing yourself right now?** ❍ Yes ❍ No

   If yes, please describe: ______________________________

Next steps:

- If patient answers "No" to all questions 1 through 4, screening is complete (not necessary to ask question #5). No intervention is necessary (**Note: Clinical judgment can always override a negative screen).*
- **If patient answers "Yes" to any of questions 1 through 4, or refuses to answer, they are considered a positive screen. Ask question #5 to assess acuity:**
  - ☐ "Yes" to question #5 = **acute positive screen** (imminent risk identified)
    - **Patient requires a STAT safety/full mental health evaluation.** Patient cannot leave until evaluated for safety.
    - Keep patient in sight. Remove all dangerous objects from room. Alert physician or clinician responsible for patient's care.
  - ☐ **"No"** to question #5 = **non-acute positive screen** (potential risk identified)
    - **Patient requires a brief suicide safety assessment to determine if a full mental health evaluation is needed.** Patient cannot leave until evaluated for safety.
    - Alert physician or clinician responsible for patient's care.

Provide resources to all patients

- 24/7 National Suicide Prevention Lifeline 1-800-273-TALK (8255) En Español: 1-888-628-9454
- 24/7 Crisis Text Line: Text "HOME" to 741-741

asQ Suicide Risk Screening Toolkit NATIONAL INSTITUTE OF MENTAL HEALTH (NIMH) NIH 6/13/2017

https://www.nimh.nih.gov/research/research-conducted-at-nimh/asq-toolkit-materials/asq-tool/screening-tool_155867.pdf

TEEN PREGNANCY/PREGNANCY PREVENTION

OVERVIEW/DEFINITION:

In 2017, there was a 7% decline in U.S. pregnancy and birth rates among teens (age 15 – 19 years) from 2016.[1] This was a record low and evidence suggested the decline was due to more teens abstaining from sexual activity and more sexually active teens using birth control than in previous years.[2]

Teen pregnancy rates were more than two times higher for Hispanic teens (28.9%) and non-Hispanic black teens (27.5%), the rate for non-Hispanic white teens was 13.2%.[3] From 2007 through 2015, the teen birth rate was lowest in large urban counties (18.9%) and highest in rural counties (30.9%).[4] Studies have found that young women who are sexual minorities are at a heightened risk for teen pregnancy. This increased risk may be due to maltreatment, bullying and early sexual initiation, in part due to gender nonconformity. [5]

There is growing recognition of the importance of multidimensional strategies to pregnancy prevention, that engages stakeholders across a community.[6] One of the approaches to reduce the incidence of teen pregnancies was comprehensive sexuality education programs that have shown positive outcomes, including delay in the initiation and reduction in the frequency of sexual intercourse, a reduction in the number of partners, and an increase in condom use.[7] Evidence-based practices in reproductive health care, such as removing medical barriers to contraception, promoting the delivery of quality family planning services, and improving the clinical environment have also impacted the teen pregnancy rate.[8] Parent conversations with their children about sexuality education have been correlated with a delay in sexual debut and increased use of condoms and contraception.[9]

The diagnosis of a pregnancy is a sensitive time for the adolescent, their families, and the sexual partner.[10] Most women are diagnosed with pregnancy after a missed menstrual cycle and a positive urine or serum human Chorionic Gonadotropin (hCG). Pregnancy tests that use the woman's blood are done by a healthcare provider to get a very early diagnosis of pregnancy or to confirm an at-home pregnancy test. Blood tests are very accurate and can determine a pregnancy by the second week after conception.[11] The pregnancy is diagnosed as viable with serial exams and normal pregnancy development, a normal dating ultrasound, or positive fetal heart tones by Doppler.[12]

Adolescent pregnancy prevention is defined as decreasing the number of unintended and intended pregnancies among teenage youth through comprehensive sexual health education, including school and community partnerships, and education about abstinence and contraception.[13]

TEEN PREGNANCY/PREGNANCY PREVENTION *(continued from previous page)*

OVERVIEW/DEFINITION *(continued)*

SOCIAL AND ENVIRONMENTAL RISKS FOR TEEN PREGANCY:

There are many factors that put teens at risk for becoming pregnant:[14]

- Cultural and family experience
- Family patterns of early sexual experience
- Socioeconomic status
- Educational attainment of the teen
- Lack of sex education programs in schools
- History of physical or sexual abuse
- Substance use
- Early pubertal development
- Living in a foster home, homeless, juvenile justice system, no linkage to a support system[15]

SIGNS AND SYMPTOMS:

- Absence of menstruation
- Extreme tiredness
- Swollen and tender breasts
- Nausea and/or vomiting
- Bloating of the belly
- Darkening in the area around the nipple

MANAGEMENT/POTENTIAL INTERVENTIONS:

- Maintain confidentiality and follow school, state and federal guidelines and applicable laws that govern care to teens.[16,17] This includes parental notification of a positive pregnancy test.
- Assist with pregnancy identification when a teen has complaints of missed periods, breast tenderness, nausea and/or vomiting, by asking about additional signs and symptoms, sexual activity, use of contraceptives and the date of the last menstrual period.[18]
- Encourage the student to seek medical attention to confirm a positive pregnancy test including when there is a positive result from a pregnancy test kit.[19]
- Provide emotional support and foster communication between the pregnant teen and family.[20]
- Provide guidance regarding healthl care (encourage to seek obstetric or gynecologic care as soon as the pregnancy is known), pregnancy counseling services and community resources, including public health agencies, making referrals as needed. [21,22]
- Consider mental health screening for depression and other disorders as indicated (positive pregnancy test, perinatal loss).[23]
- Monitor for physical and mental health complications and any history of abuse.[24]
- Help connect to academic counseling and programs for pregnant teens within the school system and community that support pregnant teens to stay in school.

TEEN PREGNANCY/PREGNANCY PREVENTION *(continued from previous page)*

MANAGEMENT/POTENTIAL INTERVENTIONS *(continued)*

- Document according to nursing standards of care for every visit.
- Provide support and education to the pregnant teen that includes nutritional counseling; discussion about smoking, illegal drugs and alcohol; seeking healthcare provider guidance about medications during pregnancy; and signs/symptoms of pregnancy complications including ectopic pregnancies during pregnancy.[25]
- Develop individualized health plans so the pregnant teen can remain in school with any needed accommodations.[26]
- Build a support network for students including the core services that include childcare, preventative health care for infants and children, case management and economic assistance.[27]
- Follow-up and refer the student for health care when there is a negative pregnancy test.
- Follow the state law regarding the age of legal consent for sexual activity and notify authorities if the student is less than that age. [28]
- Follow state and local laws regarding child abandonment.[29] Many states have enacted safe-haven laws as an incentive for mothers in crisis to safely relinquish their babies to designated locations where babies are protected and provided health care until a permanent home is found. Safe-haven laws generally allow the parent to be shielded from criminal liability and prosecution. [30]

POTENTIAL COMPLICATIONS:

Socio-economic

- Increased high school dropout for girls [31]
- More likely to have lower school achievement, more health problems, be incarcerated, give birth as a teenager and face unemployment as a young adult[32]
- More likely to rely on public assistance [33]
- More likely to live in poverty as adults [34]

Health

- Spontaneous abortion/miscarriage, ectopic pregnancy, sexually transmitted infections, hypertensive disorders, low birth weight infants, and psychosocial (substance abuse, anxiety, depression) problems[35,36]

PREGNANCY PREVENTION:

Community and School Collaboration:

- Participate in community and school efforts to provide comprehensive, evidence-based teen pregnancy prevention programming (e.g. sex education advisory board membership, policy and procedure committees).[37]
- Utilize data (Youth Risk Behavior Survey, Centers for Disease Control and Prevention (CDC), School Health Profiles) to inform school staff, school board and community stakeholders about youth risk behaviors and sub-populations most at risk for teen pregnancy.

TEEN PREGNANCY/PREGNANCY PREVENTION *(continued from previous page)*

PREGNANCY PREVENTION *(continued)*

Individual Students:

- Maintain a confidential, safe and informative health office that ensures visual and auditory privacy.
- Display teen-focused magazines, informational pamphlets and posters related to adolescent sexual health and reproduction.[38]
- Encourage teens to talk to their parents or another trusted adult about sex and relationships.[39]
- Encourage teens to talk to their healthcare provider and ask about all types of birth control and which is best for them.[40]
- Discuss with sexually active teens (if school policy and applicable state and federal laws allow) the most effective reversible methods of birth control.[41]
- Explain to teens what is meant by confidential services (their health information cannot be shared with anyone without their permission, unless the healthcare provider is concerned they might hurt themselves or someone else).[42]
- Help teens locate Title X family planning clinics if appropriate and meets school district policy and procedures and any applicable state and federal laws.[43]
- Discuss normal physical, emotional, and sexual development.[44]

NOTES:

Factors that shape the content and delivery of sexual health education include state and school district policies, state education standards, funding from state and federal sources, individual teacher comfort, knowledge and skills.[45]

CDC provides the *U.S. Selected Practice Recommendations (US SPR) for Contraceptive Use, 2016* that addresses common and complex issues regarding initiation and use of specific contraceptive methods.[46]

REFERENCES

[1] Centers for Disease Control and Prevention. (2019). *Reproductive health: Teen pregnancy.* https://www.cdc.gov/teenpregnancy/

[2] Ibid.

[3] Ibid.

[4] Ibid.

[5] Charleton, B.M., Roberts, A., Rosario, M., Katz-Wise, S.L., Calzo, J.P., Speigelman, D. & Austin, B. (2018). Teen pregnancy risk factors among young women of diverse sexual orientations. *Pediatrics, 141*(4), e2 – e10. https://doi.org/10.1542/peds.2017-2278

[6] Brindis, C.D. (2017). Advancing the field of teenage pregnancy prevention through community-wide pregnancy prevention initiatives. *Journal of Adolescent Health, 60*(3S), S1-S2. https://doi.org/10.1016/j.jadohealth.2016.11.027

TEEN PREGNANCY/PREGNANCY PREVENTION *(continued from previous page)*

[7] Breuner, C.C. & Mattson, G. (2016). Sexuality education for children and adolescents. *Pediatrics, 138*(2), e1 – e11. https://doi.org/10.1542/peds.2016-1348

[8] Barfield, W.D., Warner, L., & Kappeler, E. (2017). Why we need evidenced-based, community-wide approaches for prevention of teen pregnancy. *Journal of Adolescent Health, 60*(3S), S3 – S6. https://doi.org/10.1016/j.jadohealth

[9] Breuner, C.C. & Mattson, G. (2016). Sexuality education for children and adolescents. *Pediatrics, 138*(2), e1 – e11. https://doi.org/10.1542/peds.2016-1348

[10] Hornberger, L. (2017). Diagnosis of pregnancy and providing options counseling for the adolescent patient. *Pediatrics, 140*(3), 1-9. https://doi.org/10.1542/peds.2017 – 2273

[11] Stanford's Children's Health (2019). Signs of pregnancy/the pregnancy test. https://www.stanfordchildrens.org/en/topic/default?id=signs-of-pregnancythe-pregnancy-test-85-P01236

[12] Ibid.

[13] Centers for Disease Control and Prevention. (2019). *Reproductive health: Teen pregnancy.* https://www.cdc.gov/teenpregnancy/

[14] Beshears, V. (2019). Students who are pregnant and parenting. In J. Selekman, R. A. Shanon, & C. F. Yonkaitus (Eds.). *School nursing: A comprehensive text* (3rd ed., pp. 864-885). F.A. Davis Company.

[15] Koh, H. (2014). The teen pregnancy prevention program: An evidenced-based public health program model. Journal of Adolescent Health, 54(3), S1-S2. doi: https://doi.org/10.1016/j.jadohealth.2013.12.031

[16] Ibid.

[17] Ahern, N.R., Bramlet, T. (2016). An update on teen pregnancy. *Journal of Psychosocial Nursing*, *54*(2), 25 – 28. https://doi.org/10.3928/02793695-20160119-03

[18] Beshears, V. (2019). Students who are pregnant and parenting. In J. Selekman, R. A. Shanon, & C. F. Yonkaitus (Eds.). *School nursing: A comprehensive text* (3rd ed., pp. 864-885). F.A. Davis Company.

[19] Ibid.

[20] National Association of School Nurses. (2015). Pregnant and parenting students – The role of the school nurse (Position Statement). Author.

[21] Beshears, V. (2019). Students who are pregnant and parenting. In J. Selekman, R. A. Shanon, & C. F. Yonkaitus (Eds.). *School nursing: A comprehensive text* (3rd ed., pp. 864-885). F.A. Davis Company.

[22] Ahern, N.R., Bramlet, T. (2016). An update on teen pregnancy. *Journal of Psychosocial Nursing*, *54*(2), 25 – 28. https://doi.org/10.3928/02793695-20160119-03

[23] Ibid.

[24] Ibid.

[25] Beshears, V. (2019). Students who are pregnant and parenting. In J. Selekman, R. A. Shanon, & C. F. Yonkaitus (Eds.). *School nursing: A comprehensive text* (3rd ed., pp. 864-885). F.A. Davis Company.

[26] National Association of School Nurses (2015). *Pregnant and parenting students – The role of the school nurse* (Position Statement). Author.

[27] Ibid.

[28] Hornberger, L. (2017). Diagnosis of pregnancy and providing options counseling for the adolescent patient. *Pediatrics, 140*(3), 1-9. https://doi.org/10.1542/peds.2017 – 2273

TEEN PREGNANCY/PREGNANCY PREVENTION *(continued from previous page)*

[29] Beshears, V. (2019). Students who are pregnant and parenting. In J. Selekman, R. A. Shannon, & C. F. Yonkaitis (Eds.). School nursing: A comprehensive text (3rd ed., pp. 864-885). F.A. Davis Company.

[30] Child Welfare information Gateway (2017). *Infant safe haven laws.* https://www.childwelfare.gov/topics/systemwide/laws-policies/statutes/safehaven/

[31] Centers for Disease Control and Prevention. (2019). *Reproductive health: Teen pregnancy.* https://www.cdc.gov/teenpregnancy/

[32] Ahern, N.R., Bramlet, T. (2016). An update on teen pregnancy. *Journal of Psychosocial Nursing, 54*(2), 25 – 28. https://doi.org/10.3928/02793695-20160119-03

[33] Koh, H. (2014). The teen pregnancy prevention program: An evidenced-based public health program model. *Journal of Adolescent Health, 54*(3), S1-S2. https://doi.org/10.1016/j.jadohealth.2013.12.031

[34] Ibid.

[35] Ahern, N.R., Bramlet, T. (2016). An update on teen pregnancy. *Journal of Psychosocial Nursing, 54*(2), 25 – 28. https://doi.org/10.3928/02793695-20160119-03

[36] Beshears, V. (2019). Students who are pregnant and parenting. In J. Selekman, R. A. Shannon, & C. F. Yonkaitis (Eds.). School nursing: A comprehensive text (3rd ed., pp. 864-885). F.A. Davis Company.

[37] Rabitte, M. & Enriquez, M. (2018). The role of policy on sexual health education in schools. *Journal of School Nursing, 35*(1), 27-38. https://doi.org/10.1177/1059840518789240

[38] Centers for Disease Control and prevention (2019). *Reproductive health: Teen pregnancy.* https://www.cdc.gov/teenpregnancy/

[39] Ahern, N.R., Bramlet, T. (2016). An update on teen pregnancy. *Journal of Psychosocial Nursing, 54*(2), 25 – 28. https://doi.org/ 10.3928/02793695-20160119-03

[40] Ibid.

[41] Ibid.

[42] Ibid.

[43] Ibid.

[44] Ibid.

[45] Breuner, C.C. & Mattson, G. (2016). Sexuality education for children and adolescents. *Pediatrics, 138*(2), e1 – e11. https://doi.org/10.1542/peds.2016-1348

[46] Centers for Disease Control and Prevention. (2018). *US Selected Practice Recommendations (US SPR) for Contraceptive Use, 2016 that addresses common and complex issues.* https://www.cdc.gov/reproductivehealth/contraception/mmwr/spr/summary.html

OTHER REFERENCES CONSULTED

For teens:

Sex, etc. (2019). *By teens for teens.* https://sexetc.org/sex-ed/info-center/stories/?topic=stories-relationships

TRAUMA INFORMED CARE

OVERVIEW/DEFINITION:

An individual's history of trauma may influence his or her health, relationships and ability to adopt healthy behaviors. Trauma-informed care principles include patient empowerment, choice, collaboration, safety, and trustworthiness. A traumatic event can be a single event or the cumulation of multiple events happening over time.[1] Childhood exposure to trauma is unfortunately prevalent. Children in the United States will have increased likelihood of being exposed to violence and crime than adults.

Adverse childhood experiences (ACEs) include:

- emotional abuse
- physical abuse
- sexual abuse
- emotional neglect
- loss of a parent due to separation, divorce or death
- family member with mental illness in the home
- substance abuse in the home
- violence in the home
- incarcerated family member

The 2016 National Survey of Children's Exposure to Violence assessed a representative sample of 4,000 children under 18 years of age in the U.S. and showed that:[2]

- more than one-third of all youth surveyed (37.3%) experienced a physical assault, primarily at the hands of siblings and peers;
- five percent experienced a sexual offense in the past year and 1.4% experienced a sexual assault;
- maltreatment, defined as physical abuse, emotional abuse, neglect and custodial interference occurred 15.2 % during the previous year, lifetime 38.1 %; and
- thirty percent of youth who are exposed to a traumatic event develop symptoms of posttraumatic stress.

The recent rise in school-related violence impacts children as well.

A trauma-informed school model can assist students in dealing with concerns from trauma exposure, such as posttraumatic stress disorder, anxiety, and other physical and emotional symptoms. School nurses should be involved in wellness promotion, prevention, recognition and early identification, and reporting and management of trauma due to their close involvement and interaction with children.[3] Trauma informed care should be throughout the school environment and should not be in silos.

TRAUMA INFORMED CARE *(continued from previous page)*

ANTICIPATED CONCERNS/PROBLEMS:

Common responses to trauma include posttraumatic stress response which includes an intense emotional response, and post-traumatic stress disorder. Post traumatic stress disorder can include reminders about an unpleasant event that can last for many weeks or months or years after the event. Symptoms that can manifest are:[4,5]

- anger, low frustration, tolerance and angry outbursts
- depression, sadness, mood fluctuations, withdrawal from activities and relationships
- aggression
- self-isolation
- attentional deficits and hyperactivity difficulty focusing and sustaining attention/ concentration
- increased startle response, hypervigilance, scanning the environment looking for threats

A trauma history and its symptoms can be misdiagnosed if not viewed in a trauma-informed manner. Not every child will manifest classic symptoms. Symptoms may differ based on the age and developmental level of the child. When school staff notice inappropriate student behavior, a history of trauma should be considered as a cause. A careful assessment should be completed including input from students, teachers, and caregivers. The child's current and past behaviors, coping strategies, and symptoms of stress should be assessed.

Not everyone perceives trauma in the same way, so it is imperative that the individual's perception is taken into consideration. School nurses need to understand their own responses to visible symptoms and behaviors and recognize their own potential to misunderstand or misinterpret based on implicit bias. *(Refer to POST TRAUMATIC STRESS DISORDER).*

MANAGEMENT/POTENTIAL INTERVENTIONS:

- Physical and emotional safety and support of students must be on the forefront of the entire school community.
- A trauma-informed approach should be incorporated, creating a safe and welcoming environment. Positive and warm décor, low noise level, and an area that can provide the child privacy.[6]
- Training and education for all faculty and staff related to ACEs and positive behavioral interventions should be implemented and reinforced regularly.
- Parents and community members can be educated to understand ACEs and supported to prevent students from being exposed to additional ACEs.
- Provision of trauma informed care also requires school employees to understand their implicit biases and to explore the school environment for policies and procedures which may not support trauma informed care. The school nurse can be a leader in advocating for change to policies which are inequitable and are not aligned with trauma informed care principles.
- School nurses can also provide a safe and trusted space, learn and incorporate methods of calming, and help the student build resilience over time.

TRAUMA INFORMED CARE *(continued from previous page)*

FOLLOW-UP:

- Implementing trauma informed care requires a collaborative approach.
- Screening, recognition of symptoms and supportive care are needed.
- Faculty and staff should have an awareness of trauma,and an understanding of how trauma occurs and how trauma can affect children in the short and long term.
- A trauma specialist can help train the staff and be available for consultation.[7]
- Staff training may improve the school's ability to respond to childrens' needs.
- A multi-tiered approach may reduce the negative impact of trauma. Strong social and emotional skills as well as trust-based relationships are the greatest mediators to adversity. They should be employed universally within the school setting. Safe and supportive strategies at more intense levels should focus on coping skill development, collaborative and proactive problem solving, as well as restorative practices.[8]

NOTES:

If there are significant concerns, a referral should be made to appropriate mental health services and the child's primary healthcare provider.[9]

RESOURCES

The National Child Traumatic Stress Network. https://www.nctsn.org/

REFERENCES

[1]Substance Abuse and Mental Health Services Administration. (2014). *SAMHSA's concept of trauma and guidance for a trauma-informed approach*. HHS Publication No. (SMA) 14-4884. Substance Abuse and Mental Health Services Administration. https://store.samhsa.gov/system/files/sma15-4420.pdf

[2] Finkelhor, D., & Turner, H. (2016). *National survey of children's exposure to violence III, 1997-2014 [United States].* Inter-university Consortium for Political and Social Research [distributor). https://doi.org/10.3886/ICPSR36523.v1

[3] Kataoka, S., Vona, P., Acuna, A., Jaycox, L., Escudero, P., Rojas, C. Ramirez, E., Langley, A., & Stein, B. (2018). Applying a trauma informed school systems approach: Examples from school community-academic partnerships. *Ethnicity & Disease, 28* (2),417-426. https://doi.org/10.18865/ed.28.S2.417

[4] Substance Abuse and Mental Health Services Administration. (2014). *SAMHSA's concept of trauma and guidance for a trauma-informed approach*. HHS Publication No. (SMA) 14-4884. Substance Abuse and Mental Health Services Administration. https://store.samhsa.gov/system/files/sma15-4420.pdf

[5] Finkelhor, D., & Turner, H. (2016). *National survey of children's exposure to violence III, 1997-2014 [United States].* Inter-university Consortium for Political and Social Research [distributor). https://doi.org/10.3886/ICPSR36523.v1

[6] Centers for Health Care Strategies, Inc. (2018). *Hiring a trauma informed workforce.* http://www.traumainformedcare.chcs.org/wp-content/uploads/2018/11/Fact-Sheet-Hiring-a-TIC-Workforce.pdf

[7] Kataoka, S., Vona, P., Acuna, A., Jaycox, L., Escudero, P., Rojas, C. Ramirez, E., Langley, A., & Stein, B. (2018). Applying a trauma informed school systems approach: Examples from school community-academic partnerships. *Ethnicity & Disease, 28* (2),417-426. https://doi.org/10.18865/ed.28.S2.417

[8] Frydman, S.J., & Mayor, C. (2017). Trauma and early adolescent development: Case examples from a trauma-informed public health middle school program., *Children & Schools*, *39*(4), pp. 238–247. https://doi.org/ 10.1093/cs/cdx017

[9] Centers for Health Care Strategies, Inc. (2018). *Hiring a trauma informed workforce.* http://www.traumainformedcare.chcs.org/wp-content/uploads/2018/11/Fact-Sheet-Hiring-a-TIC-Workforce.pdf

APPENDIX

Cover your Cough

Stop the spread of germs that can make you and others sick!

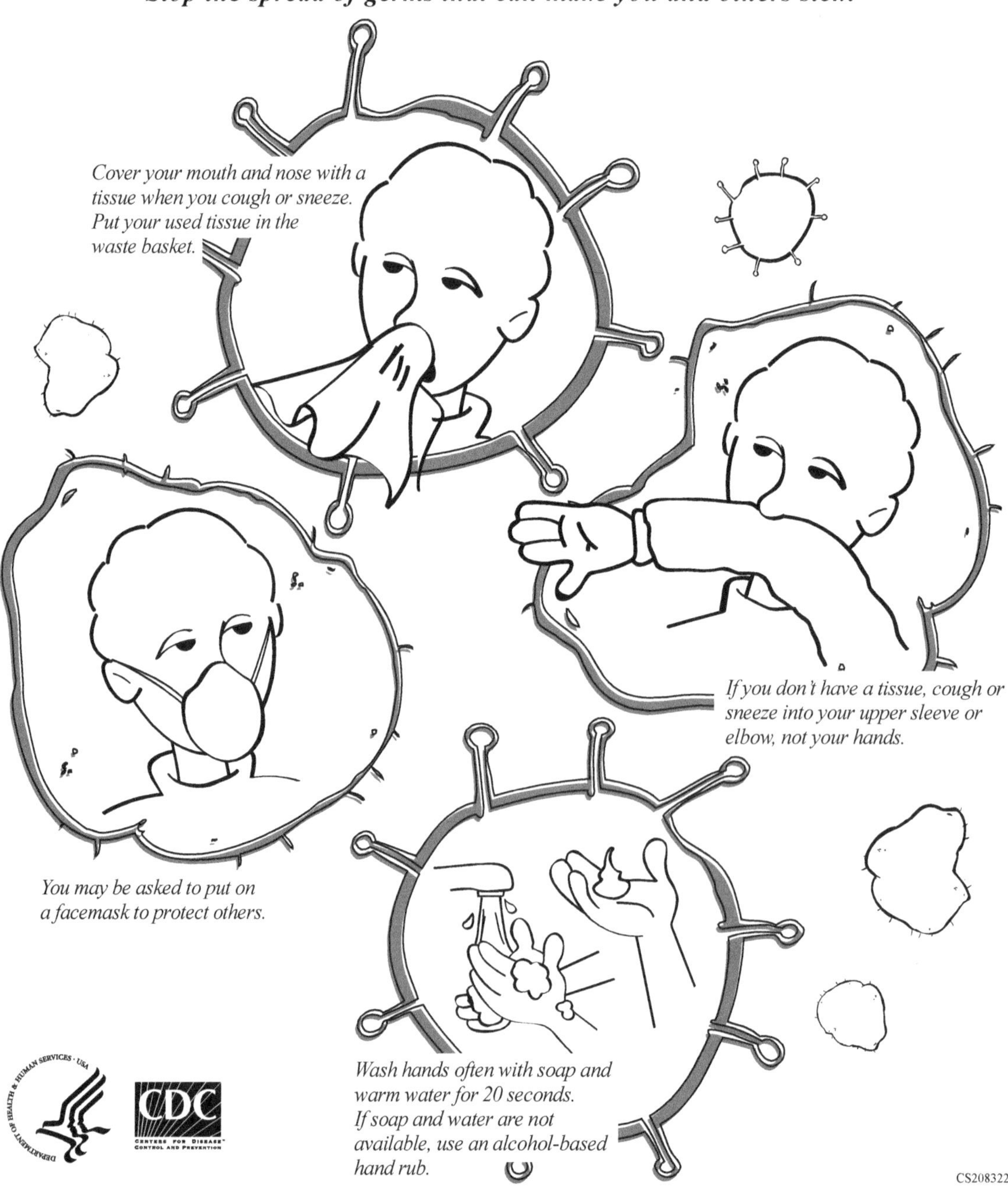

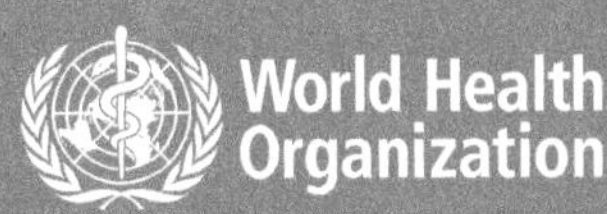

Patient Safety

A World Alliance for Safer Health Care

SAVE LIVES

Clean **Your** Hands

Hand Hygiene: Why, How & When?

WHY?

- Thousands of people die every day around the world from infections acquired while receiving health care.
- Hands are the main pathways of germ transmission during health care.
- Hand hygiene is therefore the most important measure to avoid the transmission of harmful germs and prevent health care-associated infections.
- This brochure explains how and when to practice hand hygiene.

WHO?

- Any health-care worker, caregiver or person involved in direct or indirect patient care needs to be concerned about hand hygiene and should be able to perform it correctly and at the right time.

HOW?

- Clean your hands by **rubbing them with an alcohol-based formulation**, as the preferred mean for routine hygienic hand antisepsis if hands are not visibly soiled. It is faster, more effective, and better tolerated by your hands than washing with soap and water.
- **Wash your hands with soap and water** when hands are visibly dirty or visibly soiled with blood or other body fluids or after using the toilet.
- If exposure to potential spore-forming pathogens is strongly suspected or proven, including outbreaks of *Clostridium difficile*, hand washing with soap and water is the preferred means.

WHO acknowledges the Hôpitaux Universitaires de Genève (HUG), in particular the members of the Infection Control Programme, for their active participation in developing this material.

Revised August 2009

HOW TO HANDRUB?

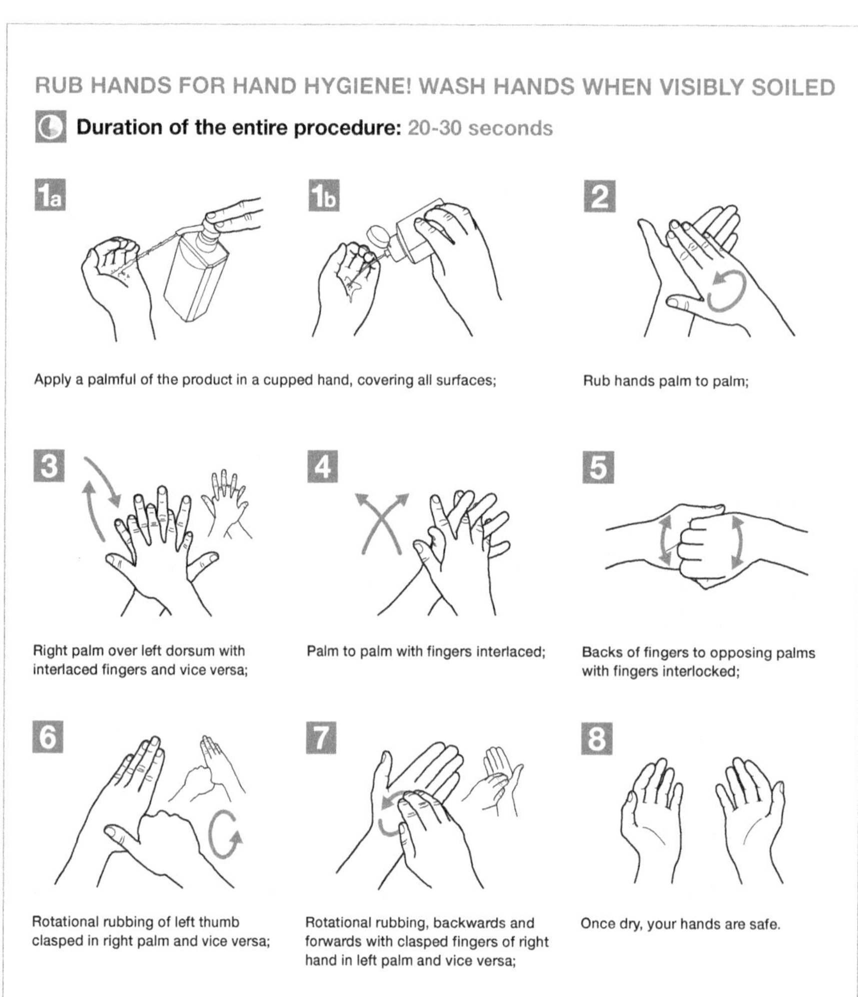

WHO acknowledges the Hôpitaux Universitaires de Genève (HUG), in particular the members of the Infection Control Programme, for their active participation in developing this material.

HOW TO HANDWASH?

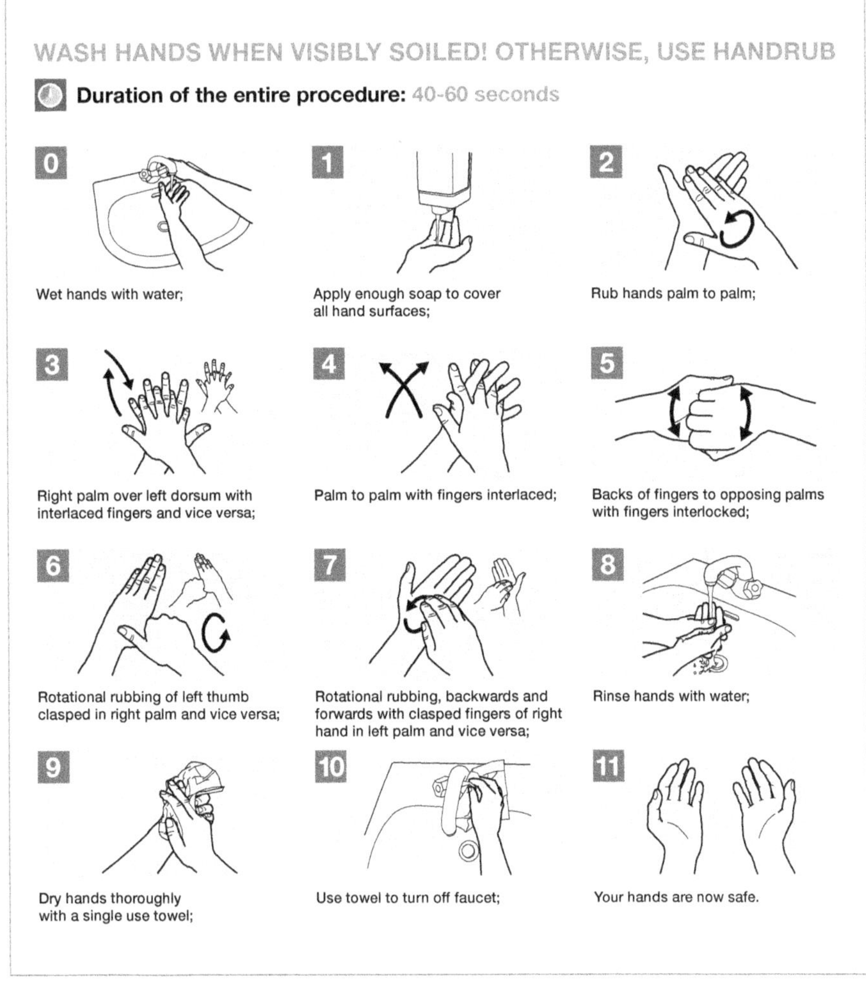

Hand care

- Take care of your hands by regularly using a protective hand cream or lotion, at least daily.
- Do not routinely wash hands with soap and water immediately before or after using an alcohol-based handrub.
- Do not use hot water to rinse your hands.
- After handrubbing or handwashing, let your hands dry completely before putting on gloves.

Please remember

- Do not wear artificial fingernails or extenders when in direct contact with patients.
- Keep natural nails short.

WHO acknowledges the Hôpitaux Universitaires de Genève (HUG), in particular the members of the Infection Control Programme, for their active participation in developing this material.

WHEN?

YOUR 5 MOMENTS FOR **HAND HYGIENE***

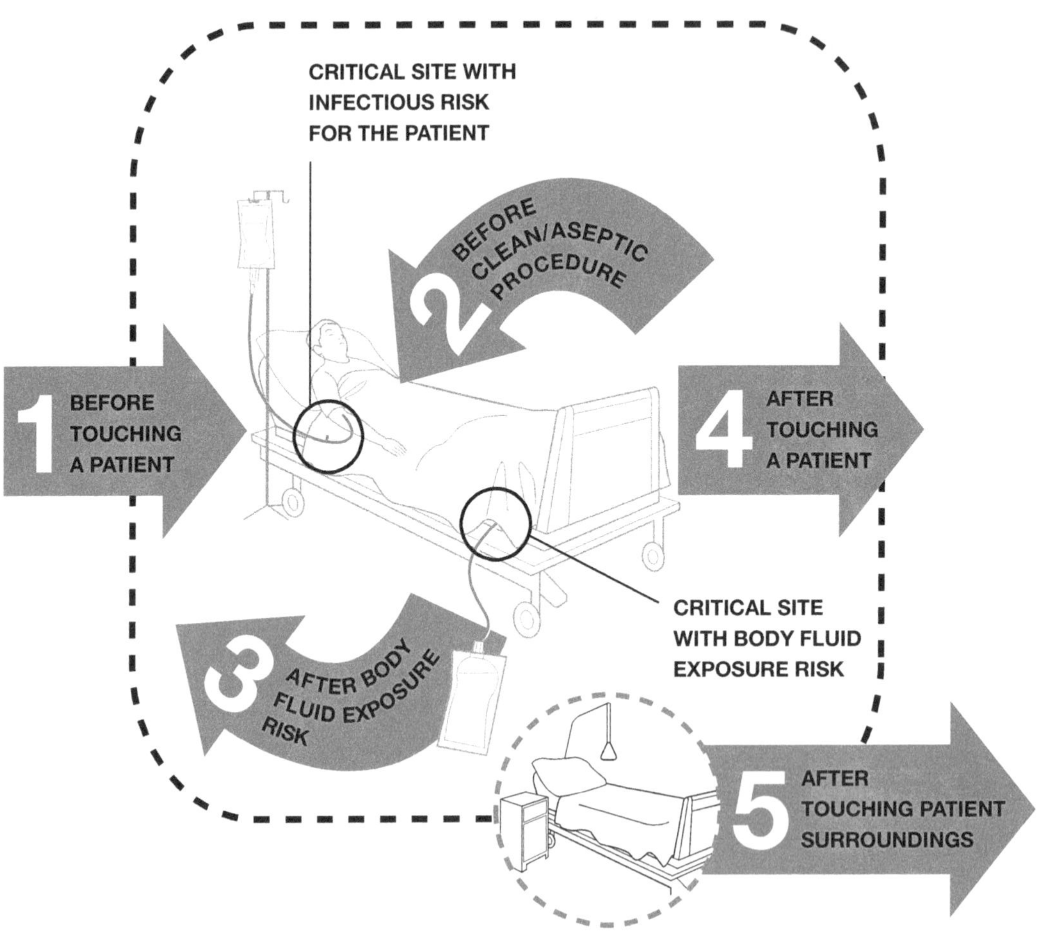

*__NOTE:__ Hand hygiene must be performed in all indications described regardless of whether gloves are used or not.

WHO acknowledges the Hôpitaux Universitaires de Genève (HUG), in particular the members of the Infection Control Programme, for their active participation in developing this material.

1 Before touching a patient

WHY? To protect the patient against colonization and, in some cases, against exogenous infection, by harmful germs carried on your hands

WHEN? Clean your hands before touching a patient when approaching him/her*

Situations when Moment 1 applies:

a) Before shaking hands, before stroking a child's forehead

b) Before assisting a patient in personal care activities: to move, to take a bath, to eat, to get dressed, etc

c) Before delivering care and other non-invasive treatment: applying oxygen mask, giving a massage

c) Before performing a physical non-invasive examination: taking pulse, blood pressure, chest auscultation, recording ECG

2 Before clean / aseptic procedure

WHY? To protect the patient against infection with harmful germs, including his/her own germs, entering his/her body

WHEN? Clean your hands immediately before accessing a critical site with infectious risk for the patient (e.g. a mucous membrane, non-intact skin, an invasive medical device)*

Situations when Moment 2 applies:

a) Before brushing the patient's teeth, instilling eye drops, performing a digital vaginal or rectal examination, examining mouth, nose, ear with or without an instrument, inserting a suppository / pessary, suctioning mucous

b) Before dressing a wound with or without instrument, applying ointment on vesicle, making a percutaneous injection / puncture

c) Before inserting an invasive medical device (nasal cannula, nasogastric tube, endotracheal tube, urinary probe, percutaneous catheter, drainage), disrupting / opening any circuit of an invasive medical device (for food, medication, draining, suctioning, monitoring purposes)

d) Before preparing food, medications, pharmaceutical products, sterile material

3 After body fluid exposure risk

WHY? To protect you from colonization or infection with patient's harmful germs and to protect the health-care environment from germ spread

WHEN? Clean your hands as soon as the task involving an exposure risk to body fluids has ended (and after glove removal)*

Situations when Moment 3 applies:

a) When the contact with a mucous membrane and with non-intact skin ends

b) After a percutaneous injection or puncture; after inserting an invasive medical device (vascular access, catheter, tube, drain, etc); after disrupting and opening an invasive circuit

c) After removing an invasive medical device

d) After removing any form of material offering protection (napkin, dressing, gauze, sanitary towel, etc)

e) After handling a sample containing organic matter, after clearing excreta and any other body fluid, after cleaning any contaminated surface and soiled material (soiled bed linen, dentures, instruments, urinal, bedpan, lavatories, etc)

4 After touching a patient

WHY? To protect you from colonization with patient germs and to protect the health-care environment from germ spread

WHEN? Clean your hands when leaving the patient's side, after having touched the patient *

Situations when Moment 4 applies, if they correspond to the last contact with the patient before leaving him / her:

a) After shaking hands, stroking a child's forehead

b) After you have assisted the patient in personal care activities: to move, to bath, to eat, to dress, etc

c) After delivering care and other non-invasive treatment: changing bed linen as the patient is in, applying oxygen mask, giving a massage

d) After performing a physical non-invasive examination: taking pulse, blood pressure, chest auscultation, recording ECG

5 After touching patient surroundings

WHY? To protect you from colonization with patient germs that may be present on surfaces / objects in patient surroundings and to protect the health-care environment against germ spread

WHEN? Clean your hands after touching any object or furniture when living the patient surroundings, without having touched the patient*

This Moment 5 applies in the following situations if they correspond to the last contact with the patient surroundings, without having touched the patient:

a) After an activity involving physical contact with the patients immediate environment: changing bed linen with the patient out of the bed, holding a bed trail, clearing a bedside table

b) After a care activity: adjusting perfusion speed, clearing a monitoring alarm

c) After other contacts with surfaces or inanimate objects (note – ideally try to avoid these unnecessary activities): leaning against a bed, leaning against a night table / bedside table

***NOTE:** Hand hygiene must be performed in all indications described regardless of whether gloves are used or not.

WHO acknowledges the Hôpitaux Universitaires de Genève (HUG), in particular the members of the Infection Control Programme, for their active participation in developing this material.

HAND HYGIENE AND MEDICAL GLOVE USE

- The use of gloves does not replace the need for cleaning your hands.
- Hand hygiene must be performed when appropriate regardless of the indications for glove use.
- Remove gloves to perform hand hygiene, when an indication occurs while wearing gloves.
- Discard gloves after each task and clean your hands – gloves may carry germs.
- Wear gloves only when indicated according to Standard and Contact Precautions (see examples in the pyramid below) – otherwise they become a major risk for germ transmission.

The Glove Pyramid – to aid decision making on when to wear (and not wear) gloves

Gloves must be worn according to **STANDARD** and **CONTACT PRECAUTIONS**. The pyramid details some clinical examples in which gloves are not indicated, and others in which clean or sterile gloves are indicated. Hand hygiene should be performed when appropriate regardless of indications for glove use.

STERILE GLOVES INDICATED

Any surgical procedure; vaginal delivery; invasive radiological procedures; performing vascular access and procedures (central lines); preparing total parental nutrition and chemotherapeutic agents.

EXAMINATION GLOVES INDICATED IN CLINICAL SITUATIONS

Potential for touching blood, body fluids, secretions, excretions and items visibly soiled by body fluids.

DIRECT PATIENT EXPOSURE: Contact with blood; contact with mucous membrane and with non-intact skin; potential presence of highly infectious and dangerous organism; epidemic or emergency situations; IV insertion and removal; drawing blood; discontinuation of venous line; pelvic and vaginal examination; suctioning non-closed systems of endotrcheal tubes.

INDIRECT PATIENT EXPOSURE: Emptying emesis basins; handling/cleaning instruments; handling waste; cleaning up spills of body fluids.

GLOVES NOT INDICATED (except for CONTACT precautions)

No potential for exposure to blood or body fluids, or contaminated environment

DIRECT PATIENT EXPOSURE: Taking blood pressure, temperature and pulse; performing SC and IM injections; bathing and dressing the patient; transporting patient; caring for eyes and ears (without secretions); any vascular line manipulation in absence of blood leakage.

INDIRECT PATIENT EXPOSURE: Using the telephone; writing in the patient chart; giving oral medications; distributing or collecting patinet dietary trays; removing and replacing linen for patient bed; placing non-invasive ventilation equipment and oxygen cannula; moving patient furniture.

WHO acknowledges the Hôpitaux Universitaires de Genève (HUG), in particular the members of the Infection Control Programme, for their active participation in developing this material.

Glossary

Alcohol-based formulation	An alcohol-containing preparation (liquid, gel or foam) designed for application to the hands for hygienic hand antisepsis.
Body fluids	Blood; excretions like urine, faeces, vomit; meconium; lochia; secretions like saliva, tears, sperm, colostrum, milk, mucous secretions, wax, vernix; exudates and transudates like lymphatic, pleural fluid cerebrospinal fluid, ascitis fluid, articular fluid, pus (except sweat); organic samples like tissues, cells, organ, bone marrow, placenta.
Clean / aseptic procedure	Any care activity that implies a direct or indirect contact with a mucous membrane, non-intact skin, an invasive medial device. During such a procedure no germs should be transmitted.
Critical site	Critical sites are associated with risk of infection. They either correspond to body sites or medical devices that have to be protected against harmful germs (called critical sites with risk of infection for the patient), or body sites or medical devices that potentially lead to hand exposure to body fluids and bloodborne pathogens (called critical sites with body fluid exposure risk).
Hand care	Actions to prevent skin irritation.
Hand hygiene	Any action of hygienic hand antisepsis in order to reduce transient microbial flora (generally performed either by handrubbing with an alcohol-based formulation or handwashing with plain or antimicrobial soap and water).
Indication for hand hygiene	Moment during health care when hand hygiene must be performed to prevent harmful germ transmission and/or infection.
Invasive medical device	Any medical device that enters the body either through a body opening or through a skin or mucous membrane breaking.

WHO acknowledges the Hôpitaux Universitaires de Genève (HUG), in particular the members of the Infection Control Programme, for their active participation in developing this material.

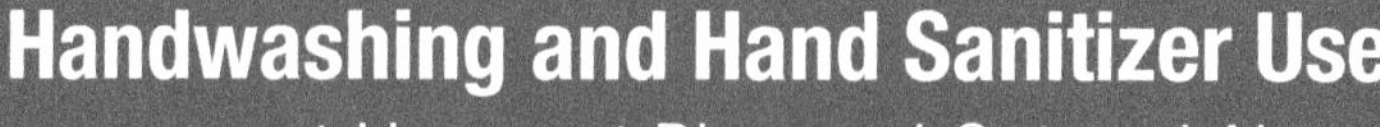

Handwashing and Hand Sanitizer Use
at Home, at Play, and Out and About

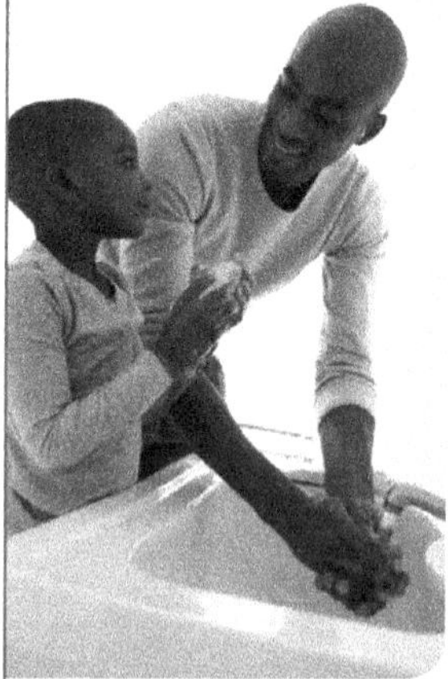

Germs are everywhere! They can get onto hands and items we touch during daily activities and make you sick. Cleaning hands at key times with soap and water or hand sanitizer is one of the most important steps you can take to avoid getting sick and spreading germs to those around you.

There are important differences between washing hands with soap and water and cleaning them with hand sanitizer. For example, alcohol-based hand sanitizers don't kill ALL types of germs, such as a stomach bug called norovirus, some parasites, and *Clostridium difficile,* which causes severe diarrhea. Hand sanitizers also may not remove harmful chemicals, such as pesticides and heavy metals like lead. Handwashing reduces the amounts of all types of germs, pesticides, and metals on hands. Knowing when to clean your hands and which method to use will give you the best chance of preventing sickness.

When should I use?

Soap and Water

- Before, during, and after preparing food
- Before eating food
- Before and after caring for someone who is sick
- Before and after treating a cut or wound
- After using the bathroom, changing diapers, or cleaning up a child who has used the bathroom
- After blowing your nose, coughing, or sneezing
- After touching an animal, animal food or treats, animal cages, or animal waste
- After touching garbage
- If your hands are visibly dirty or greasy

Alcohol-Based Hand Sanitizer

- Before and after visiting a friend or a loved one in a hospital or nursing home, unless the person is sick with *Clostridium difficile* (if so, use soap and water to wash hands).
- If soap and water are not available, use an alcohol-based hand sanitizer that contains at least 60% alcohol, and wash with soap and water as soon as you can.

* Do **NOT** use hand sanitizer if your hands are visibly dirty or greasy: for example, after gardening, playing outdoors, or after fishing or camping (unless a handwashing station is not available). Wash your hands with soap and water instead.

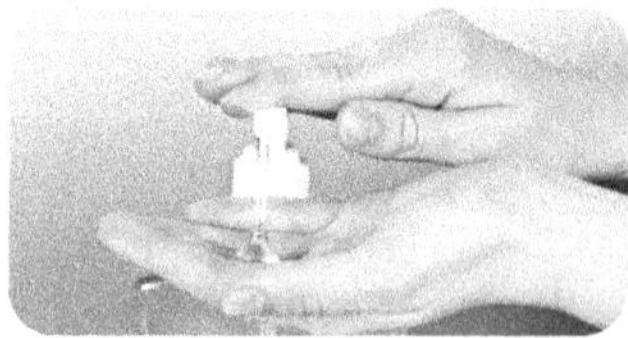

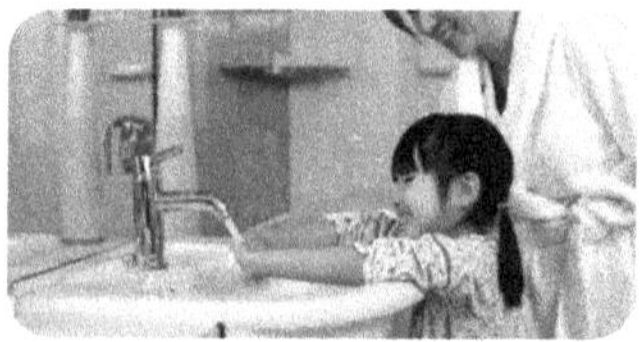

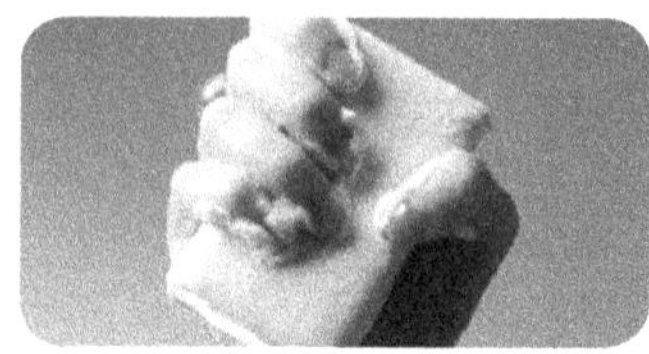

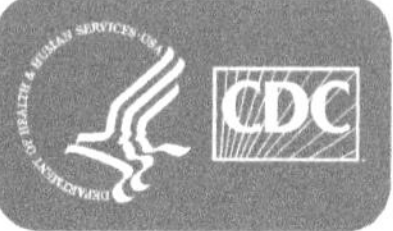

U.S. Department of Health and Human Services
Centers for Disease Control and Prevention

CS270631

Stop Germs! Wash Your Hands.

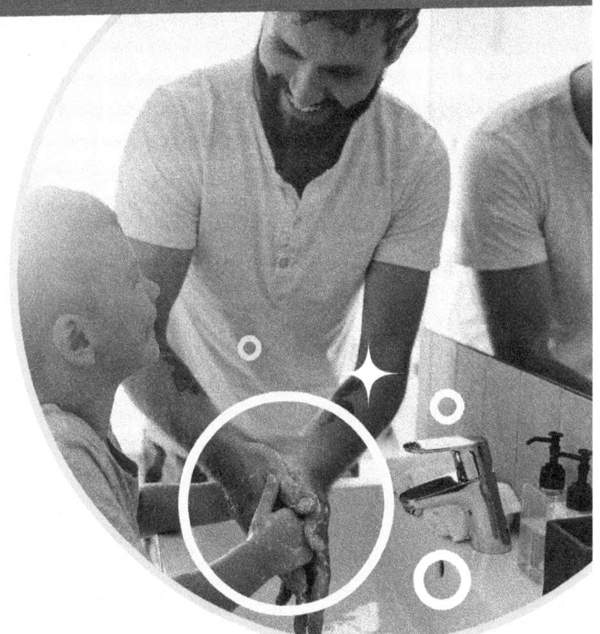

When?

- After using the bathroom
- Before, during, and after preparing food
- Before eating food
- Before and after caring for someone at home who is sick with vomiting or diarrhea
- After changing diapers or cleaning up a child who has used the toilet
- After blowing your nose, coughing, or sneezing
- After touching an animal, animal feed, or animal waste
- After handling pet food or pet treats
- After touching garbage

How?

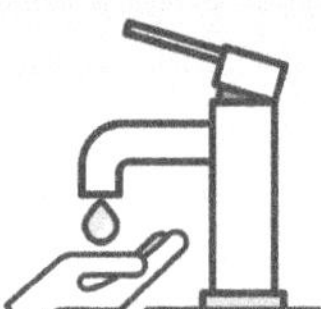

Wet your hands with clean, running water (warm or cold), turn off the tap, and apply soap.

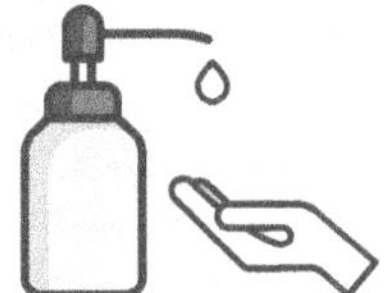

Lather your hands by rubbing them together with the soap. Be sure to lather the backs of your hands, between your fingers, and under your nails.

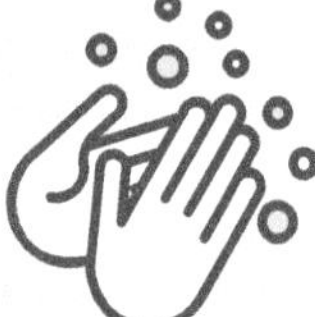

Scrub your hands for at least 20 seconds. Need a timer? Hum the "Happy Birthday" song from beginning to end twice.

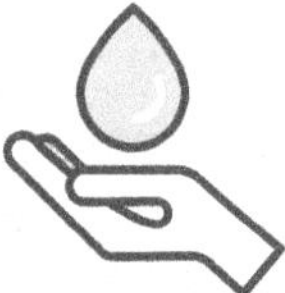

Rinse hands well under clean, running water.

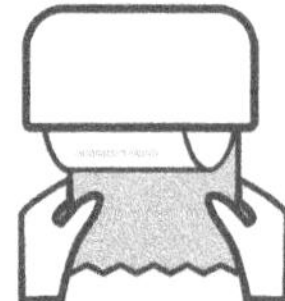

Dry hands using a clean towel or air dry them.

Keeping hands clean is one of the most important things we can do to stop the spread of germs and stay healthy.

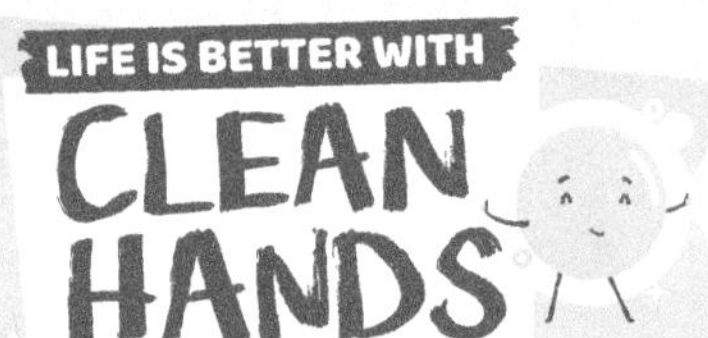

www.cdc.gov/handwashing

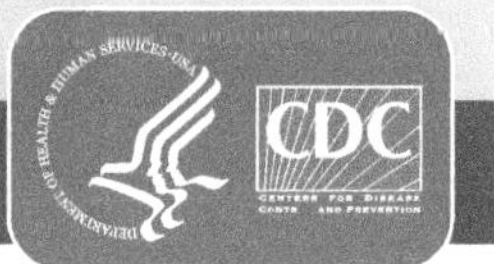

This material was developed by CDC. The Life is Better with Clean Hands Campaign is made possible by a partnership between the CDC Foundation, GOJO, and Staples. HHS/CDC does not endorse commercial products, services, or companies.

CS310027-A

Handwashing: Keeping Your Family Healthy

Handwashing is an easy, cheap, and effective way to prevent the spread of germs and keep kids and adults healthy. When your family is healthy, you don't have to worry about missing school, work, or other activities.

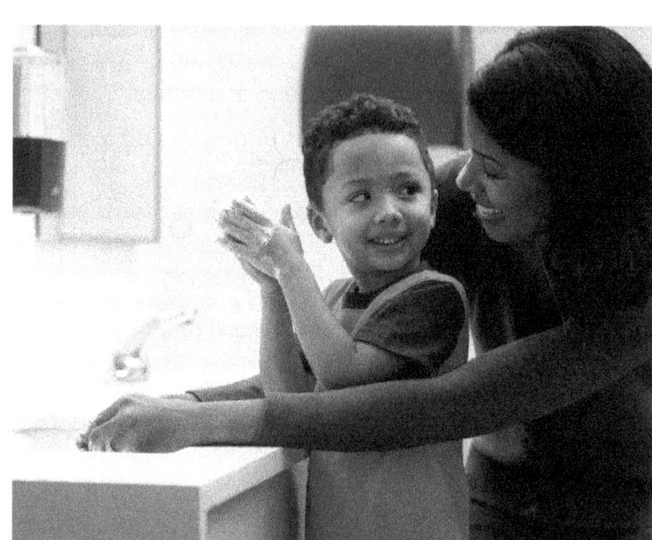

Help your child develop handwashing skills

Parents and caretakers play an important role in teaching children to wash their hands. Handwashing can become a lifelong healthy habit if you start teaching it at an early age. Teach kids the five easy steps for handwashing—wet, lather, scrub, rinse, and dry—and the key times to wash hands, such as after using the bathroom or before eating. You can find ways to make it fun, like making up your own handwashing song or turning it into a game.

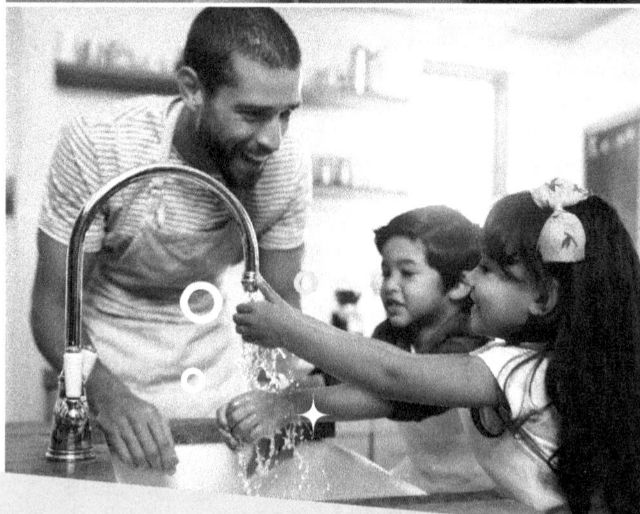

Lead by example

Young children learn by imitating the behaviors of adults in their lives. When you make handwashing part of your routine, you're setting an example for your children to follow.

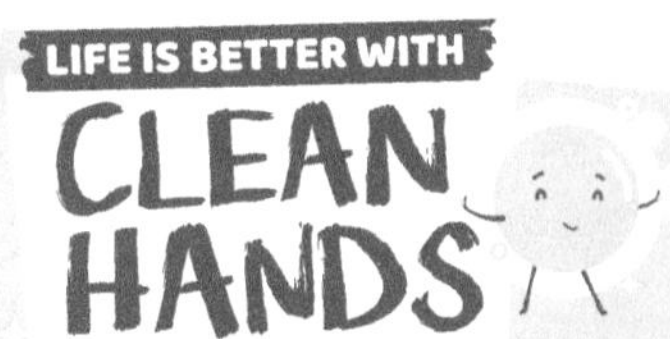

www.cdc.gov/handwashing

This material was developed by CDC. The Life is Better with Clean Hands Campaign is made possible by a partnership between the CDC Foundation, GOJO, and Staples. HHS/CDC does not endorse commercial products, services, or companies.

CS310275-A

Key Steps of Standard Precautions

You can't tell if people have infectious diseases just by looking at them. Using "Standard Precautions" means protecting yourself as if all blood, liquid, or airborne body fluids could be infected. Use these precautions whenever there is a chance of contact with blood or body fluids, including during tasks such as bathing, wound care, doing laundry, and toileting.

- Wash your hands frequently throughout your workday! Follow these steps:
  1. Get your hands wet and cover your hands and wrists with soap.
  2. Briskly rub the front and back of your hands, fingers, and under your fingernails for at least 20 seconds. (You can sing "Happy Birthday" two times.) To clean nails, put a pool of soap in your palm and, using a circular motion, work soap under the nails of your opposite hand. Repeat. Clean between your fingers.
  3. Rinse your hands thoroughly.
  4. Dry your hands with a clean paper or cloth towel. Do not shake water off your hands.
  5. Turn off the water with a clean towel, and—as necessary—open door with towel, also.
  6. Throw the paper towel away.
- Remove any blood or body waste from your skin or the client's skin by washing with soap and running water.
- Use disposable non-latex gloves!
  1. Wash and dry your hands.
  2. Make sure the gloves fit.
  3. Put disposable gloves on when you are ready to do an activity that requires them.
  4. Check for tears or holes. If you find any, do not use the gloves. Replace with a new pair.
  5. NEVER touch your mouth or eyes while wearing used gloves.
  6. After the activity, take off gloves, pulling down from inside the wrist (do not touch the outside of the gloves) so that they are inside out.
  7. Throw away gloves in a proper container.
  8. Wash and dry your hands.
- Wear an apron, mask, and eye protectors as necessary.
- Properly handle and dispose of possibly infected linens and wastes.
- Properly handle and dispose of sharps (such as needles and diabetes sticks). See http://www.cdc.gov/needledisposal/ for more information

U.S. Department of Health and Human Services, Centers for Disease Control and Prevention, National Institute for Occupational Safety and Health, 2014. *Caring for yourself while caring for others.* DHHS (NIOSH) Publication No. 2015-102. http://www.cdc.gov/niosh/docs/2015-102/default.htm

CPSIA information can be obtained
at www.ICGtesting.com
Printed in the USA
JSHW031420030520
5468JS00003B/4

9 781734 829501